Navigating Head and Neck Cancer

Navigating Head and Neck Cancer

Advances in Diagnosis and Treatment

Edited by

ZODWA DLAMINI

Founding Director, Pan African Cancer Research Institute (PACRI)
Director, SAMRC Precision Oncology Research Unit (PORU)
DSI/NRF SARChI Chair in Precision Oncology and Cancer Prevention (POCP)

OXFORD
UNIVERSITY PRESS

OXFORD
UNIVERSITY PRESS

Oxford University Press is a department of the University of Oxford.
It furthers the University's objective of excellence in research, scholarship,
and education by publishing worldwide. Oxford is a registered trade mark of
Oxford University Press in the UK and certain other countries.

Published in the United States of America by Oxford University Press
198 Madison Avenue, New York, NY 10016, United States of America.

CIP data is on file at the Library of Congress

ISBN 978–0–19–779419–7

DOI: 10.1093/med/9780197794197.001.0001

Printed by Marquis Book Printing, Canada

The manufacturer's authorized representative in the EU for product safety is
Oxford University Press España S.A., Parque Empresarial San Fernando de Henares,
Avenida de Castilla, 2 – 28830 Madrid (www.oup.es/en or product.safety@oup.com).
OUP España S.A. also acts as importer into Spain of products made by the manufacturer

MIX
Paper | Supporting responsible forestry
FSC www.fsc.org FSC® C103567

Contents

Preface

Head and neck cancer remains one of the most challenging malignancies, demanding a nuanced and comprehensive understanding of its epidemiology, diagnosis, and management. *Navigating Head and Neck Cancer: Advances in Diagnosis and Treatment* seeks to bridge existing knowledge gaps while integrating the latest advancements to address the multifaceted challenges posed by this complex disease.

This volume examines critical aspects of head and neck cancer care, including epidemiology, risk factors, and global inequalities that influence disease prevalence and outcomes. Through a detailed exploration of inequalities, we uncover how socioeconomic, environmental, and healthcare disparities shape the burden of this disease and its management across regions.

The text emphasizes innovative approaches, such as surgical innovations and precision medicine, highlighting their transformative roles in enhancing treatment outcomes. Precision medicine in particular offers a new frontier by tailoring interventions based on genetic, molecular, and biomarker data, while surgical advancements refine procedures to optimize patient recovery and function.

Recognizing the value of a multidisciplinary approach, this book underscores the importance of collaboration among oncologists, surgeons, radiologists, pathologists, and supportive care providers in delivering patient-centered care. Such teamwork is essential not only in treatment but also in addressing survivorship, quality of life, and the psychosocial impacts of head and neck cancer.

In addition, we examine biomarkers and predictive modeling as critical tools for advancing diagnostic accuracy and personalizing treatment strategies. The integration of artificial intelligence and machine learning is explored, reflecting how these technologies are revolutionizing predictive modeling and clinical decision-making in head and neck cancer care.

Health systems and organizational frameworks for managing head and neck cancer are also discussed, with particular focus on resource allocation, policy implementation, and the coordination of multidisciplinary teams to achieve equitable care delivery. Prevention strategies, including public health initiatives, risk reduction, and early detection campaigns, are presented as vital components for mitigating the global burden of head and neck cancers.

The volume's global perspectives highlight regional variations, emphasizing the unique challenges and opportunities that shape head and neck cancer care in different parts of the world. By considering cultural, environmental, and healthcare-specific factors, we aim to foster a deeper understanding of the disease's dynamics across diverse populations.

This book adopts a collaborative methodology, with contributions from leading experts in oncology, surgery, radiology, epidemiology, and public health. It reflects evidence-based insights, clinical expertise, and technological advancements, ensuring a holistic exploration of the subject matter.

Through its comprehensive approach, *Navigating Head and Neck Cancer: Advances in Diagnosis and Treatment* aims to serve as a critical resource for oncologists, researchers, surgeons, policymakers, and educators. It also empowers patients and caregivers with accessible information to navigate the complexities of head and neck cancer. Ultimately, this book aspires to inspire innovation, drive equity in care, and guide the next generation of advancements in head and neck cancer management worldwide.

Contributors

Melvin Ambele
Department of Oral and Maxillofacial Pathology, School of Dentistry, Faculty of Health Sciences
University of Pretoria
Institute for Cellular and Molecular Medicine, Department of Immunology
South African Medical Research Council, Extramural Unit for Stem Cell Research and Therapy
Faculty of Health Sciences
University of Pretoria

Oluwatoyin A. Asojo
Dartmouth Cancer Center
Dartmouth College, One Medical Center Drive

Onyemaechi O. Azu
Department of Medical Biosciences
University of the Western Cape

Jyotsna Batra
Centre for Genomics and Personalised Health
Queensland University of Technology
Translational Research Institute
Queensland University of Technology
School of Biomedical Sciences, Faculty of Health
Queensland University of Technology

Meshack Bida
Department of Anatomical Pathology, National Health Laboratory Services
University of Pretoria

Graham Chakafana
Department of Chemistry and Biochemistry
Hampton University

Aristotelis Chatziioannou
Center of Systems Biology
Biomedical Research Foundation of the Academy of Athens

Nkhensani Chauke-Malinga
Papillon Plastic Surgery

Ian C. Chikanza
Department of Rheumatology & Immunology (Adult & Paediatric), International Arthritis & Hypermobility Center
Faculty of Medicine, Catholic University
Department of Pediatrics & Child Health
University of Zimbabwe

Talent Chipiti
SAMRC Precision Oncology Research Unit (PORU), DSTI/NRF SARChI Chair in Precision Oncology and Cancer Prevention (POCP)
Pan African Cancer Research Institute (PACRI), University of Pretoria

Botle Precious Damane
Department of Surgery, Steve Biko Academic Hospital
University of Pretoria

Demetra Demetriou
SAMRC Precision Oncology Research Unit (PORU), DSTI/NRF SARChI Chair in Precision Oncology and Cancer Prevention (POCP)
Pan African Cancer Research Institute (PACRI), University of Pretoria

Dineo Disenyane
Department of Anatomical Pathology, National Health Laboratory Services: Tshwane Academic Division, Faculty of Health Sciences
University of Pretoria

Zodwa Dlamini
SAMRC Precision Oncology Research Unit (PORU), DSTI/NRF SARChI Chair in Precision Oncology and Cancer Prevention (POCP)
Pan African Cancer Research Institute (PACRI), University of Pretoria

Rupert C. Ecker
Translational Research Institute
School of Biomedical Sciences, Faculty of Health
Queensland University of Technology
TissueGnostics GmbH, R&D Department

Innocent A. Edagha
Department of Human Anatomy, School of Medicine
Moi University

Olalekan Fadebi
SAMRC Precision Oncology Research Unit (PORU), DSTI/NRF SARChI Chair in Precision Oncology and Cancer Prevention (POCP)
Pan African Cancer Research Institute (PACRI), University of Pretoria

Godfrey Grech
Department of Pathology, Faculty of Medicine and Surgery
University of Malta

Felix Holst
Department of Surgery, Faculty of Health Sciences
University of Pretoria

Rodney Hull
SAMRC Precision Oncology Research Unit (PORU), DSTI/NRF SARChI Chair in Precision Oncology and Cancer Prevention (POCP)
Pan African Cancer Research Institute (PACRI), University of Pretoria

Abidemi Paul Kappo
Molecular Biophysics and Structural Biology (MBSB) Group, Department of Biochemistry, Kingsway Campus
University of Johannesburg

Alexandre Kokoua
Laboratory of Anatomy, Experimental Surgery and Biomechanics (LANCEB)
University Felix Houphouet-Boigny

Emmanuel Konan
Laboratory of Anatomy, Experimental Surgery and Biomechanics (LANCEB)
University Felix Houphouet-Boigny

Alexis Koskan
College of Health Solutions
Arizona State University

Tsholofelo Kungoane
Department of Oral and Maxillofacial Pathology, School of Dentistry, Faculty of Health Sciences
University of Pretoria

Elisa Marie Ledet
Tulane Cancer Center's Prostate Cancer Biorepository, Tulane Cancer Center
Tulane University

Zhen Lin
Tulane Cancer Center and Tulane University Health Sciences Center

Georgios Lolas
3rd Department of Internal Medicine and Laboratory
National & Kapodistrian University of Athens
Integrate Computational & Mathematical Modelling Approaches (InCELLiA)

Thifhelimbilu Emmanuel Luvhengo
Department of Surgery
University of the Witwatersrand

Sylvester L. Lyantagaye
Department of Biochemistry, University of Dar es Salaam—Mbeya College of Health and Allied Sciences
Department of Molecular Biology and Biotechnology, College of Natural and Applied Sciences
University of Dar es Salaam

Lloyd Mabonga
SAMRC Precision Oncology Research Unit (PORU), DSTI/NRF SARChI Chair in Precision Oncology and Cancer Prevention (POCP)
Pan African Cancer Research Institute (PACRI), University of Pretoria

Mzubanzi Mabongo
Department of Maxillofacial and Oral Surgery
University of Pretoria

Ellen Mabunda
Department of Pediatric Surgery, Charlotte Maxeke Johannesburg Academic Hospital
University of Witwatersrand
Batsirai Mabvakure
Cancer Prevention and Control Program, Georgetown Lombardi Comprehensive Cancer Center
Georgetown University School of Medicine

Lorraine Tshegofatso Maebele
Botle Precious Damane, Department of Surgery, Steve Biko Academic Hospital
University of Pretoria

Ngoakoana Mahlachana
Department of Pediatrics and Child Health, Division of Hematology Oncology, Charlotte Maxeke Johannesburg Academic Hospital
University of Witwatersrand

Charles A. Maimela
Department of Mercantile Law, Faculty of Law
University of Pretoria

Stylianos Makrogkikas
Research Unit of Advanced, Composite Nano-Materials and Nanotechnology, School of Chemical Engineering
National Technical University of Athens

Arun Mankan
Fortrea Inc., Durham

Tania Maphoso
Botle Precious Damane, Department of Surgery, Steve Biko Academic Hospital
University of Pretoria

Thabang Marema
Department of Biochemistry, Microbiology and Biotechnology, School of Molecular and Life Sciences
University of Limpopo

Rahaba Marima
SAMRC Precision Oncology Research Unit (PORU), DSTI/NRF SARChI Chair in Precision Oncology and Cancer Prevention (POCP)
Pan African Cancer Research Institute (PACRI), University of Pretoria

Nelisiwe Prenate Masuku
Phytomedicine Programme, Department of Paraclinical Sciences, Faculty of Veterinary Science
University of Pretoria

Diana Mavuso
Department of Oral and Maxillofacial Pathology, School of Dentistry, Faculty of Health Sciences
University of Pretoria

Zukile Mbita
Department of Biochemistry, Microbiology and Biotechnology, School of Molecular and Life Sciences
University of Limpopo

Langanani Mbodi
Department of Obstetrics and Gynaecology, Gynaecologic Oncology Unit
University of the Witwatersrand

Ravi Mehrotra
Indian Cancer Genome Atlas
Centre for Health Innovation and Policy (CHIP) Foundation

Joseph G. Mhlanga
Department of Maxillofacial and Oral Surgery
University of Pretoria

Dunja Mihajlovic
Fortrea Inc., Durham

Sheefa Mirza
Department of Internal Medicine, School of Clinical Medicine, Faculty of Health Sciences
University of the Witwatersrand

Thabiso Victor Miya
SAMRC Precision Oncology Research Unit (PORU), DSTI/NRF SARChI Chair in Precision Oncology and Cancer Prevention (POCP)
Pan African Cancer Research Institute (PACRI), University of Pretoria

Mahlori Mkhabele
SAMRC Precision Oncology Research Unit (PORU), DSTI/NRF SARChI Chair in Precision Oncology and Cancer Prevention (POCP)
Pan African Cancer Research Institute (PACRI), University of Pretoria

Pontsho Moela
Department of Biochemistry, Genetics and Microbiology
University of Pretoria

Mohammed Alaouna
SAMRC Precision Oncology Research Unit (PORU), DSTI/NRF SARChI Chair in Precision Oncology and Cancer Prevention (POCP)
Pan African Cancer Research Institute (PACRI), University of Pretoria

Ntlotlang Mokgautsi
Department of Biochemistry, Genetics and Microbiology
University of Pretoria

Thulo Molefi
Department of Medical Oncology, Steve Biko Academic Hospital
University of Pretoria

Benny Mosoane
Department of Anatomical Pathology, National Health Laboratory Services
University of Pretoria

Thanyani Victor Mulaudzi
Botle Precious Damane, Department of Surgery, Steve Biko Academic Hospital
University of Pretoria
Thendo Netshiongolwe
Papillon Aesthetics, Netcare

Sibusiso Sizwe Nkosi
Department of Maxillofacial and Oral Surgery
University of Pretoria

Masibulele Nonxuba
Department of Medical Immunology, Centre for Neuroendocrinology
University of Pretoria

Amahle Nyalambisa
SAMRC Precision Oncology Research Unit (PORU), DSTI/NRF SARChI Chair in Precision Oncology and Cancer Prevention (POCP)
Pan African Cancer Research Institute (PACRI), University of Pretoria

Samuel O. Olojede
Department of Human Anatomy
Walter Sisulu University

Clement Penny, Department of Internal Medicine, School of Clinical Medicine, Faculty of Health Sciences
University of the Witwatersrand

Serwalo Ramagaga
Department of Head and Neck, Steve Biko Academic Hospital
University of Pretoria

Kamal S. Saini
Fortrea Inc., Durham
Addenbrooke's Hospital, Cambridge University Hospitals NHS Foundation Trust

Shobana Sampath
Department of Biotechnology
Vel Tech Rangarajan Dr Sagunthala R&D Institute of Science and Technology

Suzana Savkovic
School of Medicine
Department of Pathology & Laboratory Medicine, Diabetes Research, Tulane Cancer Center

Kenneth Segwapa
Papillon Aesthetics, Netcare

Solly Selahle
Department of Plastic, Reconstructive and Aesthetic Surgery
Steve Biko Academic Hospital University of Pretoria
Amanda Skepu
Future Production Chemicals Cluster
Council for Scientific and Industrial Research (CSIR)

Chrysis Sofianos
Division of Plastic and Reconstructive Surgery
University of the Witwatersrand

Mark Torres-Holmes
Department of Otorhinolaryngology and Head and Neck Surgery
Steve Biko Academic Hospital
Mediclinic Morningside Hospital

Stuart C. Winter
Department of Otolaryngology, Head and Neck Surgery, Nuffield Department of Surgical Sciences
University of Oxford
Blenheim Head and Neck Unit
Churchill Hospital, Oxford

Zarah Yakoob
Department of Oral and Maxillofacial Pathology, School of Dentistry, Faculty of Health Sciences
University of Pretoria

SECTION I

OVERVIEW OF HEAD AND NECK CANCER

1
Understanding Head and Neck Cancer

Zodwa Dlamini, Rodney Hull, Mahlori Mkhabele, Serwalo Ramagaga, and Ravi Mehrotra

1.1 Introduction

Head and neck cancers (HNC) is a term used to describe a variety of cancers that normally arise from squamous cells and are usually described as *head and neck squamous cell carcinoma* (HNSCC). Typically, these squamous cell carcinomas originate from the epithelial cells lining the oral cavity sinonasal tract, pharynx, larynx, and salivary glands (Pai & Westra, 2009). HNCs describe various cancers that arise from various sites in the mucosal surfaces of the head and neck region. These include sites such as the mouth, throat and voice box, salivary glands, and sinuses (Chow, 2020). More specifically, these include cancers of the oral cavity, which include cancers of the lips, front of the tongue, the gums, the lining of the cheeks, the floor of the mouth, and the hard palate. Cancers of the throat include the pharynx, which is divided into three different subtypes depending on the portion of the pharynx. The *nasopharynx* is the upper portion of the pharynx just behind the nasal cavity. The *oropharynx* can be described as the middle portion of the pharynx and includes the soft palate and back of the throat. The final part of the pharynx is the *hypopharynx*, which is the lower part of the pharynx. A third site for HNSCC is the larynx or voice box, the cartilaginous structure just below the pharynx, and it includes the epiglottis. A fourth site includes the small cavities between the bones in the nasal cavity known as the *paranasal sinuses.* This group of cancers includes those that arise in the nasal cavity. Finally, cancers arise in the salivary glands on the floor of the mouth and throughout the mouth and throat (Figure 1.1) (Chow, 2020; Son et al., 2018).

1.2 Background on Head and Neck Cancers

1.2.1 Epidemiology

It is estimated that the groups of cancers classed as HNSCC are the sixth most common group of cancers. In 2022, it was reported that worldwide there were

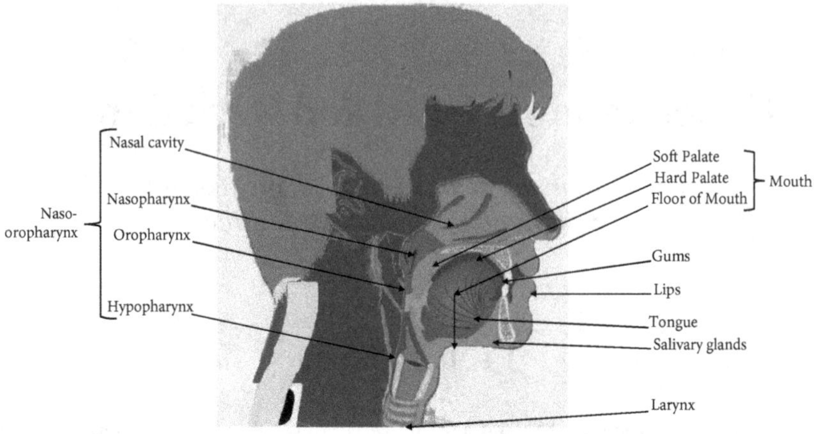

Figure 1.1 Sites of various head and neck cancers. HNCs are a collective term for all cancers that develop from the squamous mucosa of the head and neck and includes cancers of the mouth, lips, gums, tongue, salivary glands, larynx, and nasopharynx.

947,211 recorded cases, with 482,428 recorded deaths (Ferlay et al., 2024). Cancer statistics indicate that the incidence of HNSCC cases continues to rise (Siegel et al., 2020). However, in South Africa, the incidence of all types of HNSCC has remained the same over > 20 years (Figure 1.2A and 1.2B). Salivary gland cancer rates have increased slightly while the incidence of lip cancer has decreased slightly. The data seem to show wild variations in the year-by-year incidence of mouth and tongue cancer. This may be due to difficulties in the diagnosis and reporting of these types of HNSCC.

Males are more prone to develop HNSCC than are females (Figure 1.2C). The incidence ratio between the two sexes can range from 2:1 to 4:1 (Ferlay et al., 2024). Patients are normally diagnosed between the ages of 50 and 70 years (Ridge et al., 2009). The incidence of HNSCC is very high in the United States, France, Spain, Russia, Australia, India, and Namibia, with age-standardized incidence rates among males being > 10 (Figure 1.3A). Additionally, the incidence rates of stage IV HNC in these countries are on the rise (Thompson-Harvey et al., 2020). However, when compared to the mortality rates, only the high incidence in Portugal, India, and Russia translates into high mortality rates. Many low- to middle-income countries have disproportionately high mortality rates when compared to their incidence rates (Figure 1.3B). This is especially true in Africa. Treatment and screening for HNSCC have advanced in the past few decades. Despite this, the prognosis for HNSCC is still poor since the 5-year chance of

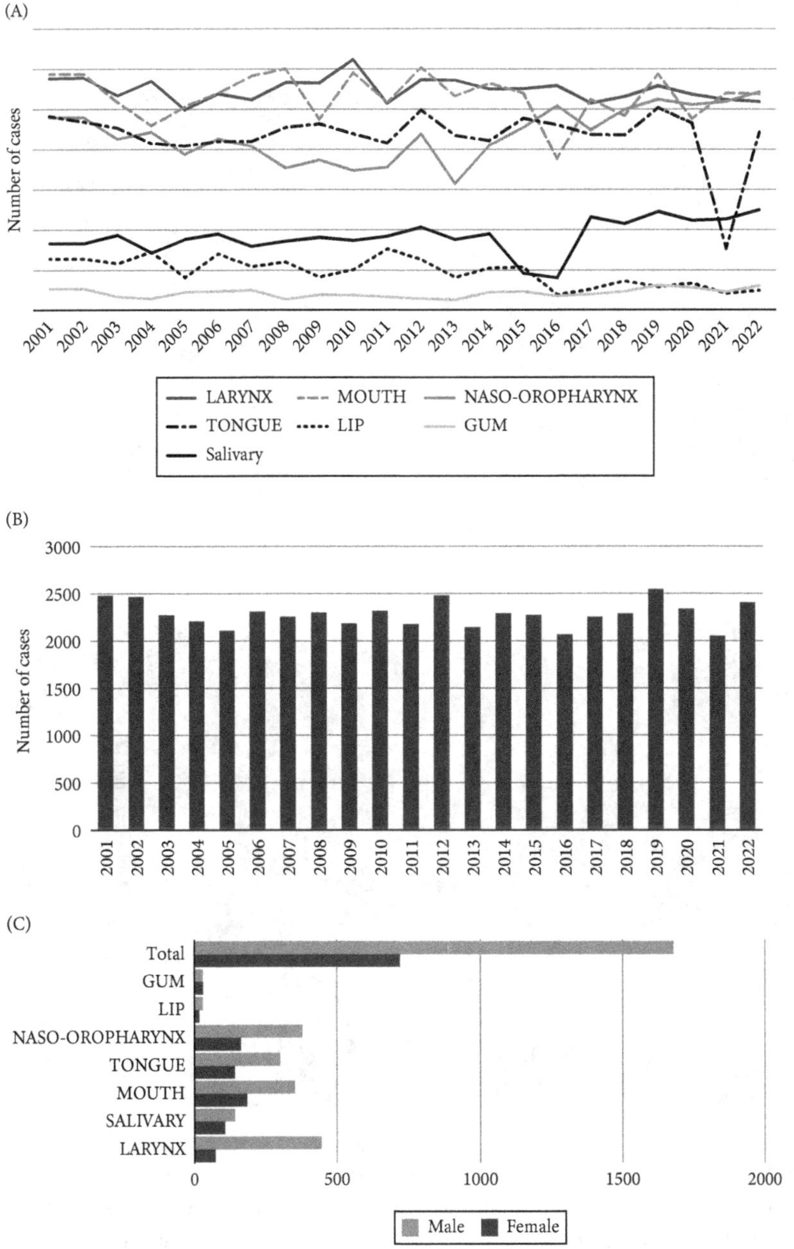

Figure 1.2 Incidence of various head and neck cancers in South Africa. (A) The incidence of various head and neck squamous cell cancers (HNSCCs) in South Africa from 2001 to 2022 using data from the South African National Cancer Registry (see references to National Cancer Registry, 2001–2020). The graph shows that the incidence of these cancers in South Africa has remained stable. This is confirmed by (B) the incidence of all HNSCC combined in South Africa over the past 20 years (C) The incidence rate of HNSCC in South Africa in 2022 separated into males and females, showing that males are far more likely to be diagnosed with all forms of HNSCC.

(A)

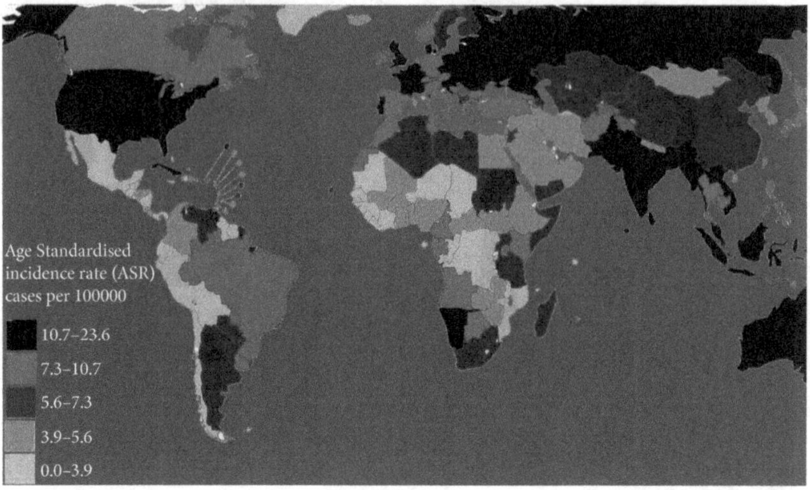

(B)

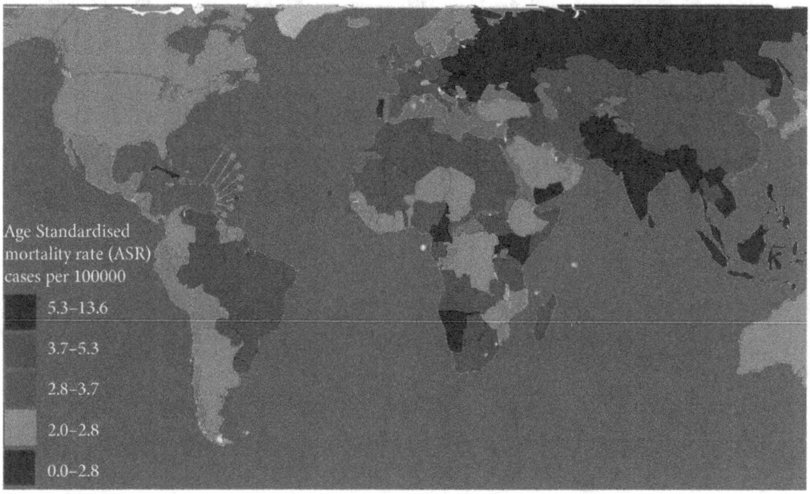

Figure 1.3 Incidence and mortality of head and neck squamous cell cancers (HNSCCs) worldwide. (A) The incidence rate of HNSCC worldwide shows the high incidence rates in many high-income countries (HICs), such as the United States, the United Kingdom, Portugal, Central Europe, and Australia. High incidence rates are also seen in Russia, Namibia, and the Indian subcontinent. (B) Mortality rates of HNSCC worldwide show a disproportionate level of mortality in low- and middle-income countries with many HICs with very high incidence rates having mid to low mortality rates. Africa in general shows a generally high mortality rate in countries where there is only a mid to low incidence of HNC.

survival is only 28–67%, depending on the stage at presentation (Hashim et al., 2019; Pulte & Brenner, 2010).

1.2.2 Risk Factors

A large body of studies exists on the risk and causal factors for HNSCC. Tobacco use is one of the strongest risk factors for HNSCC. This is followed by alcohol use. These two factors may have synergistic effects as alcohol and tobacco use commonly occur together. For instance, alcohol and tobacco use alone increases the risk of developing HNSCC by 3 to 9 times while the combined use of alcohol and tobacco increases the risk of developing HNSCC by 100 times (Neville & Day, 2002; Settle et al., 2009; Zandberg et al., 2016). In Western Europe, it is estimated that 75% of all cases of lip, mouth, and pharyngeal cancers are caused by tobacco use (Tuyns et al., 1988). Increases in the level of *p53* mutations are also associated with frequent and excessive use of alcohol and smoking, with mutations in this gene occurring at a higher rate in HNSCC patients who drink and smoke compared to those HNSCC patients who do not (Brennan et al., 1995). The use of smokeless tobacco products and snuff is associated with increased HNSCC risk (Boffetta et al., 2008). The increased risk of HNSCC caused by tobacco use is increased further in individuals with genetic alterations in metabolic enzymes (Singh et al., 2015). The ability of alcohol to contribute to HNSCC development is thought to be the result of the ability of alcohol to act as a solvent resulting in increased mucosal exposure to carcinogens as well as increased absorbance of carcinogens by cells normally protected by the mucosa (Pöschl & Seitz, 2004). Additionally, alcohol is metabolized to acetaldehyde, and acetaldehyde forms adducts with DNA, leading to mutations (Pöschl & Seitz, 2004).

Other risk factors associated with drug use include the traditional practice of areca or betel nut (*Areca catechu*) chewing. This practice originated in Southeast Asia and has both stimulant and narcotic effects due to the presence of the psychoactive compound arecoline (International Human Genome Sequencing Consortium, 2004). Consumption of the traditional Indian after-meal pan masala is also associated with increased risk of HNSCC. Analysis of the ingredients has revealed the presence of compounds whose consumption is linked to an increase in cancer risk. This includes compounds such as magnesium carbonate (Garg et al., 2015).

Environmental risk factors for HNSCC include environmental contaminants and pollutants. This includes paint fumes, plastic byproducts, and gasoline fumes (Brown et al., 1988) and formaldehyde (Luce et al., 1993). Other environmental risk factors include exposure to high-energy electromagnetic waves, including ultraviolet (UV) radiation as the result of overexposure to sunlight or gamma radiation (Azzam et al., 2020).

A history of HNSCCs in first-degree family members was found to increase the risk of developing HNSCC overall by 1.7. This risk increases depending on which family member. A parent only increases the risk slightly with an odds ratio (OR) of 1.8, while a sibling with HNSCC greatly increases the risk of developing HNSCC with an OR of 2.2 (Negri et al., 2009). Viral infections are also known to increase the risk of developing HNSCC. Infection with the human papillomavirus (HPV) seems to be a strong risk factor for HNSCC, especially oropharynx cancer. This is linked to the E6 protein of specific HPV types binding to and accelerating the degradation of P53, allowing for the evasion of apoptosis and increased cell proliferation (Gillison et al., 2000; Mork et al., 2001). Epstein-Barr virus (EBV) also increases the risk for HNSCC. EBV infection is particularly associated with oropharyngeal and nasopharyngeal cancers (Shaw & Beasley, 2016; Shotelersuk et al., 2000).

Other personal behaviors and health conditions can also be risk factors for the development of HNSCC. For instance, poor oral hygiene is associated with an increased risk for mouth and tongue cancers (Sari et al., 2024). Like esophageal cancer, gastroesophageal reflux increases the risk of developing HNSCC. This is especially true for cancer of the larynx, where reflux disease increases the risk of developing this cancer with an OR of 2.47 (Sari et al., 2024). Poor diet is also associated with an increased risk of HNSCC (Saraiya et al., 2020).

1.2.3 Inequalities in HNSCC

Factors that contribute to disparities in HNSCC include differences linked to sex, race, ethnicity, substance abuse, and socioeconomic status (Fei-Zhang et al., 2023; Islami et al., 2021). The influence of socioeconomic factors and poverty in HNSCC inequalities is exacerbated by the fact that these cancers are some of the most expensive to treat and manage. This high cost means that both patients and health systems are placed under a huge burden, one that is disproportionate in lower-income countries and poorer communities (Massa et al., 2019; Wissinger et al., 2014). A simple measure that can be used to demonstrate the contribution of social factors and inequality to HNSCC treatment, diagnosis, and outcome is known as the *social determinants of health* (SDoH) (Gruszczynski et al., 2022). A hospital study showed that patients with more of those SDoHs associated with being more vulnerable are more likely to succumb to HNSCC. Patients relying on public health systems also have a lower chance of survival. Even those more vulnerable patients who survived over an initial period showed worse outcomes as time goes on compared to patients with more advantageous SDoHs

(Menezes et al., 2023). Among adolescents and young adults (AYA) diagnosed with cancer, HNSCC is one of the more common cancers and is a major cause of cancer-related mortality. A study in India showed that, between 2011 and 2015, HNSCC was the most common cancer found among patients in the 15–29 age group (Sharma & Singh, 2016). In the United States, HNSCCs were in the top 10 leading causes of cancer-related death among AYA (Anderson & Nichols, 2020). There are also pediatric-specific SDoHs, including being male, being a member of a racial minority, poverty, and language isolation (Gruszczynski et al., 2022).

1.3 Diagnosis and Screening

Approximately 65% of cases present in an advanced state (Jemal et al., 2007; Muto et al., 2004). This is very likely because the early detection of many HNSCCs is difficult. This is due to patients not remembering their exact medical history and the fact that many vague or seemingly unimportant medical histories can contribute to HNSCC development. Another contributing factor is that many HNSCCs may lack any distinctive diagnostic features (Jemal et al., 2007; Muto et al., 2004).

1.3.1 Traditional and New Diagnosis and Screening Methods

The most common conventional means of diagnosing HNSCC relies on biopsies to prepare tissue sections and then using these sections to perform histopathology or on the use of clinical radiological and medical imaging examinations (Fuller et al., 2015; Jemal et al., 2007; Muto et al., 2004). Biopsy provides the most accurate diagnosis of HNSCCs and remains the gold standard of HNSCC diagnosis (Badvi et al., 2017). Despite biopsy being the gold standard for HNSCC diagnosis, its disadvantages include it being invasive and requiring trained clinicians to perform the removal, preparation, and analysis of the tissue. Unfortunately, biopsy is an invasive procedure involving local anaesthetization and requiring the excising of enough tissue (both width and depth). It is also complicated by requiring the correct handling and processing of the excised tissue while effectively avoiding contamination, which will ensure an accurate and definitive diagnosis (Masthan et al., 2013). These disadvantages contribute to the delayed diagnosis of HNSCC and lead to diagnosis at more advanced stages (Mascitti et al., 2018). Additionally, HNSCCs commonly undergo metastasis, which contributes to the 5-year survival rate being < 50% (Cristaldi et al., 2019). As a result, new diagnostic modalities have been developed for many HNSCCs (Badvi et al., 2017).

Biomarkers can be used for HNSCC diagnosis and monitoring. The material to be tested for the presence of these biomarkers can be obtained from a wide variety of samples, including plasma, serum, saliva, and tissue (Marakala, 2023). Another revolutionary diagnostic tool is the use of liquid biopsies to provide the material for screening for or monitoring of various HNSCCs through circulating tumor DNA (ctDNA), circulating tumor cells (CTCs), and exosomal miRNAs. These tools can be used to not only detect the presence of the cancer but also to inform treatment choice and planning as well as monitor response to treatment (Franzmann et al., 2005). Saliva is one of the most promising sources for obtaining material for testing for the presence of biomarkers for many types of HNSCC (Javaid et al., 2016). The presence of various proteins in the saliva has been suggested as a useful biomarker in HNSCC (Franzmann et al., 2005). One of the new methods used to diagnose oral cancer is *exfoliative cytology*, which uses microscopic examination of exfoliated cells in the saliva (Göregen et al., 2011).

The use of various biomarkers has improved diagnosis, precision, and sensitivity (Marakala, 2023). The highest diagnostic test accuracy (DTA) for HNSCC has been achieved using a specific combination of biomarkers that include miR-196a + miR-196b, pro\propionate+, acetone+, acetate + choline, and pGSN + sFasL (Franzmann et al., 2005). The use of circulating biomarkers still needs to be validated for HNSCC before they can be integrated into a clinical setting (Nonaka & Wong, 2018).

1.3.2 Prevention

As with other cancers, prevention of HNSCC is the best way to decrease the impact of this disease. The most effective means to prevent HNSCC is through public health programs that increase the implementation of screening programs and help to increase public awareness of the disease (Muto et al., 2004). An accumulation of genetic and epigenetic changes contributes to the development of HNSCC. These changes can be targeted to prevent the development of these cancers. Methods to counter these changes can be aimed to interrupt, delay, or reverse these changes using chemo-preventative compounds, either natural or synthetic (Hong & Sporn, 1997). High doses of retinoids have been shown to reverse early premalignant lesions in oral cancers. Unfortunately, these high doses are associated with mucocutaneous toxicity (Hong et al., 1986). A study showed that the combination of interferon-α, α-tocopherol, and 13-*cis*-retinoic acid was able to reverse dysplastic HNSCC lesions (Papadimitrakopoulou et al., 1999). This combination of drugs was able to prevent the development of laryngeal lesions into full-blown cancer of the larynx. Analyzing laryngeal tissue following treatment showed that the histology reverted to a more normal appearance following treatment. However, the genetic changes driving the initial transformation remained present (Mao et al., 1998). The contribution of HPV infection to the development of HNSCC can be negated through the institution of HPV vaccination programs (Brocklehurst et al., 2013).

The leading method for preventing the development of secondary HNSCC is to screen for high-risk patients. The highest risk factor for the development of secondary HNSCC is a previous medical history involving a primary HNSCC. A primary HNSCC increases the risk of developing secondary HNSCC by 2–7% per year (Gan et al., 2013; Kim et al., 2007). Risk factors that contribute to the development of secondary tumors include lifestyle factors such as the use of tobacco and alcohol as well as genetic and immune-related factors. The genetic basis underlying the development of secondary HNSCC includes factors such as genetic instability, mutations, and preexisting genetic susceptibilities. Immune-related factors primarily result from immunodeficiency, which can result from cancer treatments such as chemotherapy and radiotherapy as well as from immunosuppression resulting from autoimmune diseases and immunosuppressive drugs used for organ transplant. Finally, immune suppression might be the result of surgical treatment (Harris et al., 2013). The most basic screening tool for oral cancer remains routine inspection of the oral cavity. This is most effective when performed by the same primary care provider who can then identify changes earlier, resulting in an earlier diagnosis. However, the same is not true for laryngeal or pharyngeal cancers (Prout et al., 1990). Genetic tests for the prevention of secondary HNSCC include screening patients for *p53* abnormalities and *cyclin D1* polymorphisms (Izzo et al., 2003) as well as testing for aneuploidy or loss of heterozygosity at various tumor suppressor loci in those patients with premalignant lesions (Partridge et al., 2000; Rosin et al., 2000). At the same time, certain drugs can be used to prevent metastasis or the progression of HNSCC. These include selective cyclooxygenase-2 inhibitors, EGFR kinase inhibitors, and natural products such as the epigallocatechin gallate component of green tea (Deng et al., 2024).

1.4 Treating HNC

HNSCC are difficult to treat because they are a diverse group of cancers with different characteristics and require different treatment approaches. Since the cancer may affect the mouth, tongue, lips, or gums, patients may not be eating properly, resulting in malnourishment. Many comorbidities also are associated with HNSCC. Finally, treatments themselves, such as radiation therapy, surgery, and chemotherapy, may have side effects especially associated with the location of HNSCC, including difficulties in eating and breathing as well as disfigurements in the patient's appearance (Kalavacherla et al., 2024). Advances have been made in all the traditional treatments for HNSCC, including surgery, radiotherapy, chemotherapy, and targeted therapeutic agents. Advancements in surgical treatment have centered on the conservation of organ function, microsurgery, more effective reconstructive surgery, and robot-assisted surgery. Radiation therapy has advanced through the use of divided radiation doses and the use of more directed techniques with tissue segmentation. Chemotherapy drugs have been used in conjunction with other treatments to reverse the development of resistance to treatment, while new targeted therapies have been designed to target new molecules and pathways.

1.4.1 Traditional Treatments

The initial treatment for localized HNSCC takes the form of surgery in combination with chemotherapy or radiotherapy (Karabajakian et al., 2017). The most common chemotherapy drugs used to treat HNSCC are docetaxel, cisplatin, and 5-fluorouracil (5-FU). Treatment with these drugs is normally followed with radiation therapy (Pignon et al., 2009). Cisplatin-based treatment enhanced OS in patients with localized HNSCC, according to a meta-analysis of 50 trials (Pignon et al., 2009). Despite the survival advantages offered by cisplatin, especially in postoperative treatment, its use is associated with side defects. These include hematologic toxicities, mucositis, and nausea (Bernier et al., 2004). Multiagent chemotherapy in conjunction with radiation therapy has been shown to be successful in the treatment of HNSCC. Examples include a combination of radiation and various combinations of 5-FU, cisplatin, paclitaxel, and hydroxyurea (Forastiere et al., 2003; Garden et al., 2001; Vokes et al., 2000). In the late 1980s to mid-1990s, the use of chemotherapy in combination with radiotherapy led to successful treatment of laryngeal cancer while preserving the larynx. In addition to this, the survival rates achieved using this strategy were comparable to those achieved with treatment involving surgical resection and postoperative radiation (Lefebvre et al., 1996). Chemotherapy used in conjunction with radiotherapy has the added advantage of minimizing radio resistance since chemotherapy can inhibit the repair of DNA damage induced by radiation (Pignon et al., 2000). The use of chemotherapy and radiation therapy in the treatment of HNSCC also showed higher survival rates compared to radiation therapy alone (Adelstein et al., 2003; Forastiere et al., 2001) and demonstrated a greater degree of organ preservation (Forastiere et al., 2003).

Molecular targeted therapies have shown the greatest advancement in the past few decades (Kozakiewicz & Grzybowska-Szatkowska, 2018). These new targeted therapies are a strategy to treat HNSCC without the toxicity associated with chemotherapy. Some of these treatments target epidermal growth factor receptor (EGFR), tyrosine kinases, vascular endothelial growth factors (VEGF), protein farnesylation, and *p53*.

EGFR is overexpressed in 80–100% of both premalignant and malignant HNSCC lesions. This overexpression is associated with poor and adverse outcomes (Rubin Grandis et al., 1998). The binding of epidermal growth factor and transforming growth factor-α to EGFR leads to dimerization of EGFR, receptor tyrosine kinase activation, and downstream signaling cascade activation as a result of the phosphorylation of multiple substrates. This signaling pathway can then activate cell proliferation and tumor growth (Salomon et al., 1995). Multiple methods have been developed to inhibit EGFR expression or signaling. Signaling can be targeted using tyrosine kinase inhibitors, monoclonal antibodies, and ligand-linked toxin. EGFR expression can be downregulated using antisense oligonucleotides (Mendelsohn & Baselga, 2003). The blocking of EGFR expression using anti-sense EGFR DNA creates a complementary DNA sequence that binds to the *EGFR* DNA sequence, thus blocking its transcription. This therapy can be personalized by changing the sequence to suit the mutations in an individual patient. These antisense treatments can reduce the proliferation of HNSCC cells (Bauman et al., 2018).

Monoclonal antibodies targeting EGFR include those such as cetuximab, which binds to domain III of the extracellular region of EGFR (Matta et al., 2009). Not only does this antibody inhibit the binding of ligands to EGFR, but it can also block the function of EGFR by inhibiting its phosphorylation (Huang & Harari, 2000). Cetuximab has been shown to effectively increase the effectiveness of HNSCC treatment, resulting in increased survival when it is used in combination with other conventional therapies. The antibody can also be used to increase treatment effectiveness in cisplatin-resistant HNSCC (Mendelsohn & Baselga, 2003). Other monoclonal antibodies targeting EGFR include panitumumab, zalutumumab, and nimotuzumab (Subramanium et al., 2015; Vermorken et al., 2013).

Small molecules that inhibit receptor tyrosine kinase activity can bind reversibly or irreversibly and were shown to be clinically effective in treating HNSCC. These include gefitinib (Iressa) and erlotinib (Tarceva) (Soulieres et al., 2004). Use of these compounds to treat HNSCC showed response rates of 10% (gefitinib) and 4% (erlotinib) with the side effects of these compounds including acne, rash, diarrhea, and nausea (Soulieres et al., 2004).

Abnormalities in components of G1 to S-phase cell cycle transition signaling and regulation pathways are found in ~90% of all human cancers, and HNSCC is no exception. In various cancers of the head and neck, cyclin D1 is overexpressed while its inhibitor p16 is not expressed (Patel et al., 1998). The drug flavopiridol is a cyclin-dependent kinase inhibitor that was shown to decrease the expression of cyclin D1 and VEGF, leading to increased levels of apoptosis and decreased growth in HNSCC tumors (Patel et al., 1998). Ribociclib is a CDK 4/6 inhibitor that has been shown to be effective in the treatment of HPV-negative HNSCC (Goel et al., 2020). It induces cell cycle arrest in HNSCC cell lines and increases the sensitivity of HNSCC to radiotherapy (Tzong-Shyuan et al., 2019). Another CDK inhibitor, palbociclib, was used in conjunction with cetuximab to successfully treat cisplatin- and cetuximab-resistant HPV-negative HNSCC (Adkins et al., 2019).

1.4.2 Immunotherapy

The poor prognosis for HNSCC despite advances in surgery, radiotherapy, and chemotherapy has led to the development of immunotherapy for HNSCC, especially for HPV-negative HNSCC. The development of immunotherapy is based on the strategy that an immune system that functions properly can effectively combat the growth of cancer. Most immunotherapies rely on blocking signaling pathways that can downregulate immune activation against cancer cells. Alternatively, they can attempt to stimulate those immune pathways that activate the immune system against cancer cells (Bauman et al., 2017). Immunotherapy can be used in conjunction with many chemotherapy drugs such as cisplatin that can induce immunogenic changes that stimulate the immune system (de Biasi et al., 2014). Immunotherapies are effective against both HPV-positive and HPV-negative HNSCCs (Bauman et al., 2017). To be effective against HPV-positive HNSCC, immunotherapy can target virus-specific tumor antigens, such as E6 and E7 (Bauman et al., 2017).

Programmed cell death protein 1 (PD-1) and programmed death-ligand 1 (PD-L1) are common targets for immunotherapy since PD-1 is an immunoreceptor that suppresses inflammatory response once its ligands, PD-L1 and PD-L2, bind to it. PD-1 is expressed on both T and B lymphocytes, monocytes, and dendritic cells (Grzywnowicz & Giannopoulos, 2012). HNSCC cells express both the receptor and the ligand, leading to dysfunction in the immune system's response to the cancer (Dong et al., 1999). Anti-PD-1 antibodies such as nivolumab have been shown to be effective when used in conjunction with chemotherapy, resulting in increased survival rates with fewer adverse effects (Ferris et al., 2016). Cytotoxic T lymphocyte antigen 4 (CTLA4) is present on the surfaces of activated T lymphocytes, where it binds to B7 ligands on antigen-presenting cells (APCs, including tumor cells). CTLA4 competes with other receptors such as CD28 to compete for B7 ligands to prevent T-cell activation and proliferation. T cells can be activated by inhibiting CTLA-4 ligand-binding receptors, thus activating the immune response (Rotte, 2019). Ipilimumab is a CTLA-4 inhibitor that can be used in conjunction with PD-1 inhibitors to effectively treat HNSCC (Zech et al., 2020). Another receptor present on the surface of activated T, B, dendritic, and natural killer cells is the lymphocyte-activated gene-3 (LAG-3). It inhibits the interaction between T-cell receptors and MHC-II, impairing cytokine production and T-cell proliferation. The anti-LAG-3 antibody relatlimab inhibits binding of LAG-3 to MHC-II, leading to an increase in immune response to HNSCC cells (Long et al., 2018). Immune cells such as $CD4^+$ and $CD8^+$ T cells, regulatory T cells, mast cells, natural killer cells, and dendritic cells express T-cell immunoglobulin mucin-3 (TIM-3). The ligand for TIM-3, galectin-9, is produced by tumor cells and acts to suppress immune responses (Wolf et al., 2020). Anti-TIM-3 antibodies can increase the immune response against cancers including HNSCC (Sakuishi et al., 2010).

1.4.3 Precision Medicine

"Precision medicine" usually refers to the personalization of systemic therapy according to the molecular features of a tumor; however, this term should also include radiation therapy since the targeting and application of radiation can be customized to each individual patient (Fröhlich et al., 2018). In practice, personalized medicine relies on diagnostic testing using a patient's genetic makeup, molecular or cellular analyses, or imaging features (Cheng et al., 2018). HNSCCs can be analyzed through the use of genetic testing to characterize mutations that promote disease progression and treatment resistance or sensitivity (Pollock & Grandis, 2015). Changes in gene expression and transcription can be identified using transcriptomic, epigenetic, and proteomic testing (Yang et al., 2023). Current approaches to the treatment of HNSCC do not account for the clinical and molecular heterogeneity of these cancers (Grégoire et al., 2018). This commonly results in misdiagnosis and delays (Schlumpf & Haerle, 2014). Data from omics profiling studies can be used to identify subgroups of each of the various HNSCCs, but the identification of these various patterns is difficult, time-consuming, may be open to bias, and many patterns and features may be overlooked. To do this with any degree of accuracy and in a timely fashion requires the use of complex algorithms employed by artificial intelligence (AI) and machine learning. Modeling and algorithms employed by AI using machine and deep learning can be used to make accurate and efficient predictions (LeCun et al., 2015).

1.4.4 Surgical Interventions

In cases of oral, laryngeal, and hypopharyngeal squamous cell cancers where oncological resection is viable, surgical intervention is the primary approach. These surgical interventions are then followed by adjuvant therapies in the form of radiation therapy or chemotherapy (Chinn & Myers, 2015; Pfister et al., 2020). Recent advances in these types of surgical interventions include the use of transoral robotic surgery (TORS) and transoral laser microsurgery (TLM), and these advanced techniques have reduced postoperative hospital stays by 52% compared to standard open surgery. They have also resulted in a 90% reduction of patients requiring the continued use of a feeding tube at 1 year after surgery (White et al., 2013). TORS is generally reserved for small to moderately sized HNSCCs that are classed as T1–T2 staged tumors (White et al., 2013). Despite its usefulness, there has been a shift away from the use of surgery in high-volume treatment centers due to most patients requiring adjuvant therapy in conjunction with surgery. In these cases, surgery in conjunction with other treatments has been replaced with radiation alone or concurrent chemotherapy (Adelstein et al., 2017).

1.4.5 Radiation Therapy

Conventional radiation therapy relies on two or three radiation beams aimed from different directions, thus increasing the volume of radiation directed at the tissue. Advances in radiation therapy in HNSCC include three-dimensional conformal radiation therapy (3D CRT) where each of multiple beams is used to outline the target to deliver the highest dose to the tumor with the least amount of damage to surrounding tissue (Mallick & Waldron, 2009). A further development of this is intensity-modulated radiation therapy (IMRT), where, in addition to directing the beam, the strength of the beam can also be modulated. IMRT has become the standard for HNSCC treatment (Fregnani et al., 2016). Most commonly IMRT is used to treat nasopharynx and oropharynx cancers while avoiding the brain, brainstem, optic nerve, optic stem, and parotid salivary gland (Kwong et al., 2004). Another advancement linked to dosage is radiotherapy fractionation, where the radiation dosage is divided over time (Fu et al., 2000). Medical imaging can be used in conjunction with radiation therapy to guide the delivery of radiation. Image-guided radiotherapy allows the patient to be identically positioned for each treatment (Parvathaneni et al., 2012). Radiation therapy also needs to adapt as therapy progresses to account for the changes brought about by the treatment (Barker et al., 2004). Despite all attempts to minimize the effect of radiation therapy on normal tissue, radiation toxicity is a concern in the treatment of HNSCC. This is further exacerbated when radiation is used in combination with chemotherapy (Cox et al., 1995).

1.5 Prognosis and Quality of Life

The quality of life of patients undergoing or having completed treatment can be severely impacted due to both the disease and its treatments. Surgical resection may be functionally and aesthetically deforming; these deformations impact the quality of life by limiting the use of the mouth or throat as well as being psychologically damaging due to changes in appearance (Jemal et al., 2007; Muto et al., 2004). It is estimated that up to 60% of HNSCC survivors have unmet needs, and this situation will worsen as the number of survivors increases. Thus, current care models that are already inadequate will only become worse. This problem can only be resolved through the development of new care strategies and models (Agarwal et al., 2014). The same is true of those with terminal illnesses receiving palliative care. These patients may require specialized treatments and have needs unique to the consequences of HNSCC and its treatment. These needs may be both physical and social. A good—but in many cases impractical—approach is to continuously assess the patients' needs as treatment proceeds to establish their physical and psychological well-being at every step of the process. In palliative care, this will include psychological assessments, symptom management, and pain relief (Foxwell & Scott, 2011).

The Functional Assessment of Cancer Therapy Quality of Life Measurement System (FACT-H&N) is the tool most often used to assess the quality of life for HNSCC patients, as are various quality of life questionnaires (de Melo Filho et al., 2013). The FACT-H&N questionnaire contains 38 questions divided into physical well-being, social/family well-being, emotional well-being, functional well-being, and specific concerns (de Melo Filho et al., 2013). Other questionnaires examine specific domains to assess the patient's quality of life. These include pain, appearance, activity, recreation, deglutition, chewing, speech, shoulder mobility, taste, saliva production, mood, and anxiety (Fayers et al., 2001).

The quality of life for HNSCC patients may best be served by a combination of approaches including a holistic view. *Complementary and alternative medicine* (CAM) describes a collection of medical interventions that are not considered part of conventional medicine. The use of CAM is thought to be fairly prevalent and is on the increase (Barnes et al., 2008). With the adoption of CAM in the care of patients suffering from various diseases as a strategy to improve quality of life, the term "CAM" has been steadily replaced with the term "integrative medicine," with the primary difference being that integrative medicine is a collaborative approach using both CAM and conventional approaches (Milden & Stokols, 2004). The increased use of these treatments by patients is commonly found in cancer patients, including HNSCC patients. Medical professionals treating these patients must familiarize themselves with these therapies to best assist their patients in the choice and application of various CAM treatments. However, many physicians and medical personnel feel that they are not knowledgeable enough about these treatments and thus will not engage with their patients concerning them (Milden & Stokols, 2004). Additionally many health insurance and medical aid companies will not pay for these treatments (Trinidade et al., 2011). Important considerations for the use of these treatments include any potential risks or benefits they may have as well as any evidence from scientific studies showing their effectiveness. A factor that is often of greater concern to the medical professional is whether the patient intends to use these therapies in combination with standard treatments or in place of them (Miller et al., 2010).

1.6 Conclusion

This volume aims to provide readers with a comprehensive review of the current situation of HNCs, covering the epidemiology, risk factors, diagnosis, treatment, and management of these cancers. It will highlight the latest advancements in diagnostic tools, therapeutic approaches, and multidisciplinary care strategies while offering insights into global perspectives on these cancers. Finally, the volume will discuss survivorship issues, quality of life considerations, and the psychosocial impacts of HNCs on patients during diagnosis, treatment, and recovery (Figure 1.4).

Chapter 1 discusses the fundamentals of HNC. Chapter 2 examines the various risk factors associated with HNC and offers a comprehensive review encompassing both well-established and emerging risk factors. That chapter also examines the role played by socioeconomic factors in influencing the risk of HNC, highlighting the intricate interplay between socioeconomic conditions and the epidemiology of the disease. Chapter 3 investigates inequalities in the burden, treatment, and ultimate outcomes in HNC. The chapter also discusses strategies that can be employed to address and mitigate these disparities.

The next section of the volume discusses the technological advances in diagnosis and treatment of HNCs. The first chapter of this section, Chapter 4, delves into the forefront of medical technology to explore the latest breakthroughs in diagnostic tools and techniques for HNC. This includes cutting-edge imaging technologies and molecular diagnostics, and the chapter highlights how these advancements are transforming the early detection of HNCs. Chapter 5 focuses on the paradigm shift brought about by precision medicine in the realm of HNC

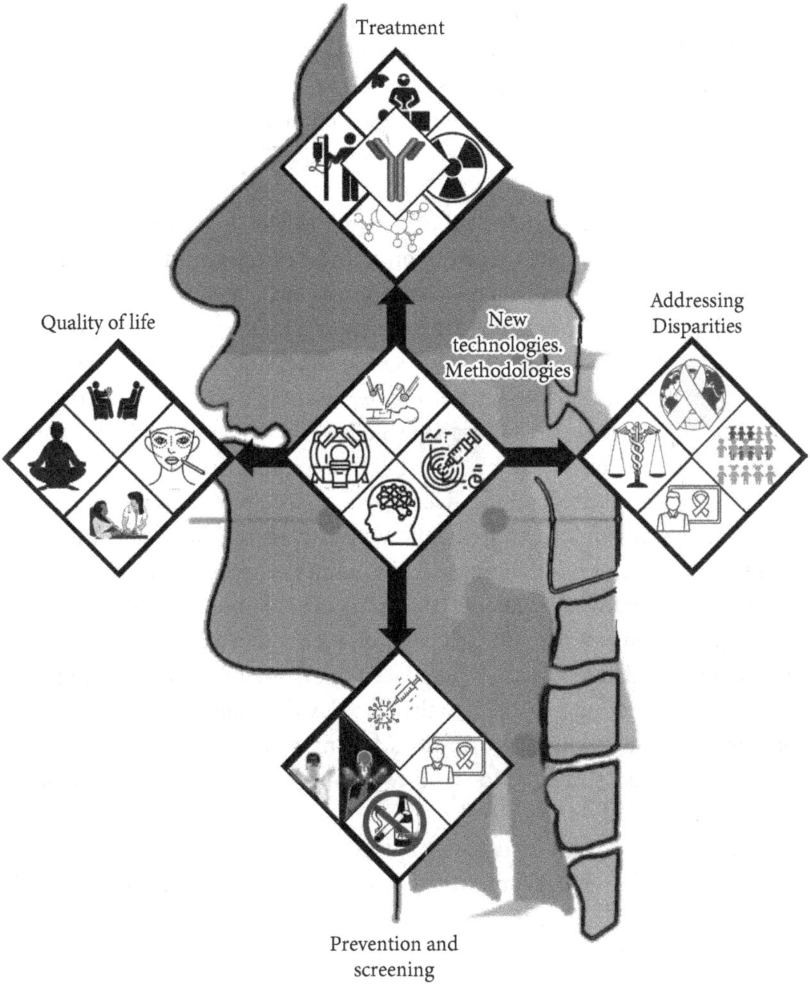

Figure 1.4 A summary of the approaches and topics covered in this book. The central theme concerns the advances in treatments, diagnosis, prevention, and screening in the management of head and neck squamous cell cancers (HNSCCs). It also encompasses the improvements in the quality of life of HNSCC patients and addresses disparities in the treatment of HNSCC by examining key developments and new technologies that promise these improvements.

treatment. It discusses the tailoring of therapeutic approaches based on individual patient characteristics, such as genetic and molecular profiles, and examines how this strategy can revolutionize clinicians' approach in personalizing the treatment of HNCs. Chapter 6 discusses the use of immunotherapy to treat HNC.

It highlights how immunotherapy and targeted therapies represent a new frontier in HNC treatment. This chapter delves into the mechanisms, successes, and challenges of these novel approaches.

The next section of the book discusses comprehensive HNC care. The first chapter in this section, Chapter 7, is a comprehensive exploration of the latest surgical innovations in HNC. It covers subjects such as minimally invasive techniques to cutting-edge robotic surgeries and intricate reconstructive procedures. It discusses the contribution of these new techniques to improved precision, reduced invasiveness, and enhanced postoperative recovery. Chapter 8 examines the evolving landscape of radiation therapy for HNC and discusses the refinement of traditional techniques and the introduction of IMRT and proton therapy. It also discusses the use of these technologies to optimize treatment outcomes while minimizing collateral damage to healthy tissues. Chapter 9 reviews the use of multidisciplinary approaches in the treatment of HNCs. These approaches include diverse medical disciplines such as surgery, radiation therapy, systemic treatments, and supportive care. The chapter highlights how healthcare teams employing these disciplines synergize to provide holistic and patient-centered care. Chapter 10 conducts a comprehensive examination of the organization and structure of health systems dedicated to managing HNC. The chapter delves into the challenges faced in organizing and delivering effective HNC care, offering insights into the complexities inherent in the healthcare landscape and identifying opportunities for improvement. It achieves this by discussing potential strategies to enhance the overall organization and delivery of care for individuals facing HNC.

Section four of this book discusses survivorship, quality of life, and holistic care in HNCs. The first chapter of this section, Chapter 11, focuses on the long-term care of HNC survivors. It reviews the effect the disease has on the physical, emotional, and social aspects of survivorship and examine rehabilitation, supportive care, and strategies to enhance the overall quality of life for patients. Chapter 12 explores emerging technologies poised to shape the trajectory of HNC diagnosis and treatment. This includes the use of AI applications to novel therapeutic modalities. The chapter provides information concerning topics at the forefront of research and innovation that will pave the way for the next generation of advancements in cancer care. Chapter 13 discusses the use of biomarkers and predictive modeling in personalized medicine for HNC and the role of these biomarkers in predicting treatment responses and prognosis and in guiding individualized therapeutic decisions. Chapter 14 reviews the integration of AI into the realm of HNC. The chapter discusses the role AI can play in image analysis for early detection and in predictive modeling for treatment response. The chapter highlights the transformative potential of AI in enhancing diagnostic accuracy, treatment planning, and, ultimately, patient outcomes.

The concluding section of this book discusses global perspectives and prevention of HNC. The first chapter of this section, Chapter 15, focuses on the unique challenges and advancements in the diagnosis and treatment of HNCs in pediatric patients. This includes discussion on age-specific considerations to tailored treatment approaches, emphasizing the importance of specialized care for young patients facing this complex disease. Chapter 16 explores comprehensive prevention strategies for HNC. It begins by examining primary prevention measures, delving into the realm of lifestyle modifications and the potential impact of vaccination. It will also discuss the use of early detection and screening programs and the crucial role they play in secondary cancer prevention efforts. Additionally, the chapter highlights the significance of public health interventions in reducing the overall incidence of HNC, providing a holistic view of preventive measures that can be employed at various levels to mitigate the impact of this complex disease. Chapter 17 delves into the often-overlooked psychological and social dimensions of living with HNC. It addresses the emotional challenges, impact on relationships, and the importance of psychosocial support for HNC patients. This chapter explores the growing significance of complementary and integrative therapies in supporting individuals with HNC. Chapter 18 discusses various holistic approaches, showcasing their role in enhancing overall well-being and complementing traditional medical treatments. The chapter also discusses palliative care in HNC, providing an in-depth exploration of supportive care tailored to all stages of the disease. The chapter also outlines strategic approaches for the integration of palliative care into the comprehensive treatment plan for HNC.

The conclusion of the book, in Chapter 19, combines insights from two perspectives: first, it explores regional variations in the prevalence, diagnosis, and treatment of HNC on a global scale. Second, in its role as a conclusion, it provides a roadmap for future research and innovation in the field. The discussion emphasizes the importance of international collaboration, highlights existing gaps in knowledge, and presents strategic recommendations to advance research initiatives and improve outcomes for individuals affected by HNC.

References

ADELSTEIN, D., GILLISON, M. L., PFISTER, D. G., SPENCER, S., ADKINS, D., BRIZEL, D. M., BURTNESS, B., BUSSE, P. M., CAUDELL, J. J., CMELAK, A. J., COLEVAS, A. D., EISELE, D. W., FENTON, M., FOOTE, R. L., GILBERT, J., HADDAD, R. I., HICKS, W. L., HITCHCOCK, Y. J., JIMENO, A., LEIZMAN, D., LYDIATT, W. M., MAGHAMI, E., MELL, L. K., MITTAL, B. B., PINTO, H. A., RIDGE, J. A., ROCCO, J., RODRIGUEZ, C. P., SHAH, J. P., WEBER, R. S., WITEK, M., WORDEN, F., YOM, S. S., ZHEN, W., BURNS, J. L., & DARLOW, S. D. 2017. NCCN guidelines insights: Head and neck cancers, Version 2.2017. *J Natl Compr Canc Netw*, 15, 761–70.

ADELSTEIN, D. J., LI, Y., ADAMS, G. L., WAGNER, H., JR., KISH, J. A., ENSLEY, J. F., SCHULLER, D. E., & FORASTIERE, A. A. 2003. An intergroup phase III comparison of standard radiation therapy and two schedules of concurrent chemoradiotherapy in patients with unresectable squamous cell head and neck cancer. *J Clin Oncol*, 21, 92–8.

ADKINS, D., LEY, J., NEUPANE, P., WORDEN, F., SACCO, A. G., PALKA, K., GRILLEY-OLSON, J. E., MAGGIORE, R., SALAMA, N. N., TRINKAUS, K., VAN TINE, B. A., STEUER, C. E., SABA, N. F., & OPPELT, P. 2019. Palbociclib and cetuximab in platinum-resistant and in cetuximab-resistant human papillomavirus-unrelated head and neck cancer: A multicentre, multigroup, phase 2 trial. *Lancet Oncology*, 20, 1295–1305.

AGARWAL, S. K., MUNJAL, M., KOUL, R., & AGARWAL, R. 2014. Prospective evaluation of the quality of life of oral tongue cancer patients before and after the treatment. *Ann Palliat Med*, 3, 238–43.

ANDERSON, C., & NICHOLS, H. B. 2020. Trends in late mortality among adolescent and young adult cancer survivors. *J Natl Cancer Inst*, 112, 994–1002.

AZZAM, P., MROUEH, M., FRANCIS, M., DAHER, A. A., & ZEIDAN, Y. H. 2020. Radiation-induced neuropathies in head and neck cancer: Prevention and treatment modalities. *Ecancermedicalscience*, 14, 1133.

BADVI, J. A., KULSOOM, J., & UJJAN, I. J. E. M. 2017. Recent techniques for diagnosis of oral squamous cell carcinoma. 5, 165–8.

BARKER, J. L., JR., GARDEN, A. S., ANG, K. K., O'DANIEL, J. C., WANG, H., COURT, L. E., MORRISON, W. H., ROSENTHAL, D. I., CHAO, K. S., TUCKER, S. L., MOHAN, R., & DONG, L. 2004. Quantification of volumetric and geometric changes occurring during fractionated radiotherapy for head-and-neck cancer using an integrated CT/linear accelerator system. *Int J Radiat Oncol Biol Phys*, 59, 960–70.

BARNES, P. M., BLOOM, B., & NAHIN, R. L. 2008. Complementary and alternative medicine use among adults and children: United States, 2007. *Natl Health Stat Report*, 1–23.

BAUMAN, J. E., COHEN, E., FERRIS, R. L., ADELSTEIN, D. J., BRIZEL, D. M., RIDGE, J. A., O'SULLIVAN, B., BURTNESS, B. A., BUTTERFIELD, L. H., CARSON, W. E., DISIS, M. L., FOX, B. A., GAJEWSKI, T. F., GILLISON, M. L., HODGE, J. W., LE, Q. T., RABEN, D., STROME, S. E., LYNN, J., & MALIK, S. 2017. Immunotherapy of head and neck cancer: Emerging clinical trials from a National Cancer Institute Head and Neck Cancer Steering Committee Planning Meeting. *Cancer*, 123, 1259–71.

BAUMAN, J. E., DUVVURI, U., THOMAS, S., GOODING, W. E., CLUMP, D. A., KARLOVITS, B., WEHBE, A., MILLER, F. R., KIM, S., SEN, M., HERON, D. E., GRANDIS, J. R., & ARGIRIS, A. 2018. Phase 1 study of EGFR-antisense DNA, cetuximab, and radiotherapy in head and neck cancer with preclinical correlatives. *Cancer*, 124, 3881–9.

BERNIER, J., DOMENGE, C., OZSAHIN, M., MATUSZEWSKA, K., LEFÈBVRE, J. L., GREINER, R. H., GIRALT, J., MAINGON, P., ROLLAND, F., BOLLA, M., COGNETTI, F., BOURHIS, J., KIRKPATRICK, A., & VAN GLABBEKE, M. 2004. Postoperative irradiation with or without concomitant chemotherapy for locally advanced head and neck cancer. *N Engl J Med*, 350, 1945–52.

BOFFETTA, P., HECHT, S., GRAY, N., GUPTA, P., & STRAIF, K. 2008. Smokeless tobacco and cancer. *Lancet Oncol*, 9, 667–75.

BRENNAN, J. A., BOYLE, J. O., KOCH, W. M., GOODMAN, S. N., HRUBAN, R. H., EBY, Y. J., COUCH, M. J., FORASTIERE, A. A., & SIDRANSKY, D. 1995. Association between cigarette smoking and mutation of the p53 gene in squamous-cell carcinoma of the head and neck. *N Engl J Med*, 332, 712–7.

BROCKLEHURST, P., KUJAN, O., O'MALLEY, L. A., OGDEN, G., SHEPHERD, S., & GLENNY, A. M. 2013. Screening programmes for the early detection and prevention of oral cancer. *Cochrane Database Syst Rev*, 2013, Cd004150.

BROWN, L. M., MASON, T. J., PICKLE, L. W., STEWART, P. A., BUFFLER, P. A., BURAU, K., ZIEGLER, R. G., & FRAUMENI, J. F., JR. 1988. Occupational risk factors for laryngeal cancer on the Texas Gulf Coast. *Cancer Res*, 48, 1960–4.

CHENG, L., LOPEZ-BELTRAN, A., MASSARI, F., MACLENNAN, G. T., & MONTIRONI, R. 2018. Molecular testing for BRAF mutations to inform melanoma treatment decisions: A move toward precision medicine. *Mod Pathol*, 31, 24–38.

CHINN, S. B., & MYERS, J. N. 2015. Oral cavity carcinoma: Current management, controversies, and future directions. *J Clin Oncol*, 33, 3269–76.

CHOW, L. Q. M. 2020. Head and neck cancer. *N Engl J Med*, 382, 60–72.

COX, J. D., STETZ, J., & PAJAK, T. F. 1995. Toxicity criteria of the Radiation Therapy Oncology Group (RTOG) and the European Organization for Research and Treatment of Cancer (EORTC). *Int J Radiat Oncol Biol Phys*, 31, 1341–6.

CRISTALDI, M., MAUCERI, R., DI FEDE, O., GIULIANA, G., CAMPISI, G., & PANZARELLA, V. 2019. Salivary biomarkers for oral squamous cell carcinoma diagnosis and follow-up: Current status and perspectives. *Front Physiol*, 10, 1476.

DE BIASI, A. R., VILLENA-VARGAS, J., & ADUSUMILLI, P. S. 2014. Cisplatin-induced antitumor immunomodulation: A review of preclinical and clinical evidence. *Clin Cancer Res*, 20, 5384–91.

DE MELO FILHO, M. R., ROCHA, B. A., DE OLIVEIRA PIRES, M. B., FONSECA, E. S., DE FREITAS, E. M., JUNIOR, H. M., & SANTOS, F. B. G. J. B. J. O. O. 2013. Quality of life of patients with head and neck cancer. 79, 82–8.

DENG, J., MISRA, V., VILASH, N., WU, W., HUA, C., SON, K., CANFORA, F., KONG, F. Y. S., PAOLINI, R., MCCULLOUGH, M., & CELENTANO, A. 2024. Can a cup a day keep cancer away? A systematic review exploring the potential of coffee constituents in preventing oral squamous cell carcinoma. *J Oral Pathol Med*, 53, 8–19.

DONG, H., ZHU, G., TAMADA, K., & CHEN, L. 1999. B7-H1, a third member of the B7 family, co-stimulates T-cell proliferation and interleukin-10 secretion. *Nat Med*, 5, 1365–9.

FAYERS, P., AARONSON, N. K., BJORDAL, K., GRØNVOLD, M., CURRAN, D., & BOTTOMLEY, A. 2001. *EORTC QLQ-C30 Scoring Manual*. Brussels, Belgium: European Organisation for Research and Treatment of Cancer.

FEI-ZHANG, D. J., CHELIUS, D. C., PATEL, U. A., SMITH, S. S., SHEYN, A. M., & RASTATTER, J. C. 2023. Assessment of social vulnerability in pediatric head and neck cancer care and prognosis in the United States. *JAMA Netw Open*, 6, e230016.

FERLAY, J., ERVIK, M., LAM, F., COLOMBET, M., MERY, L., PIÑEROS, M., ZNAOR, A., SOERJOMATARAM, I., & BRAY, F. J. L., FRANCE: INTERNATIONAL AGENCY FOR RESEARCH ON CANCER. 2024. Global cancer observatory: Cancer today. Available at: https://gco.iarc.who.int/today [Accessed April 2, 2024.]

FERRIS, R. L., BLUMENSCHEIN, G., JR., FAYETTE, J., GUIGAY, J., COLEVAS, A. D., LICITRA, L., HARRINGTON, K., KASPER, S., VOKES, E. E., EVEN, C., WORDEN, F., SABA, N. F., IGLESIAS DOCAMPO, L. C., HADDAD, R., RORDORF, T., KIYOTA, N., TAHARA, M., MONGA, M., LYNCH, M., GEESE, W. J., KOPIT, J., SHAW, J. W., & GILLISON, M. L. 2016. Nivolumab for recurrent squamous-cell carcinoma of the head and neck. *N Engl J Med*, 375, 1856–67.

FORASTIERE, A., KOCH, W., TROTTI, A., & SIDRANSKY, D. 2001. Head and neck cancer. *N Engl J Med*, 345, 1890–900.

FORASTIERE, A. A., GOEPFERT, H., MAOR, M., PAJAK, T. F., WEBER, R., MORRISON, W., GLISSON, B., TROTTI, A., RIDGE, J. A., CHAO, C., PETERS, G., LEE, D. J., LEAF, A., ENSLEY, J., & COOPER, J. 2003. Concurrent chemotherapy and radiotherapy for organ preservation in advanced laryngeal cancer. *N Engl J Med*, 349, 2091–8.

FOXWELL, K. R., & SCOTT, S. E. 2011. Coping together and apart: Exploring how patients and their caregivers manage terminal head and neck cancer. *J Psychosoc Oncol*, 29, 308–26.

FRANZMANN, E. J., REATEGUI, E. P., CARRAWAY, K. L., HAMILTON, K. L., WEED, D. T., & GOODWIN, W. J. 2005. Salivary soluble CD44: A potential molecular marker for head and neck cancer. *Cancer Epidemiol Biomarkers Prev*, 14, 735–9.

FREGNANI, E. R., PARAHYBA, C. J., MORAIS-FARIA, K., FONSECA, F. P., RAMOS, P. A., DE MORAES, F. Y., DA CONCEIÇÃO VASCONCELOS, K. G., MENEGUSSI, G.,

SANTOS-SILVA, A. R., & BRANDÃO, T. B. 2016. IMRT delivers lower radiation doses to dental structures than 3DRT in head and neck cancer patients. *Radiat Oncol*, 11, 116.

FRÖHLICH, H., BALLING, R., BEERENWINKEL, N., KOHLBACHER, O., KUMAR, S., LENGAUER, T., MAATHUIS, M. H., MOREAU, Y., MURPHY, S. A., PRZYTYCKA, T. M., REBHAN, M., RÖST, H., SCHUPPERT, A., SCHWAB, M., SPANG, R., STEKHOVEN, D., SUN, J., WEBER, A., ZIEMEK, D., & ZUPAN, B. 2018. From hype to reality: Data science enabling personalized medicine. *BMC Med*, 16, 150.

FU, K. K., PAJAK, T. F., TROTTI, A., JONES, C. U., SPENCER, S. A., PHILLIPS, T. L., GARDEN, A. S., RIDGE, J. A., COOPER, J. S., & ANG, K. K. 2000. A Radiation Therapy Oncology Group (RTOG) phase III randomized study to compare hyperfractionation and two variants of accelerated fractionation to standard fractionation radiotherapy for head and neck squamous cell carcinomas: First report of RTOG 9003. *Int J Radiat Oncol Biol Phys*, 48, 7–16.

FULLER, C., CAMILON, R., NGUYEN, S., JENNINGS, J., DAY, T., & GILLESPIE, M. B. 2015. Adjunctive diagnostic techniques for oral lesions of unknown malignant potential: Systematic review with meta-analysis. *Head Neck*, 37, 755–62.

GAN, S. J., DAHLSTROM, K. R., PECK, B. W., CAYWOOD, W., LI, G., WEI, Q., ZAFEREO, M. E., & STURGIS, E. M. 2013. Incidence and pattern of second primary malignancies in patients with index oropharyngeal cancers versus index nonoropharyngeal head and neck cancers. *Cancer*, 119, 2593–601.

GARDEN, A., PAJAK, T., VOKES, E., FORASTIERE, A., RIDGE, J., JONES, C., HORWITZ, E., GLISSON, B., NABELL, L., & COOPER, J. J. L. C. 2001. A phase II randomized trial of concurrent radiation (RT) and chemotherapy for advanced squamous cell carcinomas (SCC) of the head and neck. 34, S66–S67.

GARG, A., CHATURVEDI, P., MISHRA, A., & DATTA, S. 2015. A review on harmful effects of pan masala. 52, 663–6.

GILLISON, M. L., KOCH, W. M., CAPONE, R. B., SPAFFORD, M., WESTRA, W. H., WU, L., ZAHURAK, M. L., DANIEL, R. W., VIGLIONE, M., SYMER, D. E., SHAH, K. V., & SIDRANSKY, D. 2000. Evidence for a causal association between human papillomavirus and a subset of head and neck cancers. *J Natl Cancer Inst*, 92, 709–20.

GOEL, B., TRIPATHI, N., BHARDWAJ, N., & JAIN, S. K. J. C. T. I. M. C. 2020. Small molecule CDK inhibitors for the therapeutic management of cancer. *Curr Top Med Chem*, 20, 1535–63.

GÖREGEN, M., AKGÜL, H. M., & GÜNDOĞDU, C. J. T. J. O. M. S. 2011. The cytomorphological analysis of buccal mucosa cells in smokers. *Turk J Med Sci*, 41, 205–10.

GRÉGOIRE, V., THORWARTH, D., & LEE, J. A. 2018. Molecular imaging-guided radiotherapy for the treatment of head-and-neck squamous cell carcinoma: Does it fulfill the promises? *Semin Radiat Oncol*, 28, 35–45.

GRUSZCZYNSKI, N. R., LOW, C. M., CHOBY, G., MEISTER, K. D., SMITH, B. H., & BALAKRISHNAN, K. 2022. Effects of social determinants of health care on pediatric thyroid cancer outcomes in the United States. *Otolaryngol Head Neck Surg*, 166, 1045–54.

GRZYWNOWICZ, M., & GIANNOPOULOS, K. J. A. H. P. 2012. The role of receptor programmed death-1 and its ligands in immune system and tumors. *Acta Haematol Pol*, 43, 132–145.

HARRIS, M. S., PHILLIPS, D. R., SAYER, J. L., & MOORE, M. G. 2013. A comparison of community-based and hospital-based head and neck cancer screening campaigns: Identifying high-risk individuals and early disease. *JAMA Otolaryngol Head Neck Surg*, 139, 568–73.

HASHIM, D., GENDEN, E., POSNER, M., HASHIBE, M., & BOFFETTA, P. 2019. Head and neck cancer prevention: From primary prevention to impact of clinicians on reducing burden. *Ann Oncol*, 30, 744–56.

HONG, W. K., ENDICOTT, J., ITRI, L. M., DOOS, W., BATSAKIS, J. G., BELL, R., FOFONOFF, S., BYERS, R., ATKINSON, E. N., VAUGHAN, C., & TOTH, B. B. 1986. 13-cis-retinoic acid in the treatment of oral leukoplakia. *N Engl J Med*, 315, 1501–5.

HONG, W. K., & SPORN, M. B. 1997. Recent advances in chemoprevention of cancer. *Science*, 278, 1073–7.

HUANG, S. M., & HARARI, P. M. 2000. Modulation of radiation response after epidermal growth factor receptor blockade in squamous cell carcinomas: Inhibition of damage repair, cell cycle kinetics, and tumor angiogenesis. *Clin Cancer Res*, 6, 2166–74.

INTERNATIONAL HUMAN GENOME SEQUENCING CONSORTIUM. 2004. Finishing the euchromatic sequence of the human genome. *Nature*, 431, 931–45.

ISLAMI, F., WARD, E. M., SUNG, H., CRONIN, K. A., TANGKA, F. K. L., SHERMAN, R. L., ZHAO, J., ANDERSON, R. N., HENLEY, S. J., YABROFF, K. R., JEMAL, A., & BENARD, V. B. 2021. Annual report to the nation on the status of cancer, Part 1: National cancer statistics. *J Natl Cancer Inst*, 113, 1648–69.

IZZO, J. G., PAPADIMITRAKOPOULOU, V. A., LIU, D. D., DEN HOLLANDER, P. L., BABENKO, I. M., KECK, J., EL-NAGGAR, A. K., SHIN, D. M., LEE, J. J., HONG, W. K., & HITTELMAN, W. N. 2003. Cyclin D1 genotype, response to biochemoprevention, and progression rate to upper aerodigestive tract cancer. *J Natl Cancer Inst*, 95, 198–205.

JAVAID, M. A., AHMED, A. S., DURAND, R., & TRAN, S. D. 2016. Saliva as a diagnostic tool for oral and systemic diseases. *J Oral Biol Craniofac Res*, 6, 66–75.

JEMAL, A., SIEGEL, R., WARD, E., MURRAY, T., XU, J., & THUN, M. J. 2007. Cancer statistics, 2007. *CA Cancer J Clin*, 57, 43–66.

KALAVACHERLA, S., BERNARD, B., KIM, S. S., DORNISCH, A., BLUMENFELD, L., LINNEMEYER-RISSER, K., SANGHVI, P., & GUO, T. 2024. Early improved functional outcomes in head and neck cancer patients with primary tumor detection. *Laryngoscope*, 134, 701–7.

KARABAJAKIAN, A., TOUSSAINT, P., NEIDHARDT, E.-M., PAULUS, V., SAINTIGNY, P., & FAYETTE, J. 2017. Chemotherapy for localized head and neck squamous cell cancers. 28, 362–8.

KIM, S. Y., ROH, J. L., YEO, N. K., KIM, J. S., LEE, J. H., CHOI, S. H., & NAM, S. Y. 2007. Combined 18F-fluorodeoxyglucose-positron emission tomography and computed tomography as a primary screening method for detecting second primary cancers and distant metastases in patients with head and neck cancer. *Ann Oncol*, 18, 1698–703.

KOZAKIEWICZ, P., & GRZYBOWSKA-SZATKOWSKA, L. 2018. Application of molecular targeted therapies in the treatment of head and neck squamous cell carcinoma. *Oncol Lett*, 15, 7497–505.

KWONG, D. L., POW, E. H., SHAM, J. S., MCMILLAN, A. S., LEUNG, L. H., LEUNG, W. K., CHUA, D. T., CHENG, A. C., WU, P. M., & AU, G. K. 2004. Intensity-modulated radiotherapy for early-stage nasopharyngeal carcinoma: A prospective study on disease control and preservation of salivary function. *Cancer*, 101, 1584–93.

LECUN, Y., BENGIO, Y., & HINTON, G. 2015. Deep learning. *Nature*, 521, 436–44.

LEFEBVRE, J. L., CHEVALIER, D., LUBOINSKI, B., KIRKPATRICK, A., COLLETTE, L., & SAHMOUD, T. 1996. Larynx preservation in pyriform sinus cancer: Preliminary results of a European Organization for Research and Treatment of Cancer phase III trial. EORTC Head and Neck Cancer Cooperative Group. *J Natl Cancer Inst*, 88, 890–9.

LONG, L., ZHANG, X., CHEN, F., PAN, Q., PHIPHATWATCHARA, P., ZENG, Y., CHEN, H. J. G., & GENES CANCER. 2018. The promising immune checkpoint LAG-3: From tumor microenvironment to cancer immunotherapy. *Genes*, 9, 176.

LUCE, D., GÉRIN, M., LECLERC, A., MORCET, J. F., BRUGÈRE, J., & GOLDBERG, M. 1993. Sinonasal cancer and occupational exposure to formaldehyde and other substances. *Int J Cancer*, 53, 224–31.

MALLICK, I., & WALDRON, J. N. 2009. Radiation therapy for head and neck cancers. *Semin Oncol Nurs*, 25, 193–202.

MAO, L., EL-NAGGAR, A. K., PAPADIMITRAKOPOULOU, V., SHIN, D. M., SHIN, H. C., FAN, Y., ZHOU, X., CLAYMAN, G., LEE, J. J., LEE, J. S., HITTELMAN, W. N., LIPPMAN, S. M., & HONG, W. K. 1998. Phenotype and genotype of advanced premalignant head and neck lesions after chemopreventive therapy. *J Natl Cancer Inst*, 90, 1545–51.

MARAKALA, V. 2023. Head and neck cancer biomarkers: Systematic review and meta-analysis. *Clin Chim Acta*, 542, 117280.

MASCITTI, M., ORSINI, G., TOSCO, V., MONTERUBBIANESI, R., BALERCIA, A., PUTIGNANO, A., PROCACCINI, M., & SANTARELLI, A. 2018. An overview on current non-invasive diagnostic devices in oral oncology. *Front Physiol*, 9, 1510.

MASSA, S. T., OSAZUWA-PETERS, N., ADJEI BOAKYE, E., WALKER, R. J., & WARD, G. M. 2019. Comparison of the financial burden of survivors of head and neck cancer with other cancer survivors. *JAMA Otolaryngol Head Neck Surg*, 145, 239–49.

MASTHAN, K. M., SANKARI, S. L., BABU, N. A., & RAJGURU, J. P. 2013. How to help the oral pathologist in making an accurate diagnosis. *J Clin Diagn Res*, 7, 181–4.

MATTA, A., RALHAN, R. J. H., & ONCOLOGY, N. 2009. Overview of current and future biologically based targeted therapies in head and neck squamous cell carcinoma. *Head & Neck Oncology*, 1, 1–8.

MENDELSOHN, J., & BASELGA, J. 2003. Status of epidermal growth factor receptor antagonists in the biology and treatment of cancer. *J Clin Oncol*, 21, 2787–99.

MENEZES, F. D. S., VERZINHASSE PERES, S., DE CASTRO JUNIOR, G., ANTUNES, J. L. F., LATORRE, M., & TOPORCOV, T. N. 2023. Survival inequalities in head and neck cancers: A hospital-based cohort study. *Head Neck*, 45, 2377–93.

MILDEN, S. P., & STOKOLS, D. 2004. Physicians' attitudes and practices regarding complementary and alternative medicine. *Behav Med*, 30, 73–82.

MILLER, M. C., PRIBITKIN, E. A., DIFABIO, T., & KEANE, W. M. 2010. Prevalence of complementary and alternative medicine use among a population of head and neck cancer patients: A survey-based study. *Ear Nose Throat J*, 89, E23–7.

MORK, J., LIE, A. K., GLATTRE, E., HALLMANS, G., JELLUM, E., KOSKELA, P., MØLLER, B., PUKKALA, E., SCHILLER, J. T., YOUNGMAN, L., LEHTINEN, M., & DILLNER, J. 2001. Human papillomavirus infection as a risk factor for squamous-cell carcinoma of the head and neck. *N Engl J Med*, 344, 1125–31.

MUTO, M., NAKANE, M., KATADA, C., SANO, Y., OHTSU, A., ESUMI, H., EBIHARA, S., & YOSHIDA, S. 2004. Squamous cell carcinoma in situ at oropharyngeal and hypopharyngeal mucosal sites. *Cancer*, 101, 1375–81.

NATIONAL CANCER REGISTRY. 2001. *Summary statistics of cancer diagnosed histologically in South Africa in 2001*. National Institute for Occupational Health (NIOH) Johannesburg.

NATIONAL CANCER REGISTRY. 2002. *Summary statistics of cancer diagnosed histologically in South Africa in 2002*. National Institute for Occupational Health (NIOH) Johannesburg.

NATIONAL CANCER REGISTRY. 2003. *Summary statistics of cancer diagnosed histologically in South Africa in 2003*. National Institute for Occupational Health (NIOH) Johannesburg.

NATIONAL CANCER REGISTRY. 2004. *Summary statistics of cancer diagnosed histologically in South Africa in 2004*. National Institute for Occupational Health (NIOH) Johannesburg.

NATIONAL CANCER REGISTRY. 2005. *Summary statistics of cancer diagnosed histologically in South Africa in 2005*. National Institute for Occupational Health (NIOH) Johannesburg.

NATIONAL CANCER REGISTRY. 2006. *Summary statistics of cancer diagnosed histologically in South Africa in 2006*. National Institute for Occupational Health (NIOH) Johannesburg.

NATIONAL CANCER REGISTRY. 2007. *Summary statistics of cancer diagnosed histologically in South Africa in 2007*. National Institute for Occupational Health (NIOH) Johannesburg.

NATIONAL CANCER REGISTRY. 2008. *Summary statistics of cancer diagnosed histologically in South Africa in 2008*. National Institute for Occupational Health (NIOH) Johannesburg.

NATIONAL CANCER REGISTRY. 2009. *Summary statistics of cancer diagnosed histologically in South Africa in 2009*. National Institute for Occupational Health (NIOH) Johannesburg.

NATIONAL CANCER REGISTRY. 2010. *Summary statistics of cancer diagnosed histologically in South Africa in 2010.* National Institute for Occupational Health (NIOH) Johannesburg.

NATIONAL CANCER REGISTRY. 2011. *Summary statistics of cancer diagnosed histologically in South Africa in 2011.* National Institute for Occupational Health (NIOH) Johannesburg.

NATIONAL CANCER REGISTRY. 2012. *Summary statistics of cancer diagnosed histologically in South Africa in 2012.* National Institute for Occupational Health (NIOH) Johannesburg.

NATIONAL CANCER REGISTRY. 2013. *Summary statistics of cancer diagnosed histologically in South Africa in 2013.* National Institute for Occupational Health (NIOH) Johannesburg.

NATIONAL CANCER REGISTRY. 2014. *Summary statistics of cancer diagnosed histologically in South Africa in 2014.* National Institute for Occupational Health (NIOH) Johannesburg.

NATIONAL CANCER REGISTRY. 2015. *Summary statistics of cancer diagnosed histologically in South Africa in 2015.* National Institute for Occupational Health (NIOH) Johannesburg.

NATIONAL CANCER REGISTRY. 2016. *Summary statistics of cancer diagnosed histologically in South Africa in 2016.* National Institute for Occupational Health (NIOH) Johannesburg.

NATIONAL CANCER REGISTRY. 2017. *Summary statistics of cancer diagnosed histologically in South Africa in 2017.* National Institute for Occupational Health (NIOH) Johannesburg.

NATIONAL CANCER REGISTRY. 2018. *Summary statistics of cancer diagnosed histologically in South Africa in 2018.* National Institute for Occupational Health (NIOH) Johannesburg.

NATIONAL CANCER REGISTRY. 2019. *Summary statistics of cancer diagnosed histologically in South Africa in 2019.* National Institute for Occupational Health (NIOH) Johannesburg.

NATIONAL CANCER REGISTRY. 2020. *Summary statistics of cancer diagnosed histologically in South Africa in 2020.* National Institute for Occupational Health (NIOH) Johannesburg.

NATIONAL CANCER REGISTRY. 2021. *Summary statistics of cancer diagnosed histologically in South Africa in 2021.* National Institute for Occupational Health (NIOH) Johannesburg.

NATIONAL CANCER REGISTRY. 2022. *Summary statistics of cancer diagnosed histologically in South Africa in 2022.* National Institute for Occupational Health (NIOH) Johannesburg.

NEGRI, E., BOFFETTA, P., BERTHILLER, J., CASTELLSAGUE, X., CURADO, M. P., DAL MASO, L., DAUDT, A. W., FABIANOVA, E., FERNANDEZ, L., WÜNSCH-FILHO, V., FRANCESCHI, S., HAYES, R. B., HERRERO, R., KOIFMAN, S., LAZARUS, P., LENCE, J. J., LEVI, F., MATES, D., MATOS, E., MENEZES, A., MUSCAT, J., ELUF-NETO, J., OLSHAN, A. F., RUDNAI, P., SHANGINA, O., STURGIS, E. M., SZESZENIA-DABROWSKA, N., TALAMINI, R., WEI, Q., WINN, D. M., ZARIDZE, D., LISSOWSKA, J., ZHANG, Z. F., FERRO, G., BRENNAN, P., LA VECCHIA, C., & HASHIBE, M. 2009. Family history of cancer: Pooled analysis in the International Head and Neck Cancer Epidemiology Consortium. *Int J Cancer*, 124, 394–401.

NEVILLE, B. W., & DAY, T. A. 2002. Oral cancer and precancerous lesions. *CA Cancer J Clin*, 52, 195–215.

NONAKA, T., & WONG, D. T. W. 2018. Liquid biopsy in head and neck cancer: Promises and challenges. *J Dent Res*, 97, 701–8.

PAI, S. I., & WESTRA, W. H. 2009. Molecular pathology of head and neck cancer: Implications for diagnosis, prognosis, and treatment. *Annu Rev Pathol*, 4, 49–70.

PAPADIMITRAKOPOULOU, V. A., CLAYMAN, G. L., SHIN, D. M., MYERS, J. N., GILLENWATER, A. M., GOEPFERT, H., EL-NAGGAR, A. K., LEWIN, J. S., LIPPMAN, S. M., & HONG, W. K. 1999. Biochemoprevention for dysplastic lesions of the upper aerodigestive tract. *Arch Otolaryngol Head Neck Surg*, 125, 1083–9.

PARTRIDGE, M., PATEROMICHELAKIS, S., PHILLIPS, E., EMILION, G. G., A'HERN, R. P., & LANGDON, J. D. 2000. A case-control study confirms that microsatellite assay can identify patients at risk of developing oral squamous cell carcinoma within a field of cancerization. *Cancer Res*, 60, 3893–8.

PARVATHANENI, U., LARAMORE, G. E., & LIAO, J. J. 2012. Technical advances and pitfalls in head and neck radiotherapy. *J Oncol*, 2012, 597467.

PATEL, V., SENDEROWICZ, A. M., PINTO, D., JR., IGISHI, T., RAFFELD, M., QUINTANILLA-MARTINEZ, L., ENSLEY, J. F., SAUSVILLE, E. A., & GUTKIND, J. S.

1998. Flavopiridol, a novel cyclin-dependent kinase inhibitor, suppresses the growth of head and neck squamous cell carcinomas by inducing apoptosis. *J Clin Invest*, 102, 1674–81.

PFISTER, D. G., SPENCER, S., ADELSTEIN, D., ADKINS, D., ANZAI, Y., BRIZEL, D. M., BRUCE, J. Y., BUSSE, P. M., CAUDELL, J. J., CMELAK, A. J., COLEVAS, A. D., EISELE, D. W., FENTON, M., FOOTE, R. L., GALLOWAY, T., GILLISON, M. L., HADDAD, R. I., HICKS, W. L., HITCHCOCK, Y. J., JIMENO, A., LEIZMAN, D., MAGHAMI, E., MELL, L. K., MITTAL, B. B., PINTO, H. A., RIDGE, J. A., ROCCO, J. W., RODRIGUEZ, C. P., SHAH, J. P., WEBER, R. S., WEINSTEIN, G., WITEK, M., WORDEN, F., YOM, S. S., ZHEN, W., BURNS, J. L., & DARLOW, S. D. 2020. Head and neck cancers, Version 2.2020, NCCN clinical practice guidelines in oncology. *J Natl Compr Canc Netw*, 18, 873–98.

PIGNON, J. P., BOURHIS, J., DOMENGE, C., & DESIGNÉ, L. 2000. Chemotherapy added to locoregional treatment for head and neck squamous-cell carcinoma: Three meta-analyses of updated individual data. MACH-NC Collaborative Group. Meta-Analysis of Chemotherapy on Head and Neck Cancer. *Lancet*, 355, 949–55.

PIGNON, J. P., LE MAÎTRE, A., MAILLARD, E., & BOURHIS, J. 2009. Meta-analysis of chemotherapy in head and neck cancer (MACH-NC): An update on 93 randomised trials and 17,346 patients. *Radiother Oncol*, 92, 4–14.

POLLOCK, N. I., & GRANDIS, J. R. 2015. HER2 as a therapeutic target in head and neck squamous cell carcinoma. *Clin Cancer Res*, 21, 526–33.

PÖSCHL, G., & SEITZ, H. K. 2004. Alcohol and cancer. *Alcohol Alcohol*, 39, 155–65.

PROUT, M. N., HEEREN, T. C., BARBER, C. E., ROSE, L., MORRIS, S. G., HURLEY, C., GELLER, A. C., WITZBURG, R. A., & KOH, H. K. 1990. Use of health services before diagnosis of head and neck cancer among Boston residents. *Am J Prev Med*, 6, 77–83.

PULTE, D., & BRENNER, H. 2010. Changes in survival in head and neck cancers in the late 20th and early 21st century: A period analysis. *Oncologist*, 15, 994–1001.

RIDGE, J., GLISSON, B., LANGO, M., FEIGENBERG, S. 2009. Chapter: Head Neck Tumors. *In:* PAZDUR, R., ed. *Cancer Management: A Multidisciplinary Approach*. New York: Oncology Group, 872.

ROSIN, M. P., CHENG, X., POH, C., LAM, W. L., HUANG, Y., LOVAS, J., BEREAN, K., EPSTEIN, J. B., PRIDDY, R., LE, N. D., & ZHANG, L. 2000. Use of allelic loss to predict malignant risk for low-grade oral epithelial dysplasia. *Clin Cancer Res*, 6, 357–62.

ROTTE, A. 2019. Combination of CTLA-4 and PD-1 blockers for treatment of cancer. *J Exp Clin Cancer Res*, 38, 255.

RUBIN GRANDIS, J., MELHEM, M. F., GOODING, W. E., DAY, R., HOLST, V. A., WAGENER, M. M., DRENNING, S. D., & TWEARDY, D. J. 1998. Levels of TGF-alpha and EGFR protein in head and neck squamous cell carcinoma and patient survival. *J Natl Cancer Inst*, 90, 824–32.

SAKUISHI, K., APETOH, L., SULLIVAN, J. M., BLAZAR, B. R., KUCHROO, V. K., & ANDERSON, A. C. 2010. Targeting Tim-3 and PD-1 pathways to reverse T cell exhaustion and restore anti-tumor immunity. *J Exp Med*, 207, 2187–94.

SALOMON, D. S., BRANDT, R., CIARDIELLO, F., & NORMANNO, N. 1995. Epidermal growth factor-related peptides and their receptors in human malignancies. *Crit Rev Oncol Hematol*, 19, 183–232.

SARAIYA, V., BRADSHAW, P., MEYER, K., GAMMON, M., SLADE, G., BRENNAN, P., ABEDI-ARDEKANI, B., & OLSHAN, A. 2020. The association between diet quality and cancer incidence of the head and neck. *Cancer Causes Control*, 31, 193–202.

SARI, E. F., JOHNSON, N. W., MCCULLOUGH, M. J., & CIRILLO, N. 2024. Prevalence and risk factors of oral potentially malignant disorders in Indonesia: A cross-sectional study undertaken in 5 provinces. *Sci Rep*, 14, 5232.

SCHLUMPF, M. F., & HAERLE, S. 2014. The current role of imaging in head and neck cancer: A clinician's perspective. *Swiss Med Wkly*, 144, w14015.

SETTLE, K., POSNER, M. R., SCHUMAKER, L. M., TAN, M., SUNTHARALINGAM, M., GOLOUBEVA, O., STROME, S. E., HADDAD, R. I., PATEL, S. S., CAMBELL, E. V., 3RD,

SARLIS, N., LORCH, J., & CULLEN, K. J. 2009. Racial survival disparity in head and neck cancer results from low prevalence of human papillomavirus infection in black oropharyngeal cancer patients. *Cancer Prev Res (Phila)*, 2, 776–81.

SHARMA, D., & SINGH, G. 2016. Spectrum of cancer in adolescents and young adult: An epidemiological and clinicopathological evaluation. *Indian J Cancer*, 53, 457–9.

SHAW, R., & BEASLEY, N. 2016. Aetiology and risk factors for head and neck cancer: United Kingdom National Multidisciplinary Guidelines. *J Laryngol Otol*, 130, S9–s12.

SHOTELERSUK, K., KHORPRASERT, C., SAKDIKUL, S., PORNTHANAKASEM, W., VORAVUD, N., & MUTIRANGURA, A. 2000. Epstein-Barr virus DNA in serum/plasma as a tumor marker for nasopharyngeal cancer. *Clin Cancer Res*, 6, 1046–51.

SIEGEL, R. L., MILLER, K. D., & JEMAL, A. 2020. Cancer statistics, 2020. *CA Cancer J Clin*, 70, 7–30.

SINGH, S. A., CHOUDHURY, J. H., KAPFO, W., KUNDU, S., DHAR, B., LASKAR, S., DAS, R., KUMAR, M., & GHOSH, S. K. 2015. Influence of the CYP1A1 T3801C polymorphism on tobacco and alcohol-associated head and neck cancer susceptibility in Northeast India. *Asian Pac J Cancer Prev*, 16, 6953–61.

SON, E., PANWAR, A., MOSHER, C. H., & LYDIATT, D. 2018. Cancers of the major salivary gland. *J Oncol Pract*, 14, 99–108.

SOULIERES, D., SENZER, N. N., VOKES, E. E., HIDALGO, M., AGARWALA, S. S., & SIU, L. L. 2004. Multicenter phase II study of erlotinib, an oral epidermal growth factor receptor tyrosine kinase inhibitor, in patients with recurrent or metastatic squamous cell cancer of the head and neck. *J Clin Oncol*, 22, 77–85.

SUBRAMANIUM, S., BALASUNDARAM, V., NITHYA, S., & KIRAN, P. J. J. O. C. T. 2015. Nimotuzumab with induction chemotherapy and chemo-radiation in patients with advanced head and neck cancer. 6, 146–52.

THOMPSON-HARVEY, A., YETUKURI, M., HANSEN, A. R., SIMPSON, M. C., ADJEI BOAKYE, E., VARVARES, M. A., & OSAZUWA-PETERS, N. 2020. Rising incidence of late-stage head and neck cancer in the United States. *Cancer*, 126, 1090–101.

TRINIDADE, A., SHAKEEL, M., HURMAN, D., & HUSSAIN, A. 2011. Traditional and complementary and alternative medicines make for unwilling bedfellows in the management of cancer: A case report with a tragic outcome. *J Laryngol Otol*, 125, 1193–5.

TUYNS, A. J., ESTÈVE, J., RAYMOND, L., BERRINO, F., BENHAMOU, E., BLANCHET, F., BOFFETTA, P., CROSIGNANI, P., DEL MORAL, A., LEHMANN, W., & MERLETTI, F. 1988. Cancer of the larynx/hypopharynx, tobacco and alcohol: IARC international case-control study in Turin and Varese (Italy), Zaragoza and Navarra (Spain), Geneva (Switzerland) and Calvados (France). *Int J Cancer*, 41, 483–91.

TZONG-SHYUAN, T. A. I., PAI-MEI, L. I. N., CHING-FANG, W. U., SHIH-KAI, H., CHUNG-I, H., CHIH-CHUN, W., & YU-CHIEH, S. U. 2019. CDK4/6 inhibitor LEE011 is a potential radiation-sensitizer in head and neck squamous cell carcinoma: An in vitro study. *Anticancer Research*, 39, 713.

VERMORKEN, J. B., STÖHLMACHER-WILLIAMS, J., DAVIDENKO, I., LICITRA, L., WINQUIST, E., VILLANUEVA, C., FOA, P., ROTTEY, S., SKLADOWSKI, K., TAHARA, M., PAI, V. R., FAIVRE, S., BLAJMAN, C. R., FORASTIERE, A. A., STEIN, B. N., OLINER, K. S., PAN, Z., & BACH, B. A. 2013. Cisplatin and fluorouracil with or without panitumumab in patients with recurrent or metastatic squamous-cell carcinoma of the head and neck (SPECTRUM): An open-label phase 3 randomised trial. *Lancet Oncology*, 14, 697–710.

VOKES, E. E., KIES, M. S., HARAF, D. J., STENSON, K., LIST, M., HUMERICKHOUSE, R., DOLAN, M. E., PELZER, H., SULZEN, L., WITT, M. E., HSIEH, Y. C., MITTAL, B. B., & WEICHSELBAUM, R. R. 2000. Concomitant chemoradiotherapy as primary therapy for locoregionally advanced head and neck cancer. *J Clin Oncol*, 18, 1652–61.

WHITE, H., FORD, S., BUSH, B., HOLSINGER, F. C., MOORE, E., GHANEM, T., CARROLL, W., ROSENTHAL, E., SWEENY, L., & MAGNUSON, J. S. 2013. Salvage surgery for recurrent cancers of the oropharynx: Comparing TORS with standard open surgical approaches. *JAMA Otolaryngol Head Neck Surg*, 139, 773–8.

WISSINGER, E., GRIEBSCH, I., LUNGERSHAUSEN, J., FOSTER, T., & PASHOS, C. L. 2014. The economic burden of head and neck cancer: A systematic literature review. *Pharmacoeconomics*, 32, 865–82.

WOLF, Y., ANDERSON, A. C., & KUCHROO, V. K. 2020. TIM3 comes of age as an inhibitory receptor. *Nature Rev Immunol*, 20, 173–85.

YANG, H., ZHOU, L., YANG, F., CHEN, J., & WANG, Y. 2023. Prognostic value of O6-methylguanine-DNA methyltransferase hypermethylation and expression in head and neck cancer: A systematic review and meta-analysis. *Medicine (Baltimore)*, 102, e33472.

ZANDBERG, D. P., LIU, S., GOLOUBEVA, O., ORD, R., STROME, S. E., SUNTHARALINGAM, M., TAYLOR, R., MORALES, R. E., WOLF, J. S., ZIMRIN, A., LUBEK, J. E., SCHUMAKER, L. M., & CULLEN, K. J. 2016. Oropharyngeal cancer as a driver of racial outcome disparities in squamous cell carcinoma of the head and neck: 10-year experience at the University of Maryland Greenebaum Cancer Center. *Head Neck*, 38, 564–72.

ZECH, H. B., MOECKELMANN, N., BOETTCHER, A., MUENSCHER, A., BINDER, M., VETTORAZZI, E., BOKEMEYER, C., SCHAFHAUSEN, P., BETZ, C. S., & BUSCH, C.-J. 2020. Phase III study of nivolumab alone or combined with ipilimumab as immunotherapy versus standard of care in resectable head and neck squamous cell carcinoma. 16, 3035–43.

2

Risk Factors in Head and Neck Cancer

Demetra Demetriou, Mzubanzi Mabongo, Mark Torres-Holmes, Elisa Marie Ledet, and Zodwa Dlamini

2.1 Introduction

Head and neck cancer (HNC) ranks seventh in global cancer incidence and represents 5% of global cancer cases (Dhull et al., 2018). Common HNC are squamous cell carcinoma (SCC), which accounts for 90% of HNC, followed by lymphomas. It is believed that >70% of SCC in the head and neck region could be prevented through lifestyle modifications, specifically by significantly decreasing exposure to common risk factors like alcohol and tobacco (Cogliano et al., 2011). HNSCC encompasses various malignancies arising from the oropharynx, larynx, nasal cavity, hypopharynx, oral cavity, paranasal sinuses, and nasopharynx (Kasper et al., 2015; Rath & Mohanti, 2003). These organs play roles in breathing, swallowing, and filtering and moistening inhaled air. HNC poses a considerable global health challenge, with its occurrence and fatality rates showing notable differences among various regions and population groups. Men, older individuals, and those with lower socioeconomic status are notably vulnerable to HNC. Recognizing these epidemiological trends is crucial for tackling the impact of HNC and enacting tailored prevention strategies (Barsouk et al., 2023).

SCC originates in the flat squamous cells lining the aerodigestive tract within the head and neck. These cells form a thin layer known as the *epithelium*, below which is the lamina propria, and this is collectively called the *mucosa* or *mucous membrane*. Cancer confined to the squamous cell layer (epithelium) is termed "carcinoma in situ." Cancer beyond this layer that infiltrates deeper tissues is classified as "invasive SCC." HNCs originating from the salivary glands are regarded as a different and separate entity, with their behavior characterized by different growth and metastatic patterns compared to SCCs. Typically, these cancers are categorized as either adenocarcinoma, mucoepidermoid carcinoma, or adenoid cystic carcinoma.

Five primary HNC types are classified based on their anatomical origin. These include paranasal sinus and nasal cavity cancer, salivary gland cancer, hypopharyngeal and laryngeal cancers, nasopharyngeal cancer, oropharyngeal cancer, and oral cancer. Oral SCC is usually human papillomavirus (HPV)-negative and oropharyngeal cancers HPV-positive. Paranasal sinus and nasal cavity cancer affect the nasal passages and surrounding sinuses. Salivary gland cancer originates from glands producing saliva. Hypopharyngeal and laryngeal cancer involve the lower throat and the voice box, respectively. Nasopharyngeal cancer develops in the upper throat behind the nose. Oral cavity and oropharyngeal cancer involves the mouth and middle throat. While other cancers may occur in this region, their diagnosis and treatment differ significantly (Figure 2.1). The American Joint Committee on Cancer (AJCC) categorizes HNC into seven groups due to their different presentations and prognosis. These categories include lip and oral cancer, major salivary gland cancer, nasopharynx cancer, HPV^+ mediated oropharynx cancer, HPV^- mediated oropharynx and hypopharynx cancer, nasal cavity and paranasal sinuses cancer, and larynx cancer (Zanoni et al., 2019).

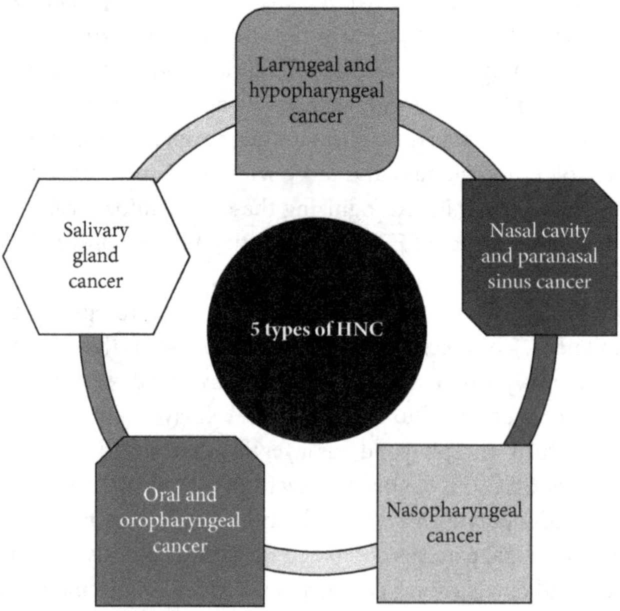

Figure 2.1 The five types of head and neck cancer (HNC). Each type of HNC is named based on its anatomical origin and includes nasal cavity and paranasal sinus cancer, salivary glands, hypopharyngeal and laryngeal cancer, nasopharyngeal cancer, oropharyngeal cancer and oral cancer.

2.2 Epidemiology

Based on the estimates from GLOBOCAN (2020), HNC ranks as the seventh most prevalent cancer, representing about 890,000 new cases annually, and it leads to approximately 450,000 deaths each year. These figures encompass around 380,000 cases affecting the oral cavity and lips, 185,000 affecting the larynx, 98,000 affecting the oropharynx, 133,000 affecting the nasopharynx, 54,000 affecting the salivary glands, and 84,000 affecting the hypopharynx (Sung et al., 2021). HNC exhibits significant variations in both mortality and incidence rates across different regions and demographic groups (Barsouk et al., 2023). Globally, there is an increased prevalence in men with an approximate ratio of 2:1, and it is more common among individuals aged 50 and older. HNC incidence rates are particularly elevated in south and southeast Asia, due to the widespread habit of chewing the carcinogenic areca or betel nut (*Areca catechu*; see Cheong et al., 2017), followed by eastern and central Europe and South America (Sung et al., 2021). Notably, India has the highest incidence rates, contributing to up to 80% of all HNC cases (Gormley et al., 2022). The global occurrence of HNC is on the rise, particularly among younger demographics, with an anticipated 30% annual surge in incidence projected by 2030 (Sung et al., 2021). This trend may be linked to shifts in lifestyle behaviors, such as tobacco use, high alcohol consumption, and increasing the prevalence of HPV-related oropharyngeal cancer. Predictions suggest that HPV will soon surpass tobacco as the primary contributor to the burden of HNC, leading to a higher incidence of oropharyngeal HNC compared to oral cancer, which is predominantly associated with tobacco use (Fitzmaurice et al., 2017; Sung et al., 2021).

There has been a notable 23% rise in cases of laryngeal cancer in the past decade (Fitzmaurice et al., 2017). Younger women in developed countries have experienced a significant increase in incidence, which is likely influenced by changing cultural norms regarding tobacco and alcohol use as well as a rising burden of HPV (Bosetti et al., 2020; Miranda-Filho & Bray, 2020). In Japan, there has been an increase in oral cavity, salivary gland, and oropharyngeal tumors, particularly among women, while incidences of nasopharyngeal associated with the Epstein-Barr virus (EBV) and laryngeal tumors have declined in East Asian populations (Kawakita et al., 2022). Similarly, in the United Kingdom, oropharyngeal HNC has risen by 7.3% in men and 6.5% in women, and oral cancer has increased by 2.8% and 3.0% in men and women, respectively, with the greatest increases observed in individuals of lower socioeconomic status (Creaney et al., 2022; Louie et al., 2015).

Low- and middle-income countries (LMICs) account for 70% of cancer-related fatalities worldwide, making it the second greatest cause of death overall. Nonetheless, there is a severe lack of data regarding cancer research in Africa

(Coutts et al., 2022; Ngoma & Ngoma, 2019). The bulk of the information on HNC originates from economically developed nations that have different patient demographics and resource availability than African nations. This has consequences for the medical, surgical, and rehabilitative care of HNC (Coutts et al., 2022). Surgery has traditionally been the primary treatment for oropharyngeal cancer, and it is still the main treatment for HNC in Africa. The lack of radiation or chemotherapy services in some areas is the main justification given for surgical intervention in Africa (Coutts et al., 2022). Only four nations—South Africa, Tanzania, Uganda, and Nigeria—have access to radiation treatment; however, the radiation waiting periods were unduly lengthy. According to reports, Nigerian patients are experiencing increasing costs of these therapies due to a lack of health insurance; patients frequently live far from treatment facilities with the necessary management resources, making poor access to hospitals a major concern. These are all relevant factors in South Africa as well (Coutts et al., 2022).

Paucity of access and low patient compliance made chemotherapy difficult as well. These difficulties included patients frequently turning to traditional medicine due to a shortage of medical oncologists providing chemotherapy and the high cost of the chemotherapy drugs (Gilyoma et al., 2015; Nabukenya et al., 2018; Passos et al., 2015). Not enough staff is available to utilize this technology due to radiation concerns, and staff members' training and dosage administration skills are insufficient (Rosenblatt & Zubizarreta, 2017). According to 84.3% of participants, traditional herbalists in western Uganda are easily accessible, reasonably priced, and sensitive to cultural beliefs, which is why they prioritized seeking treatment from them in Uganda (Coutts et al., 2022; Rosenblatt & Zubizarreta, 2017). Further research comparing traditional health-seeking management to Western approaches relevant to HNC in Africa is necessary because the continent is home to a varied range of ethnicities and cultures that could help to explain factors like delayed diagnosis. A deeper understanding of the differences between traditional and Western medicine will help to clarify the fundamental causes of the way HNC is managed, particularly in Africa (Coutts et al., 2022).

The absence of multidisciplinary team management (MDT) involvement in HNC treatment in Africa, including post-surgery rehabilitation, is worrisome (Coutts et al., 2022). Delayed access to appropriate treatment options early on leads to more complications later, affecting both medical and rehabilitative staff. The MDT should address these additional complications in both acute and chronic phases of HNC. Further exploration of this issue in the African context is necessary, along with data on practice patterns related to long-term rehabilitation. One major concern that has been brought to light is the deficient healthcare system throughout Africa. Professionals should be prompted by this to think about moving toward postsurgical follow-ups and community-based therapy, which could improve patient access to services all the way through the treatment process (King et al., 2009). In light of Africa's restricted access to medical professionals and cancer services, a transdisciplinary approach to HNC treatment may prove advantageous (Fagan, 2018). This method maximizes time and cost-effectiveness since the treatment team, irrespective of discipline, works toward the same objective and follows the same treatment plan (Beaudoin et al., 2020; Fagan, 2018). On the other hand, difficulties including inadequate initial training and the provision of superficial care could occur.

2.3 Head and Neck Cancer Risk

A risk factor increases the likelihood of cancer development, though many do not directly cause it. Understanding and discussing these factors with a healthcare provider can inform lifestyle choices. Two major risk factors for HNC are tobacco use, including smoking and chewing, and excessive alcohol intake. These substances, especially when used together, significantly elevate risk. Other factors include prolonged sun exposure for skin cancers, HPV infection, EBV exposure, genetic factors and family history of HNC, gender (men are at higher risk), age (>40), exposure to certain inhalants, poor oral hygiene, marijuana use, inadequate nutrition, gastroesophageal reflux disease (GERD), weakened immune system, radiation exposure, and a previous history of HNC, which increases the likelihood of recurrence (Figure 2.2).

2.3.1 Cigarettes and Tobacco

Tobacco harbors various cancer-causing compounds like nitrosamines, aldehydes, aromatic amines, and polycyclic aromatic hydrocarbons released during combustion at elevated temperatures. These chemicals cause DNA damage within oropharyngeal cells, thereby contributing to cancer development. Heavy smokers of cigarettes face a significantly heightened risk of HNC with a 5- to 25-fold increase compared to nonsmokers (Morita et al., 1999). Similarly, individuals who smoke pipes or cigars are also at an elevated risk, albeit to a lesser extent (Wyss et al., 2013b). Consistent use of chewing tobacco is linked to increased odds ratios (OR) of 1.7 for HNC and 3.0 for oral cancer specifically (Wyss et al., 2013a). Tobacco consumption increases the risk of HNC in a dose-dependent fashion (Maier et al., 1992). Tobacco use in South Africa is on the rise although the World Health Organization (WHO) reported a continued decline in tobacco use rates globally, trending in 2022

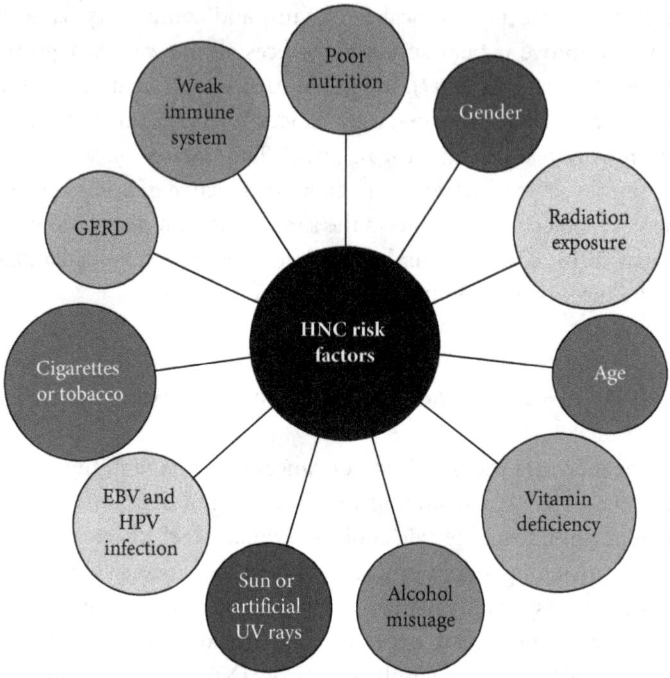

Figure 2.2 Head and neck cancer (HNC) risk factors. Numerous factors can increase the risk of HNC, including cigarettes/tobacco usage, alcohol abuse, viral infections (human papillomavirus and Epstein-Barr virus), ultraviolet radiation (sun or artificial rays), radiation exposure, genetics factors, poor nutrition, weak immune system, potential oral lesions, oral microbiome dysbiosis, chronic inflammation, necrosis, gender, age, vitamin D deficiency, and gastro-esophageal reflux disease. Men show increased risk to develop HNC.

with about 1 in 5 adults worldwide consuming tobacco compared to 1 in 3 in 2000 (Pan American Health Organization [PAHO], 2024; Reddy et al., 2015; Rossouw, 2021).

The use of electronic cigarettes (e-cigarettes) has grown over the past 10 years (Grana et al., 2014). Because they contain fewer dangerous and cancer-causing substances than traditional tobacco products, they are thought to be safer. However, this is still a controversial topic (Szukalska et al., 2020). In 2021, 4.5% of United States adults 18 years and older were e-cigarettes users. The biggest percentage of users were in the 18–24 age group (11.0%), followed by the 25–44 age group (6.5%) and the 45 and older age group (2.0%). In general and among persons aged 25–44, men were more likely to use e-cigarettes than women (Kramarow & Elgaddal, 2023). The use of multiple tobacco products in combination poses a health risk since it can lead to increased exposure to toxins and poorer respiratory results compared to the use of one product alone (Goniewicz et al., 2018; Reddy et al., 2021; Smith et al., 2021).

People with particular metabolic and genetic predispositions, such as the metabolic activation of N′-nitrosonornicotine via 2′-hydroxylation or 5′-hydroxylation leading to the formation of DNA adducts and increased glutathione S-transferase (GST) polymorphisms, alongside excessive drinking, face the greatest risk of developing HNC when combined with smoking (Fan et al., 2019; Jethwa & Khariwala, 2017; Lacko et al., 2014; Wyss et al., 2013b). Childhood exposure to secondhand smoke has an OR of 1.28 for HNC, after adjustments for HPV status, drinking, and smoking (Troy et al., 2013). According to research on cases in Western Europe, tobacco continues to be the primary risk factor for HNC, contributing to approximately 75% of all cases (Tuyns et al., 1988). As household disposable income rises due to economic advancement, tobacco consumption is on the rise in developing countries (Morojele et al., 2016; Peer, 2018; Perelman et al., 2017). While tobacco use has decreased overall in developed nations, there has been an increase in certain demographic groups, notably women (Lee et al., 2019; Wang et al., 2012).

Opium usage has been linked to a higher incidence of laryngeal cancer. The juice of the immature poppy seedpod is extracted to produce opium, an illegal drug that includes a variety of alkaloids. The International Agency for Research on Cancer states that smoking or consuming various kinds of opium is carcinogenic to humans. For instance, results from the 50,045 participants in the Golestan Cohort Study (GCS) in Iran showed that opium use was linked to an increased risk of laryngeal cancer, with the risk increasing with dosage (Basnayake et al., 2023).

2.3.2 Alcohol Misuse

Among nonsmokers, alcohol intake contributes to approximately 4% of HNC cases worldwide (Zandberg et al., 2016). The risk of HNC rises in proportion to the quantity and regularity of alcohol consumption, with a relative risk of 1.3 times for all drinkers and 2.5 times for heavy drinkers (>50 g/day). Individuals who consume more than three alcoholic beverages daily face the highest risk (Zandberg et al., 2016). The risk of HNC varies depending on the type of alcohol consumed. Spirits consumers face higher risks compared to those who consume wine or beer. However, this effect may become insignificant when adjusted for alcohol concentration (Castellsagué et al., 2004; Hashibe et al., 2007; Rumgay et al., 2021). Alcohol, acting as a solvent, increases the vulnerability of mucosal tissue to carcinogens like nitrites or smoke found in food (Barsouk et al., 2023). Acetaldehyde, a byproduct of ethanol metabolism through alcohol dehydrogenase, is mutagenic and contributes to symptoms like headaches and flushing associated with heavy alcohol consumption. Drugs like disulfiram and metronidazole inhibit acetaldehyde conversion, leading to adverse reactions when combined with alcohol (Rumgay et al., 2021; Yu et al., 2011). Notably, variants in acetaldehyde dehydrogenase, the enzyme responsible for acetaldehyde breakdown, are linked to increased HNC risk, resistance to chemoradiotherapy, and poorer prognosis, particularly in heavy alcohol consumers. These variants are also associated with the flushing response to alcohol commonly observed in East Asian populations (Yu et al., 2011).

Alcohol and tobacco used together significantly amplify the risk of HNC. The projected rise in global HNC cases in the coming years is attributed to increased consumption of alcohol and tobacco, particularly in developing countries. Research from various regions, including the United Kingdom, China, and Lebanon, links alcohol intake to 32–37% of oropharyngeal HNC cases, with approximately 90% of these cases have a history of smoking (Charafeddine et al., 2017; Parkin, 2011; Wang et al., 2012; Zandberg et al., 2016). Globally, tobacco or alcohol use contributes to 72% of HNC cases, with almost half of them (35%) associated with both factors combined (Zandberg et al., 2016). Concurrent heavy use of alcohol and tobacco escalates the risk of HNC by 40 times (Rumgay et al., 2021). Interestingly, the association between cigarette smoking and HNC in Black Americans surpasses that of White Americans, while the risk related to alcohol consumption remains consistent between the groups. This suggests potential disparities in tobacco product quality or metabolic differences based on race (Voltzke et al., 2018).

2.3.3 Viral Infections

2.3.3.1 Human Papilloma Virus

According to De Martel et al. (2012), p16 positivity on immunohistochemistry indicates that 72% of HNC cases in affluent countries are caused by HPV infection, while only 13% of cases occur in underdeveloped countries (De Martel et al., 2012). The protein capsid of > 20 high-risk HPV serotypes has allowed for their identification. In North America, 85–90% of HPV-associated oropharyngeal HNC cases are connected to HPV16; in contrast, 50–75% of cases of cervical cancer are related to both HPV16 and -18 (Varier et al., 2016). Viral oncogenesis happens when basal keratinocytes become infected; these cells are frequently exposed because of microabrasions from intercourse (Zhang et al., 2021). A history of several sexual partners, anal intercourse, and oral sex—the latter bearing the highest risk when the mouth contacts female genitalia—are risk factors for HPV-associated oropharyngeal cancer. A compromised immune system puts people at higher risk, especially if they also have HIV infection (Barsouk et al., 2023). The risk of HPV is 1.5–2.5 times higher in women living with HIV. Worldwide, the OR of getting HNC for people who have more than four oral sex partners is 2.25 (95% confidence interval [CI] 1.42–3.58) (Heck et al., 2010).

Oropharyngeal cancer linked to HPV has been more common in developing countries in recent times. In the United States, this cancer affects primarily young adults and increased by 225% between 1984 and 2004 (Chaturvedi et al., 2013). Cervical cancer has been eclipsed by HPV-related HNC as the most common HPV-associated malignancy in the United States (Berman & Schiller, 2017). The prevalence of HPV-related HNC has significantly grown in the United States across several demographic categories, especially among White men younger than 45, who saw an annual increase of 5.1% between 2008 and 2012. Conversely, Black Americans have about a 50% greater rate of HNCs that are not related to HPV (DeSantis et al., 2013). Comparably, from 1989 to 2006, the number of HPV-related HNC cases in the United Kingdom increased by 51% (Chenevert & Chiosea, 2012).

The improved prognosis and superior response to radiation may be explained by the unique features that HPV-positive HNCs display, such as fewer genetic mutations, increased B-cell infiltration into the tumor microenvironment, and a preserved apoptotic response (Elrefaey et al., 2014; Zhang et al., 2021). According to Chaturvedi et al. (2011), HPV positivity is linked to a noticeably longer median survival (130 vs. 20 months) for HNC patients (Chaturvedi et al, 2011), and, when other risk factors are considered, it independently lowers the chance of mortality by 64% (Ang et al., 2010). As a result of the significant variation in survival rates, HPV-positive HNC is currently staged differently (Fakhry et al., 2008).

2.3.3.2 Epstein-Barr Virus

Nasopharyngeal carcinoma is rare in many parts of the world but is a common cancer in southern China. Research has identified EBV as the main cause of this cancer. In another context, chronic hepatitis C virus (HCV) infection is strongly linked to hepatocellular carcinoma and other types of cancer like lymphoproliferative disorders (Barsouk et al., 2023).

2.3.4 Ultraviolet Radiation Skin Exposure

Ultraviolet A (UVA) and B (UVB) radiation are responsible for skin damage and skin cancer by altering the DNA of skin cells (D'Orazio et al., 2013). Basal cell and SCC are the two most common non-melanoma skin cancers (Cives et al., 2020). The most vulnerable areas of the head and neck skin are a bare scalp, temples, eyelids, cheeks, nose, lips, and ears (Stanienda-Sokół et al., 2017). Melanoma is also caused by UV exposure, particularly if one was exposed to blistering sunburns in one's youth. The fairer the skin, the higher the risk of skin cancer (Gupta et al., 2016). Certain genetic diseases such as retinitis pigmentosa and albinism significantly increase the risk of skin cancers (Lekalakala et al., 2015; Singh & Tripathy, 2023). It is important to note that UV ray exposure occurs even on cloudy days. The heat we feel on our skin when in sunshine is from infrared not UV rays. Recommendations to reduce skin cancer risk include wearing hats and sunglasses when outside and applying sunscreen of at least SPF 30 every day (Diffey, 2002).

2.3.5 Radiation Exposure

Radiation therapy in the past, whether for benign or malignant reasons, has been associated with an increased risk of sarcomas, salivary gland tumors, thyroid cancer, and SCC. While there is a correlation, it is crucial to understand that there is an extended period of time until any negative consequences show up and that total risk is still rather low (Barsouk et al., 2023).

2.3.6 Genetic Factors

The risk of HNC is significantly influenced by genetic factors. A hereditary genetic condition called Fanconi anemia that affects DNA repair significantly raises the risk of HNC, especially oral cavity malignancies (Velleuer & Dietrich, 2014). Changes in the genes involved in the Fanconi anemia pathway are contributory, even if the exact mechanisms are not entirely understood. Polymorphisms in genes linked to immunity and carcinogen metabolism, such as Il10, cytochrome P450 1A1 (CYP1A1), glutathione S-transferase μ1 (GSTM1), and CTLA4, have been linked through meta-analyses to an increased risk of HNC (Cadoni et al., 2012; Fang et al., 2018; Niu et al., 2015; Wang et al., 2016). As a result, compromised immunity and altered carcinogen metabolism could be factors in the development of HNC. Reducing the incidence of HNC worldwide requires a variety of strategies, such as increased oral hygiene, decreased tobacco use, and universal HPV vaccination (Chan et al., 2017). Although it is gradually increasing in women and decreasing in men, the incidence of this type of cancer is three times higher in men than in women (Hassan et al., 2007).

2.3.7 Poor Nutrition

Malnutrition is prevalent among head and neck cancer patients, often triggered by factors such as cachexia, dysphagia, treatment side effects (surgery, chemotherapy, and/or radiotherapy), and unhealthy social behaviors like heavy smoking, inadequate diet, and alcohol abuse (Caruso et al., 2021; Cravo et al., 2000, Frowen et al., 2020; Lees, 1999; Mercadante et al., 2015). Approximately half of HNC patients experience significant undernourishment, with roughly 80% of them undergoing substantial unintentional weight loss throughout their treatment (Gorenc et al., 2015; Orell-Kotikangas et al., 2017; van Bokhorst-de van der et al., 1999). As with all cancers, HNC affects the body's intake, gastrointestinal (GI) function, and nutrient storage. Malnutrition in these patients stems from various factors, including tumor-related GI abnormalities or side effects of anticancer treatments, along with tumor-induced metabolic changes (von Meyenfeldt, 2005).

More than 50% of individuals with advanced HNC experience severe malnutrition and substantial involuntary weight loss upon diagnosis (Chasen & Bhargava, 2009). Dysphagia and odynophagia are common symptoms associated with HNC, and many patients also present with chronic malnutrition due to alcohol and tobacco abuse as well as unhealthy dietary habits (Bhattacharjee et al., 2015). Specific dietary elements can either protect individuals from HNC or increase their susceptibility to certain illnesses. Numerous studies have shown a protective impact associated with increased consumption of fruits and vegetables. Conversely, case-control studies suggest that regular intake of preserved meats containing higher levels of added nitrites might elevate the risk of nasopharyngeal carcinoma (Barsouk et al., 2023).

2.3.8 Weak Immune System

The risk of HNC is increased by immunodeficiency brought on by organ transplantation or HIV infection. HIV-positive people have a two- to three-fold increased incidence of HNC and are more likely to develop other non–AIDS-defining malignancies (Barsouk et al., 2023). In a similar vein, recipients of organ transplants are more susceptible to HNC. Without typical risk factors, even those who have had bone marrow transplantation are at an increased risk of developing HNC, particularly in the oral cavity (McCarter et al., 2016).

2.3.9 Oral Potential Lesions

Oral potential lesions (OPL) are mucosal lesions that have been reported to have high tendency to undergo malignant transformation (Iocca et al., 2020; Lorini et al., 2021). These OPL affect about 4.5% of the population (Mello et al., 2018). The lesions that have been reported to undergo malignant transformation are lichen planus, leukoplakia, oral lichenoid lesions, proliferative verrucous leukoplakia, oral submucosal fibrosis, and erythroplakia (Aluckal et al., 2022). The most common lesions are leukoplakia, erythroplakia, and lichen planus. The risk for malignant transformation is histologically characterized by cellular atypia and changes in architecture of the epithelium, referred to as dysplasia. The epithelium of these OPL is described by varying levels of dysplasia, such as mild, moderate, and severe. Mild epithelial dysplasia refers to changes limited to the basal third of the oral epithelium, while dysplasia involving the lower half of the oral epithelium is referred to as moderate. When epithelial dysplasia extends from the base to the upper half of the oral epithelium, it is described as severe. The dysplasia involving the full thickness of the epithelium is referred to as carcinoma in situ (Clarkson et al., 2024). The malignant transformation rate of proliferative verrucous leukoplakia and erythroplakia is 49% and 33%, respectively (Iocca et al., 2020). OPL with moderate or severe dysplasia had 2.37 times the odds of transforming to malignant lesions than OPL with mild dysplasia (Lorini et al., 2021).

Although some of the risk factors are idiopathic, host-related and lifestyle factors are similar to those of oral SCC, mainly smoking, alcohol abuse, tobacco and tobacco-derivate chewing, and oral virus infections (HPV) have been reported as risk factors (Mello et al., 2018). These lesions are managed by close observation, surgical excision, and laser ablation. Although these lesions have high recurrence after treatment, prompt treatment is recommended to prevent malignant transformation. Obviously, changes in lifestyle could help in preventing these lesions as well.

2.3.10 Dysbiosis of Oral Microbiome

In a healthy state, the oral microbiota and host immune system exist in a symbiotic relationship, with commensal bacteria and sentinel host immune cells coexisting in the oral environment. *Oral microbiota* refers to all oral microorganisms consisting of commensal and opportunistic organisms in the healthy oral cavity. Oral microbiota comprise bacteria fungi, viruses, archaea, and protozoa (Zhang et al., 2018). The state in which the oral microbiome promotes a specific pathological state or disease is referred to as *dysbiosis*.

The first reported association between development of malignancy and bacterial infection was that of *Helicobacter pylori*, which was found to be the cause of causative agent of gastric cancers (Wroblewski et al., 2010). Subsequent studies revealed an association between members of the oral microbiome and oral squamous carcinoma, especially *Porphyromas gingivalis* (Irfan et al., 2020). The oral microbiome can be perturbed by several factors such as poor oral hygiene, tobacco use, and alcohol consumption thus resulting in dysbiosis of the microbiota

(Oyeyemi et al., 2023). Dysbiosis of the oral microbiome was also reported as a risk factor for development of cancer (La Rosa et al., 2020). Dysbiosis of oral microbiota can stimulate the release of chronic inflammatory mediators that encourage cell proliferation, mutagenesis, oncogene activation, and angiogenesis (Radaic & Kapila, 2021), and it may also promote epigenetic alterations resulting in tumor development. Some carcinogenic substances could be produced by bacteria, such as the bacterial conversion of ethanol to acetaldehyde, which is a known carcinogen (Radaic & Kapila, 2021; Zhang et al., 2018).

2.3.11 Chronic Inflammation and Necrosis

Chronic periodontitis and other oral infections and inflammations have also been linked to an increased risk of HNC (Hashim et al., 2019; Miranda-Filho & Bray, 2020). Chronic irritation of the oral mucosa may result from trauma, poor oral hygiene, poor dentition, and poorly fitting dentures (false teeth) (Singhvi et al., 2017). The site most affected by mucosal trauma occurs on the lateral border of the tongue and the area of contact with dental appliances. A Swedish study found that poor oral hygiene and ill-fitting dentures were strongly associated with oral cancer. Dentures may be colonized by candida or HPV, which causes irritation that results in chronic inflammation (Rosenquist, 2005).

2.4 Head and Neck Cancer Prevention, Screening, and Early Diagnosis

Preventing HNC involves various strategies such as encouraging HPV vaccination; reducing tobacco, alcohol, and areca nut exposure; and promoting a healthy lifestyle (Figure 2.3). Smoking cessation, alongside counseling and pharmacotherapy, has been proved effective, although challenges persist in maintaining abstinence rates (Hashim et al., 2019; Jordan & Xi, 2018; McCarter et al., 2016). Decreasing alcohol consumption, especially in vulnerable populations, is crucial, with pharmacotherapy and counseling showing promise (Bernstein et al., 2021; Kim et al., 2018; Ray et al., 2020). Ceasing areca nut consumption has demonstrated significant potential in reducing oral cancer incidence, particularly in targeted community interventions (Guha et al., 2014; Little et al., 2014; Paulino et al., 2020; Reichart et al., 2003; Tseng et al., 2021). HPV vaccination plays a pivotal role, showing promising results in reducing HPV prevalence and associated cancers (Lee et al., 2018; Markowitz et al., 2016).

Secondary prevention and oral screening involve regular oral examinations for high-risk individuals, although the efficacy of routine screening for the

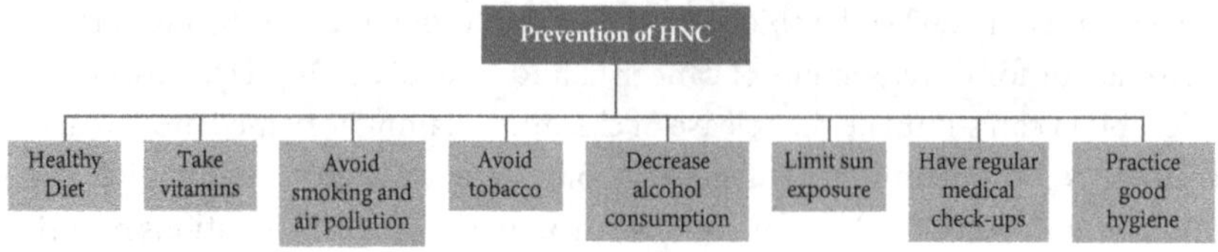

Figure 2.3 Preventative measures to decrease the risks of head and neck cancer. Follow a healthy diet, get vitamins via food or supplementation, avoid smoking or polluted areas, avoid tobacco usage, decrease alcohol consumption, limit sun exposure, have regular medical check-ups and practice good hygiene habits (e.g., washing hand regularly).

general population remains debated. Special attention is warranted for those with risk factors like prior history of HNC or premalignant conditions, as well as hereditary cancer syndromes and immunosuppression; these patients should undergo regular screening. While alternative screening methods exist, routine HPV screening is not currently recommended (Gan et al., 2013; Kim et al., 2022; Macek et al., 2003; Sankaranarayanan et al., 2005; Smith et al., 2017).

"Early diagnosis" is defined by the WHO in the Guide to Cancer Early Diagnosis 2017 as the early identification of cancer in patients who have symptoms of the disease. There are three steps to early diagnosis. The first step involves patients appraising their own symptoms well, leading to health-seeking behavior. The major barriers to this are good health literacy, cancer stigma, and limited access to primary care. The second step involves a clinical diagnosis and staging based on pathology and radiology. There is often a low index of suspicion by primary caregivers for HNC and, even if there is suspicion, adequate training and equipment such as scopes are required to examine the difficult regions of the head and neck such as the pharynx, larynx, and sinuses. Poor radiology and pathology services make diagnosis and staging difficult. Poor coordination of services and loss of follow-up is another major barrier. The third step is access to high-quality, affordable multidisciplinary team treatment in a timely manner. Financial, geographic, logistical, and sociocultural barriers reduce the chances of meeting the goal of treatment within 1 month of diagnosis.

2.5 Socioeconomic Factors Influencing the Risk of Head and Neck Cancer

The absolute or relative amounts of financial resources, authority, and position associated with an individual, group, or country's wealth are all included in the concept of socioeconomic status, which can influence early diagnoses and treatment of patients with HNC. It is a complex idea that considers several variables, including employment position, income, education, and other aspects (Braveman et al., 2005; Havranek et al., 2015). Socioeconomic factors affect a person's ability to manage stress, afford housing and healthcare, and engage in health-related activities. For example, earning money through work makes it easier to pay for things like housing, childcare, education, food, and medical care. Furthermore, poorer communities frequently do not have access to high-quality healthcare at the community level (Bruna et al., 2006; Chida et al., 2008). Furthermore, socioeconomic characteristics may skew or confound the relationships between different variables and health outcomes.

For example, the interplay of gender, race/ethnicity, and socioeconomic level might have distinct implications on health outcomes for different demographic groups. According to Conway et al. (2015), those with HNC are primarily from lower socioeconomic backgrounds. A substantial portion of South Africans live in substandard, crowded housing; have limited access to water and sanitary facilities; and face socioeconomic challenges. These situations make it harder to maintain strict dental and general hygiene and social separation. Psychological issues, such dread of going into a high-risk dental environment for treatment, can also contribute to oral health neglect (Magan, 2020). According to the international UICC-AJCC classification, stage III or IV is the advanced stage at which more than half of HNC cases are diagnosed (Conway et al., 2015). This is a worrying scenario because the prognosis of HNC is related to the stage at which it is treated; earlier intervention produces better results with fewer side effects. Delays in diagnosis, presentation, or early identification of a tumor that has progressed can all lead to late-stage diagnosis. To successfully plan public health initiatives, it is imperative to quantify the roles played by these various systems.

2.6 Limitations and Future Prospects

Early detection plays a pivotal role in the prognosis of HNC due to limited treatment options for advanced and recurrent cases (Hofmann et al., 2020). However, efficient screening methods are still lacking, thus posing challenges for pathologists in routine clinical practice (Mäkitie et al., 2020). The lack of information regarding the prevalence of oral diseases, risk factors, workforce development, and healthcare services is one of the issues affecting oral health in Africa (World Health Organization, 2023). Since many African nations lack mechanisms for monitoring oral health, it is the duty of oral health researchers and academic institutions to contribute the critical data that inform policy creation and decision-making. Data are also required because the evidence currently accessible is frequently from other nations and does not address the contextual factors that increase the likelihood of poor oral health in Africa (El Tantawi et al., 2023). Most South Africans do not have enough and adequate access to dental care facilities. The number of dentists in South Africa is 0.13 per 1,000 people, which is lower than in the majority of other middle-income nations (Strachan et al., 2011). Furthermore, disparities exist in the allocation of South Africa's oral health care workers (OHCW) (Strachan et al., 2011; World Health Organization, 2016). Only 25% of South African dentists were employed by the public sector in 2009, despite the fact that 84–90% of the country's population depends on public oral health services (Strachan et al., 2011).

The discovery of novel diagnostic biomarkers is particularly beneficial for poorly differentiated cancers or in cases where confirming cancer presence or recurrence is challenging, as after adjuvant radiotherapy (Starzyńska et al., 2021). Additionally, noninvasive methods like exhaled breath analysis show promise but require further clinical validation. The utility of liquid biopsy in HNC diagnosis remains a subject of debate but holds potential for earlier detection of metastasis and in monitoring treatment response (Kong & Birkeland, 2021). Analysis of circulating tumor DNA and other blood-based markers may offer predictive and prognostic insights (Bellairs et al., 2017; Payne et al., 2019; Schmidt et al., 2016). For instance, the analysis of p16-negative oral SCC (OSCC) revealed varying 5-year disease-free survival rates based on the number of positive lymph nodes (Li et al., 2021). Given the significance of early detection, ongoing research into efficient biomarkers and diagnostic methods is imperative to enhance outcomes for HNC patients.

The contemporary management of HNC typically involves a combination of surgery, radiotherapy, and systemic therapy (Kitamura et al., 2021). Despite advancements in cancer treatment, the 5-year survival rate for HNC patients has remained largely unchanged in recent decades, highlighting the ongoing need for new therapeutic targets (Hasnat et al., 2020). Immunotherapy, particularly pembrolizumab in combination with platinum and fluorouracil, has gained prominence for patients with recurrent or metastatic disease exhibiting positive PD-L1 expression (Cohen et al., 2019). Clinical trials investigating the efficacy of agents like nivolumab, T-cell inducible co-stimulatory receptor agonist, and monalizumab, alone or in combination, hold promise for platinum-resistant patients (Borel et al., 2020). Additionally, radiotherapy shows potential benefits even among patients with advanced or metastatic disease (Biau & Bourhis, 2020; Karam & Raben, 2019). Ongoing research and clinical trials are crucial for identifying innovative treatment strategies to improve outcomes for HNC patients.

Clinical and radiological biomarkers for assessing treatment response and radiation therapy toxicity in head and neck tumors are currently scarce and not routinely employed in clinical practice. However, the "omics" approach presents a promising avenue for research, potentially offering extensive data to predict treatment response and patient toxicity (Scott et al., 2021). Tumor genomic profiling shows potential for customizing radiation doses based on tumor radiosensitivity (Marcu & Marcu, 2021). Additionally, immune system status, particularly the neutrophil-to-lymphocyte ratio, correlates with oncologic outcomes and radiation-related side effects (Fanetti et al., 2020; Homa-Mlak et al., 2021). Further development in these areas is essential for advancing personalized radiation treatment approaches. The quest for new diagnostic, prognostic, and predictive biomarkers, along with promising treatment targets, holds the potential to enhance the prognosis of HNC patients (Starzyńska et al., 2022).

2.7 Conclusion

With rising rates of death and occurrence, head and neck malignancies are becoming more common. Preventable risk factors such alcohol use, HPV infection, tobacco use, and areca nut consumption are major contributors to this increase. It is expected that HPV-related HNC in affluent countries will surpass those cancers brought on by alcohol and tobacco use. Notwithstanding this unsettling pattern, advancements in therapy have increased patient survival rates. People with HNC in Africa face a variety of difficulties, such as limited access to quality healthcare and a shortage of trained healthcare personnel. Context-relevant data on HNC is similarly scarce in Africa, and this hinders the development of guidelines and policies that are appropriate for different contexts. Comprehensive public health initiatives are necessary to address the burden of HNC. The main goals of the intervention should be to inform people about the dangers of using substances that cause cancer and to encourage them to give up using alcohol, tobacco products, and areca nuts. Preventing HPV-related HNC requires expanding access to HPV vaccination and promoting safe sexual behavior. Additionally, early detection and intervention may result from the identification and screening of high-risk patients. By putting these diverse measures into practice, the anticipated rise in HNC cases can be effectively curbed. To change behaviors, raise awareness, and put preventive measures into place, cooperation between communities, legislators, and healthcare experts is essential. We may aim for better results and minimize the burden of this terrible disease by working together to lessen the effects of HNC.

References

ALUCKAL, E., LI, R., PEI, L., LEE, A., AL-SHMA, S., & ABRAHAM, A. 2022. Premalignant lesions of the oral cavity: An update. *J Orofacial Res*, 11, 49–55.

ANG, K. K., HARRIS, J., WHEELER, R., WEBER, R., ROSENTHAL, D. I., NGUYEN-TÂN, P. F., WESTRA, W. H., CHUNG, C. H., JORDAN, R. C., & LU, C. 2010. Human papillomavirus and survival of patients with oropharyngeal cancer. *N Engl J Med*, 363, 24–35.

BARSOUK, A., ALURU, J. S., RAWLA, P., SAGINALA, K., & BARSOUK, A. 2023. Epidemiology, risk factors, and prevention of head and neck squamous cell carcinoma. *Med Sci* [Online], 11. https://pubmed.ncbi.nlm.nih.gov/37367741/

BASNAYAKE, B. W. M. T. J., LEO, P., RAO, S., VASANI, S., KENNY, L., HAASS, N. K., & PUNYADEERA, C. 2023. Head and neck cancer patient-derived tumouroid cultures: Opportunities and challenges. *Br J Cancer*, 128, 1807–18.

BEAUDOIN, P.-L., ANCHOUCHE, S., GAFFAR, R., GUADAGNO, E., AYAD, T., & POENARU, D. 2020. Barriers in access to care for patients with head and neck cancer in resource-limited settings: A systematic review. *JAMA Otolaryngol Head Neck Surg*, 146, 291–7.

BELLAIRS, J. A., HASINA, R., & AGRAWAL, N. 2017. Tumor DNA: An emerging biomarker in head and neck cancer. *Cancer Metastasis Rev*, 36, 515–523.

BERMAN, T. A., & SCHILLER, J. T. 2017. Human papillomavirus in cervical cancer and oropharyngeal cancer: One cause, two diseases. *Cancer*, 123, 2219–29.

BERNSTEIN, E., GUO, N., GOTO, T., & ROTHBERG, M. B. 2021. Characterizing the variation of alcohol cessation pharmacotherapy in primary care. *J Gen Intern Med*, 36, 1989–96.

BHATTACHARJEE, A., BAHAR, I., & SAIKIA, A. 2015. Nutritional assessment of patients with head and neck cancer in North-East India and dietary intervention. *Indian J Palliat Care*, 21, 289–95.

BIAU, J., & BOURHIS, J. 2020. Combining immunotherapy and radiotherapy in head and neck squamous cell cancers: Which perspectives? *Curr Opin Oncol*, 32(3), 196–202. doi:10.1097/CCO.0000000000000628. PMID: 32251158.

BOREL, C., JUNG, A. C., & BURGY, M. 2020. Immunotherapy breakthroughs in the treatment of recurrent or metastatic head and neck squamous cell carcinoma. *Cancers* [Online], 12.https://pubmed.ncbi.nlm.nih.gov/32967162/

BOSETTI, C., CARIOLI, G., SANTUCCI, C., BERTUCCIO, P., GALLUS, S., GARAVELLO, W., NEGRI, E., & LA VECCHIA, C. 2020. Global trends in oral and pharyngeal cancer incidence and mortality. *Int J Cancer*, 147, 1040–9.

BRAVEMAN, P. A., CUBBIN, C., EGERTER, S., CHIDEYA, S., MARCHI, K. S., METZLER, M., & POSNER, S. 2005. Socioeconomic status in health research: One size does not fit all. *JAMA*, 294, 2879–88.

BRUNA, G., MARY, S., DEBBIE, A. L., JOHN, W. L., & GEORGE DAVEY, S. 2006. Indicators of socioeconomic position (part 1). *J Epidemiol Community Health*, 60, 7.

CADONI, G., BOCCIA, S., PETRELLI, L., DI GIANNANTONIO, P., ARZANI, D., GIORGIO, A., DE FEO, E., PANDOLFINI, M., GALLÌ, P., PALUDETTI, G., & RICCIARDI, G. 2012. A review of genetic epidemiology of head and neck cancer related to polymorphisms in metabolic genes, cell cycle control and alcohol metabolism. *Acta Otorhinolaryngol Ital*, 32, 1–11.

CARUSO, D., BARCA, I., GIOFRÈ, E., FERRAGINA, F., VARANO, A., KALLAVERJA, E., & CRISTOFARO, M. G. 2021. Maxillofacial surgical oncology during Covid-19 phase-1 and phase-2 of Italian lockdown; Single centre experience. *Ann Ital Chir*, 92, 575–81.

CASTELLSAGUÉ, X., QUINTANA, M. J., MARTÍNEZ, M. C., NIETO, A., SÁNCHEZ, M. J., JUAN, A., MONNER, A., CARRERA, M., AGUDO, A., & QUER, M. 2004. The role of type of tobacco and type of alcoholic beverage in oral carcinogenesis. *Int J Cancer*, 108, 741–9.

CHAN, K. C. A., WOO, J. K. S., KING, A., ZEE, B. C. Y., LAM, W. K. J., CHAN, S. L., CHU, S. W. I., MAK, C., TSE, I. O. L., LEUNG, S. Y. M., CHAN, G., HUI, E. P., MA, B. B. Y., CHIU, R. W. K., LEUNG, S.-F., VAN HASSELT, A. C., CHAN, A. T. C., & LO, Y. M. D. 2017. Analysis of plasma Epstein–Barr virus DNA to screen for nasopharyngeal cancer. *N Engl J Med*, 377, 513–22.

CHARAFEDDINE, M. A., OLSON, S. H., MUKHERJI, D., TEMRAZ, S. N., ABOU-ALFA, G. K., & SHAMSEDDINE, A. I. 2017. Proportion of cancer in a Middle eastern country attributable to established risk factors. *BMC Cancer*, 17, 1–11.

CHASEN, M. R., & BHARGAVA, R. 2009. A descriptive review of the factors contributing to nutritional compromise in patients with head and neck cancer. *Support Care Cancer*, 17, 1345–51.

CHATURVEDI, A. K., ANDERSON, W. F., LORTET-TIEULENT, J., CURADO, M. P., FERLAY, J., FRANCESCHI, S., ROSENBERG, P. S., BRAY, F., & GILLISON, M. L. 2013. Worldwide trends in incidence rates for oral cavity and oropharyngeal cancers. *J Clin Oncol*, 31, 4550.

CHATURVEDI, A. K., ENGELS, E. A., PFEIFFER, R. M., HERNANDEZ, B. Y., XIAO, W., KIM, E., JIANG, B., GOODMAN, M. T., SIBUG-SABER, M., COZEN, W., LIU, L., LYNCH, C. F., WENTZENSEN, N., JORDAN, R. C., ALTEKRUSE, S., ANDERSON, W. F., ROSENBERG, P. S., & GILLISON, M. L. 2011. Human papillomavirus and rising oropharyngeal cancer incidence in the United States. *J Clin Oncol*, 29, 4294–301.

CHENEVERT, J., & CHIOSEA, S. 2012. Incidence of human papillomavirus in oropharyngeal squamous cell carcinomas: now and 50 years ago. *Hum Pathol*, 43, 17–22.

CHEONG, S. C., VATANASAPT, P., YI-HSIN, Y., ZAIN, R. B., KERR, A. R., & JOHNSON, N. W. 2017. Oral cancer in South East Asia: Current status and future directions. *Transl Res Oral Oncol*, 2, 2057178X17702921.

CHIDA, Y., HAMER, M., WARDLE, J., & STEPTOE, A. 2008. Do stress-related psychosocial factors contribute to cancer incidence and survival? *Nat Clin Pract Oncol*, 5, 466–75.

CIVES, M., MANNAVOLA, F., LOSPALLUTI, L., SERGI, M. C., CAZZATO, G., FILONI, E., CAVALLO, F., GIUDICE, G., STUCCI, L. S., PORTA, C., & TUCCI, M. 2020. Non-melanoma skin cancers: Biological and clinical features. *Int J Mol Sci*, 21(15), 5394. doi:10.3390/ijms21155394. PMID: 32751327; PMCID: PMC7432795.

CLARKSON, E., HADIOONZADEH, R., & PETERS, S. M. 2024. Treatment of oral dysplasia. *Dental Clin*, 68, 133–49.

COGLIANO, V. J., BAAN, R., STRAIF, K., GROSSE, Y., LAUBY-SECRETAN, B., EL GHISSASSI, F., BOUVARD, V., BENBRAHIM-TALLAA, L., GUHA, N., & FREEMAN, C. 2011. Preventable exposures associated with human cancers. *J Nat Cancer Inst*, 103, 1827–39.

COHEN, E. E. W., BELL, R. B., BIFULCO, C. B., BURTNESS, B., GILLISON, M. L., HARRINGTON, K. J., LE, Q. T., LEE, N. Y., LEIDNER, R., LEWIS, R. L., LICITRA, L., MEHANNA, H., MELL, L. K., RABEN, A., SIKORA, A. G., UPPALURI, R., WHITWORTH, F., ZANDBERG, D. P., & FERRIS, R. L. 2019. The Society for Immunotherapy of Cancer consensus statement on immunotherapy for the treatment of squamous cell carcinoma of the head and neck (HNSCC). *J Immunother Cancer*, 7, 184.

CONWAY, D. I., BRENNER, D. R., MCMAHON, A. D., MACPHERSON, L. M. D., AGUDO, A., AHRENS, W., BOSETTI, C., BRENNER, H., CASTELLSAGUE, X., CHEN, C., CURADO, M. P., CURIONI, O. A., DAL MASO, L., DAUDT, A. W., DE GOIS FILHO, J. F., D'SOUZA, G., EDEFONTI, V., FABIANOVA, E., FERNANDEZ, L., FRANCESCHI, S., GILLISON, M., HAYES, R. B., HEALY, C. M., HERRERO, R., HOLCATOVA, I., JAYAPRAKASH, V., KELSEY, K., KJAERHEIM, K., KOIFMAN, S., LA VECCHIA, C., LAGIOU, P., LAZARUS, P., LEVI, F., LISSOWSKA, J., LUCE, D., MACFARLANE, T. V., MATES, D., MATOS, E., MCCLEAN, M., MENEZES, A. M., MENVIELLE, G., MERLETTI, F., MORGENSTERN, H., MOYSICH, K., MÜLLER, H., MUSCAT, J., OLSHAN, A. F., PURDUE, M. P., RAMROTH, H., RICHIARDI, L., RUDNAI, P., SCHANTZ, S., SCHWARTZ, S. M., SHANGINA, O., SIMONATO, L., SMITH, E., STUCKER, I., STURGIS, E. M., SZESZENIA-DABROWSKA, N., TALAMINI, R., THOMSON, P., VAUGHAN, T. L., WEI, Q., WINN, D. M., WUNSCH-FILHO, V., YU, G.-P., ZHANG, Z.-F., ZHENG, T., ZNAOR,

A., BOFFETTA, P., CHUANG, S.-C., GHODRAT, M., AMY LEE, Y.-C., HASHIBE, M., & BRENNAN, P. 2015. Estimating and explaining the effect of education and income on head and neck cancer risk: INHANCE consortium pooled analysis of 31 case-control studies from 27 countries. *Int J Cancer*, 136, 1125–39.

COUTTS, K. A., SEEDAT, J., & VLOK, E. 2022. The management of head and neck cancer in Africa: What lessons can be learned from African literature? *S Afr J Oncol*, 6, 3.

CRAVO, M. L., GLÓRIA, L. M., & CLARO, I. 2000. Metabolic responses to tumour disease and progression: Tumour-host interaction. *Clin Nutr*, 19, 459–65.

CREANEY, G., MCMAHON, A. D., ROSS, A. J., BHATTI, L. A., PATERSON, C., & CONWAY, D. I. 2022. Head and neck cancer in the UK: What was the stage before COVID-19? UK cancer registries analysis (2011–2018). *Br Dent J*, 233, 787–93.

D'ORAZIO, J., JARRETT, S., AMARO-ORTIZ, A., & SCOTT, T. 2013. UV radiation and the skin. *Int J Mol Sci*, 14, 12222–48.

DE MARTEL, C., FERLAY, J., FRANCESCHI, S., VIGNAT, J., BRAY, F., FORMAN, D., & PLUMMER, M. 2012. Global burden of cancers attributable to infections in 2008: A review and synthetic analysis. *Lancet Oncol*, 13, 607–15.

DESANTIS, C., NAISHADHAM, D., & JEMAL, A. 2013. Cancer statistics for African Americans, 2013. *CA: A Cancer J Clin*, 63, 151–66.

DHULL, A. K., ATRI, R., DHANKHAR, R., CHAUHAN, A. K., & KAUSHAL, V. 2018. Major risk factors in head and neck cancer: A retrospective analysis of 12-year experiences. *World J Oncol*, 9, 80–4.

DIFFEY, B. L. 2002. Human exposure to solar ultraviolet radiation. *J Cosmetic Dermatol*, 1(3), 124–30. doi:10.1046/j.1473-2165.2002.00060.x. PMID: 17147711.

ELREFAEY, S., MASSARO, M. A., CHIOCCA, S., CHIESA, F., & ANSARIN, M. 2014. HPV in oropharyngeal cancer: The basics to know in clinical practice. *Acta Otorhinolaryngol Ital*, 34, 299.

EL TANTAWI, M., FOLAYAN, M. O., & AYO-YUSUF, O. 2023. Editorial: Dentistry and oral health in Africa. *Front Oral Health*, 4, 1160976.

FAGAN, J. J. 2018. Workforce considerations, training, and diseases in Africa. *Otolaryngol Clin N Am*, 51, 643–9.

FAKHRY, C., WESTRA, W. H., LI, S., CMELAK, A., RIDGE, J. A., PINTO, H., FORASTIERE, A., & GILLISON, M. L. 2008. Improved survival of patients with human papillomavirus-positive head and neck squamous cell carcinoma in a prospective clinical trial. *J Natl Cancer Inst*, 100, 261–9.

FAN, T., SUN, G., ZHAO, L., CUI, X., & ZHONG, R. 2019. Metabolic activation and carcinogenesis of tobacco-specific nitrosamine n′-nitrosonornicotine (NNN): A density function theory and molecular docking study. *Int J Environ Res Public Health*, 16(2), 178. doi:10.3390/ijerph16020178. PMID: 30634532; PMCID: PMC6352179.

FANETTI, G., ALTERIO, D., MARVASO, G., GANDINI, S., ROJAS, D. P., GOBITTI, C., MINATEL, E., REVELANT, A., CAROLI, A., FRANCIA, C. M., ALESSANDRO, O., PEPA, M., GUGLIANDOLO, S. G., STARZYŃSKA, A., POLESEL, J., VACCHER, E., COSSU ROCCA, M., TAGLIABUE, M., ANSARIN, M., LUPATO, V., GIACOMARRA, V., DE PAOLI, A., ORECCHIA, R., FRANCHIN, G., & JERECZEK-FOSSA, B. A. 2020. Prognostic significance of neutrophil-to-lymphocyte ratio in HPV status era for oropharyngeal cancer. *Oral Dis*, 26, 1384–92.

FANG, M., HUANG, W., MO, D., ZHAO, W., & HUANG, R. 2018. Association of five Snps in Cytotoxic T-Lymphocyte antigen 4 and cancer susceptibility: Evidence from 67 studies. *Cell Physiol Biochem*, 47, 414–27.

FITZMAURICE, C., ALLEN, C., BARBER, R. M., BARREGARD, L., BHUTTA, Z. A., BRENNER, H., DICKER, D. J., CHIMED-ORCHIR, O., DANDONA, R., & DANDONA, L. 2017. Global, regional, and national cancer incidence, mortality, years of life lost, years lived with disability, and disability-adjusted life-years for 32 cancer groups, 1990 to 2015: A systematic analysis for the global burden of disease study. *JAMA Oncol*, 3, 524–48.

FROWEN, J., HUGHES, R., & SKEAT, J. 2020. The prevalence of patient-reported dysphagia and oral complications in cancer patients. *Support Care Cancer*, 28, 1141–50.

GAN, S. J., DAHLSTROM, K. R., PECK, B. W., CAYWOOD, W., LI, G., WEI, Q., ZAFEREO, M. E., & STURGIS, E. M. 2013. Incidence and pattern of second primary malignancies in patients with index oropharyngeal cancers versus index nonoropharyngeal head and neck cancers. *Cancer*, 119, 2593–601.

GILYOMA, J. M., RAMBAU, P. F., MASALU, N., KAYANGE, N. M., & CHALYA, P. L. 2015. Head and neck cancers: A clinico-pathological profile and management challenges in a resource-limited setting. *BMC Res Notes*, 8, 1–9.

GONIEWICZ, M. L., SMITH, D. M., EDWARDS, K. C., BLOUNT, B. C., CALDWELL, K. L., FENG, J., WANG, L., CHRISTENSEN, C., AMBROSE, B., & BOREK, N. 2018. Comparison of nicotine and toxicant exposure in users of electronic cigarettes and combustible cigarettes. *JAMA Netw Open*, 1, e185937–e185937.

GORENC, M., KOZJEK, N. R., & STROJAN, P. 2015. Malnutrition and cachexia in patients with head and neck cancer treated with (chemo)radiotherapy. *Rep Pract Oncol Radiother*, 20, 249–58.

GORMLEY, M., CREANEY, G., SCHACHE, A., INGARFIELD, K., & CONWAY, D. I. 2022. Reviewing the epidemiology of head and neck cancer: Definitions, trends and risk factors. *Br Dent J*, 233, 780–6.

GRANA, R., BENOWITZ, N., & GLANTZ, S. A. 2014. E-cigarettes. *Circulation*, 129, 1972–86.

GUHA, N., WARNAKULASURIYA, S., VLAANDEREN, J., & STRAIF, K. 2014. Betel quid chewing and the risk of oral and oropharyngeal cancers: A meta-analysis with implications for cancer control. *Int J Cancer*, 135, 1433–43.

GUPTA, A. K., BHARADWAJ, M., & MEHROTRA, R. 2016. Skin cancer concerns in people of color: Risk factors and prevention. *Asian Pac J Cancer Prev*, 17, 5257–64.

HASHIBE, M., BRENNAN, P., BENHAMOU, S., CASTELLSAGUE, X., CHEN, C., CURADO, M. P., MASO, L. D., DAUDT, A. W., FABIANOVA, E., & WÜNSCH-FILHO, V. 2007. Alcohol drinking in never users of tobacco, cigarette smoking in never drinkers, and the risk of head and neck cancer: Pooled analysis in the International Head and Neck Cancer Epidemiology Consortium. *J Nat Cancer Inst*, 99, 777–89.

HASHIM, D., GENDEN, E., POSNER, M., HASHIBE, M., & BOFFETTA, P. 2019. Head and neck cancer prevention: From primary prevention to impact of clinicians on reducing burden. *Ann Oncol*, 30, 744–56.

HASNAT, S., HUJANEN, R., NWARU, B. I., SALO, T., & SALEM, A. 2020. The prognostic value of toll-like receptors in head and neck squamous cell carcinoma: A systematic review and meta-analysis. *Int J Molec Sci* [Online], 21. https://pubmed.ncbi.nlm.nih.gov/33008143/

HASSAN, M. A., LUND, V. J., HOWARD, D. J., & SACKER, A. A. 2007. Are the demographics for squamous cell cancer in the head and neck changing in the United Kingdom? *J Laryngol Otol*, 121, 154–7.

HAVRANEK, E. P., MUJAHID, M. S., BARR, D. A., BLAIR, I. V., COHEN, M. S., CRUZ-FLORES, S., DAVEY-SMITH, G., DENNISON-HIMMELFARB, C. R., LAUER, M. S., LOCKWOOD, D. W., ROSAL, M., & YANCY, C. W. 2015. Social determinants of risk and outcomes for cardiovascular disease: A scientific statement from the American heart association. *Circulation*, 132, 873–98.

HECK, J. E., BERTHILLER, J., VACCARELLA, S., WINN, D. M., SMITH, E. M., SHAN'GINA, O., SCHWARTZ, S. M., PURDUE, M. P., PILARSKA, A., & ELUF-NETO, J. 2010. Sexual behaviours and the risk of head and neck cancers: A pooled analysis in the International Head and Neck Cancer Epidemiology (INHANCE) consortium. *Int J Epidemiol*, 39, 166–81.

HOFMANN, L., LUDWIG, S., VAHL, J. M., BRUNNER, C., HOFFMANN, T. K., & THEODORAKI, M.-N. 2020. The emerging role of exosomes in diagnosis, prognosis, and therapy in head and neck cancer. *Int J Molec Sci* [Online], 21. https://pubmed.ncbi.nlm.nih.

gov/32517240/#:~:text=Exosomes%20strongly%20contribute%20to%20the,immune%20suppression%20and%20tumor%20progression.

HOMA-MLAK, I., BRZOZOWSKA, A., MLAK, R., SZUDY-SZCZYREK, A., & MAŁECKA-MASSALSKA, T. 2021. Neutrophil-to-lymphocyte ratio as a factor predicting radiotherapy induced oral mucositis in head neck cancer patients treated with radiotherapy. *J Clin Med*, 10(19), 4444. doi:10.3390/jcm10194444. PMID: 34640462; PMCID: PMC8509431.

IOCCA, O., SOLLECITO, T. P., ALAWI, F., WEINSTEIN, G. S., NEWMAN, J. G., DE VIRGILIO, A., DI MAIO, P., SPRIANO, G., PARDIÑAS LÓPEZ, S., & SHANTI, R. M. 2020. Potentially malignant disorders of the oral cavity and oral dysplasia: A systematic review and meta-analysis of malignant transformation rate by subtype. *Head Neck*, 42, 539–55.

IRFAN, M., DELGADO, R. Z. R., & FRIAS-LOPEZ, J. 2020. The oral microbiome and cancer. *Front Immunol*, 11, 591088.

JETHWA, A. R., & KHARIWALA, S. S. 2017. Tobacco-related carcinogenesis in head and neck cancer. *Cancer Metastasis Rev*, 36, 411–23.

JORDAN, C. J., & XI, Z.-X. 2018. Discovery and development of varenicline for smoking cessation. *Exp Opin Drug Discov*, 13, 671–83.

KARAM, S. D., & RABEN, D. 2019. Radioimmunotherapy for the treatment of head and neck cancer. *Lancet Oncol*, 20, e404–16.

KASPER, D., FAUCI, A., HAUSER, S., LONGO, D., JAMESON, J., & LOSCALZO, J. 2015. *Harrison's Principles of Internal Medicine, 19e*. New York: McGraw-Hill.

KAWAKITA, D., OZE, I., IWASAKI, S., MATSUDA, T., MATSUO, K., & ITO, H. 2022. Trends in the incidence of head and neck cancer by subsite between 1993 and 2015 in Japan. *Cancer Med*, 11, 1553–60.

KIM, D. H., KIM, S. W., & HWANG, S. H. 2022. Efficacy of non-invasive diagnostic methods in the diagnosis and screening of oral cancer and precancer. *Brazil J Otorhinolaryngol*, 88, 937–47.

KIM, Y., HACK, L. M., AHN, E. S., & KIM, J. 2018. Practical outpatient pharmacotherapy for alcohol use disorder. *Drugs Context*, 7, 212308. doi:10.7573/dic.212308. PMID: 29445407; PMCID: PMC5804871.

KING, G., STRACHAN, D., TUCKER, M., DUWYN, B., DESSERUD, S., & SHILLINGTON, M. 2009. The application of a transdisciplinary model for early intervention services. *Infants Young Child*, 22, 211–23.

KITAMURA, N., SENTO, S., YOSHIZAWA, Y., SASABE, E., KUDO, Y., & YAMAMOTO, T. 2021. Current trends and future prospects of molecular targeted therapy in head and neck squamous cell carcinoma. *Int J Molec Sci* [Online], 22. https://pubmed.ncbi.nlm.nih.gov/33383632/

KONG, L., & BIRKELAND, A. C. 2021. Liquid biopsies in head and neck cancer: Current state and future challenges. *Cancers (Basel)*, 13(8), 1874. doi:10.3390/cancers13081874. PMID: 33919778; PMCID: PMC8070729.

KRAMAROW, E. A., & ELGADDAL, N. 2023. Current Electronic Cigarette Use among Adults Aged 18 and Over: United States, 2021. *NCHS Data Brief*, (475), 1–8. PMID: 37486729.

LA ROSA, G. R. M., GATTUSO, G., PEDULLÀ, E., RAPISARDA, E., NICOLOSI, D., & SALMERI, M. 2020. Association of oral dysbiosis with oral cancer development. *Oncol Lett*, 19, 3045–58.

LACKO, M., BRAAKHUIS, B. J. M., STURGIS, E. M., BOEDEKER, C. C., SUÁREZ, C., RINALDO, A., FERLITO, A., & TAKES, R. P. 2014. Genetic susceptibility to head and neck squamous cell carcinoma. *Int J Radiat Oncol Biol Physics*, 89, 38–48.

LEE, Y. C. A., LI, S., CHEN, Y., LI, Q., CHEN, C. J., HSU, W. L., LOU, P. J., ZHU, C., PAN, J., & SHEN, H. 2019. Tobacco smoking, alcohol drinking, betel quid chewing, and the risk of head and neck cancer in an East Asian population. *Head Neck*, 41, 92–102.

LEE, Y. S., JOHNSON, D. E., & GRANDIS, J. R. 2018. An update: Emerging drugs to treat squamous cell carcinomas of the head and neck. *Exp Opin Emerg Drugs*, 23, 283–99.

LEES, J. 1999. Incidence of weight loss in head and neck cancer patients on commencing radiotherapy treatment at a regional oncology centre. *Eur J Cancer Care*, 8, 133–6.

LEKALAKALA, P. T., KHAMMISSA, R. A., KRAMER, B., AYO-YUSUF, O. A., LEMMER, J., & FELLER, L. 2015. Oculocutaneous albinism and squamous cell carcinoma of the skin of the head and neck in sub-Saharan Africa. *J Skin Cancer*, 2015, 167847.

LI, P., FANG, Q., YANG, Y., CHEN, D., DU, W., LIU, F., & LUO, R. 2021. Survival significance of number of positive lymph nodes in oral squamous cell carcinoma stratified by p16. *Front Oncol*, 11, 545433. doi:10.3389/fonc.2021.545433. PMID: 33747901; PMCID: PMC7969991.

LITTLE, M. A., POKHREL, P., MURPHY, K. L., KAWAMOTO, C. T., SUGUITAN, G. S., & HERZOG, T. A. 2014. Intention to quit betel quid: A comparison of betel quid chewers and cigarette smokers. *Oral Health Dental Manage*, 13, 512.

LORINI, L., BESCÓS ATÍN, C., THAVARAJ, S., MÜLLER-RICHTER, U., ALBEROLA FERRANTI, M., PAMIAS ROMERO, J., SÁEZ BARBA, M., DE PABLO GARCÍA-CUENCA, A., BRAÑA GARCÍA, I., & BOSSI, P. 2021. Overview of oral potentially malignant disorders: From risk factors to specific therapies. *Cancers*, 13, 3696.

LOUIE, K. S., MEHANNA, H., & SASIENI, P. 2015. Trends in head and neck cancers in England from 1995 to 2011 and projections up to 2025. *Oral Oncol*, 51, 341–8.

MACEK, M. D., REID, B. C., & YELLOWITZ, J. A. 2003. Oral cancer examinations among adults at high risk: Findings from the 1998 National Health Interview Survey. *J Public Health Dentistry*, 63, 119–25.

MAGAN, A. 2020. Individual and social determinants of oral health in South Africa in the context of COVID-19. *S Afr Dental J*, 75, 440–4.

MAIER, H., DIETZ, A., GEWELKE, U., HELLER, W. D., & WEIDAUER, H. 1992. Tobacco and alcohol and the risk of head and neck cancer. *Clin Investig*, 70, 320–7.

MÄKITIE, A. A., ALMANGUSH, A., YOUSSEF, O., METSÄLÄ, M., SILÉN, S., NIXON, I. J., HAIGENTZ JR, M., RODRIGO, J. P., SABA, N. F., VANDER POORTEN, V., & FERLITO, A. 2020. Exhaled breath analysis in the diagnosis of head and neck cancer. *Head Neck*, 42, 787–93.

MARCU, L. G., & MARCU, D. C. 2021. Current omics trends in personalised head and neck cancer chemoradiotherapy. *J Personalized Med* [Online], 11. https://pmc.ncbi.nlm.nih.gov/articles/PMC8625829/

MARKOWITZ, L. E., LIU, G., HARIRI, S., STEINAU, M., DUNNE, E. F., & UNGER, E. R. 2016. Prevalence of HPV after introduction of the vaccination program in the United States. *Pediatrics*, 137(3), e20151968. doi:10.1542/peds.2015-1968. Epub 2016 Feb 22. PMID: 26908697.

MCCARTER, K., MARTÍNEZ, Ú., BRITTON, B., BAKER, A., BONEVSKI, B., CARTER, G., BECK, A., WRATTEN, C., GUILLAUMIER, A., & HALPIN, S. A. 2016. Smoking cessation care among patients with head and neck cancer: A systematic review. *BMJ Open*, 6, e012296.

MELLO, F. W., MIGUEL, A. F. P., DUTRA, K. L., PORPORATTI, A. L., WARNAKULASURIYA, S., GUERRA, E. N. S., & RIVERO, E. R. C. 2018. Prevalence of oral potentially malignant disorders: A systematic review and meta-analysis. *J Oral Pathol Med*, 47, 633–40.

MERCADANTE, S., AIELLI, F., ADILE, C., FERRERA, P., VALLE, A., FUSCO, F., CARUSELLI, A., CARTONI, C., MASSIMO, P., MASEDU, F., VALENTI, M., & PORZIO, G. 2015. Prevalence of oral mucositis, dry mouth, and dysphagia in advanced cancer patients. *Support Care Cancer*, 23, 3249–55.

MIRANDA-FILHO, A., & BRAY, F. 2020. Global patterns and trends in cancers of the lip, tongue and mouth. *Oral Oncol*, 102, 104551.

MORITA, S., YANO, M., TSUJINAKA, T., AKIYAMA, Y., TANIGUCHI, M., KANEKO, K., MIKI, H., FUJII, T., YOSHINO, K., & KUSUOKA, H. 1999. Genetic polymorphisms of drug-metabolizing enzymes and susceptibility to head-and-neck squamous-cell carcinoma. *Int J Cancer*, 80, 685–8.

MOROJELE, N. K., BROOK, J. S., & BROOK, D. W. 2016. Tobacco and alcohol use among adolescents in South Africa: Shared and unshared risks. *J Child Adolesc Ment Health*, 28, 139–52.

NABUKENYA, J., HADLOCK, T. A., & ARUBAKU, W. 2018. Head and neck squamous cell carcinoma in Western Uganda: Disease of uncertainty and poor prognosis. *Oto Open*, 2, 2473974X18761868.

NGOMA, T., & NGOMA, M. 2019. Cancer control in Africa: Is cancer research a luxury or necessity? *Ecancermedicalscience*, 13, 947.

NIU, Y.-M., DU, X.-Y., CAI, H.-X., ZHANG, C., YUAN, R.-X., ZENG, X.-T., & LUO, J. 2015. Increased risks between Interleukin-10 gene polymorphisms and haplotype and head and neck cancer: A meta-analysis. *Sci Rep*, 5, 17149.

ORELL-KOTIKANGAS, H., ÖSTERLUND, P., MÄKITIE, O., SAARILAHTI, K., RAVASCO, P., SCHWAB, U., & MÄKITIE, A. A. 2017. Cachexia at diagnosis is associated with poor survival in head and neck cancer patients. *Acta Oto-Laryngologica*, 137, 778–85.

OYEYEMI, B. F., KAUR, U. S., PARAMRAJ, A., TANDON, R., KUMAR, A., & BHAVESH, N. S. 2023. Microbiome analysis of saliva from oral squamous cell carcinoma (OSCC) patients and tobacco abusers with potential biomarkers for oral cancer screening. *Heliyon*, 9(11), e21773. doi:10.1016/j.heliyon.2023.e21773. PMID: 38034672; PMCID: PMC10685184.

PAN AMERICAN HEALTH ORGANIZATION (PAHO). 2024. Tobacco use declines despite tobacco industry efforts to jeopardize progress. Available at: https://www.paho.org/en/news/16-1-2024-tobacco-use-declines-despite-tobacco-industry-efforts-jeopardize-progress#:~:text=Trends%20in%202022%20show%20a,are%20successfully%20reducing%20tobacco%20use [Accessed April 15, 2024.]

PARKIN, D. M. 2011. 2. Tobacco-attributable cancer burden in the UK in 2010. *Br J Cancer*, 105, S6–S13.

PASSOS, G. D., ROGERS, A. D., PRICE, C. E., PIENAAR, C. H., VAN ZYL, J. E., FAGAN, J. J., & HUDSON, D. A. 2015. Loupe magnification for head and neck free flap reconstruction in a developing country. *Eur J Plastic Surg*, 38, 363–70.

PAULINO, Y. C., WILKENS, L. R., SOTTO, P. P., FRANKE, A. A., KAWAMOTO, C. T., CHENNAUX, J. S. N., MENDEZ, A. J., TENORIO, L. F., BADOWSKI, G., & POKHREL, P. 2020. Rationale and design of a randomized, controlled, superiority trial on areca nut/betel quid cessation: The Betel Nut Intervention Trial (BENIT). *Contemp Clin Trials Comm*, 17, 100544.

PAYNE, K., BROOKS, J., SPRUCE, R., BATIS, N., TAYLOR, G., NANKIVELL, P., & MEHANNA, H. 2019. Circulating tumour cell biomarkers in head and neck cancer: Current progress and future prospects. *Cancers* [Online], 11. https://pmc.ncbi.nlm.nih.gov/articles/PMC6721520/

PEER, N. 2018. Current strategies are inadequate to curb the rise of tobacco use in Africa. *S Afr Med J*, 108. https://pubmed.ncbi.nlm.nih.gov/30004340/

PERELMAN, J., ALVES, J., PFOERTNER, T. K., MOOR, I., FEDERICO, B., KUIPERS, M. A. G., RICHTER, M., RIMPELA, A., KUNST, A. E., & LORANT, V. 2017. The association between personal income and smoking among adolescents: A study in six European cities. *Addiction*, 112, 2248–56.

RADAIC, A., & KAPILA, Y. L. 2021. The oralome and its dysbiosis: New insights into oral microbiome-host interactions. *Comput Struct Biotechnol J*, 19, 1335–60.

RATH, G. K., & MOHANTI, B. K. 2003. *Textbook of Radiation Oncology: Principles and Practice*. New Delhi: BI Churchill Livingstone/Elsevier.

RAY, L. A., MEREDITH, L. R., KILUK, B. D., WALTHERS, J., CARROLL, K. M., & MAGILL, M. 2020. Combined pharmacotherapy and cognitive behavioral therapy for adults with alcohol or substance use disorders: A systematic review and meta-analysis. *JAMA Netw Open*, 3, e208279.

REDDY, K. P., SCHWAMM, E., KALKHORAN, S., NOUBARY, F., WALENSKY, R. P., & RIGOTTI, N. A. 2021. Respiratory symptom incidence among people using electronic cigarettes, combustible tobacco, or both. *Am J Respir Crit Care Med*, 204, 231–4.

REDDY, P., ZUMA, K., SHISANA, O., JONAS, K., & SEWPAUL, R. 2015. Prevalence of tobacco use among adults in South Africa: Results from the first South African National Health and Nutrition Examination Survey. *S Afr Med J*, 105, 648–55.

REICHART, P. A., DIETRICH, T., KHONGKHUNTHIAN, P., & SRISUWAN, S. 2003. Decline of oropharyngeal cancer in Chiangmai province, Thailand, between 1988 and 1999. *Oral Oncol*, 39, 569–73.

ROSENBLATT, E., & ZUBIZARRETA, E. 2017. *Radiotherapy in Cancer Care: Facing the Global Challenge*. Vienna: International Atomic Energy Agency.

ROSENQUIST, K. 2005. Risk factors in oral and oropharyngeal squamous cell carcinoma: A population-based case-control study in southern Sweden. *Swed Dental J. Supplement*, 1–66.

ROSSOUW, L. 2021. Socioeconomic status and tobacco consumption: Analyzing inequalities in China, Ghana, India, Mexico, the Russian Federation and South Africa. *Tob Prev Cessat*, 7, 47.

RUMGAY, H., MURPHY, N., FERRARI, P., & SOERJOMATARAM, I. 2021. Alcohol and cancer: Epidemiology and biological mechanisms. *Nutrients*, 13, 3173.

SANKARANARAYANAN, R., RAMADAS, K., THOMAS, G., MUWONGE, R., THARA, S., MATHEW, B., & RAJAN, B. 2005. Effect of screening on oral cancer mortality in Kerala, India: A cluster-randomised controlled trial. *Lancet*, 365, 1927–33.

SCHMIDT, H., KULASINGHE, A., KENNY, L., & PUNYADEERA, C. 2016. The development of a liquid biopsy for head and neck cancers. *Oral Oncol*, 61, 8–11.

SCOTT, J. G., SEDOR, G., ELLSWORTH, P., SCARBOROUGH, J. A., AHMED, K. A., OLIVER, D. E., ESCHRICH, S. A., KATTAN, M. W., & TORRES-ROCA, J. F. 2021. Pan-cancer prediction of radiotherapy benefit using genomic-adjusted radiation dose (GARD): A cohort-based pooled analysis. *Lancet Oncol*, 22, 1221–9.

SINGH, D., & TRIPATHY, K. 2023. Cancer associated retinopathy. *StatPearls* [Internet]. StatPearls Publishing. https://www.ncbi.nlm.nih.gov/books/NBK578183/

SINGHVI, H. R., MALIK, A., & CHATURVEDI, P. 2017. The role of chronic mucosal trauma in oral cancer: A review of literature. *Indian J Med Paediatr Oncol*, 38, 44–50.

SMITH, D. M., CHRISTENSEN, C., VAN BEMMEL, D., BOREK, N., AMBROSE, B., ERIVES, G., NIAURA, R., EDWARDS, K. C., STANTON, C. A., & BLOUNT, B. C. 2021. Exposure to nicotine and toxicants among dual users of tobacco cigarettes and e-cigarettes: Population Assessment of Tobacco and Health (PATH) study, 2013–2014. *Nicotine Tobacco Res*, 23, 790–7.

SMITH, R. A., ANDREWS, K. S., BROOKS, D., FEDEWA, S. A., MANASSARAM-BAPTISTE, D., SASLOW, D., BRAWLEY, O. W., & WENDER, R. C. 2017. Cancer screening in the United States, 2017: A review of current American Cancer Society guidelines and current issues in cancer screening. *CA: Cancer J*, 67, 100–121.

STANIENDA-SOKÓŁ, K., SALWOWSKA, N., SŁAWIŃSKA, M., WICHERSKA-PAWŁOWSKA, K., LORENC, A., WCISŁO-DZIADECKA, D., WYDMAŃSKI, J., & MAJEWSKI, W. 2017. Primary locations of malignant melanoma lesions depending on patients' gender and age. *Asian Pac J Cancer Prev*, 18, 3081–6.

STARZYŃSKA, A., SOBOCKI, B. K., & ALTERIO, D. 2022. Current challenges in head and neck cancer management. *Cancers (Basel)*, 14, 358.

STARZYŃSKA, A., SOBOCKI, B. K., SEJDA, A., SAKOWICZ-BURKIEWICZ, M., SZOT, O., & JERECZEK-FOSSA, B. A. 2021. ZNF-281 as the potential diagnostic marker of oral squamous cell carcinoma. *Cancers* [Online], 13. https://pubmed.ncbi.nlm.nih.gov/34071380/

STRACHAN, B., ZABOW, T., & VAN DER SPUY, Z. M. 2011. More doctors and dentists are needed in South Africa. *S Afr Med J*, 101, 523–8.

SUNG, H., FERLAY, J., SIEGEL, R. L., LAVERSANNE, M., SOERJOMATARAM, I., & JEMAL, A. 2021. Global cancer statistics 2020: GLOBOCAN estimates of incidence and mortality worldwide for 36 cancers in 185 countries. *Cancer J Clin*, 71.

SZUKALSKA, M., SZYFTER, K., FLOREK, E., RODRIGO, J. P., RINALDO, A., MÄKITIE, A. A., STROJAN, P., TAKES, R. P., SUÁREZ, C., SABA, N. F., BRAAKHUIS, B. J. M., & FERLITO, A. 2020. Electronic cigarettes and head and neck cancer risk: Current state of art. *Cancers (Basel)*, 12, 3274. doi:10.3390/cancers12113274. PMID: 33167393; PMCID: PMC7694366.

TROY, J. D., GRANDIS, J. R., YOUK, A. O., DIERGAARDE, B., ROMKES, M., & WEISSFELD, J. L. 2013. Childhood passive smoke exposure is associated with adult head and neck cancer. *Cancer Epidemiol*, 37, 417–23.

TSENG, M.-F., TSAI, S. C.-S., WU, C.-Y., LIN, C.-C., & WONG, R.-H. 2021. The effectiveness of betel quid cessation among workers through the adoption of the five action areas of the Ottawa charter. *Substance Use Misuse*, 56, 718–27.

TUYNS, A. J., ESTEVE, J., RAYMOND, L., BERRINO, F., BENHAMOU, E., BLANCHET, F., BOFFETTA, P., CROSIGNANI, P., MORAL, A. D., & LEHMANN, W. 1988. Cancer of the larynx/hypopharynx, tobacco and alcohol: IARC international case-control study in Turin and Varese (Italy), Zaragoza and Navarra (Spain), Geneva (Switzerland) and Calvados (France). *Int J Cancer*, 41, 483–91.

VAN BOKHORST-DE VAN DER, S., VAN LEEUWEN, P. A., KUIK, D. J., KLOP, W. M., SAUERWEIN, H. P., SNOW, G. B., & QUAK, J. J. 1999. The impact of nutritional status on the prognoses of patients with advanced head and neck cancer. *Cancer*, 86, 519–27.

VELLEUER, E., & DIETRICH, R. 2014. Fanconi anemia: Young patients at high risk for squamous cell carcinoma. *Mol Cell Pediatr*, 1, 9.

VOLTZKE, K. J., LEE, Y.-C. A., ZHANG, Z.-F., ZEVALLOS, J. P., YU, G.-P., WINN, D. M., VAUGHAN, T. L., STURGIS, E. M., SMITH, E., & SCHWARTZ, S. M. 2018. Racial differences in the relationship between tobacco, alcohol, and the risk of head and neck cancer: Pooled analysis of US studies in the INHANCE Consortium. *Cancer Causes Control*, 29, 619–30.

VON MEYENFELDT, M. 2005. Cancer-associated malnutrition: An introduction. *Eur J Oncol Nurs*, 9 Suppl 2, S35–8.

WANG, J. B., JIANG, Y., LIANG, H., LI, P., XIAO, H. J., JI, J., XIANG, W., SHI, J. F., FAN, Y. G., & LI, L. 2012. Attributable causes of cancer in China. *Ann Oncol*, 23, 2983–9.

WANG, Y., YANG, H., DUAN, G., & WANG, H. 2016. The association of the CYP1A1 Ile462Val polymorphism with head and neck cancer risk: Evidence based on a cumulative meta-analysis. *Onco Targets Ther*, 9, 2927–34.

WORLD HEALTH ORGANIZATION (WHO). 2016. Promoting oral health in Africa: Prevention and control of oral diseases and noma as part of essential noncommunicable disease interventions. Global: World Health Organization. https://www.who.int/publications/i/item/promoting-oral-health-in-africa-prevention-and-control-of-oral-diseases-and-noma-as-part-of-essential-noncommunicable-disease-interventions

WORLD HEALTH ORGANIZATION (WHO). 2023. *Global Oral Health Status Report: Towards Universal Health Coverage for Oral Health by 2030. Regional Summary of the African Region*. Geneva: World Health Organization.

WROBLEWSKI, L. E., PEEK, R. M., JR., & WILSON, K. T. 2010. Helicobacter pylori and gastric cancer: Factors that modulate disease risk. *Clin Microbiol Rev*, 23, 713–39.

WYSS, A., HASHIBE, M., CHUANG, S.-C., LEE, Y.-C. A., ZHANG, Z.-F., YU, G.-P., WINN, D. M., WEI, Q., TALAMINI, R., & SZESZENIA-DABROWSKA, N. 2013a. Cigarette, cigar, and pipe smoking and the risk of head and neck cancers: Pooled analysis in the International Head and Neck Cancer Epidemiology Consortium. *Am J Epidemiol*, 178, 679–90.

WYSS, A. B., HERRING, A. H., AVERY, C. L., WEISSLER, M. C., BENSEN, J. T., BARNHOLTZ-SLOAN, J. S., FUNKHOUSER, W. K., & OLSHAN, A. F. 2013b. Single-nucleotide polymorphisms in nucleotide excision repair genes, cigarette smoking, and the risk of head and neck cancer. *Cancer Epidemiol Biomarkers Prevent*, 22, 1428–45.

YU, C.-C., LO, W.-L., CHEN, Y.-W., HUANG, P.-I., HSU, H.-S., TSENG, L.-M., HUNG, S.-C., KAO, S.-Y., CHANG, C.-J., & CHIOU, S. H. 2011. Bmi-1 regulates snail expression and promotes metastasis ability in head and neck squamous cancer-derived ALDH1 positive cells. *J Oncol*, 2011, 609259. doi:10.1155/2011/609259. Epub 2010 Sep 27. PMID: 20936121; PMCID: PMC2948925.

ZANDBERG, D. P., LIU, S., GOLOUBEVA, O., ORD, R., STROME, S. E., SUNTHARALINGAM, M., TAYLOR, R., MORALES, R. E., WOLF, J. S., & ZIMRIN, A. 2016. Oropharyngeal cancer as a driver of racial outcome disparities in squamous cell carcinoma of the head and neck: 10-year experience at the University of Maryland Greenebaum Cancer Center. *Head Neck*, 38, 564–72.

ZANONI, D. K., PATEL, S. G., & SHAH, J. P. 2019. Changes in the 8th edition of the American Joint Committee on Cancer (AJCC) staging of head and neck cancer: Rationale and implications. *Curr Oncol Rep*, 21, 52.

ZHANG, S., WANG, B., MA, F., TONG, F., YAN, B., LIU, T., XIE, H., SONG, L., YU, S., & WEI, L. 2021. Characteristics of B lymphocyte infiltration in HPV+ head and neck squamous cell carcinoma. *Cancer Sci*, 112, 1402–16.

ZHANG, Y., WANG, X., LI, H., NI, C., DU, Z., & YAN, F. 2018. Human oral microbiota and its modulation for oral health. *Biomed Pharmacother*, 99, 883–93.

3

Inequalities in Head and Neck Cancer

Meshack Bida, Benny Mosoane, Masibulele Nonxuba, Dineo Disenyane, Stuart C. Winter, and Zodwa Dlamini

3.1 Introduction

According to the National Cancer Institute, the term "cancer disparities" refers to the measured differences in cancer incidences, prevalence, financial implication, and rates in screening, survival, morbidity and mortality (National Cancer Institute, 2024). Over the years, the empirical data expanded robustly, and the American Society of Clinical Oncology broadened the conceptualization of cancer health disparities to encompass parameters such as age, race and ethnicity, sexual orientation and gender identity, level of education, socioeconomic status, access to health insurance and the type of health insurance, and geographical and environmental exposures (Patel et al., 2020). In South Africa, however, cancer-related data are markedly underreported due to the equity gap between the private and the public healthcare sectors. The National Cancer Register, being pathology-based, faces challenges in capturing every cancer-related case since not all cases are diagnosed through pathology, thus preventing an accurate depiction of cancer incidences and mortality rates. To mitigate this limitation, the South African government, in collaboration with the private healthcare sector, has initiated a novel approach by introducing a patient-led cancer registry (Das, 2024). This initiative aims to strengthen the standards and comprehensiveness of cancer data in South Africa.

Head and neck cancer (HNC) is the seventh most commonly diagnosed cancer globally, with approximately 660,000 new cases and 325,000 deaths per year (Gormley et al., 2022). Despite being underreported in Africa due to the lack of cancer registries as a result of political issues and governmental policies, HNC continues to impose a significant burden (Adeola et al., 2018). Nearly 90% of HNC-related cases are attributed to squamous cell carcinoma (SCC), a subset of cancers that originate from the lining of the squamous epithelium of the oral cavity, pharynx, and larynx. As illustrated in Figure 3.1, these malignancies often develop from chronic exposure to irritants such as tobacco-derived carcinogens and excessive alcohol consumption, as well as infection with oncogenic strains of human papillomavirus (HPV) (Barsouk et al., 2023; Gormley et al., 2022).

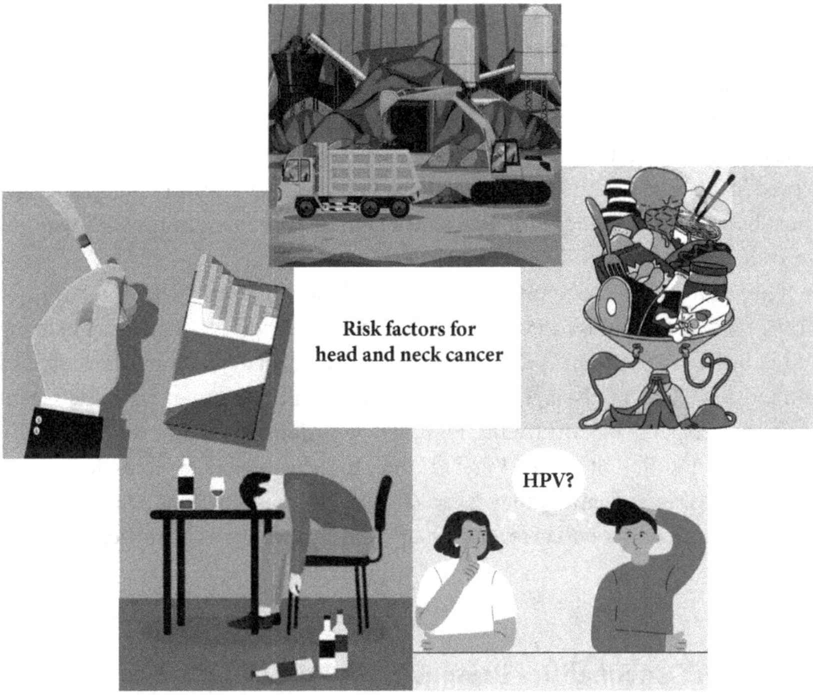

Figure 3.1 Risk factors for head and neck cancer (HNC). Chronic exposure to irritants such as tobacco-derived carcinogens, excessive alcohol consumption, and infection with oncogenic strains of human papillomavirus (HPV).

Further, known risk factors are occupation-related toxic agents (Bayer et al., 2016). Recent findings have indicated that smoking among African Americans is a significant risk factor for HNC, further compounded by experiences of discrimination and socioeconomic disparities (Mazul et al., 2023; Patangia, 2023). The association of HNC with prior exposure to tobacco and alcohol, as well as HPV infection, mirrors findings in high-income countries (Sharif & Ooi, 2024; Stransky et al., 2011). The emergence of exposomics represents a paradigm shift in cancer research, emphasizing a holistic approach that accounts for the cumulative effects of diverse exposures encountered over an individual's lifespan (Münzel et al., 2023).

It is clear that the etiology of HNC is varied; however, the role of HPV is well-studied in oropharyngeal carcinoma. A focus on the rapid rise in HPV-associated oropharyngeal cancer may, however, shift attention from the role of other factors, particularly in other structures of HNC and in underrepresented populations. While HNC subtypes involving the hypopharynx and nasopharynx are not well-studied, there seems to be an increase in oral cavity and oropharyngeal cancers and a decrease in cancers of the hypopharynx (Mazul et al., 2023). Similarly, there has been a reported rise in oral tongue-related cancer incidences among White women (Tota et al., 2017). With differing rates of smoking, sexual behavior, and HPV vaccination among different races and sexes, the rates and burden of HNC are expected to be inconsistent. To generate a practical public health intervention, population-specific trends and incidences must be well understood. A review of the demographic subgroups will help unveil relevant cancer trends and disparities.

This chapter critically investigates the inequalities present in the realm of HNC. Through a focused examination, it sheds light on the disparities existing in the burden of the disease, access to care, and ultimate outcomes for affected individuals. The analysis encompasses both within-country and between-country perspectives, unraveling complex variations in healthcare access and outcomes on different scales. Furthermore, the chapter offers strategic insights into addressing and mitigating these disparities, presenting potential avenues for interventions to enhance equity in HNC prevention, management, and outcomes.

3.2 Inequalities Present in the Realm of Head and Neck Cancer Healthcare

Inequities in HNC healthcare underscore a profound global challenge, particularly pronounced in developing nations. This issue is multifaceted, encompassing a substantial disease burden, delayed diagnoses, and limited access to both life-saving treatments and supportive care (Figure 3.2). Notably, the gap between how HNCs are addressed in developed versus developing nations continues to widen, fueled by disparities in technology, finances, and infrastructure. Addressing these inequalities demands a concerted international effort given the predominant nature of HNC in developing nations. To catalyze meaningful change on a global scale, concerted action is imperative, especially in regions such as sub-Saharan Africa, where HNC care faces formidable barriers. Initiatives aimed at enhancing access to HNC care in these areas offer valuable insights with broader applicability because the challenges confronted by African patients and healthcare providers resonate with those encountered in other developing nations' contexts. Consequently, these interventions hold promise as models for advancing equitable HNC healthcare worldwide.

In the realm of healthcare, equitable distribution of cancer treatment has long been a challenge, particularly concerning socioeconomic status. This issue, recognized since antiquity, has become more pronounced over time. Auvinen et al. highlighted the substantial influence of socioeconomic status

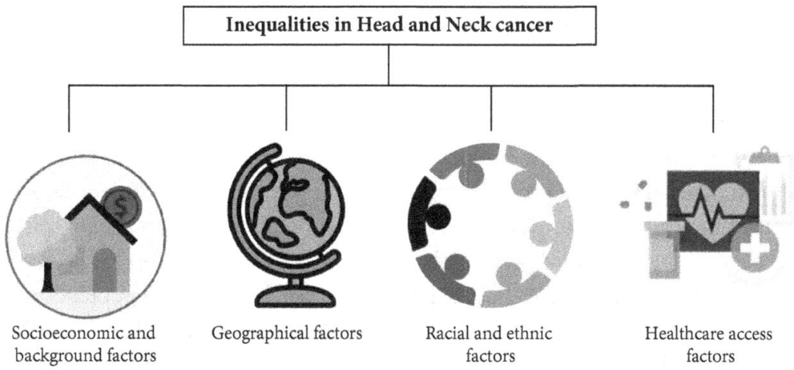

Figure 3.2 Factors that contribute to head and neck cancer (HNC). The socioeconomic background, geographic factors, race, ethnicity and health access contribute to inequalities in HNC.

on cancer survival, a theme echoed by Woods et al. in their exhaustive review that emphasized the roles of comorbidity, stage of diagnosis, and access to healthcare services in shaping socioeconomic disparities within the domain of HNC (Auvinen & Karjalainen, 1997; Woods et al., 2006). Despite the widespread acknowledgment of these determinants, they persist as complex phenomena requiring further elucidation. Numerous research endeavors have affirmed that individuals from privileged socioeconomic backgrounds enjoy higher rates of cancer survival compared to their less-advantaged counterparts (Johnson et al., 2008; Molina et al., 2008; Pagedar et al., 2019). These disparities encompass various dimensions, including income (Noel et al., 2023), occupation (Conway et al., 2021), and educational attainment (Oruç & Kaplan, 2019).

Paul Farmer introduced the concept of *structural violence* in 2004, highlighting social arrangements that expose individuals and populations to harm (Farmer, 2004). To mitigate the structural violence inherent in HNC, the International Agency for Research on Cancer has amassed empirical evidence from epidemiological studies aiming to address socioeconomic disparities in cancer mortality and morbidity. This endeavor underscores the significance of political will and targeted interventions to alleviate inequalities on a global scale (Mihor et al., 2020). Miller and Evers (2022) elucidated five primary factors contributing to nonadherence among the HNC population, including socioeconomic, condition-related, therapy-related, healthcare team- and system-related, and patient-related determinants (Miller & Evers, 2022). Previous research has also emphasized the impact of delayed HNC diagnosis and limited awareness of socioeconomic differences, with higher socioeconomic status correlating with early HNC presentation (Elwood & Gallagher, 1985; Llewellyn et al., 2004; Woolgar et al., 1999).

Geographic factors further compound disparities in HNC outcomes. Despite advancements in detection technologies and skilled healthcare providers, a significant segment of the population remains unable to access or benefit equitably from these resources, with geographical disparities playing a prominent role. Developing countries bear a disproportionate burden of HNC, with the Indian subcontinent alone accounting for a third of the global incidence (Gupta et al., 2016; Mishra & Meherotra, 2014). Research indicates that approximately 67% of the population in low- to middle-income countries are affected by HNC, contributing to at least 82% of HNC-related deaths (Patterson et al., 2020). Racial and ethnic factors further intersect with socioeconomic and geographic disparities shaping HNC prognosis and outcomes. Despite similar incidence rates between racial groups, survival rates vary significantly, with racial and ethnic minorities facing barriers to healthcare access and experiencing later-stage diagnoses (Bergmark & Sedaghat, 2017; Taylor et al., 2022). In the United States, African American HNC patients exhibit higher incidence and mortality rates, thus highlighting racial disparities in healthcare access and outcomes (Siegel et al., 2020; Yu et al., 2019).

Access to specialized care remains a critical determinant of HNC outcomes, with early detection pivotal for curative interventions. However, barriers such as travel distance, limited healthcare facilities, and shortages of healthcare professionals impede timely access to screening and treatment, particularly in developing countries (Entezami et al., 2021). Financial barriers further exacerbate disparities, with high treatment costs driving patients to bankruptcy and impeding access to care (Corry et al., 2022). Financial toxicity, encompassing both objective financial burdens and emotional distress, disproportionately affects HNC patients and their caregivers, necessitating comprehensive support mechanisms to alleviate the burden (Figure 3.3) The Comprehensive Score for Financial Toxicity (COST) was developed to evaluate this burden (Nguyen et al., 2023).

Financially, the cost of HNC treatment, including surgery, radiation therapy, chemotherapy, and supportive care, can be exorbitant, potentially leading to financial hardship and socioeconomic disparities among affected individuals. Patients from lower socioeconomic classes are faced with major financial challenges regarding the management of their HNC (Joshi et al., 2014). Scarce infrastructure, shortage of healthcare professionals, general illiteracy, and sociocultural beliefs that lead to delays in seeking healthcare services add to the challenge of cancer patients of lower socioeconomic status (Chikanda, 2005). These patients tend to present with advanced diseases.

Migration of professional healthcare workers in African countries such as Zimbabwe and South Africa have impacted healthcare services (Chikanda,

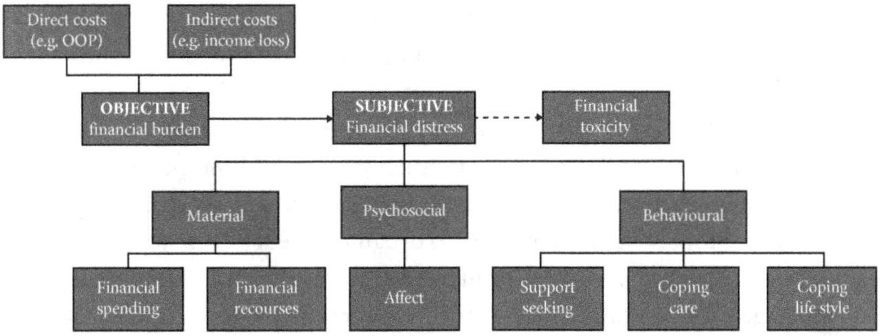

Figure 3.3 The framework of financial toxicity in head and neck cancer (HNC) care. Out-of-pocket costs and income losses are the main contributors to financial toxicity.

2005; Chintamani et al., 2011; Cooper & Aiken, 2006; Labonté et al., 2015). Developed countries like the United States that have not created sufficient educational capacity for their own needs depend on the immigration of foreign health professionals from poor countries (Polsky et al., 2007). The emigration of healthcare professionals poses a major challenge for dealing with the increase in HNC in developing regions (Adeola et al., 2018; Edwards et al., 2021; Joshi et al., 2014; Owusu et al., 2017).

Collectively, socioeconomic, geographic, racial, and ethnic factors intersect to perpetuate disparities in HNC outcomes, underscoring the need for multidimensional interventions to ensure equitable access to quality care for all populations affected by this disease. Addressing these complex determinants requires concerted efforts across healthcare systems, policy frameworks, and societal structures to achieve meaningful progress in reducing HNC-related inequities.

3.3 The Existing Burden of Disease and Ultimate Outcomes on Affected Individuals on Different Scales

The existing burden of HNC manifests across various scales, profoundly impacting affected individuals and the broader healthcare system. At the individual level, HNC inflicts substantial physical, emotional, and financial burdens on patients (Humphris & Ozakinci, 2006; Patterson et al., 2020). Physically, patients with HNC often endure debilitating symptoms such as difficulty swallowing, pain, speech impairment, and disfigurement, leading to a diminished quality of life (QoL).

Emotionally, the psychological toll of coping with a life-threatening illness, undergoing intensive treatments, and facing uncertainties about the future can be overwhelming for patients and their families (Humphris & Ozakinci, 2006; Tang et al., 2023). Major depressive disorder is a frequent mental disorder in patients with HNC and may lead to suicide (Hammermüller et al., 2021; Osazuwa-Peters et al., 2021). Higher rates of suicide are reported in patients who reside in rural areas as compared to urban dwellers (Osazuwa-Peters et al., 2021). A lack of adequate access to high-quality cancer care and mental health care and a disparate mental health care infrastructure in rural areas are regarded as factors that contribute to higher rates of suicide (Cyr et al., 2019; Morales et al., 2020).

Patil et al. (2018) regard distress as the sixth vital sign in cancer patients (Patil et al., 2018). In patients who are undergoing HNC care, distress must be monitored because patients with high distress are noncompliant with treatment and follow-up. A high level of distress has been associated with poor QoL (Thomas et al., 2009). It is therefore expected of healthcare workers to manage distress and provide counseling about disease status and its prognosis, the risks and benefits of the treatment options available, and the cost of management.

On a broader scale, the burden of HNC extends to healthcare systems, societies, and economies (Patterson et al., 2020). Healthcare systems must allocate significant resources for the diagnosis, treatment, supportive care, and development of infrastructure to address the HNC burden. Moreover, HNC contributes to productivity losses because of premature morbidity, disability, and mortality among affected individuals, leading to economic repercussions at both individual and societal levels (Patterson et al., 2020). Additionally, HNC disparities, including variations in incidence, access to care, and treatment outcomes among different demographic groups, exacerbate healthcare inequalities and social injustices.

In summary, the burden of HNC is multifaceted, impacting individuals, healthcare systems, and societies at large. Addressing this burden requires a comprehensive approach that encompasses prevention, early detection, equitable access to high-quality care, psychosocial support, and research efforts aimed at improving treatment outcomes and reducing the overall burden of the disease.

3.4 Strategic Insights into Addressing and Mitigating Head and Neck Cancer Disparities

Several prevention strategies exist, including public health initiatives aimed at raising the awareness of risk factors through community-based education campaigns to promote healthy lifestyles (Taneja, 2013). One such preventative strategy involves increasing community awareness of high-risk behaviors such as tobacco smoking and alcohol consumption through educational campaigns (Iftikhar et al., 2022). In Nigeria, an intervention program termed the Campaign for HNC Education (CHANCE) was founded in 2016 by a group of dental practitioners to promote the primary prevention of HNC. This initiative has led to the development of numerous research projects and has raised public health education programs on HNC (Kanmodi et al., 2020).

Healthcare practitioners should advocate and provide counseling for smoking cessation utilizing pharmacotherapy such as nicotine receptor agonists like varenicline and/or supportive antidepressants like bupropion. Ongoing research is currently exploring other pharmacologic agents for the treatment of smoking addiction such as GLP-1 agonists like naltrexone and semaglutide (Jordan & Xi, 2018). Other available alternative public health initiatives include promoting good oral hygiene practices and healthy diets enriched with fruits and vegetables (Taneja, 2013). Health-promoting initiatives promote quality outcomes in confirmed HNC patients who are about to undergo treatment and rehabilitation (Figure 3.4) (Bossi & Stucchi, 2023). Incorporating these initiatives and creating an assessment checklist in national guidelines for the diagnosis and treatment of HNC is recommended.

For inadequately resourced communities, expanding oral health screening and promoting HPV vaccination are recommended. HPV vaccination, approved in 2006, is routinely administered in two doses starting at ages 11–12 (adolescent females). The US Centers for Disease Control has shown that HPV vaccination promises a reduction in the prevalence rate of the high-risk oral HPV serotypes (Centers for Disease Control and Prevention [CDC], 2024). While it is still early to ascertain the full impact of vaccination programs on the incidence of SCC of the head and neck, evidence suggests that vaccination significantly reduced the prevalence of oral HPV serotypes 6, 11, 16, and 18 (the latter two being high-risk

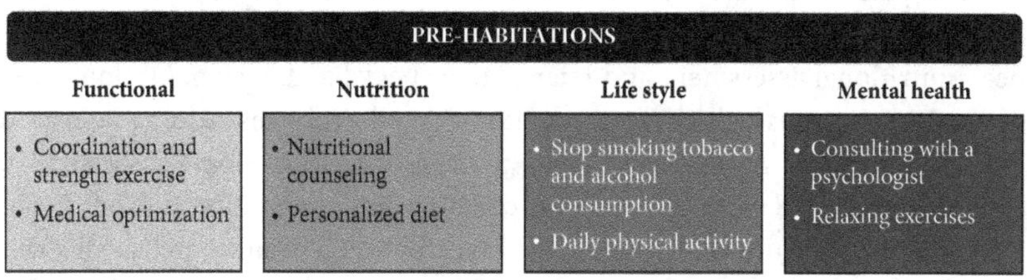

Figure 3.4 Pre-habilitation initiatives in head and neck cancer (HNC) patients. Pre-habilitation exercises that address anticipated function loss are supplemented with increased physical activity, consultations with nutrition specialists, and referrals to mental healthcare professionals.

variants) by 88.2%. Although the impact is not going to be seen for some time except in the young, this conclusion is drawn from findings reported in at least one cross-sectional study conducted in the United States (Markowitz et al., 2016a; Zhang et al., 2021).

Routine HPV screening for uterine cervix cancer is conducted through regular Pap smears, a test that samples cells from the transformation zone of the cervix to be microscopically examined for dysplastic changes. Additionally, this HPV screening test can be supplemented by molecular polymerase chain reaction (PCR) testing. Practicing safe sex and HPV vaccination can reduce transmission rates of HPV-related head and neck SCC (HNSCC; Markowitz et al., 2016b). Oral screening for HPV infection is currently not recommended as part of routine practice (Gan et al., 2013).

Secondary prevention is integral for practicing dentists, and including oral health examinations as part of general wellness checkups is recommended by the American Cancer Society. These examinations aim to detect premalignant conditions such as oral leukoplakia, which carries an estimated 12% lifetime risk of oral cavity carcinoma. Certain patient demographics are at increased hereditary genetic risk for SCC of the head and neck. These hereditary cancer syndromes include Li-Fraumeni syndrome, Plummer-Vinson, Bloom syndrome, xeroderma pigmentosum, Lynch-II syndrome, and Fanconi anemia (Báez, 2008). Immunosuppression is also associated with a higher risk of SCC of the head and neck (Nokovitch et al., 2023).

Chemoprevention strategies in HNC entail the utilization of natural products, synthetic chemical agents, or biological agents to prevent the progression of carcinogenesis (Wirth, 2014). Successful chemoprevention strategies have been implemented in high-risk populations, where primary chemoprevention was directed at individuals with premalignant lesions (erythroplakia and mucosal keratosis with atypia), and the secondary chemoprevention targeted individuals with HNC who have undergone potentially curative therapy to prevent disease recurrence or metachronous primary diseases (Figure 3.5) (Foy et al., 2013).

HNC patients often suffer nutritional deficiencies due to the location of the cancer, disease processes, and treatment (Talwar et al., 2016). These patients need nutritional assessment and referral to a specialist dietician. Optimization of nutritional status will prevent nutrition-related problems such as increased risk of infection, muscle weakness, poor QoL, depression, postoperative complications, and poor response to chemoradiotherapy (Donaldson, 2004; Gourin et al., 2014). Supportive nutritional care should be promoted at all levels of HNC management and be tailored to meet the patient's needs. As the global community embarks on the Close the Care Gap campaign (Day, 2024), the nutritional gap must receive equal attention. There is evidence that dietary strategies are important in both the prevention and treatment of HNC (Alshadwi et al.,

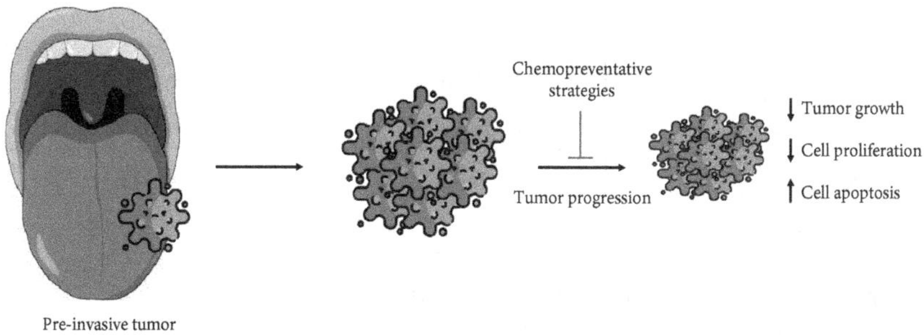

Figure 3.5 Chemopreventive strategies of head and neck cancer (HNC). Chemoprevention entails innovative strategies aimed at stopping or reversing the neoplastic process before the invasive stage. These strategies have demonstrated promising mitigation in oral squamous cell carcinoma.

2013; Haskins et al., 2020; Martinovic et al., 2023; Talwar et al., 2016; Zhang et al., 2019).

Physical exercise in patients with HNC is a supportive therapy that improves physical and psychological status and accelerates recovery (Figure 3.6) (Avancini et al., 2023). Physical exercise improves cardiorespiratory fitness, reduces post-operative complications, limits postoperative functional impairments, and shortens hospital stay (Lønbro et al., 2013; Rogers et al., 2008; Samuel et al., 2013). HNC patients receiving chemoradiotherapy and put on supervised physical exercise have demonstrated an improvement in functional capacity and QoL (Samuel et al., 2013). It is essential to explore the supportive role of physical exercise in HNC patients to improve patient outcomes.

3.5 Limitations

There is a measurable inequality in cancer healthcare between regional populations regarding the control of cancer, access to treatment, and cancer survival. These measured differences in cancer incidence, prevalence, screening and survival rates, and morbidity and mortality rates impact negatively on individuals, societies, and healthcare systems. Healthcare disparities affect individuals of different age groups, races and ethnic groups, sexual orientation and gender identity, level of education, and socioeconomic status. Parameters such as race and ethnicity may, however, be based on self-reports and clouded by societal constructs that complicate classifications.

A robust amount of data links oropharyngeal cancer to high-risk HPV infection. Safe sex and HPV vaccination can reduce transmission rates of HPV-related

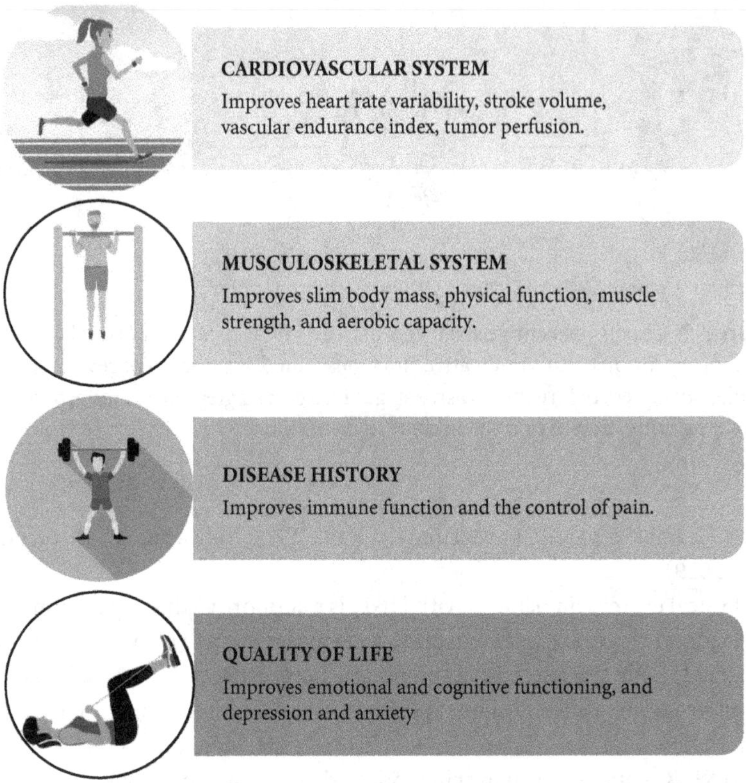

Figure 3.6 Supportive role of physical exercise in head and neck cancer (HNC) patients. Exercise improves the cardiovascular, musculoskeletal, and immune systems, and enhances overall quality of life.

cancers. The full impact of HPV vaccination programs is projected to significantly reduce the prevalence of oral HPV by 88.2%; however, the virus is known to have an extended latency period. HPV vaccine is presumed to possibly reduce the incidence of HPV-associated HNC (El Hussein & Dhaliwal, 2023; Macilwraith et al., 2023; Nassif et al., 2022; Ndon et al., 2023), although a paucity of studies provide direct evidence of this presumption.

3.6 Conclusion

In the African continent, the HNCs are predominantly driven by factors such as tobacco smoking, Western lifestyle and diet, HIV infection, HPV infection, and hostile fiscal policies. Discrimination and socioeconomic disparities have been linked to HNC in African American individuals. HNC health disparities encompass parameters such as age, race and ethnicity, level of education, socioeconomic status, access to healthcare, and geographical and environmental exposures. The shortage of healthcare professionals in developing countries drives the burden of HNC, leading to delayed diagnoses and limited access to both life-saving treatments and supportive care.

The burden of HNC is multifaceted and impacts individuals, healthcare systems, and societies at large. A comprehensive approach that encompasses prevention, early detection, equitable access to high-quality care, psychosocial support, and research efforts aimed at improving treatment outcomes and reducing the overall burden of HNC is required. The adoption of an assessment and management checklist in the national guidelines for HNC is recommended for equity of care across nations.

References

ADEOLA, H., AFROGHEH, A., & HILLE, J. 2018. The burden of head and neck cancer in Africa: The status quo and research prospects. *S Afr Dental J*, 73, 477–88.

ALSHADWI, A., NADERSHAH, M., CARLSON, E. R., YOUNG, L. S., BURKE, P. A., & DALEY, B. J. 2013. Nutritional considerations for head and neck cancer patients: A review of the literature. *J Oral Maxillofac Surg*, 71, 1853–60.

AUVINEN, A., & KARJALAINEN, S. 1997. Possible explanations for social class differences in cancer patient survival. *IARC Sci Publ*, 377–97.

AVANCINI, A., BORSATI, A., BELLUOMINI, L., GIANNARELLI, D., NOCINI, R., INSOLDA, J., SPOSITO, M., SCHENA, F., MILELLA, M., & PILOTTO, S. 2023. Effect of exercise across the head and neck cancer continuum: A systematic review of randomized controlled trials. *Support Care Cancer*, 31, 670.

BÁEZ, A. 2008. Genetic and environmental factors in head and neck cancer genesis. *J Environ Sci Health C Environ Carcinog Ecotoxicol Rev*, 26, 174–200.

BARSOUK, A., ALURU, J. S., RAWLA, P., SAGINALA, K., & BARSOUK, A. 2023. Epidemiology, risk factors, and prevention of head and neck squamous cell carcinoma. *Med Sci (Basel)*, 11(2), 42.

BAYER, O., CÁMARA, R., ZEISSIG, S. R., RESSING, M., DIETZ, A., LOCATI, L. D., RAMROTH, H., & SINGER, S. 2016. Occupation and cancer of the larynx: A systematic review and meta-analysis. *Eur Arch Otorhinolaryngol*, 273, 9–20.

BERGMARK, R. W., & SEDAGHAT, A. R. 2017. Disparities in health in the United States: An overview of the social determinants of health for otolaryngologists. *Laryngoscope Investig Otolaryngol*, 2, 187–93.

BOSSI, P., & STUCCHI, E. 2023. Exercise and nutrition interventions in head and neck cancer. *In:* VERMORKEN, J. B., BUDACH, V., LEEMANS, C. R., MACHIELS, J.-P., NICOLAI, P., & O'SULLIVAN, B., eds. *Critical Issues in Head and Neck Oncology*. Cham: Springer International, 347–54.

CENTERS FOR DISEASE CONTROL AND PREVENTION (CDC). 2024. HPV vaccination recommendations [Online]. Available at: https://www.cdc.gov/vaccines/vpd/hpv/hcp/recommendations.html#:~:text=HPV%20vaccine%20is%20recommended%20for,not%20adequately%20vaccinated%20when%20younger. [Accessed April 23, 2024.]

CHIKANDA, A. 2005. Nurse migration from Zimbabwe: Analysis of recent trends and impacts. *Nurs Inq*, 12, 162–74.

CHINTAMANI, TUTEJA, A., KHANDELWAL, R., TANDON, M., BAMAL, R., JAIN, S., NARAYAN, N., SRINIVAS, S., & KUMAR, Y. 2011. Patient and provider delays in breast cancer patients attending a tertiary care centre: A prospective study. *JRSM Short Rep*, 2, 76.

CONWAY, D. I., HOVANEC, J., AHRENS, W., ROSS, A., HOLCATOVA, I., LAGIOU, P., SERRAINO, D., CANOVA, C., RICHIARDI, L., HEALY, C., KJAERHEIM, K., MACFARLANE, G. J., THOMSON, P., AGUDO, A., ZNAOR, A., BRENNAN, P., LUCE, D., MENVIELLE, G., STUCKER, I., BENHAMOU, S., RAMROTH, H., BOFFETTA, P., VILENSKY, M., FERNANDEZ, L., CURADO, M. P., MENEZES, A., DAUDT, A., KOIFMAN, R., WUNSCH-FILHO, V., YUAN-CHIN, A. L., HASHIBE, M., BEHRENS, T., & MCMAHON, A. D. 2021. Occupational socioeconomic risk associations for head and neck cancer in Europe and South America: Individual participant data analysis of pooled case-control studies within the INHANCE Consortium. *J Epidemiol Community Health*, 75, 779–87.

COOPER, R. A., & AIKEN, L. H. 2006. Health services delivery: Reframing policies for global migration of nurses and physicians: A U.S. perspective. *Policy Polit Nurs Pract*, 7, 66s–70s.

CORRY, J., NG, W. T., MA, S. J., SINGH, A. K., DE GRAEFF, P., & OOSTING, S. F. 2022. Disadvantaged subgroups within the global head and neck cancer population: How can we optimize care? *Am Soc Clin Oncol Educ Book*, 42, 1–10.

CYR, M. E., ETCHIN, A. G., GUTHRIE, B. J., & BENNEYAN, J. C. 2019. Access to specialty healthcare in urban versus rural US populations: A systematic literature review. *BMC Health Serv Res*, 19, 974.

DAS, M. 2024. South Africa combats gaps in cancer data. *Lancet Oncol*, 25, 420.

DONALDSON, M. S. 2004. Nutrition and cancer: A review of the evidence for an anti-cancer diet. *Nutrit J*, 3, 19.

EDWARDS, R. L., PATRICIAN, P. A., BAKITAS, M., & MARKAKI, A. 2021. Palliative care integration: A critical review of nurse migration effect in Jamaica. *BMC Palliat Care*, 20, 155.

EL HUSSEIN, M. T., & DHALIWAL, S. 2023. HPV vaccination for prevention of head and neck cancer among men. *Nurse Practitioner*, 48(10), 25–32.

ELWOOD, J. M., & GALLAGHER, R. P. 1985. Factors influencing early diagnosis of cancer of the oral cavity. *Cmaj*, 133, 651–6.

ENTEZAMI, P., THOMAS, B., MANSOUR, J., ASARKAR, A., NATHAN, C. A., & PANG, J. 2021. Targets for improving disparate head and neck cancer outcomes in the low-income population. *Laryngoscope Investig Otolaryngol*, 6, 1481–8.

FARMER, P. 2004. An anthropology of structural violence. *Curr Anthropol*, 45, 305–25.

FOY, J. P., BERTOLUS, C., WILLIAM, W. N., JR., & SAINTIGNY, P. 2013. Oral premalignancy: The roles of early detection and chemoprevention. *Otolaryngol Clin North Am*, 46, 579–97.

GAN, S. J., DAHLSTROM, K. R., PECK, B. W., CAYWOOD, W., LI, G., WEI, Q., ZAFEREO, M. E., & STURGIS, E. M. 2013. Incidence and pattern of second primary malignancies in patients with index oropharyngeal cancers versus index nonoropharyngeal head and neck cancers. *Cancer*, 119, 2593–601.

GORMLEY, M., CREANEY, G., SCHACHE, A., INGARFIELD, K., & CONWAY, D. I. 2022. Reviewing the epidemiology of head and neck cancer: Definitions, trends and risk factors. *Br Dent J*, 233, 780–6.

GOURIN, C. G., COUCH, M. E., & JOHNSON, J. T. 2014. Effect of weight loss on short-term outcomes and costs of care after head and neck cancer surgery. *Ann Otol Rhinol Laryngol*, 123, 101–10.

GUPTA, B., JOHNSON, N. W., & KUMAR, N. 2016. Global epidemiology of head and neck cancers: A continuing challenge. *Oncology*, 91, 13–23.

HAMMERMÜLLER, C., HINZ, A., DIETZ, A., WICHMANN, G., PIRLICH, M., BERGER, T., ZIMMERMANN, K., NEUMUTH, T., MEHNERT-THEUERKAUF, A., WIEGAND, S.,

& ZEBRALLA, V. 2021. Depression, anxiety, fatigue, and quality of life in a large sample of patients suffering from head and neck cancer in comparison with the general population. *BMC Cancer*, 21, 94.

HASKINS, C. P., CHAMP, C. E., MILLER, R., & VYFHUIS, M. A. L. 2020. Nutrition in cancer: Evidence and equality. *Adv Radiat Oncol*, 5, 817–23.

HUMPHRIS, G. M., & OZAKINCI, G. 2006. Psychological responses and support needs of patients following head and neck cancer. *Int J Surg*, 4, 37–44.

IFTIKHAR, A., ISLAM, M., SHEPHERD, S., JONES, S., & ELLIS, I. 2022. What is behind the lifestyle risk factors for head and neck cancer? *Front Psychol*, 13, 960638.

JOHNSON, S., MCDONALD, J. T., & CORSTEN, M. J. 2008. Socioeconomic factors in head and neck cancer. *J Otolaryngol Head Neck Surg*, 37, 597–601.

JORDAN, C. J., & XI, Z. X. 2018. Discovery and development of varenicline for smoking cessation. *Expert Opin Drug Discov*, 13, 671–83.

JOSHI, P., DUTTA, S., CHATURVEDI, P., & NAIR, S. 2014. Head and neck cancers in developing countries. *Rambam Maimonides Med J*, 5, e0009.

KANMODI, K. K., OSUNRO, K. S., NWAFOR, N., & KANMODI, P. 2020. Impact of head and neck cancer (HNC) education on HNC knowledge and attitudes toward HNC peer and non-peer education: A school-based pilot study. *Yen Med J*, 2, 47–55.

LABONTÉ, R., SANDERS, D., MATHOLE, T., CRUSH, J., CHIKANDA, A., DAMBISYA, Y., RUNNELS, V., PACKER, C., MACKENZIE, A., MURPHY, G. T., & BOURGEAULT, I. L. 2015. Health worker migration from South Africa: Causes, consequences and policy responses. *Human Resources Health*, 13, 92.

LLEWELLYN, C. D., JOHNSON, N. W., & WARNAKULASURIYA, S. 2004. Factors associated with delay in presentation among younger patients with oral cancer. *Oral Surg Oral Med Oral Pathol Oral Radiol Endod*, 97, 707–13.

LØNBRO, S., DALGAS, U., PRIMDAHL, H., JOHANSEN, J., NIELSEN, J. L., AAGAARD, P., HERMANN, A. P., OVERGAARD, J., & OVERGAARD, K. 2013. Progressive resistance training rebuilds lean body mass in head and neck cancer patients after radiotherapy: Results from the randomized DAHANCA 25B trial. *Radiother Oncol*, 108, 314–19.

MACILWRAITH, P., MALSEM, E., & DUSHYANTHEN, S. 2023. The effectiveness of HPV vaccination on the incidence of oropharyngeal cancers in men: A review. *Infect Agents and*, 18, 24.

MARKOWITZ, L. E., LIU, G., HARIRI, S., STEINAU, M., DUNNE, E. F., & UNGER, E. R. 2016a. Prevalence of HPV after introduction of the vaccination program in the United States. *Pediatrics*, 137, e20151968.

MARTINOVIC, D., TOKIC, D., PUIZINA MLADINIC, E., USLJEBRKA, M., KADIC, S., LESIN, A., VILOVIC, M., LUPI-FERANDIN, S., ERCEGOVIC, S., KUMRIC, M., BUKIC, J., & BOZIC, J. 2023. Nutritional management of patients with head and neck cancer: A comprehensive review. *Nutrients*, 15(8), 1864.

MAZUL, A. L., CHIDAMBARAM, S., ZEVALLOS, J. P., & MASSA, S. T. 2023. Disparities in head and neck cancer incidence and trends by race/ethnicity and sex. *Head Neck*, 45, 75–84.

MIHOR, A., TOMSIC, S., ZAGAR, T., LOKAR, K., & ZADNIK, V. 2020. Socioeconomic inequalities in cancer incidence in Europe: A comprehensive review of population-based epidemiological studies. *Radiol Oncol*, 54, 1–13.

MILLER, J. L., & EVERS, J. 2022. Barriers to adherence to cancer treatments among head and neck cancer patients. *J Adv Pract Oncol*, 13, 515–23.

MISHRA, A., & MEHEROTRA, R. 2014. Head and neck cancer: Global burden and regional trends in India. *Asian Pacific J Cancer Prevent*, 15, 537–50.

MOLINA, M. A., CHEUNG, M. C., PEREZ, E. A., BYRNE, M. M., FRANCESCHI, D., MOFFAT, F. L., LIVINGSTONE, A. S., GOODWIN, W. J., GUTIERREZ, J. C., & KONIARIS, L. G. 2008. African American and poor patients have a dramatically worse prognosis for head and neck cancer: An examination of 20,915 patients. *Cancer*, 113, 2797–806.

MORALES, D. A., BARKSDALE, C. L., & BECKEL-MITCHENER, A. C. 2020. A call to action to address rural mental health disparities. *J Clin Transl Sci*, 4, 463–7.

MÜNZEL, T., SØRENSEN, M., HAHAD, O., NIEUWENHUIJSEN, M., & DAIBER, A. 2023. The contribution of the exposome to the burden of cardiovascular disease. *Nat Rev Cardiol*, 20, 651–69.

NASSIF, S. J., STEINWALD, P., & TRACY, J. C. 2022. Human papillomavirus vaccine and head and neck cancer. *JAMA Otolaryngol Head Neck Surg*, 148, 204.

NATIONAL CANCER INSTITUTE. 2024. Cancer disparities. Available at: https://www.cancer.gov/about-cancer/understanding/disparities#:~:text=Cancer%20disparities%20(sometimes%20called%20cancer,mortality%20(deaths) [Accessed April 16, 2024.]

NDON, S., SINGH, A., HA, P. K., ASWANI, J., CHAN, J. Y., & XU, M. J. 2023. Human papillomavirus-associated oropharyngeal cancer: Global epidemiology and public policy implications. *Cancers (Basel)*, 15(16), 4080.

NGUYEN, O. T., DONATO, U., MCCORMICK, R., REBLIN, M., KIM, L., HUME, E., OTTO, A. K., ALISHAHI TABRIZ, A., ISLAM, J. Y., HONG, Y. R., TURNER, K., & PATEL, K. B. 2023. Financial toxicity among head and neck cancer patients and their caregivers: A cross-sectional pilot study. *Laryngoscope Investig Otolaryngol*, 8, 450–7.

NOEL, C. W., HUENIKEN, K., FORNER, D., LIU, G., ENG, L., HOSNI, A., HAHN, E., IRISH, J. C., GILBERT, R., YAO, C., MONTEIRO, E., O'SULLIVAN, B., WALDRON, J., HUANG, S. H., GOLDSTEIN, D. P., & DE ALMEIDA, J. R. 2023. Association of household income at diagnosis with financial toxicity, health utility, and survival in patients with head and neck cancer. *JAMA Otolaryngol Head Neck Surg*, 149, 63–70.

NOKOVITCH, L., MAQUET, C., CRAMPON, F., TAIHI, I., ROUSSEL, L. M., OBONGO, R., VIRARD, F., FERVERS, B., & DENEUVE, S. 2023. Oral cavity squamous cell carcinoma risk factors: State of the art. *J Clin Med*, 12(9), 3264.

ORUÇ, Z., & KAPLAN, M. A. 2019. Effect of exercise on colorectal cancer prevention and treatment. *World J Gastrointest Oncol*, 11, 348–66.

OSAZUWA-PETERS, N., BARNES, J. M., OKAFOR, S. I., TAYLOR, D. B., HUSSAINI, A. S., ADJEI BOAKYE, E., SIMPSON, M. C., GRABOYES, E. M., & LEE, W. T. 2021. Incidence and risk of suicide among patients with head and neck cancer in rural, urban, and metropolitan areas. *JAMA Otolaryngol Head Neck Surg*, 147, 1045–52.

OWUSU, Y., MEDAKKAR, P., AKINNAWO, E. M., STEWART-PYNE, A., & ASHU, E. E. 2017. Emigration of skilled healthcare workers from developing countries: Can team-based healthcare practice fill the gaps in maternal, newborn and child healthcare delivery? *Int J MCH AIDS*, 6, 121–9.

PAGEDAR, N. A., DAVIS, A. B., SPERRY, S. M., CHARLTON, M. E., & LYNCH, C. F. 2019. Population analysis of socioeconomic status and otolaryngologist distribution on head and neck cancer outcomes. *Head Neck*, 41, 1046–52.

PATANGIA, B. 2023. Biopsychosocial impact of discrimination on cancer risk and outcome: A conceptual review. *Psychosom Med Res*, 5, 18.

PATEL, M. I., LOPEZ, A. M., BLACKSTOCK, W., REEDER-HAYES, K., MOUSHEY, E. A., PHILLIPS, J., & TAP, W. 2020. Cancer disparities and health equity: A policy statement from the American Society of Clinical Oncology. *J Clin Oncol*, 38, 3439–48.

PATIL, V., NORONHA, V., JOSHI, A., DEODHAR, J., GOSWAMI, S., CHAKRABORTY, S., RAMASWAMY, A., DHUMAL, S., M. V., C., KARPE, A., PANDE, N., TALREJA, V., CHANDRASEKHARAN, A., TURKAR, S., & PRABHASH, K. 2018. Distress management in patients with head and neck cancer before start of palliative chemotherapy: A practical approach. *J Global Oncol*, 1–10.

PATTERSON, R. H., FISCHMAN, V. G., WASSERMAN, I., SIU, J., SHRIME, M. G., FAGAN, J. J., KOCH, W., & ALKIRE, B. C. 2020. Global burden of head and neck cancer: Economic consequences, health, and the role of surgery. *Otolaryngol Head Neck Surg*, 162, 296–303.

POLSKY, D., SOCHALSKI, J., AIKEN, L. H., & COOPER, R. A. 2007. Medical migration to the U.S.: Trends and impact. *LDI Issue Brief*, 12, 1–4.

ROGERS, L. Q., COURNEYA, K. S., ROBBINS, K. T., MALONE, J., SEIZ, A., KOCH, L., & RAO, K. 2008. Physical activity correlates and barriers in head and neck cancer patients. *Support Care Cancer*, 16, 19–27.

SAMUEL, S. R., MAIYA, G. A., BABU, A. S., & VIDYASAGAR, M. S. 2013. Effect of exercise training on functional capacity and quality of life in head and neck cancer patients receiving chemoradiotherapy. *Indian J Med Res*, 137, 515–20.

SHARIF, R., & OOI, T. C. 2024. Understanding exposomes and its relation with cancer risk in Malaysia based on epidemiological evidence: A narrative review. *Genes Environ*, 46, 5.

SIEGEL, R. L., MILLER, K. D., & JEMAL, A. 2020. Cancer statistics, 2020. *CA Cancer J Clin*, 70, 7–30.

STRANSKY, N., EGLOFF, A. M., TWARD, A. D., KOSTIC, A. D., CIBULSKIS, K., SIVACHENKO, A., KRYUKOV, G. V., LAWRENCE, M. S., SOUGNEZ, C., MCKENNA, A., SHEFLER, E., RAMOS, A. H., STOJANOV, P., CARTER, S. L., VOET, D., CORTÉS, M. L., AUCLAIR, D., BERGER, M. F., SAKSENA, G., GUIDUCCI, C., ONOFRIO, R. C., PARKIN, M., ROMKES, M., WEISSFELD, J. L., SEETHALA, R. R., WANG, L., RANGEL-ESCAREÑO, C., FERNANDEZ-LOPEZ, J. C., HIDALGO-MIRANDA, A., MELENDEZ-ZAJGLA, J., WINCKLER, W., ARDLIE, K., GABRIEL, S. B., MEYERSON, M., LANDER, E. S., GETZ, G., GOLUB, T. R., GARRAWAY, L. A., & GRANDIS, J. R. 2011. The mutational landscape of head and neck squamous cell carcinoma. *Science*, 333, 1157–60.

TALWAR, B., DONNELLY, R., SKELLY, R., & DONALDSON, M. 2016. Nutritional management in head and neck cancer: United Kingdom National Multidisciplinary Guidelines. *J Laryngol Otol*, 130, S32–40.

TANEJA, M. K. 2013. Life style management in head and neck cancer patients. *Indian J Otolaryngol Head Neck Surg*, 65, 289–92.

TANG, Y., HUA, Y., HUANG, X., CAO, Y., & SUN, X. 2023. Psychological burden of patients with head and neck cancer undergoing radiotherapy and their family caregivers: A cross-sectional survey. *J Multidisciplinary Healthc*, 16, 927–35.

TAYLOR, D. B., OSAZUWA-PETERS, O. L., OKAFOR, S. I., BOAKYE, E. A., KUZIEZ, D., PERERA, C., SIMPSON, M. C., BARNES, J. M., BULBUL, M. G., CANNON, T. Y., WATTS, T. L., MEGWALU, U. C., VARVARES, M. A., & OSAZUWA-PETERS, N. 2022. Differential outcomes among survivors of head and neck cancer belonging to racial and ethnic minority groups. *JAMA Otolaryngol Head Neck Surg*, 148, 119–27.

THOMAS, B. C., THOMAS, I., NANDAMOHAN, V., NAIR, M. K., & PANDEY, M. 2009. Screening for distress can predict loss of follow-up and treatment in cancer patients: Results of development and validation of the Distress Inventory for Cancer Version 2. *Psychooncology*, 18, 524–33.

TOTA, J. E., ANDERSON, W. F., COFFEY, C., CALIFANO, J., COZEN, W., FERRIS, R. L., ST JOHN, M., COHEN, E. E., & CHATURVEDI, A. K. 2017. Rising incidence of oral tongue cancer among white men and women in the United States, 1973–2012. *Oral Oncol*, 67, 146–52.

WIRTH, L. J. 2014. Chemoprevention of squamous cell carcinoma of the head and neck: No time to lose momentum. *Cancer Prevent Res*, 7, 279–82.

WOODS, L. M., RACHET, B., & COLEMAN, M. P. 2006. Origins of socio-economic inequalities in cancer survival: A review. *Ann Oncol*, 17, 5–19.

WOOLGAR, J. A., ROGERS, S., WEST, C. R., ERRINGTON, R. D., BROWN, J. S., & VAUGHAN, E. D. 1999. Survival and patterns of recurrence in 200 oral cancer patients treated by radical surgery and neck dissection. *Oral Oncol*, 35, 257–65.

WORLD CANCER DAY. 2024. Close the care gap. Available at: https://www.paho.org/en/campaigns/world-cancer-day-2024-close-care-gap [Accessed April 03, 2025.]

YU, A. J., CHOI, J. S., SWANSON, M. S., KOKOT, N. C., BROWN, T. N., YAN, G., & SINHA, U. K. 2019. Association of race/ethnicity, stage, and survival in oral cavity squamous cell carcinoma: A SEER study. *OTO Open*, 3, 2473974x19891126.

ZHANG, F. F., CUDHEA, F., SHAN, Z., MICHAUD, D. S., IMAMURA, F., EOM, H., RUAN, M., REHM, C. D., LIU, J., DU, M., KIM, D., LIZEWSKI, L., WILDE, P., & MOZAFFARIAN, D. 2019. Preventable cancer burden associated with poor diet in the United States. *JNCI Cancer Spectr*, 3, pkz034.

ZHANG, Y., FAKHRY, C., & D'SOUZA, G. 2021. Projected association of human papillomavirus vaccination with oropharynx cancer incidence in the US, 2020–2045. *JAMA Oncol*, 7, e212907.

SECTION II

TECHNOLOGICAL ADVANCES IN DIAGNOSIS AND TREATMENT

4
Diagnostic Innovations for Head and Neck Cancers

Benny Mosoane, Amanda Skepu, Chrysis Sofianos, Masibulele Nonxuba, Aristotelis Chatziioannou, and Zodwa Dlamini

4.1 Introduction

The spectrum of head and neck cancers (HNC) involves malignancies of the aerodigestive tract and salivary glands. Owing to their different etiologies and clinical behaviors, tumors of the skin, thyroid, and central nervous system are not included in the discussion of HNCs. HNCs account for 3% of malignancies and 5% of cancer-related deaths (Siegel et al., 2018). These tumors are common in males, with a male-to-female ratio of 4:1 (Bray et al., 2013). Smoking and excessive alcohol intake are regarded as the dominant risk factors for the development of HNC (Ansary-Moghaddam et al., 2009). Additional risk factors include dietary factors, metabolic factors, occupational chemicals, poor oral hygiene, Epstein-Barr virus (EBV) infection, human papillomavirus (HPV) infection, and gastroesophageal reflux disease (Zabala et al., 2022). The complicated anatomy of the head and neck region perplexes the diagnosis of HNCs. Often, these cancers are present in advanced clinical stages because they adopt a stealthy pattern of progression, not causing conspicuous symptoms during the onset of the disease. Synchronous or metachronous tumors of the aerodigestive tract may present in more than one site, requiring specific examinations to be performed by HNC specialists to make an initial diagnosis (Bradley & Bradley, 2010; Chow, 2020).

The best treatment outcomes in HNCs are obtained when the tumors are treated in early stages (Glen & Botha, 2022; Pfister et al., 2014). It is thus imperative that early detection systems are set up to prompt referral, thereby offering patients a greater chance of cure. HNC patients (87%) frequently present with at least one symptom at the time of early presentation (Shuman et al., 2010). The most common symptoms, in no particular order, include dysphonia, dysphagia, odynophagia, oral pain, cervical masses, and dental and/or gingival problems.

Diagnosis of these heterogeneous groups of cancers is based on a multidisciplinary strategy and best divided into qualitative and quantitative forms of diagnosis (Figure 4.1). Histopathology provides a qualitative diagnosis that guides disease management and provides essential data for disease prognosis. Tissue diagnosis provided by histopathology uses immunohistochemistry (IHC) and molecular testing techniques to enhance diagnostic precision via the identification of prognostic and precision markers. The imaging approach is a quantitative measure that locates the mass lesion and estimates tumor volume and extension of the tumor. Imaging techniques such as ultrasound, computed tomography (CT), magnetic resonance imaging (MRI), and positron emission tomography (PET) are essential for the quantitative assessment of HNCs. The role of deep machine-learning techniques and radiomics aims to transform the diagnostic landscape.

Establishing a precise diagnosis can guide the treatment plan. This chapter delves into the forefront of medical technology and explores the latest breakthroughs in diagnostic tools and techniques for HNC. From cutting-edge imaging technologies to molecular diagnostics, discussion centers on how these advancements are transforming early detection and leading to more accurate diagnoses and improved patient outcomes.

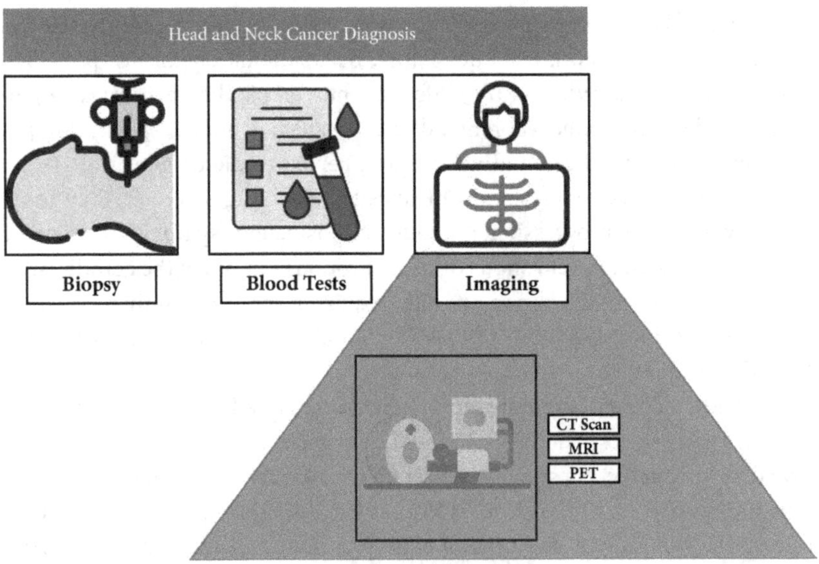

Figure 4.1 Diagnosis of head and neck cancer in clinical practice involves diagnostic imaging, blood tests, and biopsy.
CT, computed tomography scan; MRI, magnetic resonance imaging; PET, positron emission tomography.

4.2 Laboratory Diagnosis

Tissue diagnosis of HNC is crucial for an effective management plan. This essential diagnostic platform helps to exclude clinical mimickers of malignancy, such as tuberculosis and sarcoidosis. The pathologist can confirm a specific neoplasm based on cytological or tissue material, comment on prognostic factors, and assess treatment response. In addition to accurate diagnosis, the histopathology report comments on possible viral etiology, resection margin, depth of tumor invasion, lymphovascular invasion, and perineural invasion. The International Collaboration for Cancer Reporting (ICCR) provides standardized and evidence-based pathology datasets for the reporting of HNC to ascertain that all data relevant to the current state of art are contained within the report and that the presentation aligns with internationally accepted standards (International Collaboration for Cancer Reporting, 2024). Routine pathology reports should include comments on the depth of invasion, mitotic count, proliferative index in the form of Ki-67 IHC, HPV status, and programmed death ligand (PDL-1) (López et al., 2021). Initial morphological diagnosis is made on incisional biopsy and/or fine-needle aspiration cytology (FNAC). Ultrasound-guided FNAC is preferred when there is a clinical suspicion of lymph node pathology.

4.2.1 Immunohistochemistry

The role of IHC in HNC is reserved for unusual pathological neoplasms. The increased use of IHC staining in pathology workup has led to the development of digital imaging techniques that offer objective and quantifiable verification of staining. These standardized diagnostic procedures are part of laboratory quality assurance systems (Chlipala et al., 2020). Despite these innovations, the pathologist's discretion is important, particularly for very complex cases. In poorly differentiated squamous cell carcinoma (SCC) of the HNC, anti-epithelial membrane antigen (EMA), p40, p63, or pancytokeratins are used to confirm the diagnosis (Bishop et al., 2014; López et al., 2021). IHC staining plays a seminal role in the workup of poorly differentiated tumors, undifferentiated tumors, and tumors of unknown origin for accurate diagnosis and insightful therapeutic management. The recent addition of genetic markers in salivary gland and neuroendocrine cancers has refined diagnostic accuracy (López et al., 2017, 2018).

Salivary gland and neuroendocrine cancers can exhibit imprecise histomorphology, which necessitates IHC distinction. Current guidelines recommend p16 IHC for the assessment of oropharyngeal carcinoma to establish evidence of HPV. Overexpression of p16 IHC and high-risk HPV DNA in-situ hybridization are sufficient to establish HPV status (Hashmi et al., 2020). EBV early RNA in-situ hybridization (EBER-ISH) expression establishes transcriptional activity of EBV in nasopharyngeal carcinomas and other HNC (Turunen et al., 2017). PDL-1 testing using IHC is currently the standard of care in the workup of recurrent and/or metastatic SCC of the head and neck. Patients with a combined proportion score (CPS) of ≥1 are eligible for pembrolizumab treatment (Cohen et al., 2019).

IHC staining can be used to assess prognostic factors, such as the presence of TP53 gene mutations and a cell proliferation index using Ki-67. The expression of NANOG and SOX2 has been frequently observed in SCC, and, when expressed together, they suggest a higher survival rate. Loss of NANOG and SOX2 expression implies poor survival (Pedregal-Mallo et al., 2020). However, these stem cell markers have not yet been adopted in routine practice. The use of NANOG, focal adhesion kinase (FAK), and cortactin (CTTN) to stratify patients with precancerous laryngeal lesions has been proposed as a supportive marker (de Vicente et al., 2019; Grubelnik et al., 2020; Rodrigo et al., 2011). The newer and more sensitive and specific markers, such as insulinoma-associated protein 1 (INSM1), have the potential to replace regular neuroendocrine differentiation markers, such as chromogranin, synaptophysin, and CD56 (Rooper et al., 2018).

The use of immunohistochemical staining in the identification of micrometastasis and isolated tumor cells in distal sites, lymph nodes, and bone marrow is indispensable in the ultrastaging of cancers, particularly when atypical cells are not readily identifiable (Ferlito et al., 1999, 2001). The application of IHC staining on cytology material, incision biopsy, or excision biopsy material, complemented by molecular studies, renders a more accurate diagnosis of primary SCC of the oropharynx (P16 and HPV) and nasopharynx (EBV) (Broccolo et al., 2018; Mulder et al., 2020).

4.2.2 Molecular Testing

Molecular testing in HNC has shown an immense impact on the workup of neuroendocrine malignancies, hematolymphoid malignancies, and sarcoma. Tumors can now be identified based on their molecular signatures, such as the SWI/SNF chromatin remodeling complex, particularly its subunits SMARCA4 (BRG1)- and SMARCB1 (INI-1)-deficient carcinomas and nuclear protein in testis (NUT) carcinoma (Agaimy & Bishop, 2021; Thompson & Franchi, 2018). There is an increase in the number of salivary gland tumors that harbor recurrent genetic mutations, particularly translocation mutations, and the use of molecular testing to make accurate diagnoses opens avenues for the application of specific, targeted therapies.

High-throughput next-generation sequencing (NGS) techniques can detect genetic rearrangements, copy number variations (CNV), and deletions and analyze multiple DNA sequences in parallel (Kelly, 2017). NGS multigene panels can be individualized based on the tumor type and the genes being analyzed. Sánchez-Fernández et al. proposed sinonasal tumor-specific panels to analyze specific susceptibility genes (Sánchez-Fernández et al., 2021). A multigene panel can be adapted to the genes of interest and can be brought up to date with the discovery of new genes. Genomic advances allow for more precise diagnoses based on molecular profiling and open the way for the development of targeted therapies (Biankin et al., 2015). This allows the subgrouping and delineation of those patients who have a better chance of benefiting from targeted therapeutic agents. NGS tests can identify actionable driver mutations and mutations that underlie drug resistance, thereby uncovering individuals who are likely not to respond to treatment (Helman et al., 2018; Solis et al., 2022). Approval from several NGS companion molecular diagnostic assays indicates that NGS is becoming a standard of care in oncology. This fundamental change in approach from single-gene assays to NGS allows the detection of an individual's entire mutational catalogue (Allegretti et al., 2018). The interpretation of NGS results, like those of all other tests, needs to be interpreted in a clinical context and correlated with the pathological results.

Liquid biopsy (LB) in HNC serves as a biomarker for disease detection, prognostication, and therapeutic intervention where tissue acquisition is not feasible (Temilola et al., 2023). LB is a noninvasive, rapid, and repeatable tool for the detection and surveillance of cancer. LB enables the detection of mutations in circulating tumor DNA (ctDNA), which represents small fragments of DNA shed from malignant tumor cells (Martins et al., 2021; Temilola et al., 2023). Limitations in specificity, sensitivity, and overall lack of standardization remain part of an ongoing challenge in the rapid oncology application and expansion of LB.

4.3 Imaging Diagnosis

Imaging diagnostics allow for tumor identification and approximation of tumor volume. Radiologists provide quantitative diagnoses that may suggest specific differential diagnoses and can further establish whether the lesion is cystic, infiltrative, or vascular. Diagnostic imaging has seen advances and the introduction of cutting-edge technologies that have improved the diagnosis, staging, and management of HNC. Imaging modalities include ultrasound, CT, MRI, and nuclear medicine techniques such as PET.

4.3.1 Ultrasound

Ultrasound is an easily accessible, noninvasive modality that provides an excellent initial approach, particularly in the assessment of cervical masses. The ultrasound examination allows for the determination of the lesion size, location, composition, and vascular relationship. Some authors posit that ultrasound has a better sensitivity than CT for the assessment of cervical lymph node metastases (Di Martino et al., 2000; Ding et al., 2021). Ultrasound provides outstanding image resolution for thyroid gland nodules, salivary gland lesions, and lymph nodes. Ultrasound is a highly dependable imaging modality in guided, diagnostic and interventional procedures, such as core needle biopsy or fine needle aspiration. Intraoral ultrasound is currently used to assess the depth of invasion of oral cavity SCC (Noorlag et al., 2020). The shortcomings of ultrasound examination include operator skills and limited ability to assess deeper tissue structures.

4.3.2 Computed Tomography

In HNC, CT scan is used for assessment of the primary tumor, lymph node assessment, and staging of the disease (Choi et al., 2019). The high-resolution image acquisition with thin slices displays the excellent quality of multiplanar reconstructed images, which are efficacious in delineating the anatomy and planning the treatment. Generally, a slice thickness of 1–1.5 mm is used, however, high-resolution sections of 0.625 mm can be captured depending on the capability of the scanner. Iodinated contrast is used to assess blood vessels and augment the contrast between the soft tissue structures (Tshering Vogel & Thoeny, 2016).

In primary tumors, CT scans have a sensitivity of 70% and specificity of 70%, whereas in recurrent tumors the sensitivity and specificity are 65% and 80%, respectively (Cheng et al., 2017; Lell et al., 2000). For lymph node pathology, sensitivity is 85% and specificity is 95%, whereas in recurrent lymph node metastasis, sensitivity is 70% and specificity is 90% (Horváth et al., 2021; Zwittag et al., 2023). CT scan is superior to MRI in assessing the pathology of the infrahyoid region and provides excellent assessment for bone involvement by depicting calcifications. Simultaneous assessment of the head and neck pathology and thoracic cavity allows the assessment of the paratracheal lymph node, upper mediastinal lymph node, pulmonary metastases, or synchronous lung pathology.

New-generation dual-energy CT systems show enhanced detection of bone, bone marrow, and cartilage invasion by tumors (Kuno et al., 2018; Timmer et al., 2020). The major limitations of CT scan are the high dose of radiation, contrast-induced nephropathy, and allergic reactions. In the neck, the CT radiation dose from the intravenous contrast is 3.9 mSv compared to the 8 mSv of CT thorax (Smith-Bindman et al., 2009).

4.3.3 Magnetic Resonance Imaging

As a modality for the assessment of the suprahyoid region of the neck as well as the nasopharynx, oropharynx, sinuses, and oral cavity, MRI is preferred. MRI is a suitable platform for soft tissue assessment that enables the assessment of primary tumor infiltration and distinguishes edema from tumor infiltration. In addition, MRI is efficient for assessing regional lymph node and bone marrow invasion. Compared to CT, the sensitivity of MRI is estimated to be 80% with a specificity of 90% (Horváth et al., 2021).

For a high-quality assessment of anatomy, T1-weighted sequences are the best option, whereas T2-sequences are excellent in soft tissue assessment, particularly in distinguishing residual tumor from post-therapy scarring. For occult and subtle diseases, defining tumor margins and assessing perineural invasion, gadolinium sequences are exceptional. Diffusion-weighted imaging (DWI) is effective in assessing the response to treatment. For quantitative measurement, the apparent diffusion coefficient (ADC) was calculated using MRI with DWI to measure the magnitude of diffusion of water molecules within the tissues (Zakaria et al., 2023). The higher the cellular density (e.g., hypercellular tumor and pathological lymph nodes), the lower the ADC value, and the lower the cellular density, the higher the ADC value (edema, necrosis, post-treatment changes). ADC values are reliable for the post-treatment evaluation of head and neck malignancies (Bhatt et al., 2017; van der Hoorn et al., 2017).

The intravoxel incoherent motion (IVIM) DWI model, which is a biomarker for tissue microcirculation, can be used to differentiate benign and malignant salivary gland lesions and to discriminate other types of tumors in the salivary gland region (Szubert-Franczak et al., 2020). The perfusion-related parameter values are significantly different among various types of head and neck tumors, such as SCC, benign neoplasms (Warthin tumor, pleomorphic adenomas), malignant salivary gland tumors, lymphomas, and schwannomas (Sumi & Nakamura, 2013). Early changes in IVIM parameters have been found to have predictive and prognostic value in salivary gland tumors (Noij et al., 2017).

Dynamic contrast-enhanced (DCE) MRI perfusion imaging can detect and quantify tissue microvasculature to characterize HNC (Furukawa et al., 2013). DCE MRI perfusion imaging can improve the detection of unknown primary tumors and cervical lymph node metastases in SCC (Martens et al., 2020). The application of MRI spectroscopy to break down the biochemical composition and evaluate specific metabolites has the potential to differentiate between benign and malignant tissues (Abdel Razek & Poptani, 2013).

The disadvantages of MRI are related to motion artifacts, such as breathing or swallowing. Absolute contraindications to MRI are pregnancy, cardiac pacemaker, implanted cardiac defibrillator, internal pacing wires, vessel clips, and cochlear implants among others.

4.3.4 Positron Emission Tomography-Computed Tomography

PET-CT combines PET to survey hypermetabolic tissue and CT primarily to assess anatomy. 18-Flurodeoxyglucose (18-FDG) radiolabeled tracer is used to demonstrate areas of increased metabolic activity, such as cancer cells. Injected 18-FDG, which is quickly phosphorylated upon entering cells, localizes to hypermetabolic cells that use glucose for energy for several hours and allows enough time for imaging (Zampella et al., 2021). According to the National Comprehensive Cancer Network (NCCN) guidelines, PET-CT is currently indicated for the initial diagnosis of occult HNC involving the oral cavity, oropharynx, larynx, maxillary sinus, and ethmoid sinus. PET-CT is also indicated as part of staging (Fonti et al., 2019). Newer radiotracers used in HNCs to assess tumor angiogenesis include 68-Ga-NODAGA-RGD (Durante et al., 2020).

PET-CT has a high negative predictive value but a positive predictive value of 50% with high false positivity in cases of inflammatory processes. PET-CT may have poor sensitivity for lesions < 1 mm. High-density objects, such as metal implants or contrast agents, can result in falsely high standard uptake values (Mair et al., 2024).

4.4 Artificial Intelligence

A large number of studies have explored the role of artificial intelligence (AI) and machine learning (ML) in the detection of HNC by utilizing a range of testing modalities (Howard et al., 2020; Loperfido et al., 2023; Mahmood et al., 2021a; Volpe et al., 2021). AI/ML methods can make data predictions that outpace a clinician's degree of accuracy. ML utilizes computational methods to detect patterns, gather insights, and use historical information to make predictions on new data. A subfield of ML, deep learning (DL) algorithms, creates artificial neural networks (ANNs) that contain multiple hidden networks. With an increase in the volume of new data, ML algorithms have become more accurate and efficient.

DL classifies radiological and pathological images by using automated feature extraction (Figure 4.2). Owing to their relatively high levels of diagnostic accuracy, AI methods are gaining popularity. The traditional practice of tumor diagnosis based on clinical findings, examination of radiology images, and light microscopy is time-consuming and may be subjective and thus prone to errors and inconsistencies. Errors and inconsistencies in diagnosis have implications for patient management. There is a small amount of emerging data on the application of AI models to detect and grade precancerous lesions of the head and neck (Alabi et al., 2021; Mahmood et al., 2020, 2021). The accuracy of the data carries a risk of bias due to the one-centeredness of the studies.

The method of extracting a large number of quantitative features from medical images using data characterization algorithms is termed "radiomics." Radiomic features capture tissue and lesion characteristics, alone or in combination with patient demographics, histomorphology, genomic data, or proteomic data, to build predictive and prognostic models. In HNCs, radiomic algorithms can predict early patient survival and response to treatment and identify tumor subtypes (Demetriou et al., 2024; Iancu et al., 2021; Tortora et al., 2023). Radiomic experiments were conducted on retrospective data, and small samples were obtained from a few centers. Therefore, the data are not accurately reflective of the overall population, and patient selection bias remains a concern. AI techniques carry the potential to reduce present-day limitations in HNC imaging, and future efforts need to be carried out toward robust external

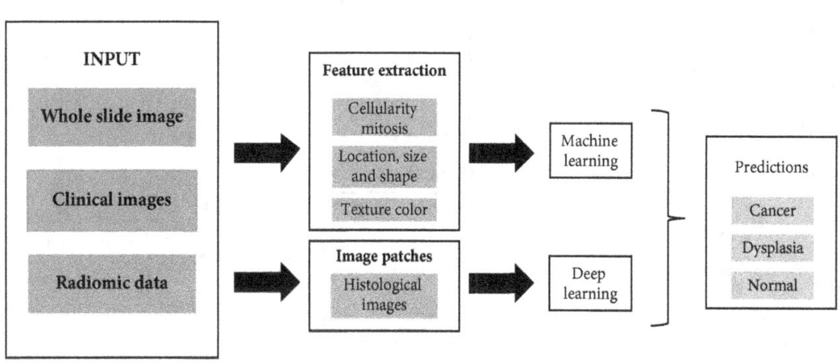

Figure 4.2 Deep learning (DL) classifies radiological and pathological images by using automated feature extraction. Feature extraction assesses cellularity, mitoses, size and shape of the lesion, as well as, and texture to aid outcome prediction.

validation efforts to standardize, refine, and finally implement radiomics and ML software in clinical practice. (Refer to Chapter 14 for more details on the role of AI.)

4.5 Summary

The diagnosis of HNC reflects the expertise of a multidisciplinary team of clinicians, radiologists, and pathologists. The multidisciplinary tumor board complements subjective assessments to limit diagnostic inaccuracy (Figure 4.3). Each diagnostic method targets a rapid and accurate diagnosis to guide the choice of treatment.

A qualitative, pathological diagnosis is a definitive diagnosis that guides prospective therapy. Many complementary advances in the molecular field are emerging to enable more specific diagnoses that apply to personalized therapy. These new technologies are still undergoing validation, and their use requires caution. Quantitative diagnostic imaging establishes the size and extent of HNC and distinguishes tumor recurrence from post-treatment changes. AI algorithms enable radiologists to perform highly specialized tasks such as radiomics, which builds predictive and prognostic models.

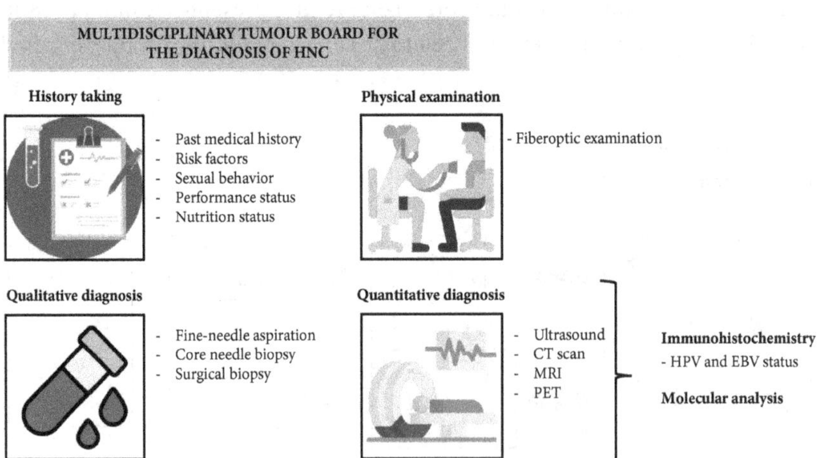

Figure 4.3 Flowchart summarizing the role of each diagnostic test or modality involved in making a diagnosis of head and neck cancer (HNC). The final diagnosis of HNC is based on clinical, radiologic, and laboratory testing.

4.6 Limitations

Establishing early and precise diagnosis will help guide the treatment plan and improve patient outcomes. Embracing the latest breakthroughs in diagnostic tools and cutting-edge techniques will gradually transform the early detection of HNC. Pathological diagnosis is regarded as the most definitive; however, despite the application of IHC and molecular testing, subjectivity remains a challenge, particularly in complex cases. LB, which can detect ctDNA, has limited specificity and sensitivity and lacks overall standardization.

Regarding diagnostic imaging, ultrasound is operator-dependent and cannot accurately assess deeper tissue structures. CT scan examination is limited by the high dose of radiation and the potential for contrast-induced nephropathy. MRI is sensitive to motion artifacts and has many contraindications. PET-CT limitations include high false positivity and poor sensitivity in smaller lesions.

The use of AI and DL in the diagnosis and prognostication of HNC has given us the opportunity to expand techniques that combine conventional approaches to improve the accurate diagnosis and detection of cancerous and precancerous lesions. This exciting avenue combines qualitative imaging modalities and quantitative pathological and molecular measurements to support disease detection, classification, and prediction. Currently, available data on HNC lack external validation and standardization. Large-scale multicenter studies are needed to pave the way for practical clinical applications.

4.7 Conclusion

HNCs are heterogeneous, have varied etiologies and clinical behaviors, and require a multidisciplinary team approach. At the forefront of medical technology, timely and accurate diagnoses are essential for HNCs, particularly with the latest advancements in diagnostic tools and techniques. Mastery of the diagnosis of HNC depends on the expertise of a multidisciplinary team of clinicians, radiologists, and pathologists, suggesting the adoption of recursive learning curves to sustain continual improvement in the decision-making process. AI brings together cutting-edge imaging technologies, histology. and molecular diagnostics to solve clinical problems.

References

ABDEL RAZEK, A. A., & POPTANI, H. 2013. MR spectroscopy of head and neck cancer. *Eur J Radiol*, 82, 982–9.

AGAIMY, A., & BISHOP, J. A. 2021. SWI/SNF-deficient head and neck neoplasms: An overview. *Semin Diagnost Pathol*, 38, 175–82.

ALABI, R. O., YOUSSEF, O., PIRINEN, M., ELMUSRATI, M., MÄKITIE, A. A., LEIVO, I., & ALMANGUSH, A. 2021. Machine learning in oral squamous cell carcinoma: Current status, clinical concerns and prospects for future: A systematic review. *Artif Intell Med*, 115, 102060.

ALLEGRETTI, M., FABI, A., BUGLIONI, S., MARTAYAN, A., CONTI, L., PESCARMONA, E., CILIBERTO, G., & GIACOMINI, P. 2018. Tearing down the walls: FDA approves next generation sequencing (NGS) assays for actionable cancer genomic aberrations. *J Exp Clin Cancer Res*, 37, 47.

ANSARY-MOGHADDAM, A., HUXLEY, R. R., LAM, T. H., & WOODWARD, M. 2009. The risk of upper aero digestive tract cancer associated with smoking, with and without concurrent alcohol consumption. *Mt Sinai J Med*, 76, 392–403.

BHATT, N., GUPTA, N., SONI, N., HOODA, K., SAPIRE, J. M., & KUMAR, Y. 2017. Role of diffusion-weighted imaging in head and neck lesions: Pictorial review. *Neuroradiol J*, 30, 356–69.

BIANKIN, A. V., PIANTADOSI, S., & HOLLINGSWORTH, S. J. 2015. Patient-centric trials for therapeutic development in precision oncology. *Nature*, 526, 361–70.

BISHOP, J. A., MONTGOMERY, E. A., & WESTRA, W. H. 2014. Use of p40 and p63 immunohistochemistry and human papillomavirus testing as ancillary tools for the recognition of head and neck sarcomatoid carcinoma and its distinction from benign and malignant mesenchymal processes. *Am J Surg Pathol*, 38, 257–64.

BRADLEY, P. J., & BRADLEY, P. T. 2010. Searching for metachronous tumours in patients with head and neck cancer: The ideal protocol! *Curr Opin Otolaryngol Head Neck Surg*, 18, 124–33.

BRAY, F., REN, J. S., MASUYER, E., & FERLAY, J. 2013. Global estimates of cancer prevalence for 27 sites in the adult population in 2008. *Int J Cancer*, 132, 1133–45.

BROCCOLO, F., CICCARESE, G., ROSSI, A., ANSELMI, L., DRAGO, F., & TONIOLO, A. 2018. Human papillomavirus (HPV) and Epstein-Barr virus (EBV) in keratinizing versus non-keratinizing squamous cell carcinoma of the oropharynx. *Infect Agents Cancer*, 13, 32.

CHENG, W., QI, Y., WANG, B., TIAN, L., HUANG, W., & CHEN, Y. 2017. Characteristics and computed tomography evaluation of primary retroperitoneal tumours: Report of 113 cases. *Ann R Coll Surg Engl*, 99, 55–9.

CHLIPALA, E. A., BENDZINSKI, C. M., DORNER, C., SARTAN, R., COPELAND, K., PEARCE, R., DOHERTY, F., & BOLON, B. 2020. An image analysis solution for quantification and determination of immunohistochemistry staining reproducibility. *Appl Immunohistochem Mol Morphol*, 28, 428–36.

CHOI, H. Y., YOON, D. Y., KIM, E. S., BAEK, S., LIM, K. J., SEO, Y. L., & YUN, E. J. 2019. Diagnostic performance of CT, MRI, and their combined use for the assessment of the direct cranial or intracranial extension of malignant head and neck tumors. *Acta Radiol*, 60, 301–7.

CHOW, L. Q. M. 2020. Head and Neck Cancer. *N Engl J Med*, 382, 60–72.

COHEN, E. E. W., BELL, R. B., BIFULCO, C. B., BURTNESS, B., GILLISON, M. L., HARRINGTON, K. J., LE, Q. T., LEE, N. Y., LEIDNER, R., LEWIS, R. L., LICITRA, L., MEHANNA, H., MELL, L. K., RABEN, A., SIKORA, A. G., UPPALURI, R., WHITWORTH, F., ZANDBERG, D. P., & FERRIS, R. L. 2019. The Society for Immunotherapy of Cancer consensus statement on immunotherapy for the treatment of squamous cell carcinoma of the head and neck (HNSCC). *J Immunother Cancer*, 7, 184.

DE VICENTE, J. C., RODRÍGUEZ-SANTAMARTA, T., RODRIGO, J. P., ALLONCA, E., VALLINA, A., SINGHANIA, A., DONATE-PÉREZ DEL MOLINO, P., & GARCÍA-PEDRERO, J. M. 2019. The emerging role of NANOG as an early cancer risk biomarker in patients with oral potentially malignant disorders. *J Clin Med*, 8(9), 1376.

DEMETRIOU, D., LOCKHAT, Z., BRZOZOWSKI, L., SAINI, K. S., DLAMINI, Z., & HULL, R. 2024. The convergence of radiology and genomics: Advancing breast cancer diagnosis with radiogenomics. *Cancers*, 16, 1076.

DI MARTINO, E., NOWAK, B., HASSAN, H. A., HAUSMANN, R., ADAM, G., BUELL, U., & WESTHOFEN, M. 2000. Diagnosis and staging of head and neck cancer: A comparison of modern imaging modalities (positron emission tomography, computed tomography, color-coded duplex sonography) with panendoscopic and histopathologic findings. *Arch Otolaryngol Head Neck Surg*, 126, 1457–61.

DING, Z., DENG, C., WANG, Z., LIU, L., MA, X., HUANG, J., WANG, X., XUAN, M., & XIE, H. 2021. Comparison of contrast-enhanced ultrasound and contrast-enhanced computed tomography for the diagnosis of cervical lymph node metastasis in squamous cell carcinoma of the oral cavity. *Int J Oral Maxillofac Surg*, 50, 294–301.

DURANTE, S., DUNET, V., GOROSTIDI, F., MITSAKIS, P., SCHAEFER, N., DELAGE, J., & PRIOR, J. O. 2020. Head and neck tumors angiogenesis imaging with (68)Ga-NODAGA-RGD in comparison to (18)F-FDG PET/CT: A pilot study. *EJNMMI Res*, 10, 47.

FERLITO, A., DEVANEY, K. O., & RINALDO, A. 2001. Is it time to develop an "ultrastaging system" for use in patients with head and neck malignancies? *Laryngoscope*, 111, 185–6.

FERLITO, A., DEVANEY, K. O., RINALDO, A., DEVANEY, S. L., & CARBONE, A. 1999. Micrometastases: Have they an impact on prognosis? *Ann Otol Rhinol Laryngol*, 108, 1185–9.

FONTI, R., CONSON, M., & DEL VECCHIO, S. 2019. PET/CT in radiation oncology. *Semin Oncol*, 46, 202–9.

FURUKAWA, M., PARVATHANENI, U., MARAVILLA, K., RICHARDS, T. L., & ANZAI, Y. 2013. Dynamic contrast-enhanced MR perfusion imaging of head and neck tumors at 3 Tesla. *Head Neck*, 35, 923–9.

GLEN, P., & BOTHA, E. 2022. Early detection and prevention of head and neck cancers. *Br Dental J*, 233, 726–30.

GRUBELNIK, G., BOŠTJANČIČ, E., PAVLIČ, A., KOS, M., & ZIDAR, N. 2020. NANOG expression in human development and cancerogenesis. *Exp Biol Med (Maywood)*, 245, 456–64.

HASHMI, A. A., YOUNUS, N., NAZ, S., IRFAN, M., HUSSAIN, Z., SHAIKH, S. T., ALI, J., FARIDI, N., NAJAM, J., SHOAIB, M., & HASHMI, S. K. 2020. p16 immunohistochemical expression in head and neck squamous cell carcinoma: Association with prognostic parameters. *Cureus*, 12, e8601.

HELMAN, E., NGUYEN, M., KARLOVICH, C. A., DESPAIN, D., CHOQUETTE, A. K., SPIRA, A. I., YU, H. A., CAMIDGE, D. R., HARDING, T. C., LANMAN, R. B., & SIMMONS, A. D. 2018. Cell-free DNA next-generation sequencing prediction of response and resistance to third-generation EGFR inhibitor. *Clin Lung Cancer*, 19, 518–30.e7.

HORVÁTH, A., PREKOPP, P., POLONY, G., SZÉKELY, E., TAMÁS, L., & DÁNOS, K. 2021. Accuracy of the preoperative diagnostic workup in patients with head and neck cancers undergoing neck dissection in terms of nodal metastases. *Eur Arch Otorhinolaryngol*, 278, 2041–6.

HOWARD, F. M., KOCHANNY, S., KOSHY, M., SPIOTTO, M., & PEARSON, A. T. 2020. Machine learning-guided adjuvant treatment of head and neck cancer. *JAMA Netw Open*, 3, e2025881.

IANCU, R. I., ZARA, A. D., MIRESTEAN, C. C., & IANCU, D. P. T. 2021. Radiomics in head and neck cancers radiotherapy: Promises and challenges. *Maedica (Bucur)*, 16, 482–8.

INTERNATIONAL COLLABORATION FOR CANCER REPORTING (ICCR). 2024. Head & neck datasets. Available at: https://www.iccr-cancer.org/datasets/published-datasets/head-neck/ [Accessed March 31, 2024.]

KELLY, P. A. 2017. Next generation sequencing and multi-gene panel testing: Implications for the oncology nurse. *Semin Oncol Nurs*, 33, 208–18.

KUNO, H., SAKAMAKI, K., FUJII, S., SEKIYA, K., OTANI, K., HAYASHI, R., YAMANAKA, T., SAKAI, O., & KUSUMOTO, M. 2018. Comparison of MR imaging and dual-energy CT for the evaluation of cartilage invasion by laryngeal and hypopharyngeal squamous cell carcinoma. *AJNR Am J Neuroradiol*, 39, 524–31.

LELL, M., BAUM, U., GREESS, H., NÖMAYR, A., NKENKE, E., KOESTER, M., LENZ, M., & BAUTZ, W. 2000. Head and neck tumors: Imaging recurrent tumor and post-therapeutic changes with CT and MRI. *Eur J Radiol*, 33, 239–47.

LOPERFIDO, A., CELEBRINI, A., MARZETTI, A., & BELLOCCHI, G. 2023. Current role of artificial intelligence in head and neck cancer surgery: A systematic review of literature. *Explor Target Antitumor Ther*, 4, 933–40.

LÓPEZ, F., HUNT, J. L., NIXON, I. J., RINALDO, A., WILLIAMS, M. D., CARDESA, A., & FERLITO, A. 2018. How phenotype guides management of the neuroendocrine carcinomas of the larynx. *J Laryngol Otol*, 132, 568–74.

LÓPEZ, F., MÄKITIE, A., DE BREE, R., FRANCHI, A., DE GRAAF, P., HERNÁNDEZ-PRERA, J. C., STROJAN, P., ZIDAR, N., STROJAN FLEŽAR, M., RODRIGO, J. P., RINALDO, A., CENTENO, B. A., & FERLITO, A. 2021. Qualitative and quantitative diagnosis in head and neck cancer. *Diagnostics (Basel)*, 11(9), 1526.

LÓPEZ, F., WILLIAMS, M. D., SKÁLOVÁ, A., HELLQUIST, H., SUÁREZ, C., NIXON, I. J., RODRIGO, J. P., CARDESA, A., STROJAN, P., QUER, M., HUNT, J. L., RINALDO, A., & FERLITO, A. 2017. How phenotype guides management of the most common malignant salivary neoplasms of the larynx? *Adv Ther*, 34, 813–25.

MAHMOOD, H., SHABAN, M., INDAVE, B. I., SANTOS-SILVA, A. R., RAJPOOT, N., & KHURRAM, S. A. 2020. Use of artificial intelligence in diagnosis of head and neck precancerous and cancerous lesions: A systematic review. *Oral Oncol*, 110, 104885.

MAHMOOD, H., SHABAN, M., RAJPOOT, N., & KHURRAM, S. A. 2021. Artificial intelligence-based methods in head and neck cancer diagnosis: An overview. *Br J Cancer*, 124, 1934–40.

MAIR, M., SINGHAVI, H., PAI, A., KHAN, M., CONBOY, P., OLALEYE, O., SALHA, R., AMEERALLY, P., VAIDHYANATH, R., & CHATURVEDI, P. 2024. A systematic review and meta-analysis of 29 studies predicting diagnostic accuracy of CT, MRI, PET, and USG in detecting extracapsular spread in head and neck cancers. *Cancers*, 16, 1457.

MARTENS, R. M., STAPPEN, R. V., KOOPMAN, T., NOIJ, D. P., COMANS, E. F., ZWEZERIJNEN, G. J., VERGEER, M. R., LEEMANS, C. R., DE BREE, R., BOELLAARD, R., CASTELIJNS, J. A., & DE GRAAF, P. 2020. The additional value of ultrafast DCE-MRI to DWI-MRI and 18F-FDG-PET to detect occult primary head and neck squamous cell carcinoma. *Cancers (Basel)*, 12(10), 2826.

MARTINS, I., RIBEIRO, I. P., JORGE, J., GONÇALVES, A. C., SARMENTO-RIBEIRO, A. B., MELO, J. B., & CARREIRA, I. M. 2021. Liquid biopsies: Applications for cancer diagnosis and monitoring. *Genes (Basel)*, 12(3), 349.

MULDER, F. J., KLUFAH, F., JANSSEN, F. M. E., FARSHADPOUR, F., WILLEMS, S. M., DE BREE, R., ZUR HAUSEN, A., VAN DEN HOUT, M., KREMER, B., & SPEEL, E. M. 2020. Presence of human papillomavirus and Epstein-Barr virus, but absence of Merkel cell polyomavirus, in head and neck cancer of non-smokers and non-drinkers. *Front Oncol*, 10, 560434.

NOIJ, D. P., MARTENS, R. M., MARCUS, J. T., DE BREE, R., LEEMANS, C. R., CASTELIJNS, J. A., DE JONG, M. C., & DE GRAAF, P. 2017. Intravoxel incoherent motion magnetic resonance imaging in head and neck cancer: A systematic review of the diagnostic and prognostic value. *Oral Oncol*, 68, 81–91.

NOORLAG, R., KLEIN NULENT, T. J. W., DELWEL, V. E. J., PAMEIJER, F. A., WILLEMS, S. M., DE BREE, R., & VAN ES, R. J. J. 2020. Assessment of tumour depth in early tongue cancer: Accuracy of MRI and intraoral ultrasound. *Oral Oncol*, 110, 104895.

PEDREGAL-MALLO, D., HERMIDA-PRADO, F., GRANDA-DÍAZ, R., MONTORO-JIMÉNEZ, I., ALLONCA, E., POZO-AGUNDO, E., ÁLVAREZ-FERNÁNDEZ, M.,

ÁLVAREZ-MARCOS, C., GARCÍA-PEDRERO, J. M., & RODRIGO, J. P. 2020. Prognostic significance of the pluripotency factors NANOG, SOX2, and OCT4 in head and neck squamous cell carcinomas. *Cancers (Basel)*, 12(7), 1794.

PFISTER, D. G., SPENCER, S., BRIZEL, D. M., BURTNESS, B., BUSSE, P. M., CAUDELL, J. J., CMELAK, A. J., COLEVAS, A. D., DUNPHY, F., EISELE, D. W., GILBERT, J., GILLISON, M. L., HADDAD, R. I., HAUGHEY, B. H., HICKS, W. L., JR., HITCHCOCK, Y. J., JIMENO, A., KIES, M. S., LYDIATT, W. M., MAGHAMI, E., MARTINS, R., MCCAFFREY, T., MELL, L. K., MITTAL, B. B., PINTO, H. A., RIDGE, J. A., RODRIGUEZ, C. P., SAMANT, S., SCHULLER, D. E., SHAH, J. P., WEBER, R. S., WOLF, G. T., WORDEN, F., YOM, S. S., MCMILLIAN, N. R., & HUGHES, M. 2014. Head and neck cancers, Version 2.2014. Clinical practice guidelines in oncology. *J Natl Compr Canc Netw*, 12, 1454–87.

RODRIGO, J. P., ÁLVAREZ-ALIJA, G., MENÉNDEZ, S. T., MANCEBO, G., ALLONCA, E., GARCÍA-CARRACEDO, D., FRESNO, M. F., SUÁREZ, C., & GARCÍA-PEDRERO, J. M. 2011. Cortactin and focal adhesion kinase as predictors of cancer risk in patients with laryngeal premalignancy. *Cancer Prev Res (Phila)*, 4, 1333–41.

ROOPER, L. M., BISHOP, J. A., & WESTRA, W. H. 2018. INSM1 is a sensitive and specific marker of neuroendocrine differentiation in head and neck tumors. *Am J Surg Pathol*, 42, 665–71.

SÁNCHEZ-FERNÁNDEZ, P., RIOBELLO, C., COSTALES, M., VIVANCO, B., CABAL, V. N., GARCÍA-MARÍN, R., SUÁREZ-FERNÁNDEZ, L., LÓPEZ, F., CABANILLAS, R., HERMSEN, M. A., & LLORENTE, J. L. 2021. Next-generation sequencing for identification of actionable gene mutations in intestinal-type sinonasal adenocarcinoma. *Sci Rep*, 11, 2247.

SHUMAN, A. G., ENTEZAMI, P., CHERNIN, A. S., WALLACE, N. E., TAYLOR, J. M., & HOGIKYAN, N. D. 2010. Demographics and efficacy of head and neck cancer screening. *Otolaryngol Head Neck Surg*, 143, 353–60.

SIEGEL, R. L., MILLER, K. D., & JEMAL, A. 2018. Cancer statistics, 2018. *CA Cancer J Clin*, 68, 7–30.

SMITH-BINDMAN, R., LIPSON, J., MARCUS, R., KIM, K. P., MAHESH, M., GOULD, R., BERRINGTON DE GONZÁLEZ, A., & MIGLIORETTI, D. L. 2009. Radiation dose associated with common computed tomography examinations and the associated lifetime attributable risk of cancer. *Arch Intern Med*, 169, 2078–86.

SOLIS, R. N., SILVERMAN, D. A., & BIRKELAND, A. C. 2022. Current trends in precision medicine and next-generation sequencing in head and neck cancer. *Curr Treat Options Oncol*, 23, 254–67.

SUMI, M., & NAKAMURA, T. 2013. Head and neck tumors: Assessment of perfusion-related parameters and diffusion coefficients based on the intravoxel incoherent motion model. *AJNR Am J Neuroradiol*, 34, 410–6.

SZUBERT-FRANCZAK, A. E., NADUK-OSTROWSKA, M., PASICZ, K., PODGÓRSKA, J., SKRZYŃSKI, W., & CIESZANOWSKI, A. 2020. Intravoxel incoherent motion magnetic resonance imaging: Basic principles and clinical applications. *Pol J Radiol*, 85, e624–35.

TEMILOLA, D. O., ADEOLA, H. A., GROBBELAAR, J., & CHETTY, M. 2023. Liquid biopsy in head and neck cancer: Its present state and future role in Africa. *Cells*, 12, 2663.

THOMPSON, L. D. R., & FRANCHI, A. 2018. New tumor entities in the 4th edition of the World Health Organization classification of head and neck tumors: Nasal cavity, paranasal sinuses and skull base. *Virchows Arch*, 472, 315–30.

TIMMER, V. C. M. L., KROONENBURGH, A. M. J. L. V., HENNEMAN, W. J. P., VAASSEN, L. A. A., ROELE, E. D., KESSLER, P. A. W. H., & POSTMA, A. A. 2020. Detection of bone marrow edema in the head and neck with dual-energy CT: Ready for clinical use? *Am J Roentgenol*, 214, 893–9.

TORTORA, M., GEMINI, L., SCARAVILLI, A., UGGA, L., PONSIGLIONE, A., STANZIONE, A., D'ARCO, F., D'ANNA, G., & CUOCOLO, R. 2023. Radiomics applications in head and neck tumor imaging: A narrative review. *Cancers (Basel)*, 15(4), 1174.

TSHERING VOGEL, D. W., & THOENY, H. C. 2016. Cross-sectional imaging in cancers of the head and neck: How we review and report. *Cancer Imaging*, 16, 20.

TURUNEN, A., RAUTAVA, J., GRÉNMAN, R., SYRJÄNEN, K., & SYRJÄNEN, S. 2017. Epstein-Barr virus (EBV)-encoded small RNAs (EBERs) associated with poor prognosis of head and neck carcinomas. *Oncotarget*, 8, 27328–27338.

VAN DER HOORN, A., VAN LAAR, P. J., HOLTMAN, G. A., & WESTERLAAN, H. E. 2017. Diagnostic accuracy of magnetic resonance imaging techniques for treatment response evaluation in patients with head and neck tumors, a systematic review and meta-analysis. *PLoS One*, 12, e0177986.

VOLPE, S., PEPA, M., ZAFFARONI, M., BELLERBA, F., SANTAMARIA, R., MARVASO, G., ISAKSSON, L. J., GANDINI, S., STARZYŃSKA, A., LEONARDI, M. C., ORECCHIA, R., ALTERIO, D., & JERECZEK-FOSSA, B. A. 2021. Machine learning for head and neck cancer: A safe bet? A clinically oriented systematic review for the radiation oncologist. *Front Oncol*, 11, 772663.

ZABALA, A., MARTÍN-ARREGUI, F. J., SAGAZOLA, J., SANTAOLALLA, F. J., & SANTAOLALLA, F. 2022. An evaluation of an innovative screening program based on risk criteria for early diagnosis of head and neck cancers. *Front Public Health*, 10, 1004039.

ZAKARIA, R., JENKINSON, M. D., RADON, M., DAS, K., POPTANI, H., RATHI, N., & RUDLAND, P. S. 2023. Immune checkpoint inhibitor treatment of brain metastasis associated with a less invasive growth pattern, higher T-cell infiltration and raised tumor ADC on diffusion weighted MRI. *Cancer Immunol Immunother*, 72, 3387–93.

ZAMPELLA, E., KLAIN, M., PACE, L., & CUOCOLO, A. 2021. PET/CT in the management of differentiated thyroid cancer. *Diagn Interv Imaging*, 102, 515–23.

ZWITTAG, P., ASEL, C., GABRIEL, M., RUBICZ, N., BAUER, B., & POIER-FABIAN, N. 2023. MRI and PET/CT in the assessment of lymph node metastases in head and neck cancer. *Sci Rep*, 13, 19347.

5
Precision Medicine in Head and Neck Cancer

Thifhelimbilu Emmanuel Luvhengo, Lloyd Mabonga, Zukile Mbita, Mark Torres-Holmes, Godfrey Grech, and Zodwa Dlamini

5.1 Introduction

Precision medicine, also known as personalized or stratified medicine, is a paradigm shift in healthcare that seeks to tailor medical interventions to the individual characteristics of each patient, including their genetic makeup, molecular profile, and environmental factors. The approach acknowledges that diseases such as cancer are heterogeneous and vary significantly between individuals (Petzschner, 2024). Precision medicine holds great promise in revolutionizing the management of HNC by offering more targeted and effective treatment strategies. It involves the use of advanced molecular profiling techniques to characterize the unique biological features of a patient's tumor (Sampson et al., 2024). Precision medicine aims to identify specific biomarkers that can guide treatment decisions and predict response to therapy by analyzing genetic mutations, gene expression patterns, and other molecular alterations (Petzschner, 2024). The goal of precision medicine is to maximize treatment efficacy while minimizing side effects and toxicity by matching patients with the most appropriate targeted therapies or treatment combinations based on their individual tumor biology. It allows for comprehensive molecular profiling of HNC tumors to identify specific genetic mutations, chromosomal aberrations, and other molecular alterations that drive tumor growth and progression (Duan et al., 2024).

With the advent of precision medicine, targeted therapies that specifically inhibit oncogenic pathways or molecular targets implicated in HNC pathogenesis have been developed (Petzschner, 2024). These include epidermal growth factor receptor (EGFR) inhibitors (e.g., cetuximab), immune checkpoint inhibitors (e.g., pembrolizumab), and small-molecule inhibitors targeting key signaling pathways (Kiran et al., 2024). Biomarkers have also been identified through molecular profiling and have been utilized as predictive and/or prognostic indicators, guiding treatment decisions and optimizing therapeutic outcomes. Human papillomavirus (HPV) infection status, EGFR expression, and TP53

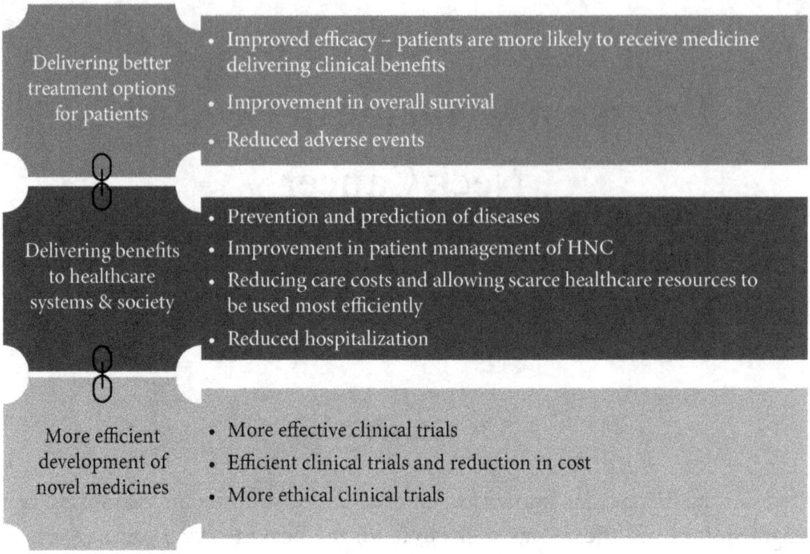

Figure 5.1 The benefits of precision medicine. Patients receive proper treatment at the right time, and it lessens the risk of harmful effects for patients while simultaneously lowering expenses and enhancing the sustainability and efficiency of healthcare systems.

mutations have been identified as potential biomarkers that may influence treatment selection and response in HNC (Kunhabdulla et al., 2024). As shown in Figure 5.1, the benefits of precision medicine have been tailored to enable the development of personalized treatment strategies according to each patient's individual characteristics. This may involve selecting the most appropriate targeted therapy, immunotherapy regimen, or combination treatment approach based on the patient's molecular profile and disease characteristics (Petzschner, 2024).

In this context, precision medicine leverages advanced "omics" technologies (shown in Figure 5.2) to comprehensively understand the molecular underpinnings of HNC and inform personalized treatment strategies (Miserocchi et al., 2022). It facilitates the integration of multiomics data into clinical practice thereby enhancing diagnostic accuracy, prognostic assessments, and therapeutic interventions, which ultimately improve patient outcomes (Duan et al., 2024). The integration of multiomics data offers a holistic view of tumor biology, capturing the complexity and heterogeneity of HNC, and enables the identification of biomarkers for early detection, prognosis, and therapeutic response, thus facilitating personalized treatment strategies (Petzschner, 2024). Precision medicine holds promise in the prevention of HNC and offers a transformative approach in the management of HNC through the identification of

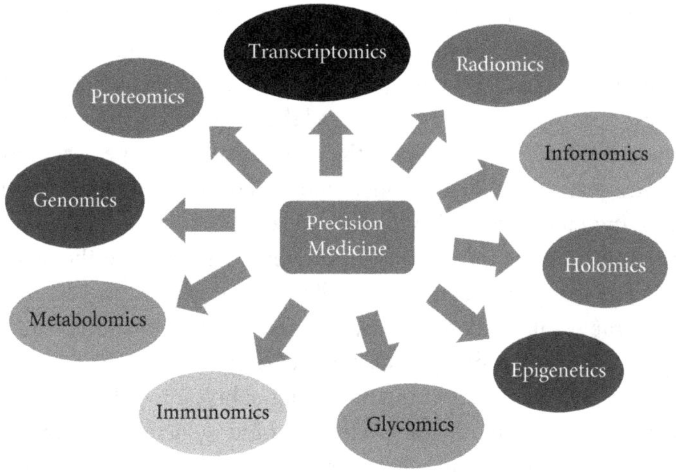

Figure 5.2 The "omic" technologies of precision medicine in head and neck cancer (HNC) management. Integration of multiple omics datasets, combined with clinical and pathological parameters, enables a comprehensive understanding of HNC biology, heterogeneity, and treatment response variability. Multidisciplinary collaborations, bioinformatics analysis, and translational research efforts are essential for leveraging omics technologies to advance precision medicine in HNC treatment and improve patient outcomes.

high-risk individuals, screening programs, and targeted interventions aimed at reducing cancer incidence and mortality (Duan et al., 2024; Petzschner, 2024). This chapter explores the use of precision medicine in HNC, focusing on the paradigm shift brought about by the various "omics" technologies in the realm of HNC management.

5.2 Genomics in Head and Neck Cancer

Precision medicine characterized by tailored treatment strategies based on an individual patient's genomic profile holds immense promise in the management of HNC (Sosinsky et al., 2024). Genomics is a cornerstone of precision oncology. It plays a pivotal role in deciphering the molecular landscape of tumors through identifying and analyzing actionable genetic alterations such as somatic mutations, copy number alterations, chromosomal rearrangements, and epigenetic modification and subsequently guiding personalized treatment decisions (Mezghani et al., 2023). Genomics also encompasses comprehensive analysis of molecular pathways involved in tumor initiation, progression, metastasis, and treatment response. The alterations affect key oncogenes, tumor suppressor genes, and DNA repair pathways, contributing to the dysregulation of cell proliferation, apoptosis, and DNA damage response (Sosinsky et al., 2024). In this context, genomic profiling helps uncover novel therapeutic targets and mechanisms of treatment resistance by elucidating the mutational landscape of head and neck tumors (Mezghani et al., 2023). Thus, genomics provides valuable insights into the underlying mechanisms driving tumorigenesis as well as the identification of potential biomarkers for diagnosis, prognosis, and targeted therapy. The integration of genomic information into clinical practice enables the delivery of targeted therapies, immunotherapies, and combination treatments tailored to the unique molecular profiles of each patient (Kemmer et al., 2018).

Genomic analysis has led to the molecular subtyping of HNC into distinct molecular subgroups, each characterized by unique genetic alterations and clinical characteristics. These subtypes, such as HPV-associated and non–HPV-associated subtypes, have important implications for patient prognosis and treatment selection (Sosinsky et al., 2024). The identification of actionable mutations and the development of personalized treatment strategies such as targeted therapies and immunotherapies tailored to individual patient profiles is enabled by genomic profiling. Patients who may benefit from specific targeted therapies or immunotherapies such as immune checkpoint inhibitors tailored to their molecular subtype can be identified through molecular subtyping (Kemmer et al., 2018). Thus, genomic profiling of head and neck tumors allows for the identification of specific genetic alterations, such as activating mutations, amplifications, or gene fusions, that drive tumor growth and progression (Sosinsky et al., 2024). Targeted therapies directed against the molecular targets offer the potential for improved treatment outcomes and reduced toxicity compared to conventional chemotherapy. For example, inhibitors targeting the EGFR, such as cetuximab, have demonstrated efficacy in patients with EGFR-amplified or overexpressed tumors (Mezghani et al., 2023).

Genomic studies have facilitated the discovery of biomarkers for early detection, prognostication, and monitoring of treatment response in HNC (Mezghani et al., 2023). Genomic biomarkers offer potential targets for noninvasive screening tests, such as liquid biopsies, saliva-based assays, and circulating tumor DNA analysis, by identifying genetic alterations associated with tumor initiation and progression. The biomarkers hold promise for improving early detection rates, enabling timely intervention, and monitoring disease recurrence in patients with HNC (Kemmer et al., 2018). Genomic biomarkers serve as valuable predictors of treatment response and prognosis in HNC, facilitating the design of biomarker-driven clinical trials. The trials aim to evaluate the efficacy of targeted therapies or novel treatment combinations in selected patient populations by enrolling patients based on specific genetic alterations or molecular subtypes. Biomarker-driven trials offer the potential for more precise patient selection, enhanced treatment response rates, and accelerated drug development (Sosinsky et al., 2024).

Table 5.1 is a list of some significant genetic biomarkers associated with HNC. Biomarkers are valuable for various aspects of cancer management, including early detection, prognosis, and tailoring individualized treatment approaches. Continuous research is leading to the discovery of new biomarkers and improving the understanding of the molecular underpinnings of HNCs (Kemmer et al., 2018). Genomic analysis helps uncover mechanisms of treatment resistance in HNC, informing strategies to overcome resistance and improve treatment efficacy. Resistance may arise due to acquired mutations, activation of alternative signaling pathways, or tumor microenvironment-mediated immune evasion (Sosinsky et al., 2024). Clinicians can develop rational combination therapies targeting multiple pathways or sequential treatment strategies to prevent or delay disease progression by identifying resistance mechanisms through genomic profiling (Mezghani et al., 2023). Ultimately, genomic information guides the development of personalized treatment plans tailored to the individual patient's tumor biology and clinical characteristics. Integrating genomic data with other omics information, such as transcriptomics, proteomics, and metabolomics, provides a comprehensive understanding of tumor behavior and treatment response (Kemmer et al., 2018). Personalized treatment plans may include a combination of targeted therapies, immunotherapies, radiation therapy, and surgery optimized to maximize efficacy while minimizing toxicity for each patient (Sosinsky et al., 2024).

However, despite its tremendous potential, genomic analysis in HNC faces challenges that include the complexity of tumor biology, the heterogeneity of patient populations, and the need for robust bioinformatics tools and data integration platforms (Kemmer et al., 2018). Future research efforts should focus on overcoming the challenges as well as translating genomic discoveries into clinical practice through collaborative research initiatives, prospective clinical trials, and the implementation of precision oncology programs in routine patient care (Sosinsky et al., 2024). The use of genomics in precision medicine revolutionizes the management of HNC by guiding personalized treatment decisions, improving treatment outcomes, and advancing our understanding of tumor biology and treatment resistance (Kemmer et al., 2018). Genomic analysis holds promise for advancing precision medicine and revolutionizing the management of HNC in the era of personalized oncology by elucidating the genetic underpinnings of tumorigenesis and treatment response. Clinicians can deliver tailored therapies that target the specific molecular drivers of each patient's cancer by leveraging genomic information, thus leading to more effective and individualized care in the era of precision oncology (Sosinsky et al., 2024).

Table 5.1 List of genetic biomarkers associated with head and neck cancer

Genetic biomarker	Role	Significance	References
TP53	Tumor suppressor gene	Mutations in TP53 are common in head and neck cancers, leading to loss of cell cycle control and increased cancer risk.	Mezghani et al., 2023
Human papillomavirus (HPV)	Oncogenic virus	The presence of high-risk HPV types (especially HPV16) is associated with a subset of head and neck cancers, particularly oropharyngeal cancers. HPV status can influence prognosis and treatment strategies.	Kemmer et al., 2018
Epidermal growth factor receptor (EGFR)	Receptor tyrosine kinase	Overexpression or amplification of EGFR is frequently observed in head and neck cancers, making it a target for therapies such as cetuximab.	Mezghani et al., 2023
Cyclin D1 (CCND1)	Cell cycle regulator	Amplification of CCND1 is associated with head and neck squamous cell carcinoma (HNSCC), promoting cell proliferation.	Mezghani et al., 2023
p16INK4A (CDKN2A)	Tumor suppressor gene	Loss or inactivation of p16INK4A is common in HPV-negative head and neck cancers. In contrast, its overexpression is a surrogate marker for HPV-associated cancers.	Sosinsky et al., 2024
PIK3CA	Gene involved in the PI3K/AKT pathway	Mutations in PIK3CA are found in a subset of head and neck cancers, contributing to cell survival and growth.	Kemmer et al., 2018
NOTCH1	Gene involved in cell differentiation	Mutations in NOTCH1 can either be oncogenic or tumor-suppressive, depending on the context. Its role in head and neck cancer is complex and under investigation.	Mezghani et al., 2023

Table 5.1 Continued

Genetic biomarker	Role	Significance	References
Fibroblast growth factor receptor 1 (FGFR1)	Receptor tyrosine kinase	Amplification of FGFR1 is observed in some head and neck cancers, offering a potential therapeutic target.	Sosinsky et al., 2024
Mesenchymal-epithelial transition factor (MET)	Receptor tyrosine kinase	Overexpression or mutations in MET are associated with poor prognosis and metastasis in head and neck cancers.	Sosinsky et al., 2024
HRAS	GTPase involved in cell signaling	Mutations in HRAS are found in a subset of head and neck cancers, contributing to tumorigenesis.	Kemmer et al., 2018
Aldehyde dehydrogenase 1 (ALDH1)	Enzyme involved in cellular detoxification	High expression of ALDH1 is associated with cancer stem cells and is a marker of poor prognosis and therapy resistance.	Mezghani et al., 2023
Matrix metalloproteinases (MMPs)	Enzymes involved in extracellular matrix remodeling	Overexpression of MMPs, particularly MMP-9, is associated with tumor invasion and metastasis in head and neck cancers.	Sosinsky et al., 2024
TWIST1 and SNAI1	Transcription factors involved in epithelial-mesenchymal transition (EMT)	Overexpression of these genes is linked to increased invasiveness and metastatic potential of head and neck cancers.	Kemmer et al., 2018
Programmed death-ligand 1 (PD-L1)	Immune checkpoint protein	Overexpression of PD-L1 can help tumors evade the immune system. PD-L1 status is used to guide immunotherapy decisions.	Sosinsky et al., 2024
CTNNB1 (β-catenin)	Gene involved in Wnt signaling pathway	Aberrations in β-catenin signaling are implicated in the progression of head and neck cancers.	Kemmer et al., 2018

5.3 Transcriptomics in Head and Neck Cancer

Transcriptomics is the study of all RNA transcripts in a cell or tissue. It offers valuable intuition into the molecular mechanisms underlying HNC and plays a crucial role in advancing precision medicine in this disease. Transcriptomics offers a comprehensive understanding of the dynamic changes in gene expression that occur during tumorigenesis, progression, and response to therapy (Lee, Roy et al., 2023; Serafini et al., 2020). Analysis of transcriptomic data in HNC has revealed molecular signatures associated with tumor subtypes, prognosis, treatment response, and therapeutic resistance, driving advancements in precision medicine and personalized treatment strategies. Transcriptomic analysis enables the identification of dysregulated genes, signaling pathways, and molecular targets that drive tumorigenesis and tumor progression in HNC (Lee, Roy et al., 2023). Researchers can pinpoint potential therapeutic targets, such as overexpressed oncogenes or downregulated tumor suppressor genes, for targeted therapy development by analyzing gene expression profiles. Moreover, transcriptomic data can inform the development of experimental therapies and preclinical models for testing novel treatment approaches in HNC. It can guide the selection of combination therapies targeting multiple pathways implicated in tumor growth and survival (Lee, Johnson et al., 2023; Serafini et al., 2020).

Transcriptomic analysis enables the molecular subtyping of HNC into distinct subgroups based on gene expression profiles (Serafini et al., 2020). The molecular subtypes exhibit unique biological features, clinical characteristics, and treatment responses. For example, studies have identified subtypes associated with HPV infection, immune infiltration, and epithelial-to-mesenchymal transition (EMT), each with implications for patient prognosis and treatment selection (Lee et al., 2023). Transcriptomics helps identify individuals who are likely to benefit from specific targeted therapies or immunotherapies, thus leading to more personalized treatment strategies by stratifying patients into molecularly defined subgroups. Transcriptomic profiling facilitates the discovery of biomarkers associated with prognosis, treatment response, and resistance in HNC (Serafini et al., 2020). Transcriptomic biomarkers have been identified for prognostication and risk stratification in HNC, aiding in patient counseling and treatment planning. Moreso, transcriptomic-based prognostic models can stratify patients into different risk groups and guide personalized treatment decisions through analyzing gene expression signatures associated with tumor aggressiveness, metastatic potential, and patient survival (Lee et al., 2023; Serafini et al., 2020).

Transcriptomic biomarkers provide valuable prognostic information beyond traditional clinical and pathological factors, enhancing risk assessment and treatment selection in clinical practice. Transcriptomic analysis allows for the development of predictive models to guide treatment decisions through identifying gene expression signatures correlated with clinical outcomes (Cavalieri et al., 2021). The models can predict patient response to chemotherapy, radiation therapy, targeted therapy, or immunotherapy, thus aiding clinicians in selecting the most effective treatment approach for individual patients. Moreover, transcriptomic profiling allows for the early detection of treatment resistance mechanisms, such as upregulation of drug efflux pumps or activation of alternative signaling pathways, enabling the development of tailored treatment strategies to overcome resistance (Lee et al., 2023). Transcriptomic analysis helps identify potential therapeutic targets for precision therapies in HNC. Transcriptomics guides the development of targeted therapies aimed at specific molecular vulnerabilities through uncovering dysregulated genes and signaling pathways driving tumorigenesis. For example, genes overexpressed in certain HNC subtypes may serve as potential targets for small-molecule inhibitors or monoclonal antibodies, leading to more tailored and effective treatment options (Lee et al., 2023; Serafini et al., 2020).

Transcriptomic studies provide acumen into the complex biology of HNC and the mechanisms underlying treatment resistance. Transcriptomics helps identify novel therapeutic targets and combination treatment strategies to overcome resistance by elucidating gene expression changes associated with drug resistance (Lee et al., 2023; Serafini et al., 2020). Decoding the molecular mechanisms driving resistance allows for the development of more effective treatment regimens and personalized approaches to combating HNC. Transcriptomic analysis informs personalized treatment planning and clinical decision-making in HNC. Ttranscriptomics helps tailor treatment strategies to individual patients by integrating gene expression data with clinical and pathological information (Serafini et al., 2020). Clinicians use transcriptomic profiling to optimize treatment selection, dosage, and sequencing, leading to improved patient outcomes and reduced treatment-related toxicity (Lee et al., 2023). Thus, transcriptomics plays a critical role in advancing precision medicine in HNC. It provides intuition into tumor biology, identifies therapeutic targets, predicts treatment responses, and guides personalized treatment strategies. Clinicians can optimize treatment decisions, improve patient outcomes, and move toward more targeted and effective therapies for HNC through leveraging transcriptomic data (Lee et al., 2023; Serafini et al., 2020).

5.4 Epigenetics: Non-coding RNA in Head and Neck Cancer

Epigenetics offers valuable insights into the molecular mechanisms underlying HNC and holds significant promise and profound implications for precision medicine approaches, including the identification of diagnostic biomarkers, prognostic indicators, and therapeutic targets (Morselli & Dieci, 2022). Epigenetics is the study of heritable changes in gene expression that do not involve alterations in the DNA sequence. Precision oncology approaches that target epigenetic regulators, such as DNA methyltransferases, histone deacetylases, and non-coding RNAs, hold promise for improving treatment outcomes and patient survival in HNC. Integrating epigenetic biomarkers into clinical decision-making processes facilitates personalized treatment selection and monitoring of treatment response, leading to more effective and individualized care for patients with HNC (Diez-Fraile et al., 2020). Epigenetic alterations, such as DNA methylation patterns and histone modifications, serve as biomarkers for HNC diagnosis and prognosis. Over the years, researchers have identified specific methylation signatures or histone modification patterns associated with HNC subtypes, disease progression, and treatment response through analyzing the epigenetic landscape of tumors. The biomarkers are used for early detection, risk stratification, and monitoring of disease recurrence in a personalized medicine approach (Duncan et al., 2021).

Epigenetic profiling allows for the identification of predictive biomarkers that can inform treatment decisions and optimize therapeutic outcomes in HNC. For example, DNA methylation status or histone modification patterns may predict the response to specific chemotherapy agents, radiation therapy, or targeted therapies (Duncan et al., 2021). Incorporating epigenetic biomarkers into clinical practice enables clinicians to tailor treatment regimens to individual patients, maximizing efficacy while minimizing toxicity (Morselli & Dieci, 2022). Decrypting the epigenetic alterations driving HNC tumorigenesis opens avenues for the development of targeted epigenetic therapies. Small molecules targeting DNA methyltransferases (DNMTs), histone deacetylases (HDACs), or other epigenetic enzymes can reverse aberrant epigenetic modifications and restore normal gene expression patterns (Duncan et al., 2021). Epigenetic therapies have the potential to synergize with conventional treatments, such as chemotherapy and radiation therapy, and overcome treatment resistance in HNC (Diez-Fraile et al., 2020).

Integrating epigenetic information into clinical decision-making allows for the development of personalized treatment strategies tailored to the individual patient's epigenetic profile. Clinicians identify specific epigenetic alterations driving tumorigenesis and select targeted therapies or combination treatments to effectively inhibit tumor growth and metastasis through profiling the epigenome of tumors (Duncan et al., 2021). Personalized epigenetic-based therapies hold promise for improving patient outcomes and long-term survival in HNC. Epigenetic biomarkers (shown in Table 5.2) have been used in monitoring treatment response and disease progression in HNC, and serial assessment of DNA

Table 5.2 Examples of epigenetic biomarkers in head and neck cancer

Epigenetic biomarker	Roles and mechanisms	Implications for HNC	References
GAS5	Regulates cell cycle progression, apoptosis, and stress response. Upregulated during growth arrest	Dysregulation is linked to altered cell cycle regulation and apoptosis. Potential role in tumor growth and survival	Fayda et al., 2016; Lambrou et al., 2020
H19	Upregulation associated with tumor growth and advancement; role as a ceRNA. Promotes tumor growth and metastasis through HMGA2 upregulation. Targets miR-148a-3p; contributes to DNA methyltransferase 1 expression	Potential diagnostic marker. Prognostic implications for metastatic tumors. Induces cellular DNA methylation	Wu et al., 2016; Kou et al., 2019
CASC9	Implicated in cancer development; interacts with proteins and regulatory molecules	Upregulation linked to cancer emergence, migration, multiplication, and spread	Sassenberg et al., 2019; Sharma et al., 2020
AFAP1-AS1	Antisense to AFAP1 gene; involved in gene expression regulation. Interaction with various cellular components	Upregulation is associated with tumor progression, invasion, and poor prognosis. Potential role in cancer cell proliferation, migration, and metastasis	Li et al., 2021; Elabd et al., 2022
p16 Gene hypermethylation (CDKN2A/INK4a)	Tumor suppressor gene; hypermethylation leads to gene inactivation; early diagnosis, prognosis, potential therapeutic target	Biomarker for early diagnosis and prognosis; potential therapeutic target	Choudhury et al., 2018
DAPK gene hypermethylation	Associated with tumor progression, prognosis, response to therapy	Diagnostic and prognostic implications; guides treatment strategies.	Reis et al., 2020

(continued)

Table 5.2 Continued

Epigenetic biomarker	Roles and mechanisms	Implications for HNC	References
MALAT1	Abundant lncRNA; prevalent upregulation in primary tumors and metastatic tissues. STAT3 binding to promoter region; transcriptional activation. Targets p21 (RAC1) -activated kinase 1 (PAK1) through suppression of miR-140-5p	Potential diagnostic and prognostic marker. Influence on metastatic progression of HNC. Facilitates proliferation, migration, and invasion of TSCC cells	Wang et al., 2018; Zhu et al., 2019
RASSF1A gene hypermethylation	Tumor suppressor gene; hypermethylation leads to inactivation; associated with uncontrolled cell growth	Biomarker for disease detection, prognosis, and treatment response; linked to more aggressive tumor behavior	Kumari et al., 2023; Yang et al., 2023
KDM6	Affects gene transcription and cellular properties	Promising for prognostic assessment and therapeutic intervention	Al Labban et al., 2018
MGMT gene methylation	DNA repair enzyme; methylation silences gene; affects repair capacity; impacts response to DNA-damaging treatments	Predicts treatment outcomes and patient prognosis; sensitivity to alkylating agents like temozolomide	Yu et al., 2020
let-7 family	Tumor suppressor miRNAs; regulate normal cell differentiation and development	Reduced expression associated with carcinogenesis; potential diagnostic and therapeutic implications	Liao et al., 2016
KDM5	Modulates gene expression and biological processes	Considered for prognostic assessment and therapeutic intervention	Su et al., 2017
miRNA-29b	Decreases levels of three β- DNA methyltransferases; reactivates E-cadherin expression	Inhibition of DNA methyltransferases may contribute to invasiveness through promoter area demethylation	Chen et al., 2016

Table 5.2 Continued

Epigenetic biomarker	Roles and mechanisms	Implications for HNC	References
miRNA-125a	Suppresses p53 protein production; enhances proliferation and migration of cancer cells	Contributes to enhanced proliferation and migration of cancer cells	Huang et al., 2020
KDM4	Influences gene transcription and cellular functions	Potential role in prognostic assessment and therapeutic intervention	Zhang et al., 2021
miRNA-101	Downregulates rap1GAP, a tumor suppressor gene; affected by oncogene EZH2	Impacts head and neck malignancies through suppression of tumor suppressor gene expression	Banerjee et al., 2011

methylation patterns or histone modifications allows for real-time monitoring of tumor dynamics and adaptation to treatment (Diez-Fraile et al., 2020). Changes in epigenetic profiles during treatment serve as early indicators of treatment response or development of resistance, prompting adjustments to therapeutic regimens for optimal patient outcomes (Morselli & Dieci, 2022). Hence, epigenetics offers a wealth of opportunities for precision medicine in HNC, from biomarker discovery and diagnostic tools to targeted therapies and personalized treatment strategies. And clinicians can optimize treatment decisions, monitor treatment response, and improve patient outcomes in HNC through leveraging epigenetic information (Diez-Fraile et al., 2020).

5.5 Proteomics in Head and Neck Cancer

The proteomic landscape of HNC tumors offers valuable acumen into the molecular mechanisms underlying HNC. It helps researchers to identify molecular signatures, therapeutic targets, and predictive biomarkers that inform personalized treatment strategies as shown in Figure 5.3 (Jain et al., 2024). Proteomics involves the large-scale analysis of proteins expressed in HNC tumors, providing intuition into protein expression levels, post-translational modifications, and protein–protein interactions (Miserocchi et al., 2022). Techniques such as mass spectrometry and protein microarrays are used to identify and quantify proteins in HNC tissues and biological fluids. Proteomic

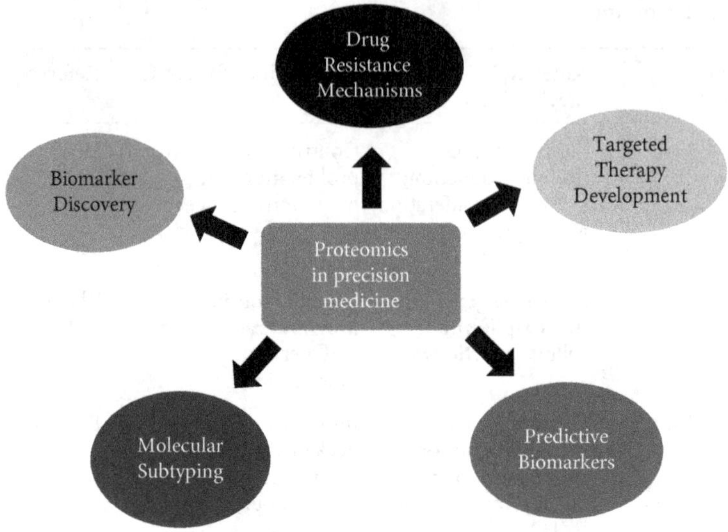

Figure 5.3 The role of proteomics in precision medicine in head and neck cancer (HNC). Proteomics plays a critical role in advancing our understanding of the molecular landscape of HNC and has important implications for diagnosis, prognosis, treatment selection, and therapeutic development. Researchers and clinicians can develop personalized treatment strategies tailored to the individual molecular profile of each patient by leveraging proteomic data, leading to improved outcomes and quality of life for HNC patients.

profiling identifies dysregulated signaling pathways and molecular targets for therapeutic intervention in HNC (Kwon et al., 2021). For example, aberrant activation of the EGFR signaling pathway in HNC has led to the development of EGFR-targeted therapies such as cetuximab. Proteomic biomarkers serve as prognostic indicators and predictors of treatment response in HNC patients, aiding in patient stratification and personalized treatment approaches (Miserocchi et al., 2022). Analysis of proteomic data enables the discovery of protein biomarkers associated with HNC diagnosis and prognosis. Researchers can identify proteins that are differentially expressed in HNC tumors through comparing the proteomic profiles of HNC patients with healthy individuals or patients with other diseases. The biomarkers are used for early detection, risk stratification, and monitoring of disease progression in HNC patients, leading to timely interventions and improved clinical outcomes (Jain et al., 2024).

Proteomic profiling in precision medicine allows for the molecular subtyping of HNC tumors based on protein expression patterns. Researchers have recently identified molecularly defined subtypes with unique biological characteristics and clinical outcomes by clustering tumors into distinct subgroups based on their proteomic profiles (Astradsson et al., 2022). Molecular subtyping facilitates personalized treatment strategies tailored to the molecular profile of individual tumors, leading to more effective and targeted therapies for HNC patients (Stögbauer et al., 2024). Proteomics provides acumen into the dysregulated signaling pathways and molecular networks driving HNC tumorigenesis and progression. Proteomic analysis guides the development of targeted therapies aimed at specific molecular targets through identifying key proteins and signaling pathways that are aberrantly activated or dysregulated in HNC (Zou et al., 2024). Targeted therapies, such as monoclonal antibodies or small-molecule inhibitors, can selectively inhibit the activity of oncogenic proteins or signaling pathways, leading to tumor regression and improved patient outcomes (Gougis et al., 2019).

Proteomic profiling in precision medicine enables the discovery of predictive biomarkers that can inform treatment decisions and predict patient responses to therapy. Over the years researchers have identified biomarkers associated with treatment response or resistance to chemotherapy, radiation therapy, targeted therapy, or immunotherapy through analyzing the protein expression profiles of HNC tumors (Mastronikolis et al., 2024). Studies identified 44 HNC-specific protein biomarkers involved in cell proliferation (STAT3, Repp86, SPARC, EGFR, CD151, CD9, VEGF, and SIRT2), cell cycle control (p53, PCNA, Ki-67, E2F1, cyclin D1, and PTEN), transcriptional repression (GLI3, Enhancer of zeste homolog 2 [EZH2], ER-β, SNAI1, and ZEB2), differentiation (extracellular matrix metalloproteinase inducer [EMMPRIN], LAMC2, and TWIST1), cell adhesion (E-CAD, CD44, and delta 1), inflammatory response (annexin A1, COX-2), binding of signaling proteins (14-3-3 γ), regulation of actin cytoskeleton (MENA), processing of tumor-associated proteins (TACE), and epithelial–mesenchymal transition (vimentin). Predictive biomarkers in precision medicine help clinicians personalize treatment regimens and optimize therapeutic outcomes for HNC patients (Kasradze et al., 2020).

Moreso, proteomic analysis provides insights into the molecular mechanisms underlying drug resistance in HNC. Researchers identify proteins or signaling pathways that mediate resistance to chemotherapy, targeted therapy, or immunotherapy by comparing the proteomic profiles of drug-sensitive and drug-resistant tumor cells (Mastronikolis et al., 2024). Deciphering the mechanisms of drug resistance allows for the development of strategies to overcome resistance and improve the efficacy of cancer treatments. Hence, proteomics holds great promise for advancing precision medicine in HNC by providing acumen into the molecular landscape of tumors and guiding personalized treatment strategies. Researchers and clinicians can develop tailored therapies that target the specific molecular vulnerabilities of individual tumors, leading to improved outcomes and quality of life for HNC patients by leveraging proteomic data (Wamsley et al., 2023).

5.6 Metabolomics in Head and Neck Cancer

Metabolomics provides a comprehensive understanding of the metabolic alterations associated with HNC. It is the study of small molecules or metabolites within biological systems. Leveraging metabolomic data significantly advances precision medicine approaches in HNC diagnosis, prognosis, treatment selection, and therapeutic development (Zhao et al., 2024). Metabolomic profiling allows for the identification of metabolic signatures or biomarkers that differentiate HNC patients from healthy individuals or those with benign conditions. Researchers can identify specific metabolites that are dysregulated in HNC by analyzing the metabolite profiles of patient samples, such as blood, saliva, or tissue (Boguszewicz et al., 2024). The metabolite biomarkers hold promise for early detection, accurate diagnosis, and monitoring of disease progression in HNC patients. Metabolomic profiling and analysis in precision medicine help predict patient responses to therapy and identify metabolic signatures associated with treatment resistance or sensitivity (Zhao et al., 2024). Researchers have identified metabolic changes that correlate with treatment response or resistance by analyzing the metabolite profiles of HNC tumors or patient biofluids before and after treatment. Thus, predictive biomarkers enable clinicians to personalize treatment regimens and optimize therapeutic outcomes for HNC patients (Chuchueva et al., 2023).

Metabolomics also provides acumen into the metabolic rewiring that occurs in HNC tumors to support their growth, survival, and metastasis. Previous research has elucidated metabolic pathways and processes that are dysregulated in HNC through profiling the metabolite composition of tumor tissues or biofluids (Zhao et al., 2024). Deciphering tumor metabolism at a molecular level allows for the identification of metabolic vulnerabilities that can be targeted for therapeutic intervention. Integrating metabolomic data with other omics data, such as genomic, transcriptomic, and proteomic data, enables the development of personalized treatment strategies for HNC patients (Chuchueva et al., 2023). Reports have highlighted that clinicians tailor treatment regimens to target specific metabolic vulnerabilities or pathways that are dysregulated in each patient's tumor by considering the metabolic profile of individual tumors. In that context, personalized metabolic therapies hold promise for improving treatment outcomes and patient survival in HNC (Boguszewicz et al., 2024).

Metabolomic studies provide mechanistic intuition into the effects of therapeutic agents on tumor metabolism and the tumor microenvironment. Research has identified novel drug targets and developed new therapeutic interventions through studying how drugs or targeted therapies modulate metabolic pathways and metabolite levels in HNC tumors (Chuchueva et al., 2023). Metabolomic approaches in precision medicine facilitate the discovery of metabolic inhibitors or modulators that selectively target metabolic vulnerabilities in HNC tumors. On that note, metabolomics offers a powerful tool for advancing precision medicine in HNC and provides acumen into tumor metabolism, identifying biomarkers for diagnosis and treatment response prediction and guiding personalized treatment strategies (Zhao et al., 2024). Researchers have developed targeted therapies that exploit the metabolic vulnerabilities of individual tumors, leading to improved outcomes and quality of life for HNC patients through leveraging metabolomic data (Boguszewicz et al., 2024).

5.7 Immunomics in Head and Neck Cancer

Immunomics offers promising avenues for HNC management. It informs personalized treatment strategies tailored to individual patient characteristics by analyzing the complex interplay between the immune system and tumors (Okano, 2024). Immunomics is the comprehensive study of the immune system and its interactions with tumors. It enables comprehensive profiling of the immune landscape within HNC tumors and the tumor microenvironment. Researchers have gained insights into the immune context of HNC tumors and identified potential targets for immunotherapy through characterization of immune cell populations, cytokine profiles, and immune checkpoint expression patterns (Wang et al., 2024). The study of the immune system and its interactions with tumors has facilitated the discovery of immune-related biomarkers that aid in HNC diagnosis, prognosis, and treatment response prediction (Table 5.3) (Sun et al., 2024).

Biomarkers that correlate with clinical outcomes and guide patient stratification for personalized treatment approaches have been identified through analyzing immune cell signatures, cytokine profiles, or immune checkpoint expression levels (Sun et al., 2024). Immunomic biomarkers improve diagnostic accuracy by providing information about the immune landscape of the tumor. These biomarkers can help predict patient outcomes and stratify patients based on their risk. Immunomic biomarkers are critical for identifying patients who are likely to benefit from immunotherapies, thus enabling personalized treatment plans. They can be used to monitor treatment response and detect early signs of recurrence, guiding clinical decision-making (Wang et al., 2024).

In precision medicine, immunomics data are used to develop predictive models for patient responses to immunotherapy in HNC (Wang et al., 2024).

Table 5.3 Examples of notable immunomic biomarkers associated with head and neck cancer

Immunomic biomarkers	Role	Significance	Reference
PD-L1 expression	Programmed death-ligand 1 (PD-L1) on tumor cells and immune cells	High PD-L1 expression is associated with immune evasion by the tumor and can predict response to immune checkpoint inhibitors like pembrolizumab and nivolumab.	Wang et al., 2024
Tumor-infiltrating lymphocytes (TILs)	Presence and types of lymphocytes within the tumor microenvironment	High levels of TILs, particularly $CD8^+$ cytotoxic T cells, are associated with better prognosis and response to immunotherapy.	Sun et al., 2024
$CD8^+$ T cells	Cytotoxic T cells involved in the anti-tumor immune response	Increased infiltration of $CD8^+$ T cells in the tumor microenvironment is linked to improved patient outcomes and response to immunotherapy.	Sun et al., 2024
$FOXP3^+$ regulatory T cells (Tregs)	Immunosuppressive T cells that regulate immune responses	High levels of $FOXP3^+$ Tregs in the tumor microenvironment are generally associated with poor prognosis due to their role in suppressing anti-tumor immunity.	Wang et al., 2024
Myeloid-derived suppressor cells (MDSCs)	Immunosuppressive cells that inhibit T cell responses	Elevated levels of MDSCs in the blood and tumor microenvironment correlate with poor prognosis and resistance to immunotherapy.	Sun et al., 2024
Immune checkpoint molecules	Proteins that regulate immune responses	Expression of molecules like CTLA-4, TIM-3, and LAG-3 can influence immune evasion and therapeutic response. They are potential targets for immune checkpoint inhibitors.	Wang et al., 2024
Cytokine profiles	Signaling proteins involved in immune responses	Elevated levels of pro-inflammatory cytokines (e.g., IL-6, IL-8, TNF-α) and anti-inflammatory cytokines (e.g., IL-10) can indicate tumor-induced immune modulation and are associated with disease progression and prognosis.	Sun et al., 2024

Table 5.3 Continued

Immunomic biomarkers	Role	Significance	Reference
Human leukocyte antigen (HLA) expression	Molecules involved in antigen presentation to T cells	Altered expression of HLA class I and II molecules can affect tumor immunogenicity and response to immunotherapy.	Sun et al., 2024
Immune gene expression signatures	Gene expression profiles related to immune responses	Specific immune-related gene signatures, such as those identified through RNA sequencing or microarray analysis, can predict patient prognosis and response to immunotherapy.	Wang et al., 2024
Exosome-derived immune biomarkers	Immune-related molecules packaged in exosomes	Exosomes containing immune checkpoint molecules (e.g., PD-L1) or immune-modulating proteins can provide insights into tumor immune evasion mechanisms and potential therapeutic targets.	Sun et al., 2024
Tumor mutational burden (TMB)	Total number of mutations within the tumor genome	High TMB is often associated with increased neoantigen load and better response to immunotherapy, serving as a predictive biomarker.	Sun et al., 2024
Neoantigens	Tumor-specific antigens resulting from somatic mutations	Presence of neoantigens can enhance tumor immunogenicity and predict response to immune-based therapies.	Sun et al., 2024
Immune cell ratios	Ratios of different immune cell types	Ratios such as $CD8^+$/Treg and $CD8^+$/MDSC can provide insights into the immune landscape of the tumor and its potential response to immunotherapy.	Wang et al., 2024
Microsatellite instability (MSI)	Genetic hypermutability resulting from impaired DNA mismatch repair	MSI-high tumors are often more responsive to immunotherapy and can serve as a predictive biomarker.	Sun et al., 2024

Researchers identify immune signatures associated with favorable or adverse responses to immunotherapy through integrating immune profiles with clinical and genomic data. These predictive models enable clinicians to select the most appropriate immunotherapy regimen for individual patients, maximizing treatment efficacy and minimizing adverse effects (Sun et al., 2024). Immunomics provides intuition into the immunosuppressive mechanisms employed by HNC tumors and informs the development of immunomodulatory therapies to enhance antitumor immune responses. Researchers can develop combination therapies that synergize with immunotherapy and overcome treatment resistance through targeting immune checkpoints, inhibitory cytokines, and regulatory immune cell populations (Wang et al., 2024).

Integrating immunomics data with other omics data, such as genomic and transcriptomic profiles, enables the development of personalized immunotherapy approaches for HNC patients. Clinicians can tailor immunotherapy regimens to maximize therapeutic efficacy and minimize adverse effects by considering the immune landscape and tumor-specific characteristics of individual patients (Wang et al., 2024). Immunomics allows for the monitoring of immune responses during treatment and disease progression in HNC patients. According to Okano (2024), clinicians can assess treatment efficacy, detect treatment resistance, and make informed decisions regarding treatment adjustments or combination therapies by tracking changes in immune cell populations, cytokine levels, or immune checkpoint expression over time. Thus, immunomics holds great promise for advancing precision medicine in HNC by providing intuition into the complex interplay between the immune system and tumors. Personalized immunotherapy approaches that target the specific immune characteristics of individual tumors and lead to improved treatment outcomes and patient survival in HNC can be developed through leveraging immunomic data (Sun et al., 2024).

5.8 Glycomics in Head and Neck Cancer

Glycomics presents a promising avenue for advancing precision medicine in HNC. It is the study of glycans or complex sugar molecules. Glycomics informs personalized treatment strategies tailored to individual patient characteristics by elucidating the glycan structures and glycosylation patterns associated with HNC (Ma et al., 2024). The analysis of glycomics profiles of HNC patients helps identify specific glycan structures or glycosylation patterns that are associated with disease progression, treatment response, or patient outcomes. It enables the identification of glycan-based biomarkers (summarized in Table 5.4) that can serve as diagnostic, prognostic, or predictive indicators in HNC (Ren et al.,

Table 5.4 Glycomic biomarkers used in head and neck cancer

Glycomic biomarker	Role	Significance
Sialylated glycans	Involved in cell–cell interactions and immune evasion	Increased sialylation, especially α2,3- and α2,6-linked sialic acids, has been observed in head and neck cancer. These modifications can facilitate tumor progression and metastasis by promoting immune evasion and altering cell adhesion.
Fucosylated glycans	Participates in cell adhesion, signaling, and immune responses	Elevated levels of fucosylation, particularly core fucosylation and Lewis antigens (e.g., sLe^x, sLe^a), are associated with head and neck cancer. These changes can enhance cell signaling and metastatic potential.
N-glycan branching	Affects protein folding, stability, and cell surface interactions	Increased branching of N-glycans, often due to upregulation of enzymes such as N-acetylglucosaminyltransferases (e.g., GnT-V), is linked to head and neck cancer. This can contribute to enhanced cell growth, migration, and invasion.
O-glycans and mucin-type glycans	Implicated in mucosal protection and signaling	Altered O-glycosylation patterns, including changes in mucin-type glycans (e.g., MUC1, MUC4), are common in head and neck cancers. These modifications can influence tumor cell adhesion, immune evasion, and metastatic behavior.
Sulfated glycans	Involved in cellular signaling and extracellular matrix interactions	Changes in sulfation patterns, particularly in glycosaminoglycans (e.g., heparan sulfate, chondroitin sulfate), have been observed in head and neck cancer. These alterations can affect tumor growth and metastasis.
Glycosyltransferase enzymes	Catalyze the addition of sugar moieties to proteins and lipids	Overexpression or altered activity of glycosyltransferases, such as ST3GAL1 (sialyltransferase) and FUT8 (fucosyltransferase), is associated with head and neck cancer. These enzymes drive the glycosylation changes seen in cancer cells.

(continued)

Table 5.4 Continued

Glycomic biomarker	Role	Significance
Gangliosides	Glycosphingolipids involved in cell signaling and membrane organization	Abnormal expression of gangliosides (e.g., GM3, GD2) is linked to head and neck cancer. These molecules can modulate cell signaling pathways and immune responses.
Lectin binding patterns	Reflects the glycan composition of cells	Changes in lectin binding patterns, detected using glycan microarrays or lectin histochemistry, can serve as biomarkers for head and neck cancer. These patterns reveal alterations in glycan structures on cancer cells.
Glycoproteins	Proteins with attached glycans that play roles in cell-cell communication and signaling	Altered glycosylation of specific glycoproteins, such as EGFR and integrins, is linked to head and neck cancer. These changes can influence receptor function and downstream signaling pathways.
Aberrant glycosylation of tumor antigens	Can be recognized by the immune system as abnormal	Tumor-associated glycoforms of antigens, such as CA19-9 (a sialyl-Lewis antigen) and Tn antigen, are found in head and neck cancer. These can serve as biomarkers for disease detection and monitoring.

Source: Carnielli et al., 2023.

2024). Glycan biomarkers also have the potential to improve early detection, risk stratification, and monitoring of disease progression in HNC patients (Ma et al., 2024). They enhance the accuracy of cancer diagnosis through blood tests, tissue biopsies, and noninvasive imaging techniques. Certain glycomic changes correlate with tumor aggressiveness, metastatic potential, and patient outcomes. Glycans and glycosylation enzymes offer potential targets for novel therapeutic strategies, including glycan-based vaccines and inhibitors of glycosylation pathways (Lin et al., 2024). Glycomics research provides intuition into the aberrant glycosylation patterns observed in HNC tumors, which can serve as therapeutic targets for personalized treatment approaches (Rasheduzzaman et al., 2020).

Researchers develop glycan-targeted therapies aimed at inhibiting tumor growth, metastasis, or immune evasion through targeting tumor-specific glycans or glycoproteins. Glycan-targeted therapies have the potential to complement existing treatment modalities and improve treatment outcomes for HNC patients (Ren et al., 2024). Glycomics allows for the comprehensive characterization of the glycan profiles of HNC tumors and the surrounding microenvironment. Researchers elucidate glycomic changes associated with tumor progression, metastasis, and treatment resistance by profiling the expression levels and structures of glycans on tumor cells (Lin et al., 2024). Deciphering the tumor glycan profile may reveal novel therapeutic targets and mechanisms underlying HNC pathogenesis (Carnielli et al., 2023). Glycomics studies uncover immunomodulatory glycan structures that regulate immune responses within the tumor microenvironment of HNC. Aberrant glycosylation patterns on tumor cells influence immune cell interactions and immune evasion mechanisms. Targeting immunomodulatory glycans enhances antitumor immune responses and improves immunotherapy outcomes in HNC (Rasheduzzaman et al., 2022).

The integration of glycomic data with other omics data, such as genomic, proteomic, and metabolomic profiles, enables the development of personalized treatment strategies for HNC patients (Xie et al., 2024). Clinicians can tailor treatment regimens to target specific glycan-related vulnerabilities or pathways that are dysregulated in each patient's tumor through considering the glycomic profile of individual tumors. Personalized glycan-targeted therapies improve treatment efficacy and patient outcomes in HNC (Rasheduzzaman et al., 2022). Thus, glycomics holds great promise for advancing precision medicine in HNC, leading to improved outcomes and quality of life for HNC patients (Carnielli et al., 2023).

5.9 Microbiomics in Head and Neck Cancer

Microbiomics, the study of microbial communities within the human body, offers promising opportunities for advancing precision medicine in HNC. Microbiomic approaches inform personalized treatment strategies tailored to individual patient characteristics by examining the complex interactions between the oral microbiome and HNC development (Desai, 2023). Microbiomic analysis allows for comprehensive profiling of the oral microbiome in HNC patients, identifying specific microbial taxa, community structures, and functional gene pathways associated with disease progression. Microbial signatures that correlate with tumor stage, grade, or clinical outcomes are identified by comparing the oral microbiome composition of HNC patients with healthy individuals (Dorobisz et al., 2023). Microbiomic studies uncover microbial biomarkers that serve as diagnostic, prognostic, or predictive indicators in HNC. Researchers have identified microbial signatures that distinguish HNC patients from healthy individuals or predict treatment responses by analyzing microbial taxa or gene expression patterns (Desai, 2023).

Over the years, microbial biomarkers have been exploited to complement existing clinical parameters and imaging modalities, improving HNC diagnosis and treatment decision-making (Desai, 2023). Table 5.5 provides a list of microbiomic biomarkers in HNC. Microbiomic biomarkers enhance diagnostic accuracy through noninvasive sampling of saliva, oral swabs, or tissue biopsies (Yalamarty et al., 2024). Specific microbial signatures can provide prognostic information regarding tumor aggressiveness, metastatic potential, and patient outcomes. Modulating the microbiome through probiotics, antibiotics, or microbiome transplants could offer novel therapeutic strategies for head and neck cancer (Godbole & Singh, 2023).

Microbiomics provides intuition into the dynamic interactions between the oral microbiome, host immune system, and tumor microenvironment in HNC. Microbiomic studies inform the development of immunomodulatory interventions or combination therapies for HNC through elucidating microbial factors that modulate immune responses, tumor cell proliferation, and treatment outcomes (Makarewicz et al., 2024). Decrypting microbiome–host interactions may reveal novel therapeutic targets and mechanisms underlying HNC pathogenesis. Manipulation of the oral microbiome holds therapeutic potential for preventing or treating HNC (Dorobisz et al., 2023). Probiotics, prebiotics, antibiotics, or microbial-based therapies are utilized to modulate the composition and function of the oral microbiome to promote host immune responses, suppress pathogenic bacteria, or enhance treatment efficacy in HNC. Moreso, microbiome-targeted approaches are a vital arsenal to inform the development of microbiome-targeted interventions as adjuvant or complementary therapies for HNC management (Galeana-Patiño et al., 2023).

On that note, integrating microbiomic data with other omics and clinical parameters enables the development of personalized treatment strategies for HNC patients (Makarewicz et al., 2024). Clinicians have tailored treatment regimens to target specific microbial vulnerabilities or pathways that are dysregulated in each patient's tumor by considering the oral microbiome profile of individual patients (Galeana-Patiño et al., 2023). Personalized microbiome-targeted therapies have the potential to improve treatment outcomes and patient survival in HNC (Dorobisz et al., 2023). Thus, microbiomics holds great promise for advancing precision medicine in HNC by providing insights into the role of the oral microbiome in HNC development and progression (Dorobisz et al., 2023). Personalized treatment strategies that target the specific microbial characteristics of individual tumors by leveraging microbiomic data have been developed, leading to improved outcomes and quality of life for HNC patients (Makarewicz et al., 2024).

Table 5.5 List of microbiomic biomarkers in head and neck cancer

Microbial biomarkers	Role	Significance	References
Human papillomavirus (HPV)	Oncogenic virus	HPV, especially types 16 and 18, is strongly associated with oropharyngeal cancers. HPV status is a key biomarker for prognosis and treatment planning.	Yalamarty et al., 2024
Fusobacterium nucleatum	Gram-negative anaerobic bacterium	Increased presence of *Fusobacterium nucleatum* is associated with head and neck squamous cell carcinoma (HNSCC). It may promote inflammation, immune evasion, and tumor progression	Makarewicz et al., 2024
Porphyromonas gingivalis	Gram-negative anaerobic bacterium involved in periodontal disease	Elevated levels of *Porphyromonas gingivalis* have been found in oral squamous cell carcinoma (OSCC) and are linked to chronic inflammation and carcinogenesis.	Makarewicz et al., 2024
Treponema denticola	Spirochete bacterium associated with periodontal disease	Increased abundance of *Treponema denticola* has been observed in head and neck cancers, potentially contributing to carcinogenesis through chronic inflammation and tissue damage.	Yalamarty et al., 2024
Candida species	Fungal organisms, particularly *C. albicans*	Overgrowth of *Candida* species is common in head and neck cancer patients, potentially contributing to carcinogenesis through inflammatory pathways and the production of carcinogenic byproducts.	Yalamarty et al., 2024
Capnocytophaga species	Gram-negative bacteria involved in periodontal health	Changes in *Capnocytophaga* species levels have been associated with head and neck cancers, suggesting a role in the oral microbiome's shift towards a pathogenic state.	Makarewicz et al., 2024
Streptococcus species	Gram-positive bacteria	Certain *Streptococcus* species, like *S. anginosus*, have been linked to head and neck cancers, possibly due to their ability to induce inflammation and DNA damage	Yalamarty et al., 2024

(*continued*)

Table 5.5 Continued

Microbial biomarkers	Role	Significance	References
Prevotella species	Gram-negative anaerobic bacteria	Altered levels of *Prevotella* species are associated with head and neck cancers, likely through mechanisms involving inflammation and immune modulation.	Makarewicz et al., 2024
Veillonella species	Gram-negative anaerobic bacteria	Increased abundance of *Veillonella* species has been noted in head and neck cancers, potentially playing a role in modulating the immune environment and promoting carcinogenesis.	Yalamarty et al., 2024
Actinomyces species	Gram-positive bacteria involved in oral health	Shifts in *Actinomyces* species populations have been observed in head and neck cancer patients, possibly contributing to a carcinogenic oral environment	Yalamarty et al., 2024
Neisseria species	Gram-negative bacteria	Certain *Neisseria* species have shown altered levels in head and neck cancer patients, indicating a potential role in the microbial dysbiosis associated with cancer development.	Makarewicz et al., 2024
Lactobacillus species	Gram-positive bacteria commonly found in the oral cavity	Decreased levels of beneficial *Lactobacillus* species have been linked to head and neck cancer, suggesting that a loss of protective oral microbiota may facilitate carcinogenesis.	Yalamarty et al., 2024
Pseudomonas aeruginosa	Opportunistic pathogen	Presence of *Pseudomonas aeruginosa* in the oral microbiome has been associated with head and neck cancers, potentially through mechanisms involving biofilm formation and chronic infection.	Makarewicz et al., 2024

5.10 Fluidomics in Head and Neck Cancer

Advancing precision medicine through fluidomics has been a promising avenue in HNC management. Fluidomics is the comprehensive analysis of biomolecules in body fluids. It provides valuable acumen into disease biology, patient stratification, and treatment response by examining molecular signatures present in blood, saliva, urine, and other fluids (Kaczor-Urbanowicz et al., 2017). The analysis of biomolecules in body fluids enables the discovery of biomolecules, such as proteins, nucleic acids, metabolites, and extracellular vesicles, that serve as diagnostic, prognostic, and predictive markers in HNC (Liu et al., 2023). Fluidomics guides personalized treatment decisions and improves patient outcomes by identifying specific biomolecular signatures associated with disease status, progression, or treatment response (Patel et al., 2022).

Fluidomics offers noninvasive methods for monitoring disease dynamics and treatment response through liquid biopsies. Liquid biopsies can detect circulating tumor DNA (ctDNA), circulating tumor cells (CTCs), and tumor-derived exosomes containing nucleic acids and proteins shed from primary and metastatic HNC lesions (Liu et al., 2023). Detection of molecular alterations such as mutations, copy number variations, and epigenetic changes in ctDNA and other circulating tumor components aid in early cancer detection, especially in cases where tissue biopsy is challenging or inconclusive. Analysis of ctDNA and CTCs in liquid biopsies provides valuable prognostic information, including tumor burden, disease stage, and risk of recurrence or metastasis (Aulakh et al., 2022). Molecular profiling of circulating tumor components is an indispensable tool to identify biomarkers associated with aggressive tumor behavior, treatment resistance, and poor clinical outcomes, thus enabling risk stratification and personalized management strategies (Patel et al., 2022).

Fluidomic biomarkers offer a noninvasive or minimally invasive approach to cancer detection and monitoring, improving patient comfort and compliance (Patel et al., 2022). Table 5.6 provides a list of notable fluidomic biomarkers associated with HNC. Early detection through fluid biomarkers can lead to better outcomes by allowing timely intervention. Biomarkers help tailor personalized treatment plans based on the molecular characteristics of the cancer. Regular monitoring of biomarkers can provide insights into disease progression, treatment response, and recurrence (Wishart et al., 2024). Liquid biopsies have also been utilized in real-time monitoring of tumor dynamics and treatment response during the course of therapy, facilitating early detection of treatment resistance and disease progression (Patel et al., 2022).

Molecular profiling of ctDNA and other circulating tumor components guide treatment selection by identifying actionable mutations, predicting response to targeted therapies, and monitoring the emergence of resistance mutations (Huang et al., 2023). Serial analysis of liquid biopsies over time helps optimize treatment regimens, adjust therapeutic interventions, and improve patient outcomes by adapting treatment strategies based on evolving tumor biology (Iams et al., 2024). Huang and coworkers highlighted that liquid biopsies offer minimally invasive approaches for serial monitoring of disease progression and treatment response, reducing the need for repeated tissue biopsies and

Table 5.6 List of notable fluidomic biomarkers associated with head and neck cancer

Fluidomic biomarkers	Role	Significance
Circulating tumor DNA (ctDNA)	Fragments of DNA released from tumor cells into the bloodstream	ctDNA can carry specific mutations, such as those in TP53, EGFR, or PIK3CA, providing a noninvasive way to detect and monitor head and neck cancer
Human papillomavirus (HPV) DNA	Viral DNA from oncogenic HPV types, especially HPV16 and HPV18	Presence of HPV DNA in saliva or blood is a significant biomarker for HPV-related oropharyngeal cancers, aiding in diagnosis and prognosis.
Exosomes	Small extracellular vesicles containing proteins, RNAs, and lipids	Exosomes from head and neck cancer patients can contain tumor-specific proteins and RNAs, providing insights into tumor biology and potential targets for therapy.
MicroRNAs (miRNAs)	Small non-coding RNAs involved in gene regulation	Altered levels of specific miRNAs (e.g., miR-21, miR-31, miR-99a) in blood or saliva are associated with head and neck cancer, serving as potential diagnostic and prognostic biomarkers.
Circulating tumor cells (CTCs)	Cancer cells that have shed from the primary tumor into the bloodstream	Detection and enumeration of CTCs can provide information on the presence and progression of head and neck cancer, and their genetic analysis can guide treatment decisions
Cytokines and chemokines	Signaling molecules involved in inflammation and immune responses	Elevated levels of cytokines (e.g., IL-6, TNF-α) and chemokines in blood can indicate an inflammatory response associated with head and neck cancer, potentially serving as biomarkers for disease activity and prognosis.
Proteomic biomarkers	Specific proteins detectable in bodily fluids	Proteins such as SCC antigen, CYFRA 21-1, and matrix metalloproteinases (MMPs) in blood or saliva are associated with head and neck cancer, aiding in diagnosis and monitoring.
Metabolomic biomarkers	Small molecules (metabolites) involved in metabolism	Altered levels of metabolites like lactate, glutamine, and amino acids in blood or saliva can reflect metabolic changes in head and neck cancer, serving as potential biomarkers for diagnosis and prognosis.

Table 5.6 Continued

Fluidomic biomarkers	Role	Significance
Cell-free RNA (cfRNA)	RNA molecules released from tumor cells into the bloodstream	Detection of tumor-specific cfRNA in blood can provide insights into gene expression profiles of head and neck cancers, offering potential for diagnosis and monitoring.
Autoantibodies	Antibodies produced by the immune system against tumor-associated antigens	Presence of specific autoantibodies in blood can indicate an immune response to head and neck cancer, providing potential biomarkers for early detection and prognosis.
Tumor markers	Substances produced by cancer cells or by the body in response to cancer	Elevated levels of squamous cell carcinoma antigen (SCC-Ag) in blood correlate with tumor burden and prognosis. Increased levels of carcinoembryonic antigen (CEA) can indicate presence and progression of head and neck cancers. Cytokeratin fragment 21-1 (CYFRA 21-1) is associated with squamous cell carcinoma of the head and neck.
Salivary biomarkers	Various molecules detectable in saliva	The presence of HPV DNA indicates HPV-related oropharyngeal cancer. Changes in levels of specific miRNAs can be used for diagnosis and monitoring. Specific protein profiles in saliva can indicate head and neck cancer.

Source: Kunhabdulla et al., 2024.

associated patient discomfort in HNC (Huang et al., 2023). Regular surveillance using liquid biopsies enables early detection of recurrence, metastasis, or treatment-related complications, facilitating timely intervention and improving patient outcomes. Fluidomics provides real-time information on tumor burden, genetic alterations, and treatment resistance in HNC patients by analyzing ctDNA, CTCs, or tumor-derived exosomes in peripheral blood or other body fluids (Huang et al., 2023; Iams et al., 2024).

Fluidomic profiling allows for the characterization of molecular alterations in HNC tumors and the systemic effects of tumor–host interactions (Huang et al., 2023). It can identify dysregulated pathways, molecular subtypes, and therapeutic targets that inform personalized treatment strategies for HNC patients by analyzing the proteomic, genomic, transcriptomic, and metabolomic profiles of body fluids (Huang et al., 2023; Iams et al., 2024). Fluidomics facilitates the monitoring of treatment response and disease progression in HNC patients. The changes in the abundance or composition of biomolecules in body fluids serve as surrogate endpoints for assessing treatment efficacy, detecting disease recurrence, and guiding therapeutic interventions (Iams et al., 2024). Thus, the utilization of fluidomic biomarkers is vital to tailor treatment regimens based on individual patient responses and disease dynamics (Rapado-González et al., 2023).

Personalized treatment approaches for HNC patients have been further improved over the years by integrating fluidomic data with other omics and clinical parameters. Clinicians have optimized treatment selection, dosage, and timing to maximize therapeutic efficacy and minimize adverse effects by considering the molecular profile of body fluids (Rapado-González et al., 2023). Fluidomics-guided precision medicine improves treatment outcomes and enhances patient care in HNC. Hence, fluidomics holds great promise for advancing precision medicine in HNC by providing insights into disease biology, patient stratification, and treatment response (Huang et al., 2023). Fluidomic analysis enables personalized treatment strategies tailored to individual patient characteristics, ultimately improving patient outcomes and quality of life in HNC by leveraging the diverse array of biomolecules present in body fluids (Huang et al., 2023; Iams et al., 2024).

5.11 Infornomics in Head and Neck Cancer

Infornomics offers a powerful approach to advancing precision medicine in HNC. It is the integration of information science, bioinformatics, and computational biology. Infornomics enables the analysis of complex datasets from multiple sources, including genomics, imaging, clinical records, and population-level data through harnessing the power of big data analytics, machine learning algorithms, and computational modeling techniques (Miserocchi et al., 2022). This comprehensive approach holds immense promise for improving diagnosis, prognosis, and treatment planning in HNC. Infornomics facilitates the integration of multiomics data, including genomics, transcriptomics, proteomics, metabolomics, and microbiomics, to provide a comprehensive understanding of tumor biology and heterogeneity. It enables the identification of key genetic alterations, signaling pathways, and molecular subtypes associated with HNC progression and treatment response by analyzing multiple layers of molecular information (Kaidar-Person et al., 2018).

Infornomics-driven approaches facilitate the discovery and validation of biomarkers for early detection, prognostication, and treatment response prediction in HNC (Lee, Johnson et al., 2023). Infornomics identifies candidate biomarkers associated with tumor biology, immune status, and treatment outcomes by analyzing large-scale datasets from patient cohorts and public repositories. The biomarkers (Table 5.7) serve as valuable predictors of patient prognosis and guide personalized treatment decisions in clinical practice (Jayawickrama et al., 2024). Infornomics enables the development of predictive models and risk stratification algorithms to identify patients at high risk of disease progression, recurrence, or treatment resistance. Infornomics-driven models predict patient outcomes, such as overall survival, progression-free survival, and treatment response, thus facilitating personalized treatment planning and patient counseling by integrating clinical, molecular, and imaging data (Lee et al., 2023).

Infornomics-driven approaches accelerate drug discovery and development by identifying novel therapeutic targets, predictive biomarkers, and combination treatment strategies for HNC (Lee et al., 2023). Infornomic biomarkers enable tailored treatment strategies based on the molecular profile of the patient's tumor. Advanced bioinformatics approaches can identify biomarkers for early detection, thus improving survival rates (Jayawickrama et al., 2024). Infornomic biomarkers provide insights into disease progression and treatment response, aiding in prognosis and monitoring. Identification of molecular targets through infornomic biomarkers can lead to the development of targeted therapies, improving treatment efficacy and reducing side effects (Lee et al., 2023). Hence, infornomic biomarkers represent a powerful tool in the management of HNC, leveraging the capabilities of computational biology and bioinformatics to extract meaningful insights from complex biological data (Jayawickrama et al., 2024).

The integration of information science, bioinformatics, and computational biology facilitates the selection of targeted therapies, immunotherapies, and precision medicine approaches tailored to individual patient characteristics and tumor biology through analyzing molecular pathways, drug interactions, and drug response profiles (Jayawickrama et al., 2024; Lee et al., 2023). It contributes to the development of clinical decision support systems (CDSS) that integrate multidimensional data to assist clinicians in making evidence-based treatment decisions (Lee et al., 2023). CDSS improves treatment planning, optimizes resource allocation, and enhances patient outcomes in HNC care through providing real-time access to patient-specific information, treatment guidelines, and predictive analytics (Miserocchi et al., 2022). Thus, infornomics holds great promise for advancing precision medicine in HNC by integrating multidimensional data, identifying biomarkers, predicting patient outcomes, and guiding personalized treatment decisions (Lee et al., 2023). It transforms the way we understand, diagnose, and treat HNC, ultimately improving patient outcomes

Table 5.7 List of infornomic biomarkers associated with head and neck cancer

Infornomic biomarkers	Role	Significance
Genomic alterations identified by NGS (next-generation sequencing)	Somatic mutations, copy number variations, and structural rearrangements	Comprehensive genomic profiling can identify key mutations (e.g., TP53, PIK3CA, EGFR) that drive head and neck cancer. These alterations can serve as diagnostic, prognostic, and therapeutic biomarkers.
Transcriptomic signatures from RNA-Seq	Differentially expressed genes and splicing variants	RNA sequencing can reveal gene expression patterns specific to head and neck cancer. Overexpression of genes like CCND1, CDK6, and HPV-related transcripts can serve as biomarkers for diagnosis and prognosis.
MicroRNA profiles from miRNA-Seq	Small noncoding RNAs involved in gene regulation	Altered microRNA expression profiles (e.g., miR-21, miR-31, miR-375) identified through high-throughput sequencing can be used as biomarkers for early detection, prognosis, and therapeutic targets.
Proteomic patterns from mass spectrometry	Protein expression and post-translational modifications	Mass spectrometry-based proteomics can identify protein expression signatures and modifications unique to head and neck cancer. Proteins like MMPs, EGFR, and p16 can serve as biomarkers for disease characterization and treatment response.
Epigenomic alterations from methylation sequencing	DNA methylation and histone modifications	Changes in DNA methylation patterns (e.g., hypermethylation of tumor suppressor genes like CDKN2A) can be identified through bisulfite sequencing and serve as biomarkers for diagnosis, prognosis, and therapeutic strategies.
Metabolomic profiles from mass spectrometry or NMR	Metabolites and metabolic pathways	Metabolomic analyses can identify altered metabolic pathways in head and neck cancer. Specific metabolites, such as lactate, glutamine, and certain amino acids, can serve as biomarkers for disease progression and treatment response.
Network biomarkers from systems biology approaches	Interaction networks and pathway analysis	Systems biology approaches can integrate multiomics data to identify key regulatory networks and pathways involved in head and neck cancer. Dysregulated pathways like PI3K/AKT/mTOR and EGFR signaling can serve as biomarkers for targeted therapies.

Table 5.7 Continued

Infornomic biomarkers	Role	Significance
Liquid biopsy data integration	ctDNA, exosomes, and CTCs in blood or saliva	Integrative analysis of liquid biopsy data using computational tools can provide comprehensive biomarkers for real-time monitoring of tumor dynamics and treatment efficacy.
Multiomics integration	Combined analysis of genomics, transcriptomics, proteomics, and metabolomics	Integrating data from multiple omics layers can reveal holistic biomarkers that capture the complexity of head and neck cancer biology. Multi-omics approaches can identify robust biomarkers for personalized medicine.
Artificial intelligence and machine learning models	Predictive models and pattern recognition	AI and machine learning algorithms can analyze large-scale omics data to identify predictive biomarkers for head and neck cancer. These models can enhance diagnostic accuracy, prognostic assessments, and treatment planning.

Source: Basheeth & Patil, 2019.

and quality of life in the era of precision oncology by leveraging big data analytics, machine learning algorithms, and computational modeling techniques (Jayawickrama et al., 2024).

5.12 Radiomics in Head and Neck Cancer

Radiomics, a burgeoning field at the intersection of medical imaging, computational biology, and machine learning, has emerged as a powerful tool in the management of HNC. Radiomics enables the noninvasive characterization of tumor phenotype, microenvironment, and treatment response through extracting quantitative imaging features from standard medical images, such as computed tomography (CT), magnetic resonance imaging (MRI), and positron emission tomography (PET) (Alabi et al., 2024; Peng et al., 2021). It holds immense promise for improving diagnosis, prognosis, and treatment planning in HNC. According to Gonçalves and coworkers, head and neck tumors exhibit significant intratumoral and intertumoral heterogeneity in terms of morphology, texture, vascularity, and cellular composition (Gonçalves et al., 2022). Radiomics allows for the quantitative characterization of tumor phenotype and heterogeneity based on imaging features extracted from medical images. Thus, radiomics can capture the spatial and functional complexities of head and neck tumors through analyzing texture, shape, and intensity patterns within the tumor region. This phenotypic characterization provides valuable insights into tumor biology, aggressiveness, and treatment response, thus facilitating personalized treatment planning (Gonçalves et al., 2022; Peng et al., 2021).

Radiomics-based predictive models stratify patients into different risk groups based on their likelihood of responding to specific treatment modalities, such as radiation therapy, chemotherapy, or immunotherapy (Gonçalves et al., 2022). And by correlating imaging features extracted from baseline scans with clinical outcomes, radiomics models identify patients who are more likely to benefit from a particular treatment regimen and those who may require alternative approaches (Alabi et al., 2024; Peng et al., 2021). Additionally, radiomics can track changes in tumor phenotype over time, allowing for early detection of treatment response or disease progression. Radiomics-derived biomarkers have shown promise in predicting patient outcomes, such as overall survival, progression-free survival, and locoregional recurrence, in HNC (Table 5.8) (Gonçalves et al., 2022). Radiomic biomarkers can improve the accuracy of diagnosing HNC by providing detailed tumor characterization. Quantitative radiomic features can predict patient outcomes, such as survival rates and likelihood of recurrence. Radiomic biomarkers help tailor treatment strategies by identifying patients who are likely to respond to specific therapies. Radiomic features can be used to monitor treatment response and detect early signs of recurrence, thus aiding in timely intervention (Gonçalves et al., 2022).

Radiomics-based prognostic models can stratify patients into different risk categories and guide personalized treatment decisions through integrating imaging features with clinical and molecular data (Alabi et al., 2024). The models provide valuable prognostic information beyond traditional clinical and pathological factors, enabling more precise risk stratification and patient counseling (Alabi et al., 2024; Peng et al., 2021). Radiomics offers a noninvasive method for assessing treatment response and monitoring disease progression in HNC (Alabi et al., 2024). Radiomics-based response assessment tools can evaluate treatment efficacy, identify residual disease, and detect early signs of recurrence through quantifying changes in imaging features pre- and post-treatment. This enables clinicians to tailor treatment strategies based on individual patient response and adjust therapy accordingly to optimize outcomes (Peng et al., 2021). Moreso, radiomics guides the development of personalized treatment plans tailored to the individual patient's tumor phenotype and clinical characteristics. Ultimately, clinicians can optimize treatment selection and delivery through integrating radiomic data with other patient-specific information, such as genomics, histopathology, and clinical staging (Alabi et al., 2024).

Table 5.8 List of notable radiomic biomarkers associated with head and neck cancer

Radiomic biomarkers	Roles	Significance	References
Tumor shape and size	Geometric features of the tumor	Features such as volume, surface area, sphericity, and compactness can indicate tumor aggressiveness and potential for spread.	Lu et al., 2024
Tumor texture	Statistical measures of tumor heterogeneity	Texture features such as entropy, contrast, homogeneity, and correlation reflect the heterogeneity within the tumor, which is associated with tumor grade and aggressiveness.	Ling et al., 2024
Intensity histogram features	Distribution of voxel intensities within the tumor	Features like mean intensity, standard deviation, skewness, and kurtosis provide information about the overall intensity distribution, correlating with tumor cellularity and necrosis.	Ling et al., 2024; Lu et al., 2024
Gray-level co-occurrence matrix (GLCM) features	Second-order statistical measures of voxel intensity pairs	Features such as energy, correlation, entropy, and homogeneity derived from GLCM describe spatial relationships between voxel intensities, offering insights into tumor texture and heterogeneity.	Lu et al., 2024
Gray-level run-length matrix (GLRLM) features	Measures of consecutive voxels with the same intensity	Features like short-run emphasis, long-run emphasis, and gray-level non-uniformity characterize texture patterns that are indicative of tumor heterogeneity and structure.	Ling et al., 2024
Gray-level size zone matrix (GLSZM) features	Measures of homogeneous zones within the tumor	Features such as zone size non-uniformity, large area emphasis, and zone percentage provide information about the size and uniformity of homogeneous regions within the tumor.	Lu et al., 2024
Wavelet transform features	Decomposition of the image into different frequency components	Wavelet features capture multiscale texture and edge information, which can reflect underlying tumor heterogeneity and microenvironment.	Ling et al., 2024; Lu et al., 2024

(continued)

Table 5.8 Continued

Radiomic biomarkers	Roles	Significance	References
Fractal dimension	Measure of the complexity of the tumor boundary	Higher fractal dimension values indicate more complex and irregular tumor shapes, which can correlate with invasive potential.	Ling et al., 2024
Radiomic signature scores	Composite scores derived from multiple radiomic features	Radiomic signature scores, developed through machine learning models, can predict clinical outcomes such as overall survival, disease-free survival, and response to therapy.	Lu et al., 2024
Radiomic risk scores	Quantitative risk assessment based on radiomic features	Radiomic risk scores can stratify patients into different risk categories, aiding in personalized treatment planning and prognostication.	Lu et al., 2024
Peritumoral features	Radiomic features extracted from the peritumoral region	Characteristics of the peritumoral area, such as edema and invasion, can provide additional prognostic information and insights into tumor spread and local invasion.	Ling et al., 2024; Lu et al., 2024

Hence, personalized treatment plans include a combination of surgery, radiation therapy, chemotherapy, targeted therapy, and immunotherapy tailored to maximize efficacy while minimizing toxicity for each patient (Gonçalves et al., 2022).

However, despite its potential, radiomics faces several challenges, including standardization of imaging protocols, reproducibility of feature extraction methods, and validation of predictive models across diverse patient cohorts (Alabi et al., 2024). Future research efforts should focus on addressing the challenges as well as integrating radiomics into clinical workflows and multicenter studies to further validate its clinical utility and facilitate its widespread adoption in routine practice (Gonçalves et al., 2022). Thus, radiomics holds great promise as a noninvasive, quantitative imaging approach for characterizing tumor phenotype, predicting treatment response, and guiding personalized treatment decisions in HNC. And with the ongoing advancements in imaging technology, computational methods, and multicenter collaborations, radiomics is poised to revolutionize the management of HNC and improve patient outcomes in the era of precision oncology (Alabi et al., 2024).

5.13 Holomics in Head and Neck Cancer

Holomics is an interdisciplinary field that integrates holistic approaches to cancer research and treatment. It offers a comprehensive framework for advancing precision medicine in HNC (Lee, Johnson et al., 2023). Holomics enables a deeper understanding of the complex molecular mechanisms underlying tumor biology and treatment response by integrating data from multiple "-omics" platforms such as genomics, transcriptomics, proteomics, metabolomics, and microbiomics with clinical data and patient-centered outcomes. The holistic approach facilitates comprehensive molecular profiling of head and neck tumors and holds immense promise for improving diagnosis, prognosis, and personalized treatment strategies in HNC (Lee, Roy et al., 2023; Ribeiro et al., 2022). Holomics provides a comprehensive view of tumor biology, heterogeneity, and microenvironment interactions through analyzing genomic alterations, gene expression patterns, protein profiles, metabolite signatures, and microbial compositions. It enables the identification of key molecular drivers, pathways, and therapeutic targets for personalized treatment planning (Ribeiro et al., 2022).

Holomics-driven approaches enable the selection of personalized treatment strategies tailored to the individual patient's molecular profile and clinical characteristics. Holomics guides treatment decisions, including surgery, radiation therapy, chemotherapy, targeted therapy, immunotherapy, or combination regimens through integrating multiomics data with clinical parameters, such as tumor stage, histology, and patient preferences. The personalized approach optimizes treatment efficacy while minimizing toxicity and treatment-related complications (Jayawickrama et al., 2024). It facilitates the development of predictive models and prognostic algorithms to assess patient outcomes and treatment responses in HNC. Holomics-driven models predict patient survival, disease progression, and treatment response probabilities through analyzing multidimensional data, including molecular, clinical, and imaging features. The predictive tools enable risk stratification, treatment optimization, patient counseling, enhanced clinical decision-making, and personalized care delivery (Lee et al., 2023; Ribeiro et al., 2022). Holomics accelerates the discovery and validation of biomarkers for early detection, prognostication, and treatment response prediction in HNC. It identifies candidate biomarkers associated with tumor progression, recurrence risk, and treatment resistance by integrating multiomics data with clinical outcomes and patient follow-up data. The biomarkers serve as valuable tools for patient stratification, clinical trial design, and targeted therapy selection in precision oncology (Jayawickrama et al., 2024; Lee, Johnson et al., 2023; Ribeiro et al., 2022).

According to Jayawickrama and coworkers, holomics employs systems biology and network analysis approaches to elucidate the complex interactions between molecular pathways, cellular processes, and tumor microenvironment components in HNC (Jayawickrama et al., 2024). It reveals the interconnectedness of biological systems and identifies potential therapeutic vulnerabilities and druggable targets by constructing molecular networks, pathway maps, and interaction diagrams (Jayawickrama et al., 2024; Lee, Johnson et al., 2023). This systems-level understanding informs the development of combination therapies and personalized treatment strategies tailored to the individual patient's molecular profile. Thus, holomics offers a holistic framework for advancing precision medicine in HNC by integrating multiomics data, predictive modeling, biomarker discovery, and systems biology approaches (Ribeiro et al., 2022). It transforms the way we diagnose, treat, and manage HNC, ultimately improving patient outcomes and quality of life in the era of precision oncology by leveraging the power of holistic analysis, personalized treatment selection, and predictive modeling (Jayawickrama et al., 2024; Ribeiro et al., 2022).

5.14 Limitations and Outlook

While precision medicine holds great promise for improving outcomes in HNC, several limitations and challenges need to be addressed to fully realize its potential. Additionally, ongoing research efforts and emerging technologies offer promising opportunities to overcome these limitations and advance precision medicine in HNC (Taylor et al., 2024). HNC is characterized by significant intratumoral and intertumoral heterogeneity, posing challenges for targeted therapy selection and treatment response prediction. Comprehensive molecular profiling of tumors and longitudinal monitoring of disease evolution are needed to capture and address tumor heterogeneity effectively (Baudrexl et al., 2024). Many potential biomarkers identified through genomic, transcriptomic, proteomic, and other omics analyses require rigorous validation to confirm their clinical utility and predictive value. Large-scale prospective studies and multicenter collaborations are essential to validate biomarkers and establish standardized protocols for their clinical implementation (Anderson et al., 2021).

Limited access to molecular testing facilities, high costs, and logistical challenges may hinder widespread adoption of precision medicine approaches in HNC (Taylor et al., 2024). Efforts to improve accessibility, affordability, and scalability of molecular testing platforms are needed to ensure equitable access to precision oncology for all patients. Acquired resistance to targeted therapies remains a significant challenge in HNC precision medicine (Baudrexl et al., 2024). Better understanding of the molecular mechanisms underlying treatment resistance and the development of novel therapeutic strategies to overcome resistance are critical for improving long-term treatment outcomes (Warinner et al., 2022). Integrating data from multiple omics disciplines (genomics, transcriptomics, proteomics, metabolomics, microbiomics) and clinical parameters presents computational and analytical challenges. Development of robust bioinformatics tools and machine learning algorithms for data integration, interpretation, and predictive modeling is essential for deriving meaningful insights from multiomics data (Taylor et al., 2024).

Tailoring treatment strategies based on individual patient characteristics, including tumor biology, molecular profile, and clinical factors, requires comprehensive patient stratification and personalized treatment algorithms (Bhat et al., 2021). Implementation of multidisciplinary tumor boards, decision support systems, and treatment guidelines based on molecular profiling can facilitate personalized treatment planning and optimization of therapeutic outcomes. Despite the challenges, significant progress has been made in precision medicine for HNC with the identification of novel biomarkers, development of targeted therapies, and implementation of molecularly guided treatment strategies (Baudrexl et al., 2024). Ongoing advances in genomic sequencing technologies, computational biology, immunotherapy, and liquid biopsy approaches hold promise for overcoming existing limitations and further improving precision medicine outcomes in HNC (Bhat et al., 2021). Collaborative research efforts, interdisciplinary collaborations, and patient-centered approaches are essential for advancing precision oncology and transforming the landscape of HNC treatment in the future (Taylor et al., 2024).

5.15 Conclusion

Precision medicine holds great promise in revolutionizing the management of HNC, offering personalized and targeted approaches to diagnosis, treatment, and patient care. The integration of molecular profiling techniques, such as next-generation sequencing (NGS), gene expression profiling, and proteomics, allows for the identification of biomarkers associated with tumor biology, treatment response, and prognosis. Clinicians can tailor treatment strategies to individual patients, thereby optimizing therapeutic efficacy while minimizing treatment-related toxicity by leveraging these biomarkers. The advent of targeted therapies, including immune checkpoint inhibitors, EGFR inhibitors, and other molecularly targeted agents, has expanded treatment options for patients with HNC, particularly those with recurrent or metastatic disease. The targeted therapies disrupt specific oncogenic pathways, offering selective and potent anticancer effects while sparing healthy tissues.

Furthermore, immunotherapy has emerged as a promising approach in HNC treatment, harnessing the power of the immune system to recognize and eliminate cancer cells. Immune checkpoint inhibitors, such as pembrolizumab and nivolumab, have demonstrated significant clinical benefit in a subset of patients with advanced HNC, leading to durable responses and improved survival outcomes. Despite the advancements, challenges remain in the implementation of precision medicine in HNC. Access to molecular profiling technologies, biomarker validation, and treatment affordability are barriers that need to be addressed to ensure equitable access to precision oncology for all patients. Additionally, ongoing research is needed to identify novel biomarkers, elucidate mechanisms of treatment resistance, and optimize treatment combinations to further improve patient outcomes. Thus, precision medicine represents a transformative approach in HNC care, offering personalized and targeted therapies tailored to individual patient characteristics. Through continued research, innovation, and collaboration, precision oncology has the potential to revolutionize cancer treatment paradigms, leading to improved outcomes and quality of life for patients with HNC.

References

AL LABBAN, D., JO, S-H., OSTANO, P., SAGLIETTI, C., BONGIOVANNI, M., PANIZZON, R. & DOTTO, G. P. 2018. Notch-effector CSL promotes squamous cell carcinoma by repressing histone demethylase KDM6B. *J Clin Invest*, 128(6), 2581–99.

ALABI, R. O., ELMUSRATI, M., LEIVO, I., ALMANGUSH, A., & MÄKITIE, A. A. 2024. Artificial intelligence-driven radiomics in head and neck cancer: Current status and future prospects. *Int J Med Inform*, 188, 105464.

ANDERSON, G., EBADI, M., VO, K., NOVAK, J., GOVINDARAJAN, A., & AMINI, A. 2021. An updated review on head and neck cancer treatment with radiation therapy. *Cancers* (Basel), 13(19), 4912.

ASTRADSSON, T., SELLBERG, F., EHRSSON, Y. T., SANDSTRÖM, K., & LAURELL, G. 2022. Serum proteomics in patients with head and neck cancer: Peripheral blood immune response to treatment. *Int J Mol Sci*, 23(11), 6304.

AULAKH, S. S., SILVERMAN, D. A., YOUNG, K., DENNIS, S. K., & BIRKELAND, A. C. 2022. The promise of circulating tumor DNA in head and neck cancer. *Cancers* (Basel), 14(12), 2968.

BANERJEE, R., MANI, R. S., RUSSO, N., SCANLON, C. S., TSODIKOV, A., JING, X., CAO, Q., PALANISAMY, N., METWALLY, T., INGLEHART, R. C., TOMLINS, S., BRADFORD, C., CAREY, T., WOLF, G., KALYANA-SUNDARAM, S., CHINNAIYAN, A. M., VARAMBALLY, S., & D'SILVA, N. J. 2011. The tumor suppressor gene rap1gap is silenced by mir-101-mediated EZH2 overexpression in invasive squamous cell carcinoma. *Oncogene*, 30(42), 4339–49.

BASHEETH, N., & PATIL, N. 2019. Biomarkers in head and neck cancer an update. *Indian J Otolaryngol Head Neck Surg*, 71(Suppl 1), 1002–11. doi:10.1007/s12070-019-01683-1.

BAUDREXL, J., SAKKAS, A., PIETZKA, S., DERKA, S., VAIRAKTARI, G., SCHEURER, M., SCHRAMM, A., WILDE, F., & EBELING, M. 2024. Evaluation of five-year overall survival rates among 18,331 head and neck cancer patients exposed to different targeted therapies through real-world data in a case-controlled study. *Anticancer Res*, 44(3), 1247–70.

BHAT, G. R., HYOLE, R. G., & LI, J. 2021. Head and neck cancer: Current challenges and future perspectives. *Adv Cancer Res*, 152, 67–102.

BOGUSZEWICZ, Ł., HEYDA, A., CISZEK, M., BIELEŃ, A., SKORUPA, A., MROCHEM-KWARCIAK, J., SKŁADOWSKI, K., & SOKÓŁ, M. 2024. Metabolite biomarkers of prolonged and intensified pain and distress in head and neck cancer patients undergoing radio- or chemoradiotherapy by means of NMR-based metabolomics: A preliminary study. *Metabolites*, 14(1), 60.

CARNIELLI, C. M., MELO DE LIMA MORAIS, T., MALTA DE SÁ PATRONI, F., PRADO RIBEIRO, A. C., BRANDÃO, T. B., SOBROZA, E., MATOS, L. L., KOWALSKI, L. P., PAES LEME, A. F., KAWAHARA, R., & THAYSEN-ANDERSEN, M. 2023. Comprehensive glycoprofiling of oral tumors associates n-glycosylation with lymph node metastasis and patient survival. *Mol Cell Proteomics*, 22(7), 100586.

CAVALIERI, S., DE CECCO, L., BRAKENHOFF, R. H., SERAFINI, M. S., CANEVARI, S., ROSSI, S., LANFRANCO, D., HOEBERS, F. J. P., WESSELING, F. W. R., KEEK, S., SCHECKENBACH, K., MATTAVELLI, D., HOFFMANN, T., LÓPEZ PÉREZ, L., FICO, G., BOLOGNA, M., NAUTA, I., LEEMANS, C. R., TRAMA, A., KLAUSCH, T., BERKHOF, J. H., TOUNTOPOULOS, V., SHEFI, R., MAINARDI, L., MERCALLI, F., POLI, T., & LICITRA, L. 2021. Bd2decide consortium. Development of a multiomics database for personalized prognostic forecasting in head and neck cancer: The big data to decide EU project. *Head Neck*, 43(2), 601–12.

CHEN, L. H., HSU, W. L., TSENG, Y. J., LIU, D. W., & WENG, C. F. 2016. Involvement of DNMT 3b promotes epithelial-mesenchymal transition and gene expression profile of invasive head and neck squamous cell carcinomas cell lines. *BMC Cancer*, 16(1), 431.

CHOUDHURY, J. H., DAS, R., LASKAR, S., et al. 2018. Detection of p16 promoter hypermethylation by methylation-specific PCR. *Methods Mol Biol*, 1726, 111–22.

CHUCHUEVA, N., CARTA, F., NGUYEN, H. N., LUEVANO, J., LEWIS, I. A., RIOS-CASTILLO, I., FANOS, V., KING, E., SWISTUSHKIN, V., RESHETOV, I., RUSETSKY, Y., SHESTAKOVA, K., MOSKALEVA, N., MARIANI, C., CASTILLO-CARNIGLIA, A., GRAPOV, D., FAHRMANN, J., LA FRANO, M. R., PUXEDDU, R., APPOLONOVA, S. A., & BRITO, A. 2023. Metabolomics of head and neck cancer in biofluids: An integrative systematic review. *Metabolomics*, 19(9), 77.

DESAI, S. 2023. Influence of pathogens on host genome and epigenome in development of head and neck cancer. *Cancer Rep* (Hoboken), 6(11), e1846.

DIEZ-FRAILE, A., CEULAER, J., DERPOORTER, C., SPAAS, C., BACKER, T., LAMORAL, P., ABELOOS, J., & LAMMENS, T. 2020. Circulating non-coding RNAs in head and neck cancer: Roles in diagnosis, prognosis, and therapy monitoring. *Cells*, 10(1), 48.

DOROBISZ, K., DOROBISZ, T., & ZATOŃSKI, T. 2023. The microbiome's influence on head and neck cancers. *Curr Oncol Rep*, 25(3), 163–71.

DUAN, X. P., QIN, B. D., JIAO, X. D., LIU, K., WANG, Z., & ZANG, Y. S. 2024. New clinical trial design in precision medicine: Discovery, development and direction. *Signal Transduct Target Ther*, 9(1), 57.

DUNCAN, L., SHAY, C., & TENG, Y. 2021. Multifaceted roles of long non-coding RNAs in head and neck cancer. *Adv Exp Med Biol*, 1286, 107–14.

ELABD, N. S., SOLIMAN, S. E., ELHAMOULY, M. S., GOHAR, S. F., ELGAMAL, A., ALABASSY, M. M., SOLIMAN, H. A., GADALLAH, A. A., ELBAHR, O. D., SOLIMAN, G., & SALEH, A. A. 2022. Long non-coding RNAs asb16-as1 and afap1-as1: Diagnostic, prognostic impact and survival analysis in colorectal cancer. *Appl Clin Genet*, 15(August), 97–109.

FAYDA, M., ISIN, M., TAMBAS, M., GUVELI, M., MERAL, R., ALTUN, M., SAHIN, D., OZKAN, G., SANLI, Y., ISIN, H., OZGUR, E., & GEZER U. 2016. Do circulating long non-coding RNAs (LNCRNAS) (LINCRNA-P21, GAS 5, HOTAIR) predict the treatment response in patients with head and neck cancer treated with chemoradiotherapy? *Tumor Biol*, 37(3), 3969–78.

GALEANA-PATIÑO, C. E., ORTIZ, M. I., CARIÑO-CORTÉS, R., LÓPEZ-SANTILLÁN, I. C., CASTRO-ROSAS, J., GÓMEZ-ALDAPA, C. A., & MUÑOZ-PÉREZ, V. M. 2023. Probiotics, as adjuvant therapy and preventive measure on progression, and complications of head and neck cancer. *Curr Pharm Biotechnol*, 24(12), 1504–14.

GODBOLE, M. S., & SINGH, V. 2023. Deciphering the impacts of gut and tissue microbiome on human cancers. *Cancer Rep* (Hoboken), 6(11), e1924.

GONÇALVES, M., GSAXNER, C., FERREIRA, A., LI, J., PULADI, B., KLEESIEK, J., EGGER, J., & ALVES, V. 2022. Radiomics in head and neck cancer outcome predictions. *Diagnostics* (Basel), 12(11), 2733.

GOUGIS, P., MOREAU BACHELARD, C., KAMAL, M., GAN, H. K., BORCOMAN, E., TOROSSIAN, N., BIÈCHE, I., & LE TOURNEAU, C. 2019. Clinical development of molecular targeted therapy in head and neck squamous cell carcinoma. *JNCI Cancer Spectr*, 3(4), pkz055.

HUANG, C., WANG, Z., ZHANG, K., DONG, Y., ZHANG, A., LU, C., & LIU, L. 2020. Microrna-107 inhibits proliferation and invasion of laryngeal squamous cell carcinoma cells by targeting CACNA2D1 in vitro. *Anticancer Drugs*, 31(3), 260–271.

HUANG, X., DUIJF, P. H. G., SRIRAM, S., PERERA, G., VASANI, S., KENNY, L., LEO, P., & PUNYADEERA, C. 2023. Circulating tumour DNA alterations: Emerging biomarker in head and neck squamous cell carcinoma. *J Biomed Sci*, 30(1), 65.

IAMS, W. T., MACKAY, M., BEN-SHACHAR, R., DREWS, J., MANGHNANI, K., HOCKENBERRY, A. J., CRISTOFANILLI, M., NIMEIRI, H., GUINNEY, J., & BENSON, A. B. 3rd. 2024. Concurrent tissue and circulating tumor DNA molecular profiling to detect guideline-based targeted mutations in a multicancer cohort. *JAMA Netw Open*, 7(1), e2351700.

JAIN, A. P., GHOSE, V., MUNSHI, S., BHAT, F. A., DEY, G., & NANJAPPA, V. 2024. Mass spectrometry-based proteomic analysis to characterize cisplatin induced early signaling events in head and neck squamous cell carcinoma. *Mol Cell Oncol*, 11(1), 2328873.

JAYAWICKRAMA, S. M., RANAWEERA, P. M., PRADEEP, R. G. G. R., JAYASINGHE, Y. A., SENEVIRATHNA, K., HILMI, A. J., RAJAPAKSE, R. M. G., KANMODI, K. K., & JAYASINGHE, R. D. 2024. Developments and future prospects of personalized medicine in head and neck squamous cell carcinoma diagnoses and treatments. *Cancer Rep* (Hoboken), 7(3), e2045.

KACZOR-URBANOWICZ, K. E., MARTIN CARRERAS-PRESAS, C., ARO, K., TU, M., GARCIA-GODOY, F., & WONG, D. T. 2017. Saliva diagnostics: Current views and directions. *Exp Biol Med* (Maywood), 242(5), 459–72.

KAIDAR-PERSON, O., GIL, Z., & BILLAN, S. 2018. Precision medicine in head and neck cancer. *Drug Resist Update*, 40, 13–16.

KASRADZE, D., JUODZBALYS, G., GUOBIS, Z., GERVICKAS, A., & CICCIÙ, M. 2020. Genetic and proteomic biomarkers of head-and-neck cancer: A systematic review. *J Cancer Res Ther*, 16(3), 410–24.

KEMMER, J. D., JOHNSON, D. E., & GRANDIS, J. R. 2018. Leveraging genomics for head and neck cancer treatment. *J Dent Res*, 97(6), 603–13.

KIRAN, N. S., YASHASWINI, C., MAHESHWARI, R., BHATTACHARYA, S., & PRAJAPATI, B. G. 2024. Advances in precision medicine approaches for colorectal cancer: From molecular profiling to targeted therapies. *ACS Pharmacol Transl Sci*, 7(4), 967–90.

KOU, N., LIU, S., LI, X., et al. 2019. H19 facilitates tongue squamous cell carcinoma migration and invasion via sponging MIR-LET-7. *Oncol Res*, 27(2), 173–82.

KUMARI, S., MISHRA, S., ANAND, N., HADI, R., RASTOGI, M., & HUSAIN, N. 2023. Circulating free DNA integrity index and promoter methylation of tumor suppressor gene p16, DAPK and RASSF1A as a biomarker for oropharyngeal squamous cell carcinoma. *Pathol – Res Pract*, 246, 154489.

KUNHABDULLA, H., MANAS, R., SHETTIHALLI, A. K., REDDY, C. R. M., MUSTAK, M. S., JETTI, R., ABDULLA, R., SIRIGIRI, D. R., RAMDAN, D., & AMMARULLAH, M. I. 2024. Identifying biomarkers and therapeutic targets by multiomic analysis for HNSCC: Precision medicine and healthcare management. *ACS Omega*, 9(11), 12602–10.

KWON, Y. W., JO, H. S., BAE, S., SEO, Y., SONG, P., SONG, M., & YOON, J. H. 2021. Application of proteomics in cancer: Recent trends and approaches for biomarkers discovery. *Front Med* (Lausanne), 8, 747333.

LAMBROU, G. I., HATZIAGAPIOU, K., & ZARAVINOS, A. 2020. The non-coding RNA GAS5 and its role in tumor therapy-induced resistance. *Int J Mol Sci*, 21(20), 1–18.

LEE, R. H., JOHNSON, D. E., & GRANDIS, J. R. 2023. To tip or not to tip: A new combination for precision medicine in head and neck cancer. *Cancer Res*, 83(19), 3162–4.

LEE, R. H., ROY, R., LI, H., HECHMER, A., ZHU, T. R., IZGUTDINA, A., OLSHEN, A. B., JOHNSON, D. E., & GRANDIS, J. R. 2023. Therapeutic implications of transcriptomics in head and neck cancer patient-derived xenografts. *PLoS One*, 18(3), e0282177.

LI, T., LIU, D., LI, C., RU, L., & WANG, X. 2021. Silencing of LNCRNA AFAP1-AS1 inhibits cell proliferation in oral squamous cancer by suppressing ccna2. *Cancer Manag Res*, 13, 7897–908.

LIAO, T. T., HSU, W. H., HO, C. H., HWANG, W. L., LAN, H. Y., LO, T., CHANG, C. C., TAI, S. K., & YANG, M. H. 2016. LET-7 modulates chromatin configuration and target gene repression through regulation of the ARID3B complex. *Cell Rep*, 14(3), 520–33.

LIN, M. C., CHUANG, Y. T., WU, H. Y., HSU, C. L., LIN, N. Y., HUANG, M. C., & LOU, P. J. 2024. Targeting tumor o-glycosylation modulates cancer-immune-cell crosstalk and enhances anti-pd-1 immunotherapy in head and neck cancer. *Mol Oncol*, 18(2), 350–68.

LING, X., ALEXANDER, G. S., MOLITORIS, J., CHOI, J., SCHUMAKER, L., TRAN, P., MEHRA, R., GAYKALOVA, D., & REN, L. 2024. Radiomic biomarkers of locoregional recurrence: Prognostic insights from oral cavity squamous cell carcinoma preoperative CT scans. *Front Oncol*, 14, 1380599. doi:10.3389/fonc.2024.1380599.

LIU, M., YU, X., BU, J., XIAO, Q., MA, S., CHEN, N., & QU, C. 2023. Comparative analyses of salivary exosomal MIRNAs for patients with or without lung cancer. *Front Genet*, 14, 1249678.

LU, H. J., SHEN, C. Y., CHIU, Y. W., LIN, W. L., PENG, C. Y., TSENG, H. C., HSIN, C. H., CHUANG, C. Y., CHEN, C. C., WU, M. F., HUANG, W. S., & SHEN, W. C. 2024. Radiomic biomarkers for platinum-refractory head and neck cancer in the era of immunotherapy. *Oral Dis*, doi:10.1111/odi.14854

MA, H., XIONG, L., ZHAO, B., HAHAN, Z., WEI, M., SHI, H., YANG, S., & REN, Q. 2024. Comprehensive investigation into the influence of glycosylation on head and neck squamous cell carcinoma and development of a prognostic model for risk assessment and anticipating immunotherapy. *Front Immunol*, 15, 1364082.

MAKAREWICZ, J., KAŹMIERCZAK-SIEDLECKA, K., SOBOCKI, B. K., DOBRUCKI, I. T., KALINOWSKI, L., & STACHOWSKA, E. 2024. Anti-cancer management of head and neck cancers and oral microbiome: What can we clinically obtain? *Front Cell Infect Microbiol*, 14, 1329057.

MASTRONIKOLIS, N. S., DELIDES, A., KYRODIMOS, E., PIPERIGKOU, Z., SPYROPOULOU, D., GIOTAKIS, E., TSIAMBAS, E., & KARAMANOS, N. K. 2024. Insights into metastatic roadmap of head and neck cancer squamous cell carcinoma based on clinical, histopathological and molecular profiles. *Mol Biol Rep*, 51(1), 597.

MEZGHANI, N., YAO, A., VASILYEVA, D., KAPLAN, N., SHACKELFORD, A., YOON, A., PHILLIPONE, E., DUBEY, S., SCHWARTZ, G. K., TAYLOR, A. M., & MOMEN-HERAVI, F. 2023. Molecular subtypes of head and neck cancer in patients of African ancestry. *Clin Cancer Res*, 29(5), 910–20.

MISEROCCHI, G., SPADAZZI, C., CALPONA, S., DE ROSA, F., USAI, A., DE VITA, A., LIVERANI, C., COCCHI, C., VANNI, S., CALABRESE, C., BASSI, M., DE LUCA, G., MECCARIELLO, G., IBRAHIM, T., SCHIAVONE, M., & MERCATALI, L. 2022. Precision medicine in head and neck cancers: Genomic and preclinical approaches. *J Pers Med*, 12(6), 854.

MORSELLI, M & DIECI, G. 2022. Epigenetic regulation of human non-coding RNA gene transcription. *Biochem Soc Trans*, 50(2), 723–36.

OKANO, S. 2024. Immunotherapy for head and neck cancer: Fundamentals and therapeutic development. *Auris Nasus Larynx*, 51(4), 684–695.

PATEL, A., PATEL, S., PATEL, P., & TANAVDE, V. 2022. Saliva based liquid biopsies in head and neck cancer: How far are we from the clinic? *Front Oncol*, 12, 828434.

PENG, Z., WANG, Y., WANG, Y., JIANG, S., FAN, R., ZHANG, H., & JIANG, W. 2021. Application of radiomics and machine learning in head and neck cancers. *Int J Biol Sci*, 17(2), 475–86.

PETZSCHNER, F. H 2024. Practical challenges for precision medicine. *Science*, 3836679, 149–50.

RAPADO-GONZÁLEZ, Ó., RODRÍGUEZ-CES, A. M., LÓPEZ-LÓPEZ, R., & SUÁREZ-CUNQUEIRO, M. M. 2023. Liquid biopsies based on cell-free DNA as a potential biomarker in head and neck cancer. *Jpn Dent Sci Rev*, 59, 289–302.

RASHEDUZZAMAN, M., KULASINGHE, A., DOLCETTI, R., KENNY, L., JOHNSON, N. W., KOLARICH, D., & PUNYADEERA, C. 2020. Protein glycosylation in head and neck cancers: From diagnosis to treatment. *Biochim Biophys Acta Rev Cancer*, 1874(2), 188422.

RASHEDUZZAMAN, M., MURUGAN, A. V. M., ZHANG, X., OLIVEIRA, T., DOLCETTI, R., KENNY, L., JOHNSON, N. W., KOLARICH, D., & PUNYADEERA, C. 2022. Head and neck cancer n-glycome traits are cell line and HPV status-dependent. *Anal Bioanal Chem*, 414(29–30), 8401–11.

REIS, R. S. D., SANTOS, J. A. D., ABREU, P. M., DETTOGNI, R. S., SANTOS, E. V. W. D., STUR, E., AGOSTINI, L. P., ANDERS, Q. S., ALVES, L. N. R., VALLE, I. B. D., LIMA, M. A., SOUZA, E. D., PODESTÁ, J. R. V., ZEIDLER, S. V. V., CORDEIRO-SILVA, M. F., & LOURO, I. D. 2020. Hypermethylation status of DAPK, MGMT and RUNX3 in HPV negative oral and oropharyngeal squamous cell carcinoma. *Genet Mol Biol*, 43(3), 1–9.

REN, X., LIN, S., GUAN, F., & KANG, H. 2024. Glycosylation targeting: A paradigm shift in cancer immunotherapy. *Int J Biol Sci*, 20(7), 2607–21.

RIBEIRO, I. P., ESTEVES, L., CARAMELO, F., CARREIRA, I. M., & MELO, J. B. 2022. Integrated multi-omics signature predicts survival in head and neck cancer. *Cells*, 11(16), 2536.

SAMPSON, K., SORENSON, C., & ADAMALA, K. P. 2024. Preparing for the future of precision medicine: Synthetic cell drug regulation. *Synth Biol (Oxf)*, 9(1), ysae004.

SASSENBERG, M., DROOP, J., SCHULZ, W. A., DIETRICH, D., LOICK, S. M., WIEK, C., SCHECKENBACH, K., GAISA, N. T., & HOFFMANN, M. J. 2019. Upregulation of the long non-coding RNA CASC9 as a biomarker for squamous cell carcinoma. *BMC Cancer*, 19(1), 1–14.

SERAFINI, M. S., LOPEZ-PEREZ, L., FICO, G., LICITRA, L., DE CECCO, L., & RESTEGHINI, C. 2020. Transcriptomics and epigenomics in head and neck cancer: Available repositories and molecular signatures. *Cancers Head Neck*, 5, 2.

SHARMA, U., BARWAL, T. S., ACHARYA, V., TAMANG, S., VASQUEZ, K. M., & JAIN, A. 2020. Cancer susceptibility candidate 9 (CASC9): A novel targetable long noncoding RNA in cancer treatment. *Transl Oncol*, 13(8), 100774.

SOSINSKY, A., AMBROSE, J., CROSS, W., TURNBULL, C., HENDERSON, S., JONES, L., HAMBLIN, A., ARUMUGAM, P., CHAN, G., CHUBB, D., NOYVERT, B., MITCHELL, J., WALKER, S., BOWMAN, K., PASKO, D., BUONGERMINO PEREIRA, M., VOLKOVA, N., RUEDA-MARTIN, A., PEREZ-GIL, D., LOPEZ, J., PULLINGER, J., SIDDIQ, A., ZAINY, T., CHOUDHURY, T., YAVORSKA, O., FOWLER, T., BENTLEY, D., KINGSLEY, C., HING, S., DEANS, Z., RENDON, A., HILL, S., CAULFIELD, M., & MURUGAESU, N. 2024. Insights for precision oncology from the integration of genomic and clinical data of 13,880 tumors from the 100,000 genomes cancer programme. *Nat Med*, 30(1), 279–89.

STÖGBAUER, F., OTTO, R., JÖHRENS, K., TINHOFER, I., KEILHOLZ, U., POREMBA, C., KELLER, U., LESER, U., WEICHERT, W., BOXBERG, M., & KLINGHAMMER, K. 2024. Molecular subtyping of head and neck cancer: Clinical applicability and correlations with morphological characteristics. *Oral Oncol*, 149, 106678.

SU, Y., YU, Q. H., WANG, X. Y., YU, L. P., WANG, Z. F., CAO, Y. C., & LI, J. D. 2017. JMJD2A promotes the Warburg effect and nasopharyngeal carcinoma progression by transactivating LDHA expression. *BMC Cancer*, 17(1), 477.

SUN, A., XING, Z., LV, R., NIU, P., ZHAO, B., MA, S., & LI, H. 2024. Research progress of immunotherapy for advanced head and neck cancer. *Med Oncol*, 41(6), 133.

TAYLOR, K. J., AMDAL, C. D., BJORDAL, K., ASTRUP, G. L., HERLOFSON, B. B., DUPREZ, F., GAMA, R. R., JACINTO, A., HAMMERLID, E., SCRICCIOLO, M., JANSEN, F., VERDONCK-DE LEEUW, I. M., FANETTI, G., GUNTINAS-LICHIUS, O., INHESTERN, J., DRAGAN, T., FABIAN, A., BOEHM, A., WÖHNER, U., KIYOTA, N., KRÜGER, M., BONOMO, P., PINTO, M., NUYTS, S., SILVA, J. C., STROMBERGER, C., SPECENIER, P., TRAMACERE, F., BUSHNAK, A., PEROTTI, P., PLATH, M., PADERNO, A., STEMPLER, N., KOURI, M., GRÉGOIRE, V., & SINGER, S. 2024. EORTC quality of life group and the EORTC head and neck group. Long-term health-related quality of life in head and neck cancer survivors: A large multinational study. *Int J Cancer*, 154(10), 1772–85.

WAMSLEY, N. T., WILKERSON, E. M., GUAN, L., LAPAK, K. M., SCHRANK, T. P., HOLMES, B. J., SPRUNG, R. W., GILMORE, P. E., GERNDT, S. P., JACKSON, R. S., PANIELLO, R. C., PIPKORN, P., PURAM, S. V., RICH, J. T., TOWNSEND, R. R., ZEVALLOS, J. P., ZOLKIND, P., LE, Q. T., GOLDFARB, D., & MAJOR, M. B. 2023. Targeted proteomic quantitation of NRF2 signaling and predictive biomarkers in HNSCC. *Mol Cell Proteomics*, 22(11), 100647.

WANG, C. W., BISWAS, P. K., ISLAM, A., CHEN, M. K., & CHUEH, P. J. 2024. The use of immune regulation in treating head and neck squamous cell carcinoma (HNSCC). *Cells*, 13(5), 413.

WANG, Y., WU, C., ZHANG, C., LI, Z., ZHU, T., CHEN, J., REN, Y., WANG, X., ZHANG, L., & ZHOU, X. 2018. TGF-β-induced STAT3 overexpression promotes human head and neck squamous cell carcinoma invasion and metastasis through MALAT1/MIR-30a interactions. *Cancer Lett*, 436, 52–62.

WARINNER, C. B., BERGMARK, R. W., SETHI, R., & RETTIG, E. M. 2022. Cancer-related activity limitations among head and neck cancer survivors. *Laryngoscope*, 132(3), 593–9.

WISHART, G., TEMPLEMAN, A., HENDRY, F., MILLER, K., & PAILHES-JIMENEZ, A. S. 2024. Molecular profiling of circulating tumour cells and circulating tumour DNA: Complementary insights from a single blood sample utilising the Parsortix® system. *Curr Issues Mol Biol*, 46(1), 773–87.

WU, T., QU, L., HE, G., TIAN, L., LI, L., ZHOU, H., JIN, Q., REN, J., WANG, Y., WANG, J., KAN, X., LIU, M., SHEN, J., GUO, M., & SUN, Y. 2016. Regulation of laryngeal squamous cell cancer progression by the LNCRNA H19/MIR-148A-3P/DNMT1 axis. *Oncotarget*, 7(10), 11553–66.

XIE, Y., LIU, X., ZHAO, C., CHEN, S., WANG, S., LIN, Z., ROBISON, F. M., GEORGE, B. M., FLYNN, R. A., LEBRILLA, C. B., & GARCIA, B. A. 2024. Development and application of glycandia workflow for glycomic analysis. *BioRxiv* [Preprint], 2024.03.12.584702.

YALAMARTY, R., MAGESH, S., JOHN, D., CHAKLADAR, J., LI, W. T., BRUMUND, K. T., WANG-RODRIGUEZ, J., & ONGKEKO, W. M. 2024. The intratumor microbiome varies by geographical location and anatomical site in head and neck squamous cell carcinoma. *Curr Probl Cancer*, 50, 101100.

YANG, H., ZHOU, L., YANG, F., CHEN, J., & WANG, Y. 2023. Prognostic value of o6-methylguanine-DNA methyltransferase hypermethylation and expression in head and neck cancer: A systematic review and meta-analysis. *Medicine*, 102(14), E33472.

YU, W., ZHANG, L., WEI, Q., & SHAO, A. 2020. O6-methylguanine-DNA methyltransferase (MGMT): Challenges and new opportunities in glioma chemotherapy. *Front Oncol*, 9(January), 1–11.

ZHANG, W., LIU, W., JIA, L., CHEN, D., CHANG, I., LAKE, M., BENTOLILA, L. A., & WANG, C. Y. 2021. Targeting KDM4A epigenetically activates tumor-cell-intrinsic immunity by inducing DNA replication stress. *Mol Cell*, 81(10), 2148–65.e9.

ZHAO, H., SHI, C., HAN, W., LUO, G., HUANG, Y., FU, Y., LU, W., HU, Q., SHANG, Z., & YANG, X. 2024. Advanced progress of spatial metabolomics in head and neck cancer research. *Neoplasia*, 47, 100958.

ZHU, M., ZHANG, C., CHEN, D., CHEN, S., & ZHENG, H. 2019. LNCRNA MALAT1 potentiates the progression of tongue squamous cell carcinoma through regulating MIR-140-5P-PAK1 pathway. *Onco Targets Ther*, 12, 1365–77.

ZOU, J., DAI, Y., XU, G., KAI, Y., LAN, L., ZHANG, J., & WANG, Y. 2024. Identification of two distinct head and neck squamous cell carcinoma subtypes based on fatty acid metabolism-related signatures: Implications for immunotherapy and chemotherapy. *Medicine (Baltimore)*, 103(16), e37824.

6
Immunotherapy and Targeted Therapy in Head and Neck Cancer

Botle Precious Damane, Lorraine Tshegofatso Maebele, Tania Maphoso, Thanyani Victor Mulaudzi, Felix Holst, Graham Chakafana, and Zodwa Dlamini

6.1 Introduction

Head and neck cancers (HNCs) rank as the seventh most prevalent cancer globally, with >660,000 new cases and 325,000 mortalities recorded annually. The incidence of HNC disease is projected to steadily increase largely due to the increasing rates of oropharyngeal cancer. Risk factors for HNC include alcohol and tobacco use, both independently and in combination, as well as human papillomavirus (HPV) infection, especially for oropharyngeal cancers (Gormley et al., 2022). Epstein-Barr virus (EBV) infection is also implicated in the development of nasopharyngeal carcinomas (NPC) (Li et al., 2023). These tumors develop within the oral cavity, pharynx, sinuses, larynx, salivary gland, and nasal cavity (Fasano et al., 2021). Head and neck squamous cell carcinoma (HNSCC) accounts for > 90% of HNCs (Fasano et al., 2021; Pereira et al., 2022), with an incidence that is projected to increase to 1.08 million new cases annually by 2030 (Li et al., 2023).

More than 50% of patients are initially diagnosed at an advanced stage (stage III or IV), and, in 10% of cases, metastasis has already occurred (Pereira et al., 2022). HNC is a prominent heterogeneous disease, and its treatment remains challenging (Li et al., 2023). Systemic therapies for HNC aim not only to extend survival but also to preserve the quality of life and essential functions of the head and neck region, including swallowing, speaking, and breathing (Nakano, 2021). Treatment of HNC requires aggressive multimodal approaches such as surgery followed by radiotherapy alone or chemoradiotherapy for oral cavity cancers and primary chemoradiotherapy for pharynx and larynx cancers (Li et al., 2023). Despite these interventions, the reported 5-year overall survival rate for HNSCC patients is < 50% (Khadela et al., 2023), indicating a challenging prognosis. Moreover, approximately 50% of patients experience relapse following surgery and chemoradiotherapy (Borel et al., 2020), often accompanied by adverse side effects from concurrent chemoradiotherapy (Goel et al., 2022). Considering the poor prognosis, toxic side effects, and low survival rate reported, it is evident that there is a critical need to explore novel therapies for HNC.

Targeted therapies are currently promising treatment agents that can accurately identify and eliminate cancer cells (Li et al., 2023) with high selectivity and reduced adverse effects. Cetuximab is currently approved by the US Food and Drug Administration (FDA) for targeting epidermal growth factor receptor (EGFR). Other therapies targeting vascular endothelial growth factor (VEGF) and its receptor (VEGFR), phosphatidylinositol-4,5-bisphosphate 3-kinase (PI3K), and others are under investigation (Roden et al., 2021). Immunotherapy is another promising therapeutic strategy that focuses on restoring antitumor immunity (Ishii et al., 2015) by promoting the destruction of tumor cells with less damage to normal cells (Pereira et al., 2022). The FDA has currently approved immune checkpoint inhibitors (ICIs) such as pembrolizumab and nivolumab for treating recurrent or distal metastatic HNSCC (Gavrielatou et al., 2020). These ICIs target the programmed cell death protein 1 (PD-1).

Targeted therapies and immunotherapies have been shown to have complementary therapeutic effects, paving the way for exploring combination therapy (Yang et al., 2022). In this chapter, we delve into the realm of immunotherapy and targeted treatments for managing HNCs. We explore how combining these approaches can help surmount therapy resistance, and we discuss the challenges involved. Furthermore, we will peer into the future to envision how these strategies may evolve to better eradicate cancer.

6.2 Drivers of HNC Pathogenesis and Their Roles in Disease Prognosis and Response to Treatment

Detection of HNCs is multifaceted, categorized into three main groups: (1) HPV-positive tumors, comprising the overexpression of p16 protein and circulating tumor HPV DNA (ctHPVDNA); (2) EBV-positive tumors, comprising EBV and anti-EBV antibodies; and (3) non–virally induced tumors, which include p53, EGFR, and programmed cell death ligand 1 (PD-L1) (Eberly et al., 2024). However, detection at an advanced stage and the limited success rates of targeted therapy (Mishra et al., 2022b) and immunotherapy (Rodrigo et al., 2024) contribute to the modest clinical benefits observed with these monotherapies. Furthermore, challenges such as the absence of reliable biomarkers, high costs, and drug-related toxicities hinder their widespread implementation (Mishra et al., 2022b; van Harten & Brakenhoff, 2021). This prompts the need to explore novel therapies to optimize treatment strategies

(Gavrielatou et al., 2020). Among these, PD-L1 provides potential effective future improvements for HNC therapeutic endeavors (Trigo et al., 2022).

6.2.1 Programmed Cell Death Ligand 1

PD-L1 is a co-inhibitory ligand of PD-1 capable of inhibiting cytokine secretion, reducing cell proliferation, and inducing apoptosis in PD-1-positive T cells (Han et al., 2020). The interaction of PD-L1 expressed on tumor cells with PD-1 promotes various mechanisms that contribute to immune suppression. This interaction leads to effector T-cell exhaustion, natural killer (NK) cell dysfunction, inhibition of apoptotic signals on tumor cells, and immune suppression when PD-L1 binds to PD-1 on regulatory T cells (Tregs) (Qiao et al., 2020). The expression of PD-L1 is usually detected by immunohistochemistry (IHC) in the tumor microenvironment (TME) and quantified using scoring algorithms. These are tumor proportion score (TPS), tumor-infiltrating immune cells (IC), and combined positive score (CPS) scoring systems. TPS and IC indicate the percentage of viable cancer cells or ICs, respectively, exhibiting partial or complete PD-L1 membrane staining at any intensity (Park et al., 2022).

The CPS analyses both tumor and infiltrating immune cells showing partial or complete PD-L1 membrane staining at any intensity (Park et al., 2022). Determining PD-L1 status through the use of IHC allows the identification of patients suitable for future immunotherapies (Cui et al., 2023; Mishra et al., 2022a) and prognostic purposes (Cui et al., 2023). The prognostic role of PD-L1 in survival seems to depend on the cell type since the high expression of PD-L1 on immune cells was associated with longer survival in localized and locoregionally advanced HNSCC patients as compared to patients with PD-L1 expressed on tumor cells (Blažek et al., 2023; Figure 6.1). The same results were reported in hepatocellular carcinoma (Liu et al., 2018). The expression of PD-L1 is associated with unfavorable prognosis in various solid tumors such as melanoma, lung, and renal cancers (Ciciola et al., 2020). Overexpression of PD-L1 in HNSCC located within the larynx, oral cavity, oropharynx, and hypopharynx was associated with the presence of distant metastases and a lower overall survival rate. This increase in PD-L1 expression was also associated with a highly aggressive tumor phenotype regardless of tumor origin, stage, or grade (Müller et al., 2017).

PD-L1-positive tumors are associated with better response rates with anti-PD-1/PD-L1 therapies. A similar trend was observed in recurrent or metastatic (RM) HNSCCs (Gavrielatou et al., 2020; Oliva et al., 2019; Park et al., 2022). Nivolumab improved overall survival regardless of PD-L1 expression. However, preliminary evidence suggested that patients with tumors expressing 1% PD-L1 or more experienced an improved response to nivolumab compared to patients with tumors expressing < 1% PD-L1 (Ferris et al., 2016). Contrary to these findings, the KEYNOTE-048 phase III randomized trial of RM-HNSCC found an increasing CPS value in patients to be directly proportional to favorable prognosis and longer overall survival. The study proposed pembrolizumab as a suitable first-line treatment for PD-L1-positive R/M HNSCC patients (Burtness et al., 2019). These studies suggest that the overexpression of PD-L1 is mostly associated with improved response to ICI therapy and favorable prognosis when expressed on immune cells rather than on cancer cells (Figure 6.1).

6.2.2 Epidermal Growth Factor Receptor

EGFR is also known as human epidermal growth factor receptor 1 (HER1) and belongs to the HER family consisting of HER2, HER3, and HER4. It is a 170 kDa receptor of ligands, EGF, amphiregulin, transforming growth factor-α (TGF-α), betacellulin, heparin-binding EGF-like growth factor (HB-EGF), epiregulin, epigen, and neuregulin. Since HER2 does not have a ligand and HER3 lacks an active tyrosine kinase domain, these receptors heterodimerize with EGFR to initiate signal transduction cascades (Kang et al., 2023). The interaction between EGFR with its ligands leads to dimerization with other HER family members, resulting in autophosphorylation on tyrosine kinase domains, which initiates downstream signaling cascades: the Ras-Raf–mitogen-activated protein kinase (MAPK)/extracellular signal-regulated kinase (ERK) pathway, the PI3K/protein kinase B (AKT) pathway, the phospholipase C γ-protein kinase C (PLCγ-PKC) pathway, the Janus kinase 2(JAK2)/signal transducer and activator of transcription 3 (STAT3) pathway, and the nuclear factor kappa-light-chain-enhancer of activated B cells (NF-κB) pathway (Kang et al., 2023).

EGFR is widely studied as a biomarker in HNSCC. The prognostic role of EGFR is mostly evaluated according to mutation, polymorphisms, EGFR variant III (vIII) expression, EGFR protein expression levels, protein activation, and EGFR ligand expression (Fasano et al., 2021). EGFR is overexpressed or mutated in > 90% of HNCs (Nair et al., 2022). This protein influences tumor cell proliferation, angiogenesis, metastasis, and inhibition of apoptosis (Rehmani & Issaeva, 2020) (Figure 6.1). Overexpression of EGFR in HNCs was associated with tumor stage (Hashmi et al., 2018), higher risk of neck lymph node metastasis, development of poorly differentiated tumors (Cívico-Ortega et al., 2023), and uncontrolled tumor growth (Verma et al., 2018). Furthermore, an increased EGFR expression was also correlated with lower overall survival (Cívico-Ortega et al., 2023; Keren et al., 2014; Zhu et al., 2013) and disease-free survival in HNSCC patients (Hashmi et al., 2018). However, according to a meta-analysis study in HNC patients, EGFR overexpression was inversely correlated with disease-free survival (Keren et al., 2014).

EGFR is not yet validated for use as a predictive marker of EGFR-targeted therapies (Milano et al., 2024). This is because the predictive value of EGFR is still contradictory according to results obtained to date for HNSCC treatments including anti-EGFR drugs (Fasano et al., 2021). For example, it was shown that the survival rate was improved in RM-HNSCC patients after adding cetuximab to chemotherapy regardless of EGFR expression (Licitra et al., 2013). Additionally, no correlation was found between EGFR and improved survival in patients taking cetuximab plus platinum-based chemotherapy or chemotherapy alone according to EGFR fluorescence in situ hybridization (FISH) score (Bossi et al., 2016). An overexpression of EGFR could not predict patient sensitivity to cetuximab in HNSCC patients (Leblanc et al., 2020). In contrast, in lung cancers, EGFR mutations predict sensitivity to tyrosine kinase inhibitors (Marret et al., 2023). Additionally, EGFR genotyping could have diverse predictive effects in EGFR-targeted therapies for HNCs (Nair et al., 2022).

The use of IHC for determining EGFR expression could be unreliable (Hutchinson et al., 2015; Milano et al., 2024). This is because IHC scoring only considers EGFR on the cell surface while there are endosomal and nuclear compartments that may be underestimated (Thariat et al., 2012). The prediction of drug efficacy relies on the accuracy and robustness of biomarker detection methods that can generate reproducible and reliable results (Gaber et al., 2018). It was suggested that the use of approaches that could evaluate EGFR IHC expression both on the membrane and in cytoplasm or dual methods (e.g., EGFR IHC and EGFR silver enhanced in situ hybridization [SISH]) rather than IHC alone should be used for determining patients who could benefit from targeted therapies (Hutchinson et al., 2015). Thus, EGFR is associated with poor prognosis, and its predictive value remains controversial (Figure 6.1). The protein expression of EGFR does not correlate with response to targeted therapies but exhibits a variable association with targeted therapy response at the genetic level. This warrants further studies comparing the predictive role of EGFR at both genetic and protein levels while using multiple methods of detection to address these discrepancies.

6.2.3 Vascular Endothelial Growth Factor

VEGF is a signaling molecule responsible for the processes of angiogenesis and vasculogenesis (Schlüter et al., 2018). Oral cavity tumors usually express high VEGF immunostaining as compared to tumors situated in the lower lip (Kyzas et al., 2005). Increased expression of VEGF promotes the growth and migration of endothelial cells, thus generating a network of blood vessels around the tumor and enabling the supply of nutrients and oxygen required for tumor growth. VEGF is one of the potential biomarkers in head and neck tumors that still requires further validation and standardization to implement its use in routine clinical practice (Dumitru & Raica, 2023). A strong VEGF expression was linked to poor prognosis and an elevated risk of laryngeal cancer recurrence (Schlüter et al., 2018). The expression levels of VEGF detected in the serum of HNSCC patients were high when compared to healthy controls (Srivastava et al., 2014).

This heightened expression of VEGF has been linked to several unfavorable clinical factors including the presence of positive lymph nodes and advanced disease as well as poor radiotherapy and chemoradiotherapy response rates (Srivastava et al., 2014). Elevated VEGF levels also correlate with a high tumor grade (Harmankaya et al., 2022), higher clinical stage, lymph node metastasis at diagnosis (Kyzas et al., 2005), and worse overall survival (Harmankaya et al., 2022; Kyzas et al., 2005). Another study demonstrated that the high expression of VEGF in tumors is associated with an increased infiltration of both tumor-promoting immune cells such as Tregs, myeloid-derived suppressor cells, and immature dendritic cell and antitumor cells such as NK, $CD4^+$ T, and $CD8^+$ T cells. This immune cell infiltration generates an immunologically "hot" tumor, which is associated with overall survival. This was coupled with the high expression of immune checkpoints such as cytotoxic T-lymphocyte antigen 4 (CTLA-4), PD-L1, PD-L2, PD-1, V-domain immunoglobulin suppressor of T cell activation (VISTA), T-cell immunoglobulin and mucin domain 3 (TIM-3), and T-cell immunoreceptor with Ig and ITIM domains (TIGIT). This immune-inflamed tumor is more likely to respond to immunotherapy (Zhu et al., 2021) (Figure 6.1).

6.2.4 Human Papillomavirus Status

An infection with several HPV genotypes is associated with benign or malignant tumors. It has been shown that the high-risk HPV strains 16 and rarely 18, 33, and others are prevalent in HNCs. Among the primary HNC patient cohort, 43.2% tested positive for salivary HR-HPV whereas the HPV 16 strain was detected in 95% of HPV-positive saliva samples (Ekanayake Weeramange et al., 2021). The DNA molecule of a high-risk HPV strain can be incorporated into the host cell genome leading to an overexpression of viral oncogenes, namely E6 and E7 (Figure 6.1) that target intracellular pathways involved in the regulation of cell cycle, DNA repair, maintenance of genomic integrity, and apoptosis, thus resulting in an uncontrolled cell growth and proliferation (Julian et al., 2021). Furthermore, HPV-positive HNSCCs are also associated with aberrant EGFR amplification and activation of the PI3K/AKT/mammalian target of rapamycin (mTOR) signaling pathways (Sun et al., 2021). High-risk HPV positivity was found to be associated with a favorable prognosis as compared to high-risk HPV-negative saliva samples (Ekanayake Weeramange et al., 2021). The prognostic ability of HPV seems to depend on its location because it was found to be strongly associated with overall survival in the oropharynx and hypopharynx, moderately associated with improved survival in the oral cavity and larynx subsites, and to have no association in the nasopharynx and sinonasal tract subsites (Li et al., 2018). HPV-positive HNSCCs exhibit greater susceptibility to treatment, often resulting in more favorable survival outcomes. Studies have indicated that monoclonal antibodies targeting PD-1/PD-L1 are more effective in HPV-positive HNSCC patients as compared to HPV-negative patients (Wang et al., 2019). The reason could be an increased expression of co-inhibitory molecules such as CTLA-4, lymphocyte-activation gene 3 (LAG-3), TIGIT, and TIM-3 (Julian et al., 2021) and an increased immune cell infiltration in HPV-positive tumors (Sun et al., 2021). In summary, HPV infections have a good prognostic and predictive value for HNC depending on their location (Figure 6.1).

6.3 Targeted Therapies/Immunotherapies and Their Mechanism of Action

6.3.1 Targeted Therapies and Their Mechanism of Action

6.3.1.1 Monoclonal Antibodies

Monoclonal antibodies are therapeutic agents widely used in treating malignancies. They commonly act by blocking a specific ligand-receptor interaction on the cell surface (Padma, 2015). Several antibodies are in clinical evaluation while others are approved by the FDA for the treatment of HNSCC (Lee et al., 2009). Cetuximab was approved by the FDA in 2006 for the treatment of HNSCC (Kang et al., 2023) as a single modality for RM-HNSCC patients who failed prior platinum-based therapy. Additionally, cetuximab was also approved in combination with radiotherapy for locoregionally advanced HNSCC or platinum-based therapy and 5-fluorouracil for first-line treatment of RM-HNSCC (Boeckx et al., 2013; De Pauw et al., 2021). Cetuximab is an anti-EGFR monoclonal antibody with a higher affinity than EGF and TGF-α (Taberna et al., 2019).

The binding of cetuximab to the extracellular domain of the EGFR prevents ligands from binding and activating EGFR, consequently inhibiting receptor homodimerization or heterodimerization with other HER molecules as well as promoting antibody-EGFR receptor complex internalization and degradation

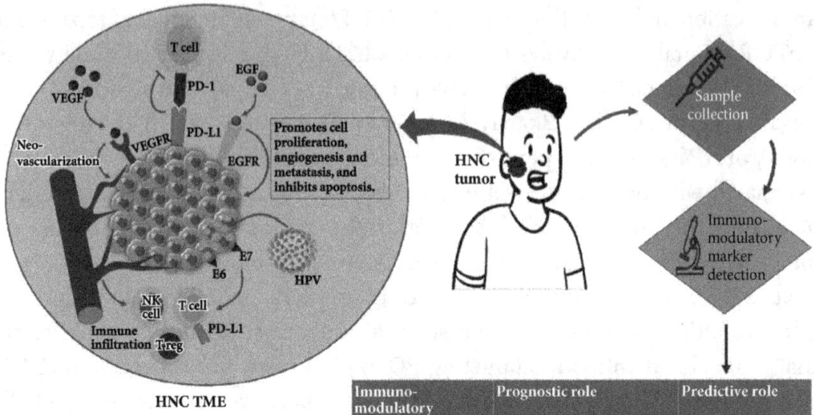

Immuno-modulatory markers	Prognostic role	Predictive role
PD-L1	Favorable prognosis when expressed on immune cells. Poor prognosis when expresed on tumor cells.	Therapy response
HPV	Favorable prognosis for oropharyngeal and hypopharyngeal tumors	Therapy response
EGFR	Poor prognosis	Unclear
VEGF	Poor prognosis	Therapy response

Figure 6.1 Immunomodulatory markers play a critical role as predictors of therapeutic response. Samples obtained from head and neck cancer (HNC) patients offer valuable insights into detecting immune markers with diverse predictive and prognostic roles. These markers serve as crucial indicators of disease progression and treatment response. Programmed cell death protein 1 (PD-1) ligand, PD-L1, human papillomavirus (HPV) status, and vascular endothelial growth factor (VEGF) expression are associated with favorable responses to therapy, whereas the predictive role of epidermal growth factor receptor (EGFR) is not yet clear. EGFR, a receptor for epidermal growth factor (EGF), and VEGF, a ligand for VEGF receptor (VEGFR), play pivotal roles in tumor progression. The VEGF/VEGFR interaction in particular contributes to neovascularization, fostering tumor growth and metastasis. The presence of HPV in the tumor microenvironment of head and neck cancers (HNCs) correlates with increased infiltration of immune cells expressing immune checkpoints. Notably, the interaction between co-inhibitory molecules like PD-1 and its ligand PD-L1 serves to dampen the activity of cytotoxic T cells, facilitating immune evasion by tumor cells. For instance, PD-L1 expression on immune cells correlates with a favorable prognosis, while its expression on tumor cells suggests a poorer outcome. Thus, understanding the intricate interplay of these immunomodulatory markers is critical for tailoring effective treatment strategies and improving patient outcomes in HNC management.

(De Pauw et al., 2021; Fasano et al., 2021). This diminishes angiogenesis and proliferation of tumor cells and promotes apoptosis (Rodríguez-Nava et al., 2023) (Figure 6.2). Cetuximab also prompts antitumor immunity via its immunoglobulin G1 (IgG1) backbone capable of binding CD16 fragment crystallizable (Fc) receptors on granulocytes, macrophages, and NK cells.

The interaction between tumor and NK cells via IgG1-CD16 generates an antibody-dependent cellular cytotoxicity (ADCC) on tumor cells by NK cells interceded by perforins and granzymes (Cai et al., 2020; De Pauw et al., 2021),

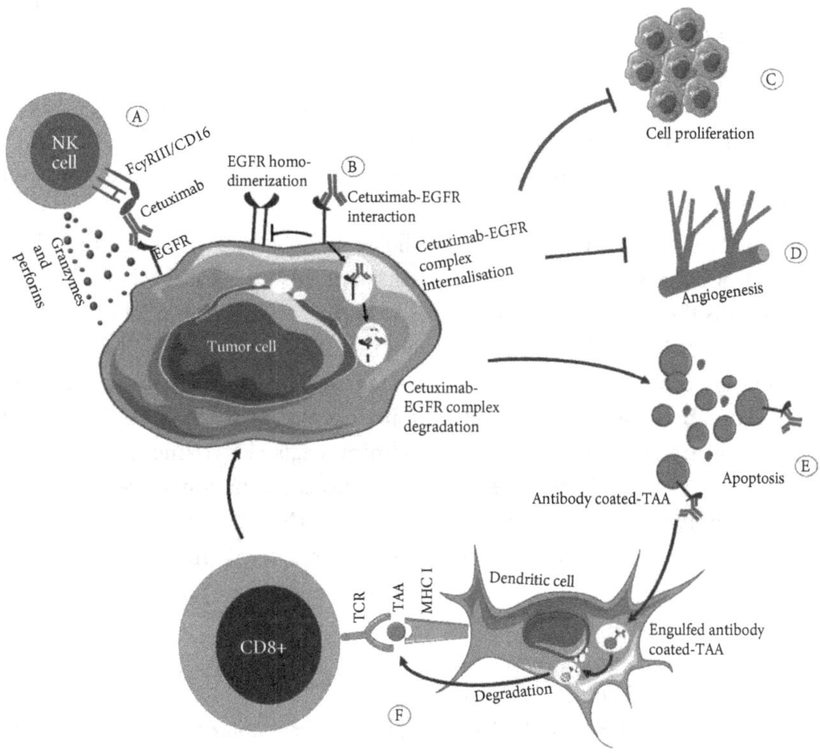

Figure 6.2 Mechanism of action of cetuximab: A) Cetuximab binds simultaneously to EGFR on tumor cells and FcγRIII (CD16) receptors on natural killer (NK) cells, triggering antibody-dependent cellular cytotoxicity (ADCC) mediated by perforin and granzyme release, ultimately leading to tumor cell apoptosis. (B) Additionally, cetuximab binding to EGFR monomers inhibits receptor dimerization, promoting internalization and degradation of the cetuximab-EGFR complex. This results in (C) suppression of tumor cell proliferation, (D) inhibition of angiogenesis, and (E) induction of apoptosis. (F) Subsequently, antibody-coated tumor-associated antigens (TAAs) derived from tumor cell debris are phagocytosed by dendritic cells (DCs) and presented on major histocompatibility complex class I (MHC I) molecules to CD8+ T cells, leading to their activation and the exertion of a cytotoxic response against remaining tumor cells.

which then perforates the tumor cell membrane and cause apoptosis (Campbell & Hasegawa, 2013) (Figure 6.2). Antibody-coated tumor-associated antigens (TAA) from cell death are engulfed by antigen-presenting cells (e.g., dendritic cells) resulting in antigen cross-presentation and stimulation of $CD8^+$ T cells (Schmitt & Ferris, 2020).

Other monoclonal antibodies that have been evaluated for treating HNSCC in clinical trials include zalutumumab, nimotuzumab, panitumumab (Taberna et al., 2019), and bevacizumab (Kordbacheh & Farah, 2021). Among all these antibodies, panitumumab is the only one that has reached phase III clinical trials. The use of panitumumab did not show any improvements in survival rate compared to the standard of care (Taberna et al., 2019). Panitumumab is not yet FDA approved (Ghosh et al., 2022) and exhibits lower binding affinity toward EGFR and CD16 compared to cetuximab (Kang et al., 2023). This human IgG2 is therefore unable to stimulate ADCC mediated by cytotoxic T or NK cells but induces ADCC promoted by monocytes and neutrophils (Rodríguez-Nava et al., 2023).

Bevacizumab (Avastin) can bind to all five varieties of VEGF and block their interaction with VEGFR on the endothelial cell surface (Kordbacheh & Farah, 2021). This then can decrease the invasive and migratory potential of HNSCC cells as well as the establishment of distant metastasis (Dumitru & Raica, 2023). Currently, there are no FDA-approved anti-VEGF monoclonal antibodies. Bevacizumab is the most studied anti-angiogenic monoclonal antibody and has demonstrated promising results in clinical trials (Hyytiäinen et al., 2021). However, a phase III study revealed that the combination of bevacizumab with chemotherapy in recurrent or metastatic HNSCC patients did not improve overall survival. Nonetheless, it demonstrated enhanced response rates and progression-free survival, albeit with an increased incidence of grade 3–5 bleeding events (Argiris et al., 2019).

6.3.1.2 Tyrosine Kinase Inhibitors

Receptor tyrosine kinases (RTKs) possess an intracellular tyrosine kinase domain that plays a crucial role in generating signals. When bound by receptors, RTKs undergo dimerization, resulting in the transfer of a phosphate group from adenosine triphosphate (ATP) to the cytoplasmic region and consequently initiating downstream signaling (Huang et al., 2020; Sola et al., 2019). In HNSCC cells, RTKs belonging to several families including HER, fibroblast growth factor receptor (FGFR), VEGFR, and platelet-derived growth factor receptor (PDGFR) and C-Met are commonly overexpressed, leading to the activation of signal transducers and activators of transcription (STAT), rat sarcoma virus (Ras)/rapidly accelerated fibrosarcoma (Raf)/mitogen-activated protein kinase (MEK)/extracellular signal-regulated kinase (ERK) and PI3K/

AKT/mTOR signaling pathways. These signaling pathways trigger the expression of genes driving the proliferation, survival, invasion, migration, and metastasis of tumor cells (Long et al., 2022). Tyrosine kinase inhibitors (TKIs) are low-molecular-weight molecules capable of passing through a cell membrane to compete with ATP for binding on oncogenic tyrosine kinases (Huang et al., 2020; Sola et al., 2019).

They have either single or multiple targets and a high selectivity for tumor cells, thereby minimizing toxicities. A total of 42 TKIs are approved as indications for various malignancies. However, there are currently no FDA-approved TKIs for the treatment of HNSCC (Sola et al., 2019). Anlotinib is a potent TKI that targets multiple receptors including VEGFR2, PDGFRα/β, c-Kit, Ret, Aurora-B, c-FMS, and the discoid region of domain receptor 1 (DDR1). It was shown to inhibit tumor cell proliferation and promote apoptosis in patient-derived xenografts (Hu et al., 2021). Sorafenib is another TKI with multiple targets such as Raf, PDGFR, VEGFR2, and VGFR3 (Kordbacheh & Farah, 2021). This TKI was evaluated as a single agent that showed a low response rate in RM-HNSCC (Micaily et al., 2020) or in combination with other therapies such as cetuximab, carboplatin, and paclitaxel and with both cisplatin and docetaxel (Kordbacheh & Farah, 2021).

Sunitinib is a multikinase inhibitor of VEGFR1, 2, and 3; PDGFRs; c-KIT; and RET (Kordbacheh & Farah, 2021) that has demonstrated a low response rate in HNSCC patients and is associated with adverse events such as bleeding (Kordbacheh & Farah, 2021; Micaily et al., 2020) and skin ulceration/fistula formation (Micaily et al., 2020). Vatalanib, cediranib, pazopanib, and nilotinib are some of the TKIs currently in clinical trial evaluations for targeting VEGFR (Micaily et al., 2020).

6.3.2 Immunotherapies and Their Mechanism of Action

6.3.2.1 Immune Checkpoint Inhibitors

The co-inhibitory receptor–ligand interaction in tumor microenvironment suppresses host immunity and as a result facilitates tumor immune escape (Yasuma-Mitobe & Matsuoka, 2018). Immune checkpoint inhibitors act by blocking the interactions between co-inhibitory receptors and their ligands thus overcoming this tumor-mediated immune inhibition and leading to a pro-inflammatory tumor microenvironment that potentially increases disease control (Iranzo et al., 2022). Pembrolizumab and nivolumab are monoclonal antibodies targeting the PD-1 pathway by binding to PD-1 and blocking its interaction with its receptors (e.g., PD-L1 and PD-L2) (Peters et al., 2018). These checkpoint inhibitors were FDA-approved in 2016 for advanced RM-HNSCC patients who have progressed following platinum-based chemotherapy irrespective of the expression of PD-L1 (Julian et al., 2021). This approval was granted after impressive survival outcomes were obtained from the Checkmate 141 and Keynote-012 randomized phase III trials for nivolumab and pembrolizumab, respectively (Kao & Lou, 2019).

6.3.2.2 Adoptive Cell Therapy

6.3.2.2.1 Chimeric Antigen Receptor T-Cell Therapy

Chimeric antigen receptor (CAR) T-cell therapy is the genetic modification and manipulation of a patient's T cells to target specific tumor antigens (Ayala Ceja et al., 2024; Cheng et al., 2021). These cells can thus accurately target and produce an antitumor effect without requiring the MHC mechanism of antigen presentation (Dong et al., 2018). Within the TME, CAR T cells bind to their specific tumor antigens through the single-chain variable fragment recognition domain, thus prompting an antitumor immune response via the secretion of pro-inflammatory cytokines, namely interleukin (IL)-2, interferon (IFN)-γ, and tumor necrosis factor (TNF)-α and through perforin- and granzyme-mediated cytolytic activity (Alnefaie et al., 2022). The antitumor effect of EGFR-specific CAR T cells was observed in a hypopharyngeal SCC in vitro model as they targeted EGFR overexpressing tumor cells (Dong et al., 2018). CAR T-cell therapy was combined with binary oncolytic adenovirus, which then disrupted the immune suppressive tumor microenvironment while HER-2-specific CAR T cells target local and metastatic disease in HNSCC xenograft and orthotopic mouse models. This approach significantly increased patient survival to over 100 days compared to the 25 days achieved by monotherapies (Rosewell Shaw et al., 2017).

6.3.2.2.2 Vaccines

HPV-positive HNSCC tumor cells express foreign antigens, including E6 and E7 proteins specific to HPV-positive cells (Julian et al., 2021). The HPV virus induces the expression of E6 and E7, and these oncoproteins are required for the maintenance of the abnormal phenotype (Meliante et al., 2023). As non-self antigens, E6 and E7 oncoproteins are recognized by the host immune system. The MEDI0457 vaccine targets E6 and E7 proteins of the HPV16 and 18 strains. The administration of this vaccine in HPV16-positive HNSCC patients resulted in an increased ratio of infiltration of cytotoxic T cells (Aggarwal et al., 2019). ISA101 is a HPV16 vaccine consisting of E6 and E7 long peptides, among which there are epitopes for cytotoxic and helper T cells to fully elicit HPV16 immunity. This vaccine generated a strong HPV16 immunity but was still ineffective for an invasive cancer treatment. AMV002 is a DNA vaccine that was evaluated in a phase I study for HPV-positive patients who had previously received treatment; it was found to be well tolerated at all doses with an augmented immunity to virus-derived tumor-specific antigens. DPX-E7 is another vaccine that is still under clinical evaluation for HPV16-positive head and neck, cervical, and anal cancers (Julian et al., 2021). Axalimogene filolisbac (AXAL or ADXS11-001) is a live-vector vaccine that utilizes an attenuated strain of Listeria monocytogenes (Lm) fused to the nonhemolytic fragment of listeriolysin O (LLO) and secretes the Lm-LLO-HPV E7 fusion protein. The administration of AXAL in HNSCC patients resulted in $CD8^+$ T-cell infiltration and the induction of TNF-α and IFN-γ (Zhou et al., 2022). However, systemic *Listeria* infections led to an early termination of other *Listeria*-based HPV E6 vaccines. Talimogene laherparepvec is an oncolytic virus-based vaccine with deleted key virulence genes essential for replication in the normal host. The evaluation of this vaccine in combination with pembrolizumab in RM-HNSCC patients refractory to platinum-based chemotherapy generated a 14% response similar to that of pembrolizumab monotherapy (Wise-Draper et al., 2022).

6.4 Potential Combinations of Immunotherapy and Targeted Therapy for Enhancing Therapy Response in Head and Neck Cancer

Despite the improved survival outcomes associated with targeted therapies, there are concerns, such as an increased tumor recurrence and side effects, linked to this treatment strategy (Yang et al., 2022). On the other hand, immunotherapy is also faced with a low response rate in a subset of patients (Hua et al., 2022) who later develop acquired drug resistance and ultimately stop responding. Moreover, patients may experience hyperprogression and immune-related adverse effects (Dobosz et al., 2022). Targeted therapy might overcome these challenges by enhancing tumor antigen presentation, producing an in situ vaccination effect through the release of antigens from dying cells that could trigger the activation of antigen-presenting cells and possibly augment the priming of tumor-specific $CD8^+$ T cells (Yu et al., 2019). Additionally, EGFR is a major target of targeted therapies and is associated with the signaling pathways that contribute to immunotherapy resistance (Kang et al., 2023). Thus, the combination of immunotherapy with targeted therapy can potentially provide synergistic and sustained management of head and neck tumors (Yang et al., 2022). This approach potentially diminishes drug resistance while concurrently generating anticancer effects such as inducing apoptosis and reducing the growth of tumor, metastatic potential, and cancer stem cell populations (Bayat Mokhtari et al., 2017). Table 6.1 shows an update on clinical trials for targeted-ICI combination therapies for head and neck tumors.

Table 6.1 Clinical trials evaluating the combination of immunotherapy with targeted therapy

Clinical trial	Status	Trial number
A prospective clinical study to evaluate the efficacy and safety of pembrolizumab combined with anlotinib in first-line treatment for patients with of recurrent metastatic R-M HNSCC PD-L1 CPS≥1	Recruiting	NCT04999800
A phase II trial of induction and maintenance pembrolizumab and olaparib in locally advanced HNSCC	Recruiting	NCT05366166
Open-label, randomized phase II trial of ramucirumab in combination with pembrolizumab versus pembrolizumab alone as first-line treatment of PD-L1 positive, RM-HNSCC	Recruiting	NCT05980000
A phase II, randomized, open-label three-arm clinical study to evaluate the safety and efficacy of lenvatinib (E7080/MK-7902) in combination with pembrolizumab (MK-3475) versus standard of care chemotherapy and lenvatinib monotherapy in participants with R-M HNSCC who have progressed after platinum therapy and immunotherapy (PD-1/PD-L1 inhibitors) (LEAP-009)	Recruiting	NCT04428151
An open-label, nonrandomized, multiarm, phase II trial to evaluate the efficacy of pembrolizumab combined with cetuximab in patients with RM-HNSCC	Active, not recruiting	NCT03082534
A prospective phases I and II trial of abemaciclib + nivolumab in patients with RM-HNSCC that progressed or recurred within 6 months after platinum-based chemotherapy	Terminated	NCT03655444
A phase II, single-arm open-label study of the combination of atezolizumab and bevacizumab in rare solid tumors	Active, not recruiting	NCT03074513
A study to evaluate the safety and efficacy of copanlisib in combination with nivolumab in patients with advanced solid tumors	Completed	NCT03735628
EACH: a randomized phase II study evaluating the safety and anti-tumor activity of the combination of avelumab and cetuximab relative to avelumab monotherapy in RM-HNSCC	Active, not recruiting	NCT03494322

6.4.1 Using Immune Checkpoint Inhibitors and Anti-VEGF Combination Therapy to Enhance Therapeutic Response

The combination of ICIs with anti-angiogenesis monoclonal antibodies holds great potential in overcoming drug resistance and enhancing patient survival due to their anticipated synergy. Angiogenesis is the formation of new blood vessels from preexisting ones and is essential for tumor growth and metastasis. It promotes an immunosuppressive tumor microenvironment by reducing tumor-infiltrating lymphocyte (TIL) infiltration and upregulation of immunosuppressive signals such as indoleamine 2, 3-dioxygenase (IDO), IL-6, IL-10, and PD-L1 (Yi et al., 2019). VEGF and its receptor VEGFR are the essential regulators of angiogenesis (Yasuda et al., 2013). Targeting their interaction normalizes tumor vascularization thereby restoring blood flow, which then increases the delivery of drugs, oxygen, and immune cells (e.g., cytotoxic T cells) to the tumor (Shrimali et al., 2010; Yasuda et al., 2013) (Figure 6.3). Combining VEGF inhibitors with anti-PD-1 in preclinical studies using a murine cancer model suppressed tumor growth in vivo with minimized side effects (Yasuda et al., 2013).

The PD-1 blockade in this study enhanced the recruitment of T cells to the tumor and local immune activation, as observed by an increased expression of pro-inflammatory cytokines, namely IFN-γ, TNF-α, and granzyme B, whereas VEGF blockade suppressed tumor neovascularization but could not promote immune activation (Yasuda et al., 2013). The administration of bevacizumab biosimilar and sintilimab combination therapy in Chinese patients with previously untreated hepatitis B virus (HBV)-associated hepatocellular carcinoma generated a significant progression-free and overall survival benefit compared to sorafenib monotherapy (Ren et al., 2021). A randomized phase II–III study investigated ICI–anti-VEGF combination therapies in RM-HNSCC patients consisting of anti-VEGF agents (namely, anlotinib, apatinib, and bevacizumab) and anti-PD-1 agents (camrelizumab, toripalimab, tislelizumab, sintilimab, and nivolumab). The results of this study demonstrated an improved 1-year overall survival rate of 87.7% with tolerable side effects (Hua et al., 2022).

A phase II trial investigating the combination of afatinib plus pembrolizumab in locally advanced/metastatic lung SCC showed limited efficacy; patients discontinued the treatments, and the study was discontinued (Levy et al., 2022). The integration of ICIs with anti-VEGF indeed demonstrated the complementary effects necessary for improving drug efficacy and patient benefit in HNC. Further studies are required to fully understand their mechanism of action and effect on patient survival and quality of life.

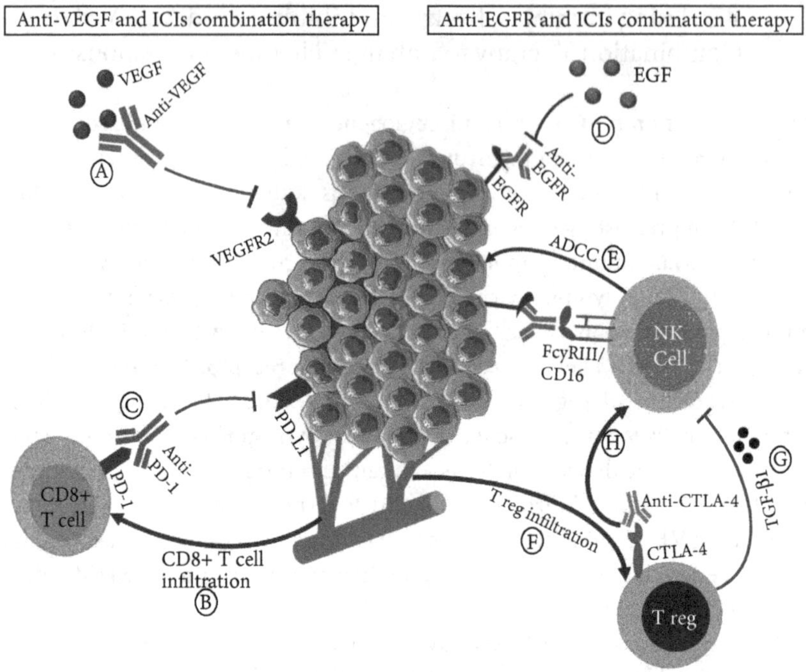

Figure 6.3 Targeted therapies and ICIs combination therapy: In the anti-VEGF and ICI combination therapy, (A) anti-VEGF antibodies bind to VEGF, preventing its interaction with VEGFR2. (B) This inhibition leads to vascular normalization, facilitating the infiltration of cytotoxic CD8+ T cells into the tumor microenvironment. (C) Concurrently, the administration of anti-PD-1 monoclonal antibodies enhances the immune response by binding to PD-1 receptors on CD8+ T cells, thereby blocking PD-1/PD-L1 interactions and restoring T cell-mediated cytotoxicity. In the anti-EGFR and ICI combination therapy, (D) anti-EGFR antibodies, such as cetuximab, bind to EGFR, blocking its activation by ligands like EGF. (E) Additionally, cetuximab can bind FcγRIII (CD16) receptors on NK cells via its IgG1 backbone, promoting antibody-dependent cellular cytotoxicity (ADCC). (F) However, cetuximab presence in the tumor microenvironment can induce infiltration of CTLA-4-expressing regulatory T cells (Tregs), which (G) suppress NK cell-mediated ADCC. (H) To counteract this immunosuppression, anti-CTLA-4 antibodies, such as ipilimumab, are administered to inhibit Tregs through CTLA-4 blockade, thereby restoring NK cell-driven ADCC.

6.4.2 Using Immune Checkpoint Inhibitors and Anti-EGFR Combination Therapy to Enhance Therapeutic Response

EGFR has surfaced as a central focal point for therapeutic interventions (Ayati et al., 2021). Monoclonal antibody–targeted therapies (e.g., cetuximab) have a better survival benefit than do EGFR-specific tyrosine kinase inhibitors. Nonetheless, they are effective in only 15–20% of HNC patients (Jie et al., 2015). This low efficacy can be resolved by supplementing with ICIs (Yang et al., 2022). The combination of pembrolizumab and afatinib demonstrated a clinical benefit greater than that of their monotherapies in a retrospective analysis of HNSCC patients (Lizotte et al., 2018). Pembrolizumab combined with cetuximab also showed promising clinical activity in R/M HNSCC (Sacco et al., 2021). Cetuximab and ICIs generated an improved response rate and a higher survival but only if ICIs were administered first because prior administration of cetuximab before ICIs resulted in poor survival and disease progression (Park et al., 2020). The treatment of head and neck tumors with cetuximab enhanced the presence of intratumoral CTLA-4^{+} Foxp3^{+} Treg. This affected the therapeutic activity of cetuximab by suppressing the expression of NKG2D in NK cells and impairing NK cell-mediated cytotoxicity and DC maturation. Incorporating ipilimumab, anti-CTLA-4 monoclonal antibodies suppressed Tregs while restoring the cytolytic effects of NK cell-mediated ADDC (Jie et al., 2015) (Figure 6.3).

6.5 Limitations and Challenges Encountered in Immuno- and Targeted Therapies

6.5.1 Immunotherapy

The advances in immunotherapy have resulted in substantial success when treating cancers; these come, however, with significant limitations. Investigating these challenges helps researchers understand the mechanism of action with regard to patient response. Resistance, whether primary or acquired, has resulted in reduced response to immunotherapies (Sharma et al., 2017). Furthermore, adverse effects from environmental modifiers of immunity contribute to this resistance (Dobosz et al., 2022). Environmental factors such as genomic composition, immune system cells, tumor microenvironment, and the host cell environment contribute to the effectiveness of these treatments (Kluger et al., 2020).

The initial exposure to antitumor therapies targets multiple biological mechanisms: priming of T cells, recognition of antigen-presenting cells, cell invasion by T cells, and elimination of cancer cells by T cells. These therapies target immune checkpoints and the structure of the immunological synapse (Kluger et al., 2020). Resistance to this process can influence various factors including antigen expression, metabolism, the presence or absence of inflammatory factors, angiogenesis, and tumor neovascularization (Haibe et al., 2020). The mechanisms of resistance at a molecular level include the absence of antigen expression, constitutive expression of PD-L1 or other co-inhibitory molecules, abnormalities in EGF/EGFR expression, loss of HLA expression or presentation, aberrant activation of the MAPK pathway, and activation of the WNT/β-catenin pathway. Additionally, the loss of the phosphatase and tensin homolog deleted on chromosome 10 (PTEN) expression leads to enhanced PI3K pathway activity and disrupts interferon pathway signaling, particularly INF and JAK/STAT signaling pathway abnormalities, and contributes to resistance (Li & Zhang, 2022).

6.5.1.1 Primary Resistance in Immunotherapy

Primary resistance in HNSCC presents as an evasion of immune surveillance and induction of immunosuppression (Dos Santos et al., 2021). To consider primary resistance in a clinical setting the following conditions need to be met: a minimum of 6 weeks of administration of the drug, either stable disease or progressive disease sustained for < 6 months in response, and confirmation of disease progression through a follow-up scan at least 4 weeks after the initial progression (Li & Zhang, 2022). In addition, an existing mechanism of primary resistance is observed in patients receiving anti-PD-1 treatment, which can further develop acquired resistance (Dos Santos et al., 2021). The loss of function in β2-microglobulin (B2M) and Janus kinases 1 and 2 (JAK1/2) are linked to the evasion of anti-PD-1 (Zhang et al., 2022). In HNSCC, research in the process of immunotherapy administration through the design of combination therapies or sequential approaches is restricted, however, preclinical studies from treatment of other cancers can provide new insights that may be relevant to HNSCC (Dos Santos et al., 2021). This is observed in metastatic melanomas, where variations in B2M immune response can lead to the loss of expression to HLA-1 (Zaretsky et al., 2016).

A study by Zhang et al. confirmed primary resistance to anti-PD-1 therapy, which represents a pivotal cause of treatment failure in colorectal carcinomas, although the precise mechanism remains uncertain (Zhang et al., 2022). In addition, HPV-positive patients with HNSCC demonstrated more diverse T-cell repertoires with impaired HLA-1 expression as compared to HPV-negative patients (Saloura et al., 2017). Immunosuppression identified in primary resistance was also observed with the inactivation of PTEN, related to the activation of PI3K pathway (Conciatori et al., 2020). A study by Zhoa et al. demonstrated the effects of nivolumab or pembrolizumab on glioblastoma patients, revealing immunosuppressive expression signatures as well as enriched PTEN variations in nonresponders (Zhao et al., 2019).

6.5.1.2 Secondary Resistance in Immunotherapy

Secondary resistance to immunotherapy develops when a previously effective drug no longer yields results despite prior successful administration to specific patients. For this to apply, a minimum of 6 months of progression-free survival must be observed (Kluger et al., 2020). Furthermore, this can be categorized by two groups: *adaptive immune resistance* and *acquired resistance* (Sharma et al., 2017). Adaptive immune resistance occurs when cancer cells are identified by the immune system but develop adaptations to defend themselves against immune attacks (Bai et al., 2020). There occurs an evolving interaction between the immune system and cancer cells that may clinically present as primary resistance, mixed response, or acquired resistance (Sharma et al., 2017). Acquired resistance is observed with patients who become unresponsive to treatments after previous success (Dos Santos et al., 2021). Acquired resistance to immunotherapy is observed in metastatic melanomas, with a clinical presentation of variations in JAK1 and JAK 2 that exhibit cancer progression after initial response to anti-PD-1 therapies (Zaretsky et al., 2016).

A study by Kakavand et al. demonstrated the effects of administering anti-PD-1 immunotherapy (nivolumab or pembrolizumab) or a combination of anti-PD-1 and anti-CTLA-4 inhibitors (nivolumab or pembrolizumab with ipilimumab) to 16 patients, with results showing an initial response to both single-target and combination therapy. However, progression was observed, and PTEN loss was identified in five of the patients within the post-progression group (Kakavand et al., 2017).

Another challenge facing immunotherapy is the lack of information regarding immune-related adverse events (Connolly et al., 2019). Although ICIs improve survival outcomes, there is also a growing consequence of adverse events (Miao et al., 2020). Moreover, as these therapies have been developed in recent years, the production of personalized cellular products can incur significant expense. For instance, patients using pembrolizumab have to be willing to pay $150,000 per quality-adjusted life-years (Chiang et al., 2021). As a result, a minority of patients may experience significantly greater benefits compared to the median outcome (Green, 2021).

6.5.2 Targeted Therapy

Despite resistance in cancer cells, other factors contribute to the limitations of targeted and combination therapy (Zhang & Zhang, 2020). The primary concerns include their lack of efficacy across all cancers, the presence of toxicity during treatment, difficulty in identifying the molecular target, and the high costs associated with this therapy (Balik et al., 2019). The difficulties encountered during ongoing early-phase dose-finding trials underscore the negative impacts associated with PI3K inhibitors, such as hyperglycemia, nausea, fatigue, rash, and gastrointestinal problems. Similarly, rash, diarrhea, and dermatitis are associated with MEK inhibition (Lopez & Banerji, 2017).

At cellular level, toxicity can be on- or off-target. On-target toxicity occurs when targeted agents that are assumed to have relatively low toxicity to normal cells have a negative effect on the normal cells (Rivera-Concepcion et al., 2022). These on-target toxicities demonstrate a class effect wherein all drugs within the same class exhibit similar toxicity, as observed in the inhibition of PI3K, which can result in hyperglycemia (Khan et al., 2016). Off-target toxicity occurs when a specific drug inhibits a nontarget protein, resulting in adverse side effects. Unlike on-target toxicity, this phenomenon typically does not demonstrate a class effect and is believed to be associated with the pharmacology of the individual drug (Rivera-Concepcion et al., 2022). This is seen with the use of osimertinib, which targets tyrosine kinase receptors belonging to the HER2 family, which has the potential for cardiotoxicity (Patel et al., 2020).

6.5.3 Environmental Modifiers Related to Cancer Stemness

The heterogeneity of tumors represents an important limitation in developing effective cancer therapies (Janku, 2014). Factors affecting the host cell, such as age, diet, gut microbiome, and comorbidities, as well as hormones can influence how cells metastasize and develop resistance (Dobosz et al., 2022). Cancer stem cells (CSCs) and their ability to preserve lineage, differentiate, and interact with other cells are modulated by their microenvironment (Ponomarev et al., 2022). Malignant transformation of stem cells develops into heterogenous tumors that are considered phenotypically different subclones (Marusyk et al., 2020). The formation of CSCs drives the survival of heterogeneous cell populations that demonstrate high plasticity and high resistance to stress factors (Ponomarev et al., 2022). In addition, CSCs' key survival mechanisms can result in tumor survival and recurrence after therapy administration (Aponte & Caicedo, 2017). The molecular and structural complexity of CSCs influence intratumor heterogeneity by activating signaling pathways to ensure self-renewal and chemoresistance (Ponomarev et al., 2022). CSCs can adapt to therapeutic interventions by altering signaling molecules that govern the metabolism of therapies (Chen et al., 2021). In cases where multiple drug resistance occurs, CSCs overexpress binding transporters, mediating the efflux of therapies and resulting in reduced intracellular drug concentration (Xiao et al., 2021).

6.5.4 Monitoring Resistance in Head and Neck Cancer Therapy Response

The critical effort of identifying resistance in HNC will ultimately result in a targeted and personalized treatment strategy (Sharma et al., 2017). To facilitate effective treatment in the presence of resistance, early detection is essential. Non–target-specific methods of detection in HNC in advanced or progressive states have been used to diagnose resistance. However, more precise predictive biomarkers in resistance ensure early detection, facilitate accurate drug administration, and reduce the disease burden (Ren et al., 2020). Monoclonal bodies are being used as predictive biomarkers because they can detect tumor-specific antigens. However, they have difficulty penetrating solid tumors due to the complex nature of the tumor microenvironment (Rodríguez-Nava et al., 2023). The use of monoclonal antibodies might be a more effective immunotherapy; however, the integrity of their Fc region triggers an immune response resulting in anti-drug antibodies (Both et al., 2013).

Single-chain variable fragments developed from recombinant technology overcame this problem: they can be modified to either be mono- or multispecific and have shown a greater affinity for tissue retention (Petersson et al., 2014). In HNSCC, predictive markers used to monitor drug resistance include P-glycoprotein, BCL-2 GST-pi, p53, bax expression HNSCC (detecting pathological response and prognosis), C-erb2 (recurring HNSCC), and TGF-α (adverse survival) (Basheeth & Patil, 2019). Advances in biomarker technology are using predictive behavior to determine the progressive nature of tumors; in HNSCC, automated miniature chips are used to analyze saliva samples, ensuring several markers are detected to determine metastasis (Lutzky et al., 2008). In addition, for the tumor marker to be considered a valid screening tool, its sensitivity and specificity must exceed 95% to avoid false positives (Basheeth & Patil, 2019).

6.6 Future Perspectives

Despite the remarkable success in recent immunotherapy clinical trials, a significant challenge that persists is the low response rate observed in some patients (Dobosz et al., 2022). Novel approaches are being developed to augment responses to immunotherapy, leveraging emerging insights into T-cell and broader immune system functionality (Riley et al., 2019). Efforts are currently under way to develop actionable solutions to combat immunotherapeutic resistance (Guo et al., 2021). Most of these treatments utilize combination strategies to overcome this plight. Moreover, the combined approach, supported by compelling clinical and preclinical evidence, entails the utilization of molecularly targeted therapy alongside immunotherapy (Robert et al., 2016). Targeted therapies sensitize tumor cells to immunotherapy, thus providing a synergistic antitumor effect (Guo et al., 2021).

Combination therapies may bring benefits such as a reduction in toxic effects, which can be achieved through the use of reduced dosages while maintaining efficacy as compared to monotherapies (Yasuda et al., 2013). Furthermore, the use of bispecific antibodies targeting EGFR and PD-1 may provide a novel and promising approach to treating HNC. These antibodies utilize a simultaneous targeting approach and have delivered more potent antitumor effects compared to monotherapies or their combination (Li et al., 2021). The combination of drugs, however, may also increase the costs of clinical care (Boshuizen & Peeper, 2020). Therefore, investigating approaches that combine therapies with repurposed pharmaceutical agents should be explored because they have previously demonstrated a potential to mitigate cancer burden. Repurposing immunotherapy or targeted therapy drugs that are used to treat other diseases, especially if they are FDA approved for similar targets as in cancer, could lower the overall cost of HNC combination therapies. As a result, this could increase therapy cost efficiency and benefit medically underserved patients (Bayat Mokhtari et al., 2017).

6.7 Conclusion

Targeted therapies and immunotherapy have significantly improved survival rates in patients with HNC. These treatments work by targeting specific molecules involved in tumorigenesis and progression, such as EGFR and other receptors, and by modulating the immune system to enhance its ability to fight cancer. For instance, drugs like cetuximab target EGFR, while ICIs such as pembrolizumab and nivolumab block proteins that inhibit the immune response, thereby allowing T cells to attack cancer cells more effectively. This dual approach not only inhibits cancer growth directly but also boosts the body's natural defenses against the tumor. Biomarkers play a vital role in tracking therapy response and have demonstrated that immunotherapies are more effective in immunologically "hot" tumors due to an increased immune cell infiltration.

Despite these beneficial clinical outcomes, drug resistance, costs, and drug-associated toxicities create a bottleneck in their clinical application. Combining targeted therapies with immunotherapy provides a more promising therapeutic approach because these therapies were shown to synergically target more than one driver of HNC pathogenesis in preclinical and clinical studies. This has thus established a basis prompting more research to explore the best ways of integrating targeted therapy and immunotherapy to elevate the current clinical response and accomplish HNC disease-free survival.

References

AGGARWAL, C., COHEN, R. B., MORROW, M. P., KRAYNYAK, K. A., SYLVESTER, A. J., KNOBLOCK, D. M., BAUML, J. M., WEINSTEIN, G. S., LIN, A., BOYER, J., SAKATA, L., TAN, S., ANTON, A., DICKERSON, K., MANGROLIA, D., VANG, R., DALLAS, M., OYOLA, S., DUFF, S., ESSER, M., KUMAR, R., WEINER, D., CSIKI, I., & BAGARAZZI, M. L. 2019. Immunotherapy targeting HPV16/18 generates potent immune responses in HPV-associated head and neck cancer. *Clin Cancer Res*, 25, 110–24.

ALNEFAIE, A., ALBOGAMI, S., ASIRI, Y., AHMAD, T., ALOTAIBI, S. S., AL-SANEA, M. M., & ALTHOBAITI, H. 2022. Chimeric antigen receptor t-cells: An overview of concepts, applications, limitations, and proposed solutions. *Front Bioeng Biotechnol*, 10, 797440.

APONTE, P. M., & CAICEDO, A. 2017. Stemness in cancer: Stem cells, cancer stem cells, and their microenvironment. *Stem Cells Int*, 2017, 5619472.

ARGIRIS, A., LI, S., SAVVIDES, P., OHR, J. P., GILBERT, J., LEVINE, M. A., CHAKRAVARTI, A., HAIGENTZ, M., JR., SABA, N. F., IKPEAZU, C. V., SCHNEIDER, C. J., PINTO, H. A., FORASTIERE, A. A., & BURTNESS, B. 2019. Phase III randomized trial of chemotherapy with or without bevacizumab in patients with recurrent or metastatic head and neck cancer. *J Clin Oncol*, 37, 3266–74.

AYALA CEJA, M., KHERICHA, M., HARRIS, C. M., PUIG-SAUS, C., & CHEN, Y. Y. 2024. Car-T cell manufacturing: Major process parameters and next-generation strategies. *J Experiment Med*, 221(2), e20230903.

AYATI, A., MOGHIMI, S., TOOLABI, M., & FOROUMADI, A. 2021. Pyrimidine-based EGFR TK inhibitors in targeted cancer therapy. *Eur J Med Chem*, 221, 113523.

BAI, R., CHEN, N., LI, L., DU, N., BAI, L., LV, Z., TIAN, H., & CUI, J. 2020. Mechanisms of cancer resistance to immunotherapy. *Front Oncol*, 10, 1290.

BALIK, K., MODRAKOWSKA, P., MAJ, M., KAźMIERSKI, Ł., & BAJEK, A. 2019. Limitations of molecularly targeted therapy. *Med Res J*, 4, 99–105.

BASHEETH, N., & PATIL, N. 2019. Biomarkers in head and neck cancer an update. *Indian J Otolaryngol Head Neck Surg*, 71, 1002–11.

BAYAT MOKHTARI, R., HOMAYOUNI, T. S., BALUCH, N., MORGATSKAYA, E., KUMAR, S., DAS, B., & YEGER, H. 2017. Combination therapy in combating cancer. *Oncotarget*, 8, 38022–43.

BLAŽEK, T., PETRáš, M., KNYBEL, L., CVEK, J., & SOUMAROVá, R. 2023. Programmed cell death ligand 1 expression on immune cells and survival in patients with nonmetastatic head and neck cancer: A systematic review and meta-analysis. *JAMA Netw Open*, 6, e236324.

BOECKX, C., BAAY, M., WOUTERS, A., SPECENIER, P., VERMORKEN, J. B., PEETERS, M., & LARDON, F. 2013. Anti-epidermal growth factor receptor therapy in head and neck squamous cell carcinoma: Focus on potential molecular mechanisms of drug resistance. *Oncologist*, 18, 850–64.

BOREL, C., JUNG, A. C., & BURGY, M. 2020. Immunotherapy breakthroughs in the treatment of recurrent or metastatic head and neck squamous cell carcinoma. *Cancers (Basel)*, 12(9), 2691.

BOSHUIZEN, J., & PEEPER, D. S. 2020. Rational cancer treatment combinations: An urgent clinical need. *Mol Cell*, 78, 1002–18.

BOSSI, P., RESTEGHINI, C., PAIELLI, N., LICITRA, L., PILOTTI, S., & PERRONE, F. 2016. Prognostic and predictive value of EGFR in head and neck squamous cell carcinoma. *Oncotarget*, 7, 74362–79.

BOTH, L., BANYARD, A. C., VAN DOLLEWEERD, C., WRIGHT, E., MA, J. K. C., & FOOKS, A. R. 2013. Monoclonal antibodies for prophylactic and therapeutic use against viral infections. *Vaccine*, 31, 1553–9.

BURTNESS, B., HARRINGTON, K. J., GREIL, R., SOULIÈRES, D., TAHARA, M., DE CASTRO, G., JR., PSYRRI, A., BASTÉ, N., NEUPANE, P., BRATLAND, Å., FUEREDER, T., HUGHES, B. G. M., MESÍA, R., NGAMPHAIBOON, N., RORDORF, T., WAN ISHAK, W. Z., HONG, R. L., GONZÁLEZ MENDOZA, R., ROY, A., ZHANG, Y., GUMUSCU, B., CHENG, J. D., JIN, F., & RISCHIN, D. 2019. Pembrolizumab alone or with chemotherapy versus cetuximab with chemotherapy for recurrent or metastatic squamous cell carcinoma of the head and neck (Keynote-048): A randomised, open-label, phase 3 study. *Lancet*, 394, 1915–28.

CAI, W. Q., ZENG, L. S., WANG, L. F., WANG, Y. Y., CHENG, J. T., ZHANG, Y., HAN, Z. W., ZHOU, Y., HUANG, S. L., WANG, X. W., PENG, X. C., XIANG, Y., MA, Z., CUI, S. Z., & XIN, H. W. 2020. The latest battles between EGFR monoclonal antibodies and resistant tumor cells. *Front Oncol*, 10, 1249.

CAMPBELL, K. S., & HASEGAWA, J. 2013. Natural killer cell biology: An update and future directions. *J Allergy Clin Immunol*, 132, 536–44.

CHEN, P., HSU, W. H., HAN, J., XIA, Y., & DEPINHO, R. A. 2021. Cancer stemness meets immunity: From mechanism to therapy. *Cell Rep*, 34, 108597.

CHENG, G., DONG, H., YANG, C., LIU, Y., WU, Y., ZHU, L., TONG, X., & WANG, S. 2021. A review on the advances and challenges of immunotherapy for head and neck cancer. *Cancer Cell Int*, 21, 406.

CHIANG, C.-L., CHAN, S.-K., LEE, S.-F., WONG, I. O.-L., & CHOI, H. C.-W. 2021. Cost-effectiveness of pembrolizumab as a second-line therapy for hepatocellular carcinoma. *JAMA Network Open*, 4, e2033761–e2033761.

CICIOLA, P., CASCETTA, P., BIANCO, C., FORMISANO, L., & BIANCO, R. 2020. Combining immune checkpoint inhibitors with anti-angiogenic agents. *J Clin Med*, 9(3), 675.

CÍVICO-ORTEGA, J. L., GONZÁLEZ-RUIZ, I., RAMOS-GARCÍA, P., CRUZ-GRANADOS, D., SAMAYOA-DESCAMPS, V., & GONZÁLEZ-MOLES, M. Á. 2023. Prognostic and clinicopathological significance of epidermal growth factor receptor (EGFR) expression in oral squamous cell carcinoma: Systematic review and meta-analysis. *Int J Molec Sci*, 24, 11888.

CONCIATORI, F., BAZZICHETTO, C., FALCONE, I., CIUFFREDA, L., FERRETTI, G., VARI, S., FERRARESI, V., COGNETTI, F., & MILELLA, M. 2020. PTEN function at the interface between cancer and tumor microenvironment: Implications for response to immunotherapy. *Int J Molec Sci*, 21, 5337.

CONNOLLY, C., BAMBHANIA, K., & NAIDOO, J. 2019. Immune-related adverse events: A case-based approach. *Front Oncol*, 9, 530.

CUI, Q., LI, W., WANG, D., WANG, S., & YU, J. 2023. Prognostic significance of blood-based PD-L1 analysis in patients with non-small cell lung cancer undergoing immune checkpoint inhibitor therapy: A systematic review and meta-analysis. *World J Surg Oncol*, 21, 318.

DE PAUW, I., BOECKX, C., & WOUTERS, A. 2021. Mechanisms of cetuximab resistance and how to overcome it. *In:* VERMORKEN, J. B., BUDACH, V., LEEMANS, C. R., MACHIELS, J.-P., NICOLAI, P., & O'SULLIVAN, B., eds. *Critical Issues in Head and Neck Oncology*. Cham: Springer International, 21–51.

DOBOSZ, P., STĘPIEŃ, M., GOLKE, A., & DZIECIĄTKOWSKI, T. 2022. Challenges of the immunotherapy: Perspectives and limitations of the immune checkpoint inhibitor treatment. *Int J Mol Sci*, 23(5), 2847.

DONG, Y. H., DING, Y. M., GUO, W., HUANG, J. W., YANG, Z., ZHANG, Y., & CHEN, X. H. 2018. The functional verification of EGFR-car T-cells targeted to hypopharyngeal squamous cell carcinoma. *Onco Targets Ther*, 11, 7053–9.

DOS SANTOS, L. V., ABRAHÃO, C. M., & WILLIAM, W. N., JR. 2021. Overcoming resistance to immune checkpoint inhibitors in head and neck squamous cell carcinomas. *Front Oncol*, 11, 596290.

DUMITRU, C. S., & RAICA, M. 2023. Vascular endothelial growth factor family and head and neck squamous cell carcinoma. *Anticancer Res*, 43, 4315–26.

EBERLY, H. W., SCISCENT, B. Y., LORENZ, F. J., RETTIG, E. M., & GOYAL, N. 2024. Current and emerging diagnostic, prognostic, and predictive biomarkers in head and neck cancer. *Biomedicines*, 12(2), 415.

EKANAYAKE WEERAMANGE, C., LIU, Z., HARTEL, G., LI, Y., VASANI, S., LANGTON-LOCKTON, J., KENNY, L., MORRIS, L., FRAZER, I., TANG, K. D., & PUNYADEERA, C. 2021. Salivary high-risk human papillomavirus (HPV) DNA as a biomarker for HPV-driven head and neck cancers. *J Mol Diagn*, 23, 1334–42.

FASANO, M., DELLA CORTE, C. M., VISCARDI, G., DI LIELLO, R., PARAGLIOLA, F., SPARANO, F., IACOVINO, M. L., CASTRICHINO, A., DORIA, F., SICA, A., MORGILLO, F., COLELLA, G., TARTARO, G., CAPPABIANCA, S., TESTA, D., MOTTA, G., & CIARDIELLO, F. 2021. Head and neck cancer: The role of anti-EGFR agents in the era of immunotherapy. *Ther Adv Med Oncol*, 13, 1758835920949418.

FERRIS, R. L., BLUMENSCHEIN, G., JR., FAYETTE, J., GUIGAY, J., COLEVAS, A. D., LICITRA, L., HARRINGTON, K., KASPER, S., VOKES, E. E., EVEN, C., WORDEN, F., SABA, N. F., IGLESIAS DOCAMPO, L. C., HADDAD, R., RORDORF, T., KIYOTA, N., TAHARA, M., MONGA, M., LYNCH, M., GEESE, W. J., KOPIT, J., SHAW, J. W., & GILLISON, M. L. 2016. Nivolumab for recurrent squamous-cell carcinoma of the head and neck. *N Engl J Med*, 375, 1856–67.

GABER, R., GOLDMANN, T., BORSTEL, S., CLINICAL, BORSTEL, ALEXAANDRIA, EGYPT & BLOCKQUOTE 2018. Mini review: Immunohistochemistry using EGFR-mutant specific antibodies in non-small cell lung carcinoma: Accuracy and reliability. *J Cancer Treat Diagn*. Available at: https://www.cancertreatmentjournal.com/articles/mini-review-immunohistochemistry-using-egfrmutant-specific-antibodies-in-nonsmall-cell-lung-carcinoma-accuracy-and-reliability.html (Accessed: 03 April 2015).

GAVRIELATOU, N., DOUMAS, S., ECONOMOPOULOU, P., FOUKAS, P. G., & PSYRRI, A. 2020. Biomarkers for immunotherapy response in head and neck cancer. *Cancer Treat Rev*, 84, 101977.

GHOSH, S., SHAH, P. A., & JOHNSON, F. M. 2022. Novel systemic treatment modalities including immunotherapy and molecular targeted therapy for recurrent and metastatic head and neck squamous cell carcinoma. *Int J Mol Sci*, 23(14), 7889.

GOEL, B., TIWARI, A. K., PANDEY, R. K., SINGH, A. P., KUMAR, S., SINHA, A., JAIN, S. K., & KHATTRI, A. 2022. Therapeutic approaches for the treatment of head and neck squamous cell carcinoma-an update on clinical trials. *Transl Oncol*, 21, 101426.

GORMLEY, M., CREANEY, G., SCHACHE, A., INGARFIELD, K., & CONWAY, D. I. 2022. Reviewing the epidemiology of head and neck cancer: Definitions, trends and risk factors. *Br Dental J*, 233, 780–6.

GREEN, A. 2021. Challenges in assessing the cost-effectiveness of cancer immunotherapy. *JAMA Netw Open*, 4, e2034020.

GUO, C. X., HUANG, X., XU, J., ZHANG, X. Z., SHEN, Y. N., LIANG, T. B., & BAI, X. L. 2021. Combined targeted therapy and immunotherapy for cancer treatment. *World J Clin Cases*, 9, 7643–7652.

HAIBE, Y., KREIDIEH, M., EL HAJJ, H., KHALIFEH, I., MUKHERJI, D., TEMRAZ, S., & SHAMSEDDINE, A. 2020. Resistance mechanisms to anti-angiogenic therapies in cancer. *Front Oncol*, 10, 221.

HAN, Y., LIU, D., & LI, L. 2020. PD-1/PD-L1 pathway: Current researches in cancer. *Am J Cancer Res*, 10, 727–42.

HARMANKAYA, I., ÇALOĞLU, V. Y., TAŞTEKIN, E., TÜRKKAN, G., ÇALOĞLU, M., & UZAL, C. 2022. Prognostic importance of microvessel density, VEGF expression and perineural invasion in laryngeal cancer treated with adjuvant radiotherapy. *Indian J Pathol Microbiol*, 65, 521–6.

HASHMI, A. A., HUSSAIN, Z. F., AIJAZ, S., IRFAN, M., KHAN, E. Y., NAZ, S., FARIDI, N., KHAN, A., & EDHI, M. M. 2018. Immunohistochemical expression of epidermal growth factor receptor (EGFR) in South Asian head and neck squamous cell carcinoma: Association with various risk factors and clinico-pathologic and prognostic parameters. *World J Surg Oncol*, 16, 118.

HU, F., GUO, L., YU, J., DAI, D., XIONG, Y., HE, Y., & ZHOU, W. 2021. Using patient-derived xenografts to explore the efficacy of treating head-and-neck squamous cell carcinoma with anlotinib. *Pathol Oncol Res*, 27, 1610008.

HUA, Y., DONG, R., JIN, T., JIN, Q., & CHEN, X. 2022. Anti-PD-1 monoclonal antibody combined with anti-VEGF agent is safe and effective in patients with recurrent/metastatic head and neck squamous cancer as second-line or beyond treatment. *Front Oncol*, 12, 781348.

HUANG, L., JIANG, S., & SHI, Y. 2020. Tyrosine kinase inhibitors for solid tumors in the past 20 years (2001-2020). *J Hematol Oncol*, 13, 143.

HUTCHINSON, R. A., ADAMS, R. A., MCART, D. G., SALTO-TELLEZ, M., JASANI, B., & HAMILTON, P. W. 2015. Epidermal growth factor receptor immunohistochemistry: New opportunities in metastatic colorectal cancer. *J Translat Med*, 13, 217.

HYYTIÄINEN, A., WAHBI, W., VÄYRYNEN, O., SAARILAHTI, K., KARIHTALA, P., SALO, T., & AL-SAMADI, A. 2021. Angiogenesis inhibitors for head and neck squamous cell carcinoma treatment: Is there still hope? *Front Oncol*, 11, 683570.

IRANZO, P., CALLEJO, A., ASSAF, J. D., MOLINA, G., LOPEZ, D. E., GARCIA-ILLESCAS, D., PARDO, N., NAVARRO, A., MARTINEZ-MARTI, A., CEDRES, S., CARBONELL, C., FRIGOLA, J., AMAT, R., & FELIP, E. 2022. Overview of checkpoint inhibitors mechanism of action: Role of immune-related adverse events and their treatment on progression of underlying cancer. *Front Med (Lausanne)*, 9, 875974.

ISHII, H., TANAKA, S., & MASUYAMA, K. 2015. Therapeutic strategy for cancer immunotherapy in head and neck cancer. *Adv Cell Molec Otolaryngol*, 3, 27690.

JANKU, F. 2014. Tumor heterogeneity in the clinic: Is it a real problem? *Ther Adv Med Oncol*, 6, 43–51.

JIE, H. B., SCHULER, P. J., LEE, S. C., SRIVASTAVA, R. M., ARGIRIS, A., FERRONE, S., WHITESIDE, T. L., & FERRIS, R. L. 2015. CTLA-4$^+$ regulatory T cells increased in cetuximab-treated head and neck cancer patients suppress NK cell cytotoxicity and correlate with poor prognosis. *Cancer Res*, 75, 2200–10.

JULIAN, R., SAVANI, M., & BAUMAN, J. E. 2021. Immunotherapy approaches in HPV-associated head and neck cancer. *Cancers (Basel)*, 13(23), 5889.

KAKAVAND, H., JACKETT, L. A., MENZIES, A. M., GIDE, T. N., CARLINO, M. S., SAW, R. P. M., THOMPSON, J. F., WILMOTT, J. S., LONG, G. V., & SCOLYER, R. A. 2017. Negative immune checkpoint regulation by vista: A mechanism of acquired resistance to anti-pd-1 therapy in metastatic melanoma patients. *Mod Pathol*, 30, 1666–76.

KANG, J. J., KO, A., KIL, S. H., MALLEN-ST CLAIR, J., SHIN, D. S., WANG, M. B., & SRIVATSAN, E. S. 2023. EGFR pathway targeting drugs in head and neck cancer in the era of immunotherapy. *Biochim Biophys Acta Rev Cancer*, 1878, 188827.

KAO, H. F., & LOU, P. J. 2019. Immune checkpoint inhibitors for head and neck squamous cell carcinoma: Current landscape and future directions. *Head Neck*, 41 Suppl 1, 4–18.

KEREN, S., SHOUDE, Z., LU, Z., & BEIBEI, Y. 2014. Role of EGFR as a prognostic factor for survival in head and neck cancer: A meta-analysis. *Tumour Biol*, 35, 2285–95.

KHADELA, A., SHAH, Y., MISTRY, P., BODIWALA, K., & AVINASH, C. B. 2023. Immunomodulatory therapy in head and neck squamous cell carcinoma: Recent advances and clinical prospects. *Technol Cancer Res Treat*, 22, 15330338221150559.

KHAN, K. H., WONG, M., RIHAWI, K., BODLA, S., MORGANSTEIN, D., BANERJI, U., & MOLIFE, L. R. 2016. Hyperglycemia and phosphatidylinositol 3-kinase/protein kinase b/

mammalian target of rapamycin (PI3K/AKT/MTOR) inhibitors in phase I trials: Incidence, predictive factors, and management. *Oncologist*, 21, 855–60.

KLUGER, H. M., TAWBI, H. A., ASCIERTO, M. L., BOWDEN, M., CALLAHAN, M. K., CHA, E., CHEN, H. X., DRAKE, C. G., FELTQUATE, D. M., FERRIS, R. L., GULLEY, J. L., GUPTA, S., HUMPHREY, R. W., LAVALLEE, T. M., LE, D. T., HUBBARD-LUCEY, V. M., PAPADIMITRAKOPOULOU, V. A., POSTOW, M. A., RUBIN, E. H., SHARON, E., TAUBE, J. M., TOPALIAN, S. L., ZAPPASODI, R., SZNOL, M., & SULLIVAN, R. J. 2020. Defining tumor resistance to PD-1 pathway blockade: Recommendations from the first meeting of the SITC immunotherapy resistance taskforce. *J ImmunoTher Cancer*, 8, e000398.

KORDBACHEH, F., & FARAH, C. S. 2021. Current and emerging molecular therapies for head and neck squamous cell carcinoma. *Cancers (Basel)*, 13(21), 5471.

KYZAS, P. A., STEFANOU, D., BATISTATOU, A., & AGNANTIS, N. J. 2005. Prognostic significance of VEGF immunohistochemical expression and tumor angiogenesis in head and neck squamous cell carcinoma. *J Cancer Res Clin Oncol*, 131, 624–30.

LEBLANC, O., VACHER, S., LECERF, C., JEANNOT, E., KLIJANIENKO, J., BERGER, F., HOFFMANN, C., CALUGARU, V., BADOIS, N., CHILLES, A., LESNIK, M., KRHILI, S., BIECHE, I., LE TOURNEAU, C., & KAMAL, M. 2020. Biomarkers of cetuximab resistance in patients with head and neck squamous cell carcinoma. *Cancer Biol Med*, 17, 208–17.

LEE, S. C., LÓPEZ-ALBAITERO, A., & FERRIS, R. L. 2009. Immunotherapy of head and neck cancer using tumor antigen-specific monoclonal antibodies. *Curr Oncol Rep*, 11, 156–62.

LEVY, B., BARLESI, F., PAZ-ARES, L., BENNOUNA, J., ERMAN, M., FELIP, E., ISLA, D., RYUN KIM, H., KIM, S. W., MADELAINE, J., MOLINIER, O., ÖZGÜROĞLU, M., RODRÍGUEZ ABREU, D., ADENIJI, A., LORENCE, R. M., VOCCIA, I., CHISAMORE, M. J., & RIESS, J. W. 2022. Phase II study of afatinib plus pembrolizumab in patients with squamous cell carcinoma of the lung following progression during or after first-line chemotherapy (LUX-LUNG-IO). *Lung Cancer*, 166, 107–13.

LI, H., TORABI, S. J., YARBROUGH, W. G., MEHRA, S., OSBORN, H. A., & JUDSON, B. 2018. Association of human papillomavirus status at head and neck carcinoma subsites with overall survival. *JAMA Otolaryngol Head Neck Surg*, 144, 519–25.

LI, L., DENG, L., MENG, X., GU, C., MENG, L., LI, K., ZHANG, X., MENG, Y., XU, W., ZHAO, L., CHEN, J., ZHU, Z., & HUANG, H. 2021. Tumor-targeting anti-EGFR x anti-PD1 bispecific antibody inhibits EGFR-overexpressing tumor growth by combining EGFR blockade and immune activation with direct tumor cell killing. *Translat Oncol*, 14, 100916.

LI, Q., TIE, Y., ALU, A., MA, X., & SHI, H. 2023. Targeted therapy for head and neck cancer: Signaling pathways and clinical studies. *Signal Transduction Targeted Ther*, 8, 31.

LI, Y.-Z., & ZHANG, H.-M. 2022. Recent advances in primary resistance mechanisms against immune checkpoint inhibitors. *Curr Opin Oncol*, 34, 95–106.

LICITRA, L., STöRKEL, S., KERR, K. M., VAN CUTSEM, E., PIRKER, R., HIRSCH, F. R., VERMORKEN, J. B., VON HEYDEBRECK, A., ESSER, R., CELIK, I., & CIARDIELLO, F. 2013. Predictive value of epidermal growth factor receptor expression for first-line chemotherapy plus cetuximab in patients with head and neck and colorectal cancer: Analysis of data from the extreme and crystal studies. *Eur J Cancer*, 49, 1161–8.

LIU, C. Q., XU, J., ZHOU, Z. G., JIN, L. L., YU, X. J., XIAO, G., LIN, J., ZHUANG, S. M., ZHANG, Y. J., & ZHENG, L. 2018. Expression patterns of programmed death ligand 1 correlate with different microenvironments and patient prognosis in hepatocellular carcinoma. *Br J Cancer*, 119, 80–8.

LIZOTTE, P. H., HONG, R. L., LUSTER, T. A., CAVANAUGH, M. E., TAUS, L. J., WANG, S., DHANESHWAR, A., MAYMAN, N., YANG, A., KULKARNI, M., BADALUCCO, L., FITZPATRICK, E., KAO, H. F., KURAGUCHI, M., BITTINGER, M., KIRSCHMEIER, P. T., GRAY, N. S., BARBIE, D. A., & JÄNNE, P. A. 2018. A high-throughput immune-oncology screen identifies EGFR inhibitors as potent enhancers of antigen-specific cytotoxic T-lymphocyte tumor cell killing. *Cancer Immunol Res*, 6, 1511–23.

LONG, Z., GRANDIS, J. R., & JOHNSON, D. E. 2022. Emerging tyrosine kinase inhibitors for head and neck cancer. *Expert Opin Emerg Drugs*, 27, 333–44.

LOPEZ, J. S., & BANERJI, U. 2017. Combine and conquer: Challenges for targeted therapy combinations in early phase trials. *Nat Rev Clin Oncol*, 14, 57–66.

LUTZKY, V. P., MOSS, D. J., CHIN, D., COMAN, W. B., PARSONS, P. G., & BOYLE, G. M. 2008. Biomarkers for cancers of the head and neck. *Clin Med Ear Nose Throat*, 1, CMENT. S1051.

MARRET, G., TEMAM, S., KAMAL, M., EVEN, C., DELORD, J. P., HOFFMANN, C., DOLIVET, G., MALARD, O., FAYETTE, J., CAPITAIN, O., VERGEZ, S., GEOFFROIS, L., ROLLAND, F., ZROUNBA, P., LACCOURREYE, L., SAADA-BOUZID, E., AIDE, N., BÉNAVENT, V., KLIJIANENKO, J., LAMY, C., GIRARD, E., VACHER, S., MASLIAH-PLANCHON, J., DE KONING, L., PUARD, V., BORCOMAN, E., JIMENEZ, M., BIÈCHE, I., GAL, J., & LE TOURNEAU, C. 2023. Randomized phase II study of preoperative afatinib in untreated head and neck cancers: Predictive and pharmacodynamic biomarkers of activity. *Sci Rep*, 13, 22524.

MARUSYK, A., JANISZEWSKA, M., & POLYAK, K. 2020. Intratumor heterogeneity: The Rosetta stone of therapy resistance. *Cancer Cell*, 37, 471–84.

MELIANTE, P. G., PETRELLA, C., FIORE, M., MINNI, A., & BARBATO, C. 2023. Head and neck squamous cell carcinoma vaccine: Current landscape and perspectives. *Curr Issues Mol Biol*, 45, 9215–33.

MIAO, R., CHEN, H. H., DANG, Q., XIA, L. Y., YANG, Z. Y., HE, M. F., HAO, Z. F., & LIANG, Y. 2020. Beyond the limitation of targeted therapy: Improve the application of targeted drugs combining genomic data with machine learning. *Pharmacol Res*, 159, 104932.

MICAILY, I., JOHNSON, J., & ARGIRIS, A. 2020. An update on angiogenesis targeting in head and neck squamous cell carcinoma. *Cancers Head Neck*, 5, 5.

MILANO, G., GAL, J., & BENSADOUN, R. J. 2024. Molecular and nutritional markers in head and neck cancer. *Curr Opin Oncol*, 5, 5.

MISHRA, P. S., SIDHU, A., DWIVEDI, G., MULAJKER, D. S., & AWASTHI, S. 2022a. Determining PD-L1 expression in head and neck squamous cell carcinoma using immunohistochemistry. *Indian J Cancer*, 59, 474–9.

MISHRA, V., SINGH, A., CHEN, X., ROSENBERG, A. J., PEARSON, A. T., ZHAVORONKOV, A., SAVAGE, P. A., LINGEN, M. W., AGRAWAL, N., & IZUMCHENKO, E. 2022b. Application of liquid biopsy as multi-functional biomarkers in head and neck cancer. *Br J Cancer*, 126, 361–70.

MÜLLER, T., BRAUN, M., DIETRICH, D., AKTEKIN, S., HÖFT, S., KRISTIANSEN, G., GÖKE, F., SCHRÖCK, A., BRÄGELMANN, J., HELD, S. A. E., BOOTZ, F., & BROSSART, P. 2017. PD-L1: A novel prognostic biomarker in head and neck squamous cell carcinoma. *Oncotarget*, 8, 52889–900.

NAIR, S., BONNER, J. A., & BREDEL, M. 2022. EGFR mutations in head and neck squamous cell carcinoma. *Int J Mol Sci*, 23(7), 3818.

NAKANO, K. 2021. Progress of molecular targeted therapy for head and neck cancer in clinical aspects. *Mol Biomed*, 2, 15.

OLIVA, M., SPREAFICO, A., TABERNA, M., ALEMANY, L., COBURN, B., MESIA, R., & SIU, L. L. 2019. Immune biomarkers of response to immune-checkpoint inhibitors in head and neck squamous cell carcinoma. *Ann Oncol*, 30, 57–67.

PADMA, V. V. 2015. An overview of targeted cancer therapy. *Biomedicine (Taipei)*, 5, 19.

PARK, J. C., DURBECK, J., CLARK, J. R., & FADEN, D. L. 2020. Treatment sequence of cetuximab and immune checkpoint inhibitor in head and neck squamous cell carcinoma differentially affects outcomes. *Oral Oncol*, 111, 105024.

PARK, J. C., KRISHNAKUMAR, H. N., & SALADI, S. V. 2022. Current and future biomarkers for immune checkpoint inhibitors in head and neck squamous cell carcinoma. *Curr Oncol*, 29, 4185–98.

PATEL, S. R., BROWN, S. N., KUBUSEK, J. E., MANSFIELD, A. S., & DUMA, N. 2020. Osimertinib-induced cardiomyopathy. *JACC Case Rep*, 2, 641–5.

PEREIRA, D., MARTINS, D., & MENDES, F. 2022. Immunotherapy in head and neck cancer: When, how, and why? *Biomedicines*, 10(9), 2151.

PETERS, S., KERR, K. M., & STAHEL, R. 2018. PD-1 blockade in advanced NSCLC: A focus on pembrolizumab. *Cancer Treat Rev*, 62, 39–49.

PETERSSON, L., STÄDE, L. W., BROFELTH, M., GÄRTNER, S., FORS, E., SANDGREN, M., VALLKIL, J., OLSSON, N., LARSEN, K. L., BORREBAECK, C. A. K., DUROUX, L., & WINGREN, C. 2014. Molecular design of recombinant SCFV antibodies for site-specific photocoupling to β-cyclodextrin in solution and onto solid support. *Biochimica et Biophysica Acta (BBA) - Proteins and Proteomics*, 1844, 2164–73.

PONOMAREV, A., GILAZIEVA, Z., SOLOVYEVA, V., ALLEGRUCCI, C., & RIZVANOV, A. 2022. Intrinsic and extrinsic factors impacting cancer stemness and tumor progression. *Cancers*, 14, 970.

QIAO, X. W., JIANG, J., PANG, X., HUANG, M. C., TANG, Y. J., LIANG, X. H., & TANG, Y. L. 2020. The evolving landscape of PD-1/PD-L1 pathway in head and neck cancer. *Front Immunol*, 11, 1721.

REHMANI, H. S., & ISSAEVA, N. 2020. EGFR in head and neck squamous cell carcinoma: Exploring possibilities of novel drug combinations. *Ann Transl Med*, 8, 813.

REN, D., HUA, Y., YU, B., YE, X., HE, Z., LI, C., WANG, J., MO, Y., WEI, X., CHEN, Y., ZHOU, Y., LIAO, Q., WANG, H., XIANG, B., ZHOU, M., LI, X., LI, G., LI, Y., ZENG, Z., & XIONG, W. 2020. Predictive biomarkers and mechanisms underlying resistance to PD1/PD-L1 blockade cancer immunotherapy. *Molec Cancer*, 19, 19.

REN, Z., XU, J., BAI, Y., XU, A., CANG, S., DU, C., LI, Q., LU, Y., CHEN, Y., GUO, Y., CHEN, Z., LIU, B., JIA, W., WU, J., WANG, J., SHAO, G., ZHANG, B., SHAN, Y., MENG, Z., WU, J., GU, S., YANG, W., LIU, C., SHI, X., GAO, Z., YIN, T., CUI, J., HUANG, M., XING, B., MAO, Y., TENG, G., QIN, Y., WANG, J., XIA, F., YIN, G., YANG, Y., CHEN, M., WANG, Y., ZHOU, H., & FAN, J. 2021. Sintilimab plus a bevacizumab biosimilar (IBI305) versus sorafenib in unresectable hepatocellular carcinoma (Orient-32): A randomised, open-label, phase 2-3 study. *Lancet Oncol*, 22, 977–90.

RILEY, R. S., JUNE, C. H., LANGER, R., & MITCHELL, M. J. 2019. Delivery technologies for cancer immunotherapy. *Nat Rev Drug Disc*, 18, 175–96.

RIVERA-CONCEPCION, J., UPRETY, D., & ADJEI, A. A. 2022. Challenges in the use of targeted therapies in non-small cell lung cancer. *Cancer Res Treat*, 54, 315–29.

ROBERT, L., RIBAS, A., & HU-LIESKOVAN, S. 2016. Combining targeted therapy with immunotherapy. Can 1+1 equal more than 2? *Semin Immunol*, 28(1), 73–80. doi:10.1016/j.smim.2016.01.001. Epub 2016 Feb 6.

RODEN, D. F., JOHNSON, J. M., SZTURZ, P., BOSSI, P., & ARGIRIS, A. 2021. New and promising targeted therapies in first and second-line settings. *In:* VERMORKEN, J. B., BUDACH, V., LEEMANS, C. R., MACHIELS, J.-P., NICOLAI, P., & O'SULLIVAN, B., eds. *Critical Issues in Head and Neck Oncology*. Cham: Springer International, 277–96.

RODRIGO, J. P., SÁNCHEZ-CANTELI, M., OTERO-ROSALES, M., MARTÍNEZ-CAMBLOR, P., HERMIDA-PRADO, F., & GARCÍA-PEDRERO, J. M. 2024. Tumor mutational burden predictability in head and neck squamous cell carcinoma patients treated with immunotherapy: Systematic review and meta-analysis. *J Transl Med*, 22, 135.

RODRÍGUEZ-NAVA, C., ORTUÑO-PINEDA, C., ILLADES-AGUIAR, B., FLORES-ALFARO, E., LEYVA-VÁZQUEZ, M. A., PARRA-ROJAS, I., DEL MORAL-HERNÁNDEZ, O., VENCES-VELÁZQUEZ, A., CORTÉS–SARABIA, K., & ALARCÓN-ROMERO, L. D. C. 2023. Mechanisms of action and limitations of monoclonal antibodies and single chain fragment variable (SCFV) in the treatment of cancer. *Biomedicines*, 11(6), 1610.

ROSEWELL SHAW, A., PORTER, C. E., WATANABE, N., TANOUE, K., SIKORA, A., GOTTSCHALK, S., BRENNER, M. K., & SUZUKI, M. 2017. Adenovirotherapy delivering cytokine and checkpoint inhibitor augments Car T cells against metastatic head and neck cancer. *Mol Ther*, 25, 2440–51.

SACCO, A. G., CHEN, R., WORDEN, F. P., WONG, D. J. L., ADKINS, D., SWIECICKI, P., CHAI-HO, W., OPPELT, P., GHOSH, D., BYKOWSKI, J., MOLINOLO, A., PITTMAN,

E., ESTRADA, M. V., GOLD, K., DANIELS, G., LIPPMAN, S. M., NATSUHARA, A., MESSER, K., & COHEN, E. E. W. 2021. Pembrolizumab plus cetuximab in patients with recurrent or metastatic head and neck squamous cell carcinoma: An open-label, multi-arm, non-randomised, multicentre, phase 2 trial. *Lancet Oncol*, 22, 883–92.

SALOURA, V., FATIMA, A., ZEWDE, M., KIYOTANI, K., BRISSON, R., PARK, J.-H., IKEDA, Y., VOUGIOUKLAKIS, T., BAO, R., KHATTRI, A., SEIWERT, T., CIPRIANI, N., LINGEN, M., VOKES, E., & NAKAMURA, Y. 2017. Characterization of the T-cell receptor repertoire and immune microenvironment in patients with locoregionally advanced squamous cell carcinoma of the head and neck. *Clin Cancer Res*, 23, 4897–907.

SCHLÜTER, A., WELLER, P., KANAAN, O., NEL, I., HEUSGEN, L., HÖING, B., HAẞKAMP, P., ZANDER, S., MANDAPATHIL, M., DOMINAS, N., ARNOLDS, J., STUCK, B. A., LANG, S., BANKFALVI, A., & BRANDAU, S. 2018. CD31 and VEGF are prognostic biomarkers in early-stage, but not in late-stage, laryngeal squamous cell carcinoma. *BMC Cancer*, 18, 272.

SCHMITT, N. C., & FERRIS, R. L. 2020. Immunotherapeutic approaches in HNSCC. *In:* ST. JOHN, M. A., & PARK, N.-H., eds. *Novel Therapies in Head and Neck Cancer: Beyond the Horizon* (pp. 117–142). New York: Academic Press.

SHARMA, P., HU-LIESKOVAN, S., WARGO, J. A., & RIBAS, A. 2017. Primary, adaptive, and acquired resistance to cancer immunotherapy. *Cell*, 168, 707–23.

SHRIMALI, R. K., YU, Z., THEORET, M. R., CHINNASAMY, D., RESTIFO, N. P., & ROSENBERG, S. A. 2010. Antiangiogenic agents can increase lymphocyte infiltration into tumor and enhance the effectiveness of adoptive immunotherapy of cancer. *Cancer Res*, 70, 6171–80.

SOLA, A. M., JOHNSON, D. E., & GRANDIS, J. R. 2019. Investigational multitargeted kinase inhibitors in development for head and neck neoplasms. *Expert Opin Investig Drugs*, 28, 351–63.

SRIVASTAVA, V. K., GARA, R. K., RASTOGI, N., MISHRA, D. P., AHMED, M. K., GUPTA, S., GOEL, M. M., & BHATT, M. L. 2014. Serum vascular endothelial growth factor-A (VEGF-A) as a biomarker in squamous cell carcinoma of head and neck patients undergoing chemoradiotherapy. *Asian Pac J Cancer Prev*, 15, 3261–5.

SUN, Y., WANG, Z., QIU, S., & WANG, R. 2021. Therapeutic strategies of different HPV status in head and neck squamous cell carcinoma. *Int J Biol Sci*, 17, 1104–18.

TABERNA, M., OLIVA, M., & MESÍA, R. 2019. Cetuximab-containing combinations in locally advanced and recurrent or metastatic head and neck squamous cell carcinoma. *Front Oncol*, 9, 383.

THARIAT, J., ETIENNE-GRIMALDI, M. C., GRALL, D., BENSADOUN, R. J., CAYRE, A., PENAULT-LLORCA, F., VERACINI, L., FRANCOUAL, M., FORMENTO, J. L., DASSONVILLE, O., DE RAUCOURT, D., GEOFFROIS, L., GIRAUD, P., RACADOT, S., MORINIèRE, S., MILANO, G., & VAN OBBERGHEN-SCHILLING, E. 2012. Epidermal growth factor receptor protein detection in head and neck cancer patients: A many-faceted picture. *Clin Cancer Res*, 18, 1313–22.

TRIGO, J., GARCÍA-COSÍO, M., GARCÍA-CASTAÑO, A., GOMÀ, M., MESIA-NIN, R., RUIZ-BRAVO, E., SORIA-RIVAS, A., CASTILLO, P., BRAÑA-GARCÍA, I., & ALBEROLA-FERRANTI, M. 2022. Recommendations for the use of biomarkers for head and neck cancer, including salivary gland tumours: A consensus of the Spanish Society of Medical Oncology and the Spanish Society of Pathology. *Clin Transl Oncol*, 24, 1890–1902.

VAN HARTEN, A. M., & BRAKENHOFF, R. H. 2021. Targeted treatment of head and neck (pre)cancer: Preclinical target identification and development of novel therapeutic applications. *Cancers (Basel)*, 13(11), 2774.

VERMA, J., DHINGRA, V., SRIVASTAVA, S., MISRA, V., VARMA, K., & SINGH, S. 2018. Evaluation of epidermal growth factor receptor expression by a new scoring system in head-and-neck squamous cell carcinoma and its association with various pathological prognostic factors. *J Oral Maxillofac Pathol*, 22, 11–17.

WANG, J., SUN, H., ZENG, Q., GUO, X. J., WANG, H., LIU, H. H., & DONG, Z. Y. 2019. HPV-positive status associated with inflamed immune microenvironment and improved response to anti-PD-1 therapy in head and neck squamous cell carcinoma. *Sci Rep*, 9, 13404.

WISE-DRAPER, T. M., BAHIG, H., TONNEAU, M., KARIVEDU, V., & BURTNESS, B. 2022. Current therapy for metastatic head and neck cancer: Evidence, opportunities, and challenges. *Am Soc Clin Oncol Educ Book*, 42, 1–14.

XIAO, H., ZHENG, Y., MA, L., TIAN, L., & SUN, Q. 2021. Clinically-relevant ABC transporter for anti-cancer drug resistance. *Front Pharmacol*, 12, 648407.

YANG, T. K., YU, Y. F., TSAI, C. L., LI, H. J., YANG, P. S., HUANG, K. W., & CHENG, J. C. 2022. Efficacy and safety of combined targeted therapy and immunotherapy versus targeted monotherapy in unresectable hepatocellular carcinoma: A systematic review and meta-analysis. *BMC Cancer*, 22, 1085.

YASUDA, S., SHO, M., YAMATO, I., YOSHIJI, H., WAKATSUKI, K., NISHIWADA, S., YAGITA, H., & NAKAJIMA, Y. 2013. Simultaneous blockade of programmed death 1 and vascular endothelial growth factor receptor 2 (VEGFR2) induces synergistic anti-tumour effect in vivo. *Clin Exp Immunol*, 172, 500–6.

YASUMA-MITOBE, K., & MATSUOKA, M. 2018. The roles of coinhibitory receptors in pathogenesis of human retroviral infections. *Front Immunol*, 9, 2755.

YI, M., JIAO, D., QIN, S., CHU, Q., WU, K., & LI, A. 2019. Synergistic effect of immune checkpoint blockade and anti-angiogenesis in cancer treatment. *Mol Cancer*, 18, 60.

YU, C., LIU, X., YANG, J., ZHANG, M., JIN, H., MA, X., & SHI, H. 2019. Combination of immunotherapy with targeted therapy: Theory and practice in metastatic melanoma. *Front Immunol*, 18(1), 60.

ZARETSKY, J. M., GARCIA-DIAZ, A., SHIN, D. S., ESCUIN-ORDINAS, H., HUGO, W., HU-LIESKOVAN, S., TORREJON, D. Y., ABRIL-RODRIGUEZ, G., SANDOVAL, S., BARTHLY, L., SACO, J., MORENO, B. H., MEZZADRA, R., CHMIELOWSKI, B., RUCHALSKI, K., SHINTAKU, I. P., SANCHEZ, P. J., PUIG-SAUS, C., CHERRY, G., SEJA, E., KONG, X., PANG, J., BERENT-MAOZ, B., COMIN-ANDUIX, B., GRAEBER, T. G., TUMEH, P. C., SCHUMACHER, T. N. M., LO, R. S., & RIBAS, A. 2016. Mutations associated with acquired resistance to PD-1 blockade in melanoma. *N Engl J Med*, 375, 819–29.

ZHANG, C., LI, D., XIAO, B., ZHOU, C., JIANG, W., TANG, J., LI, Y., ZHANG, R., HAN, K., HOU, Z., ZHANG, L., SUI, Q., LIAO, L., PAN, Z., ZHANG, X., & DING, P. 2022. B2m and JAK1/2–mutated MSI-H colorectal carcinomas can benefit from anti-PD-1 therapy. *J Immunother*, 45, 187–93.

ZHANG, Y., & ZHANG, Z. 2020. The history and advances in cancer immunotherapy: Understanding the characteristics of tumor-infiltrating immune cells and their therapeutic implications. *CellMolec Immunol*, 17, 807–21.

ZHAO, J., CHEN, A. X., GARTRELL, R. D., SILVERMAN, A. M., APARICIO, L., CHU, T., BORDBAR, D., SHAN, D., SAMANAMUD, J., MAHAJAN, A., FILIP, I., ORENBUCH, R., GOETZ, M., YAMAGUCHI, J. T., CLONEY, M., HORBINSKI, C., LUKAS, R. V., RAIZER, J., RAE, A. I., YUAN, J., CANOLL, P., BRUCE, J. N., SAENGER, Y. M., SIMS, P., IWAMOTO, F. M., SONABEND, A. M., & RABADAN, R. 2019. Immune and genomic correlates of response to anti-PD-1 immunotherapy in glioblastoma. *Nat Medicine*, 25, 462–9.

ZHOU, J. Z., JOU, J., & COHEN, E. 2022. Vaccine strategies for human papillomavirus-associated head and neck cancers. *Cancers*, 14, 33.

ZHU, C., GU, L., LIU, Z., LI, J., YAO, M., & FANG, C. 2021. Correlation between vascular endothelial growth factor pathway and immune microenvironment in head and neck squamous cell carcinoma. *BMC Cancer*, 21, 836.

ZHU, X., ZHANG, F., ZHANG, W., HE, J., ZHAO, Y., & CHEN, X. 2013. Prognostic role of epidermal growth factor receptor in head and neck cancer: A meta-analysis. *J Surg Oncol*, 108, 387–97.

SECTION III
COMPREHENSIVE CARE

7
Surgical Innovations in Head and Neck Cancers

Serwalo Ramagaga, Lloyd Mabonga, Mzubanzi Mabongo, Joseph G. Mhlanga, Sibusiso Sizwe Nkosi, Zhen Lin, and Zodwa Dlamini

7.1 Introduction

Surgical management is a cornerstone in the multidisciplinary approach in treating head and neck cancers (HNCs), encompassing a diverse array of procedures aimed at achieving optimal tumor resection while preserving essential functions and maximizing quality of life for patients (Ritter et al., 2024). The earliest reported surgical technique for disease control, radical neck dissection (RND), was reported by Jawdynski in 1888, in Polish literature (Ferlito et al., 2006a). Crile published a seminal work on RND in 1905, which was followed by a landmark second publication on the same topic (Crile, 1906). Over the years, surgical innovations in HNC have evolved significantly, driven by advancements in surgical techniques, technologies, and perioperative care strategies. These innovations have revolutionized the field, enabling more precise, minimally invasive, and function-sparing approaches to tumor removal and reconstruction (Mastronicola et al., 2023). Minimally invasive surgical techniques, such as transoral robotic surgery (TORS) and endoscopic approaches, have emerged as transformative innovations in HNC management (Wojtera et al., 2024). Advances in imaging modalities, such as intraoperative navigation systems, fluorescence-guided surgery, and 3D-printed patient-specific models, have enhanced surgical precision and decision-making in HNC surgery (Karnatz et al., 2022).

The integration of molecular profiling and precision oncology approaches has allowed for personalized treatment strategies tailored to the individual characteristics of each tumor. Innovative reconstructive techniques, including microvascular free tissue transfer, tissue engineering, and virtual surgical planning, have revolutionized the field of head and neck reconstruction, enabling restoration of speech, swallowing, and facial aesthetics with remarkable precision and success (Ritter et al., 2024). Advances in flap design, microsurgical techniques, and perioperative care have led to improved outcomes and reduced complication rates in reconstructive surgery, allowing for more comprehensive and successful rehabilitation of patients following tumor resection. The concept of adaptive and multidisciplinary care has become increasingly important in HNC surgery, emphasizing collaboration among surgical, medical, and radiation oncologists, as well as other allied healthcare professionals, to optimize treatment planning, delivery, and postoperative care (Wojtera et al., 2024).

Multidisciplinary tumor boards, comprehensive preoperative assessments, and coordinated perioperative management protocols are integral components of modern HNC care, ensuring a holistic and patient-centered approach to treatment that addresses not only the oncologic goals but also the functional and psychosocial needs of patients (Fagan, 2021). Thus, surgical innovations hold immense promise for improving treatment outcomes, enhancing patient quality of life, and shaping the future of HNC care (Mastronicola et al., 2023). As technology continues to evolve, the field of surgical oncology will undoubtedly continue to push the boundaries of what is possible, offering hope to patients and clinicians alike in the fight against HNCs (Ritter et al., 2024; Wojtera et al., 2024). This chapter explores the latest surgical innovations in HNC, from minimally invasive techniques to cutting-edge robotic surgeries and intricate reconstructive procedures. It showcases how these innovations contribute to improved precision, reduced invasiveness, and enhanced postoperative recovery.

7.2 Functional Neck Dissection

Since HNC have propensity to metastases to the lymph nodes in the neck, a diagnosis of palpable nodes in the neck decreases the overall survival by half (Almangush et al., 2020). The clinical significance and the implications of neck nodes in both spread and management of HNC was known as early as the 19th century. This knowledge led to the development of RND as a standard surgical technique for removal of fibrofatty tissue along with the associated lymph nodes and some nonlymphatic structures for regional control of the disease. The earliest reported RND surgical technique was by Jawdynski, in 1888, in Polish literature (Ferlito et al., 2006a). The initial surgical technique expected the surgeons to completely remove the neck nodes from all levels of the neck, together with the fascia, lymph vessels, the primary tumor, and several nonlymphatic tissue such as sternocleidomastoid muscles (SCM), submandibular gland, accessory nerve, and internal jugular vein (IJV). The RND procedure was regarded as an absolute minimum requirement for disease control in the neck (Crile, 1906).

Although patients undergoing RND had a four times higher survival rate than patients who did not, high morbidity was reported in patients who had undergone RND (Robbins et al., 2002). These included mainly shoulder dysfunction, frozen shoulder syndrome, winging of the scapula, massive facial edema with bilateral neck dissections, anesthesia/paresthesia of the skin, limitation of arm movement, discoloration of the lower half of the face, and disfigurement of the neck. These complications led to the development of other neck dissection techniques such as functional neck dissection (FND) and modified RND (Bocca, 1975).

FND is a surgical procedure originally described in Spanish literature by Osvaldo Suárez as a less aggressive procedure and was based purely on anatomy. The known pathogenesis of HNCs is that these tumors tend to metastasize to the neck lymph nodes via the lymph vessels. These lymph nodes are in a fibrofatty tissue that occupies the lateral aspect of the neck from the base of the skull, superiorly, to the level of the clavicle inferiorly. Posteriorly, the border is formed by the mastoid process and the anterior border of trapezius muscle, while the anterior border is the midline. This fibrofatty tissue contains both the lymph vessels and the lymph nodes and is closely adherent to the cervical fascia but does not perforate it. The philosophy of FND is based on the knowledge that the lymphatic drainage of the oral cavity, oropharynx, pharynx, and larynx is into the lymphatic system in the neck, which lies between the prevertebral fascia and the investing layer of the deep cervical fascia (Gavilán et al., 2004; Lassaletta et al., 2002). The lymphatic system is made up of lymph vessels and lymph nodes, which are within the fibrofatty tissue that runs in close vicinity to the cervical fascia. Thus, removing the fascia with the adjacent fibrofatty tissue will remove the disease and preserve anatomic structures like muscles, nerves, and glands (Bocca et al., 1984).

The pattern of nodal metastasis from the oral cavity cancers metastasize to the submental, submandibular, upper jugulodigastric, and mid-jugulodigastric nodes depending on the site of lesion (levels I, II, and III). Oropharyngeal, laryngeal, and tracheal cancers tend to spread to upper, mid, and lower jugulodigastric lymph nodes (levels II, III, and IV) (Harish, 2005). This guides the targeting of nodes in various modified neck procedures for management and staging of HNCs. Level I was subdivided into level IA, the submental group of nodes; and level IB, the submandibular lymph nodes. Level II was also subdivided by the spinal accessory nerve into IIA and IIB, both comprising the jugulodigastric lymph nodes; and level V was subdivided into level VA and VB (Robbins et al. 2002). Figure 7.1 shows the lymph node levels in the neck (Robbins et al., 2002).

FND is a unique procedure in that some anatomical structures that are not part of the lymphatic system, like the IJV, the spinal accessory nerve, the SCM, and the submandibular gland, are preserved (Gavilán et al., 1993), while these anatomical structures are sacrificed in RDN. Thus, FND reduces the morbidity associated with RND. In addition, outcomes for RND and FND were found to be similar in cNo, cN1, and cN2 (Orhan et al., 2007). This suggested that FND

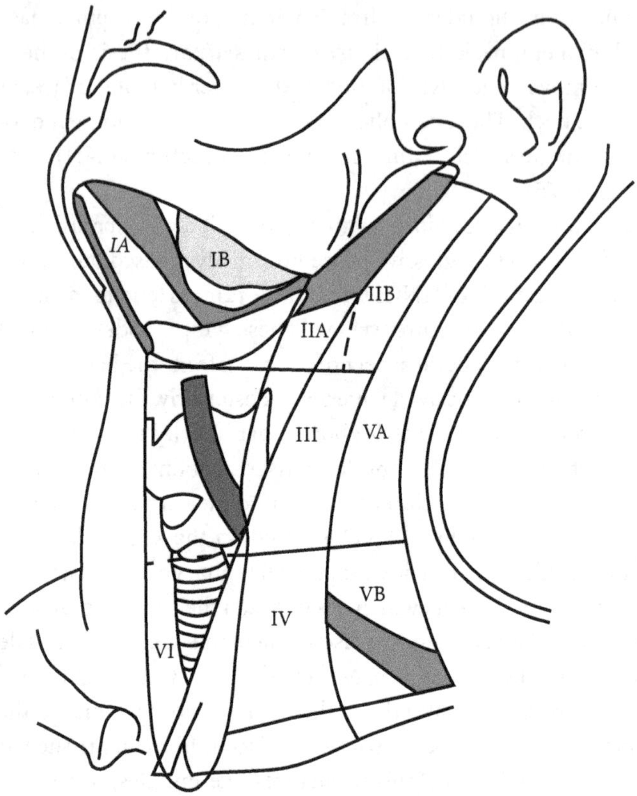

Figure 7.1 Lymph node levels in the neck. Understanding the levels of lymph nodes in the neck is crucial for the accurate staging and treatment of head and neck cancers. Each level is associated with specific anatomical landmarks and has clinical significance related to types of cancers. Accurate identification and assessment of these lymph node levels help guide surgical approaches, radiation therapy, and overall management of patients with head and neck malignancies.
Figure adapted from Robbins et al., 2002.

is equally effective in disease control as RND with less morbidity. However, shoulder dysfunction, which is a complication of accessory spinal nerve injury, was also reported after FND (Chiesa-Estomba et al., 2021). Unfortunately, this study does not indicate if the nerve injuries were transient or permanent. To address the confusion caused by the number of surgical procedures that were being developed to avoid the complications associated with RND and the accompanying challenges presented by the new nomenclature referring to these new procedures, Medina et al. developed a classification system in 1989 (Table 7.1). In this classification, FND corresponds with "modified neck dissection

Table 7.1 Classification of neck dissection

Medina classification (1989)	**AAO-HNS first update 2002 (Robbins et al., 2002)**	**2011 classification proposed by Ferlito et al. and Members of International Head and Neck Scientific Group (Ferlito et al., 2011)**
1. Radical neck dissection	Radical neck dissection	
2. Modified neck dissection • Type I (only accessory nerve preserved) • Type II (CNXI and SCM are preserved) • Type III (CN XI SCM and IJV are preserved)	Modified neck dissection	Any neck dissection is designated as "ND" and the removed lymph node levels or sublevels and/or nonlymphatic structures are denoted in parentheses
Selective neck dissection	Selective neck dissection	
Extended neck dissection	Extended neck dissection	

type III." Subsequent standardization by the American Head and Neck Society (AHNS) and the American Academy of Otolaryngology-Head and Neck Surgery (AAO-HNS) resulted in a classification for neck dissection in 1991, updated in 2001 (Robbins et al., 2002).

In both the 1991 classification and its later update, the ANHS committee abandoned the use of "functional neck dissection" in favor of "modified radical neck dissection" (MRND) Ferlito et al., 2006a). The committee distinguished four types of neck dissection: radical neck dissection, MRND, selective neck dissection, and extended RND. This classification did not differ much from Medina's classification (Table 7.1) (Medina, 1989). *Extended RND* implied that, in addition to RND, additional structures such as the skin, platysma, hypoglossal nerve, posterior belly of the digastric muscle, external or common carotid artery, and vagus nerve might be sacrificed. The simplest of these classifications was developed in 2011 (Table 7.1) (Ferlito et al., 2011); it is important to note that this committee used "modified RND" instead of FND. In summary, FDN is less aggressive yet produces equally good results with minimal mutilation (Bocca & Pignataro, 1968; Ferlito et al., 2006b; Minghua et al., 2005).

FND is indicated when the disease is confined within the lymphatic nodes or before metastases occur. Thus, this approach is ideal for patients with a high risk of occult metastasis because it can be done as an elective procedure (Ragos et al., 2016). Another additional advantage of FND is that it may be performed on both sides of the neck without increasing morbidity. When FND is performed when there is evidence of palpable and mobile neck lymph nodes it is referred to as "therapeutic FND" (Bocca et al., 1984; Ragos et al., 2016). FND may be performed as an elective or therapeutic procedure depending on the cN status. FND is contraindicated in cases with extracapsular spread, characterized by a fixed, palpable node and nodes that become mobile after radiotherapy. The actual surgical procedure is described in detail elsewhere (Bocca et al., 1984; Gavilán et al., 2004; Murchite et al., 2021).

Like the FND, MFND is one surgical technique used to manage cN0 lymph nodes and small mobile lymph nodes. However, MFND also preserves the nerves that supply the skin, such as the supraclavicular nerve, great auricular nerve, transversus colli nerve, IJV, external jugular vein (EJV), SCM, and omohyoid muscle (Minghua et al., 2005).

7.3 Surgical Techniques

As in all major surgical procedures, patients must be thoroughly selected and prepared to avoid unnecessary complications (Minghua et al., 2005). Preoperative assessment by the anesthesiologist is also important for intra operative and post operative care. The patient lies in a supine position. The patient's neck must be fully extended; this can be further achieved by putting the patient into the anti-Trendelenburg position. An endotracheal tube or tracheostomy is used to manage the airway both intraoperatively and postoperatively (Minghua et al., 2005).

7.3.1 Neck Incisions and Flaps

There are several approaches for accessing a metastatic tumor in the neck. These incisions must allow good access to the surgical site, ensure a good blood supply to the flap for good healing, and result in an aesthetically acceptable scar (Agrawal et al., 2018). The incisions must have a low incidence of complications such as wound dehiscence, flaps necrosis, and scar contracture. The most used incisions are Gluck, Conley, MacFee, transverse, and Schrodinger incisions and their modifications (Agrawal et al., 2018).

7.3.1.1 Gluck Incision

The Gluck incision is an apron flap that can be used for bilateral functional dissection of the neck metastatic tumor. When bilateral FND is going to be performed, the incision extends as shown in Figure 7.2 (Agrawal et al., 2018).

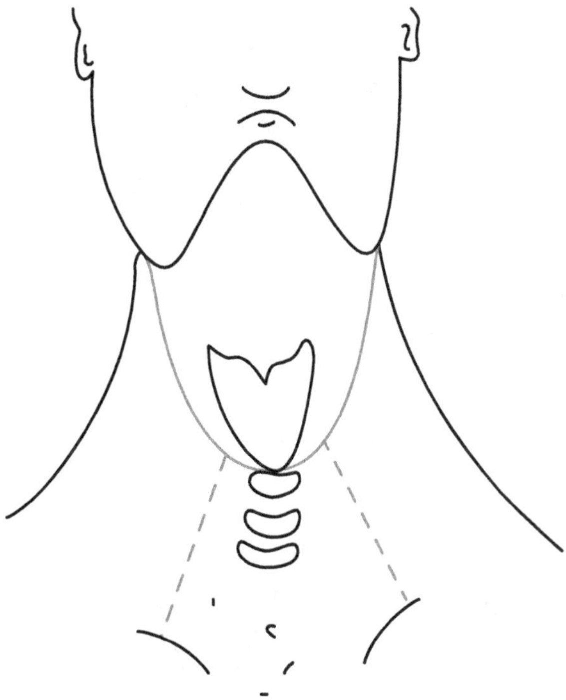

Figure 7.2 Apron flap between both mastoid tips, crossing the midline at the level of the cricoid arch. Gluck incision affords good exposure to the neck for partial and total laryngectomy. This incision can be part of tracheostomy if needed.
Figure adapted from Murchite et al., 2021.

7.3.1.2 Conley Incision

The Conley incision starts from the submental region and runs posteriorly and inferiorly. As it runs inferiorly, it runs 2 cm posterior to the anterior margin of the trapezius muscle (shown Figure 7.3) (Agrawal et al., 2018; Odate et al., 2012). The incision is typically made along the anterior border of the SCM, extending from the level of the thyroid cartilage superiorly to the sternal notch inferiorly. It may also incorporate a horizontal component along the supraclavicular fossa if additional exposure is required. The Conley incision pattern allows for excellent access to the larynx, thyroid gland, and cervical lymph nodes while minimizing disruption to the surrounding tissue planes and preserving the blood supply to the skin flap. It is a valuable surgical technique in HNC surgery, providing optimal exposure, preservation of function, and cosmetically favorable outcomes for patients undergoing laryngeal and cervical procedures (Agrawal et al., 2018).

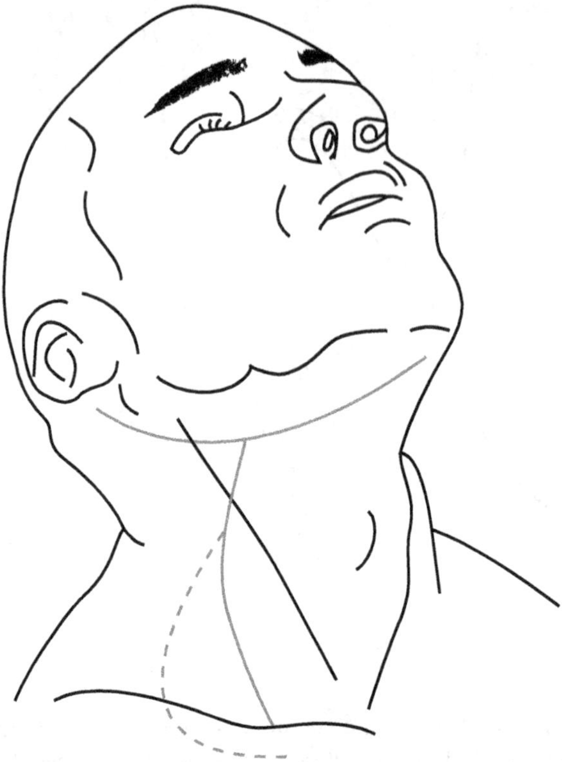

Figure 7.3 The Conley incision crosses the clavicle and turns anteriorly just below the clavicle. The submandibular part meets the curvature of the main incision below the earlobe. The flap provides access to all five levels of functional dissection. This incision has been used post-radiation without complications. Figure adapted from Lasaridis et al., 1994.

7.3.1.3 Transverse Incision

The transverse incision is made horizontally across the anterior aspect of the neck, typically along a natural skin crease or in a predetermined location to optimize cosmetic outcomes and minimize scar visibility (Figure 7.4) (Kerawala &Heliotos, 2009). The use of transverse neck incisions in NHC surgery represents a valuable technique for achieving optimal oncological outcomes while minimizing aesthetic impact and preserving functional integrity. While transverse neck incisions offer several advantages, they may not be suitable for all patients or surgical procedures. Factors such as tumor location, size, and extent of surgical resection, as well as individual patient anatomy and comorbidities, may influence the choice of incision type (Odate et al., 2012).

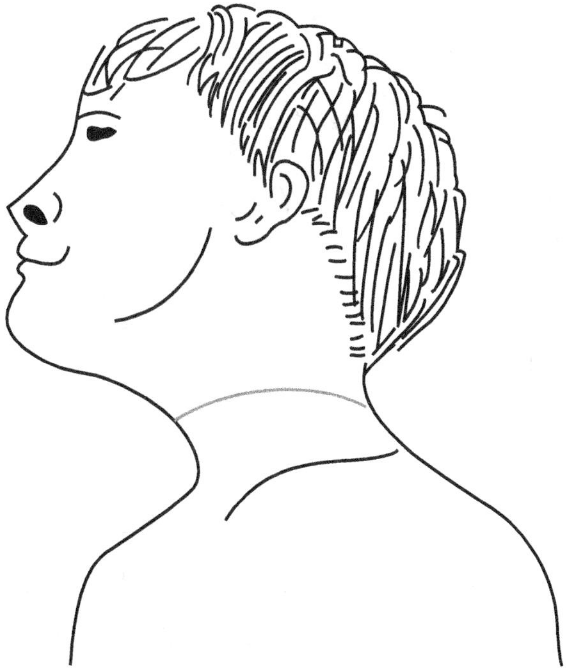

Figure 7.4 Transverse incision. This is made up of a single neck incision. The incision provides good access and is aesthetically acceptable to the patients. Figure adapted from Murchite et al., 2021.

7.3.1.4 Macfee Incision

The MacAfee incision is typically performed by making a horizontal incision along the lower border of the lower lip, extending from one commissure to the other, as shown in Figure 7.5. This incision is then extended vertically along the mental crease, which runs from the lower lip to the chin. The resulting flap of tissue is elevated to provide access to the oral cavity, floor of the mouth, and mandibular region (Kerawala & Heliotos, 2009). The incision consists of two parallel transverse incisions. The blood supply to the flaps is excellent. The MacFee incision is a preferred incision in patients who have undergone radiation. It is a valuable surgical technique in HNC surgery, providing optimal exposure, preservation of function, and cosmetically favorable outcomes for patients undergoing procedures involving the oral cavity, floor of the mouth, and mandibular region (Kerawala & Heliotos, 2009).

7.3.1.5 Weber-Ferguson Incision

The Weber-Fergusion incision is typically performed by making a curved incision along the gingivobuccal sulcus, starting from the maxillary tuberosity and

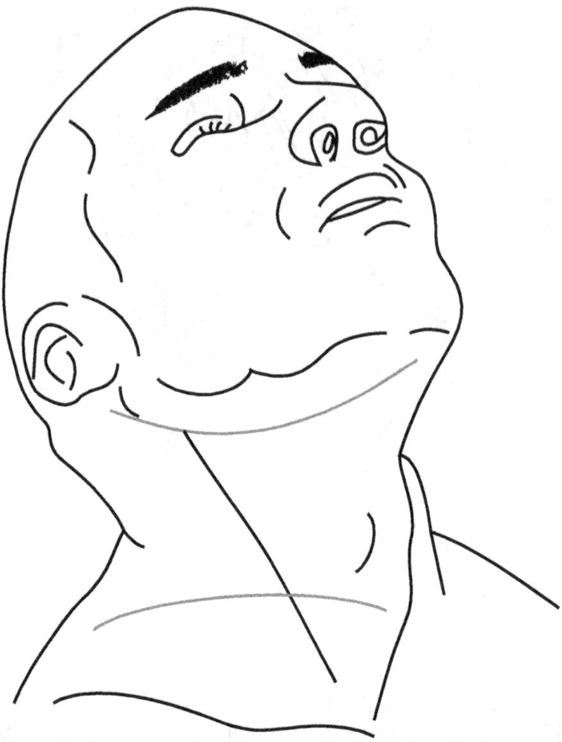

Figure 7.5 MacFee incision. This incision provides access for adequate to the lymphatic system in the neck. However, access may be a challenge to inexperienced surgeons and in patients with short neck length.
Figure adapted from Murchite et al., 2021.

extending anteriorly toward the midline of the upper lip. The incision is then extended vertically along the nasal sidewall, following the nasolabial fold, and can be extended further into the infraorbital crease as needed to provide additional exposure to the surgical site. This incision is excellent for midface exposure for access to nasal, maxillary sinus, and maxilla pathology. The incision is aesthetically acceptable (Osborne et al., 1987).

7.3.1.6 Schrodinger Incision

The Schrodinger incision commences from the midline in the submental region and curves slightly toward the mastoid process. From here a vertical incision at 90 degrees to the horizontal incision runs along the anterior border of the trapezium muscle. The Schrodinger incision is a valuable surgical technique in head and neck surgery, providing optimal exposure, preservation of function, and

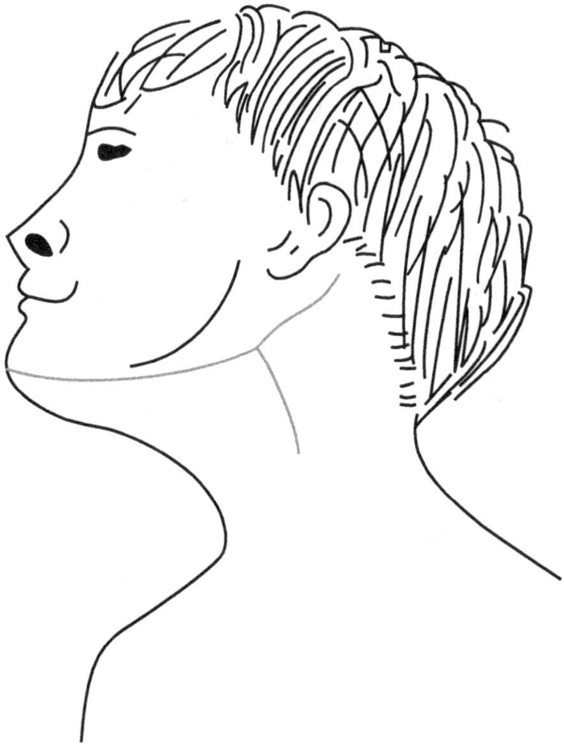

Figure 7.6 The Schobinger incision. The Schobinger incision is a surgical approach commonly utilized in head and neck surgery, particularly for procedures involving access to all surgical levels of the neck including the posterior triangle and mandible. The incision is designed to provide optimal exposure to the surgical site while minimizing cosmetic impact and preserving important anatomical structures. Figure adapted from Murchite et al., 2021.

cosmetically favorable outcomes for patients undergoing procedures involving the maxilla, mandible, and midface (Figure 7.6) (Roy et al., 2019).

7.3.1.7 Single Y Incision

The single Y incision creates a single trifurcate access and is typically performed by making a single, curved incision along the gingivobuccal sulcus of the affected side, starting from the maxillary tuberosity and extending anteriorly toward the midline of the upper lip. From this point, the incision is extended vertically along the nasal sidewall, following the nasolabial fold, and can be extended further as needed to provide additional exposure to the surgical site (Figure 7.7). (Roy et al., 2019). The single Y incision is a valuable surgical technique in head and

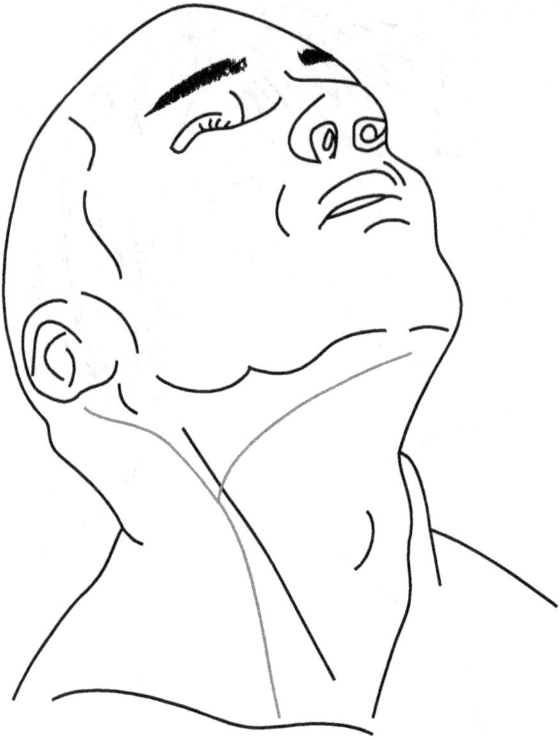

Figure 7.7 Single Y-approach. The incision provides excellent exposure to the maxilla, mandible, and midface, facilitating precise dissection and tumor excision while minimizing the risk of injury to vital structures (i.e., nerves and blood vessels). Figure adapted from Murchite et al., 2021.

neck surgery, providing optimal exposure, preservation of function, and cosmetically favorable outcomes for patients undergoing procedures involving the maxilla, mandible, and midface (Roy et al., 2019).

7.3.1.8 Double Y Incision of Martin

The double Y incision of Martin, also known as the "double-chevron" or "butterfly" incision, is a double trifurcate incision characterized by two Y-shaped incisions on both sides of the neck, with the arms of the Y extending superiorly toward the mandible and inferiorly toward the clavicle. The incisions meet at the midline of the neck, forming a butterfly-shaped pattern and offering good access to the ipsilateral side of the neck, as shown in Figure 7.8 (Roy et al., 2019). This configuration allows for extensive exposure of the oral cavity, floor of the mouth, mandible, and neck, facilitating precise dissection and tumor removal while minimizing the risk of injury to vital structures such as nerves and blood vessels.

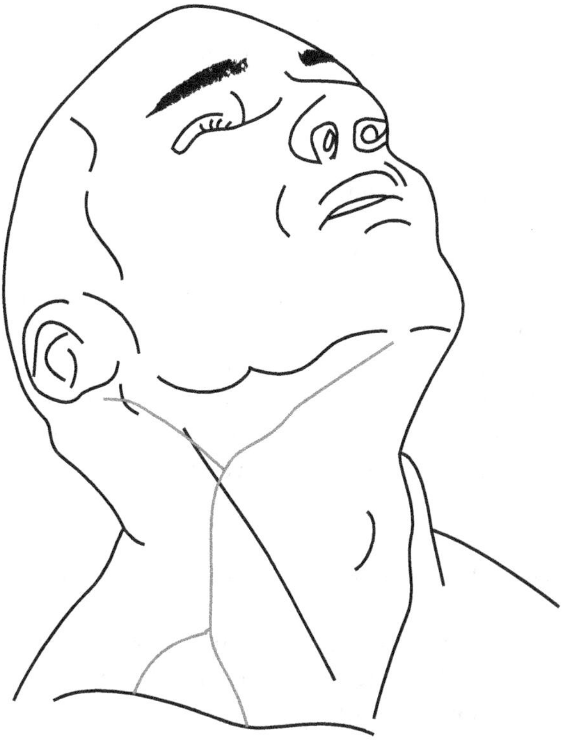

Figure 7.8 The double-Y incision of Martin. This incision is commonly employed in head and neck surgery, particularly for procedures involving access to the mandible, oral cavity, and neck. It is designed to provide optimal exposure to the surgical site while minimizing cosmetic impact and preserving important anatomical structures. Figure adapted from Murchite et al., 2021.

The tips may undergo necrosis. The double Y incision of Martin is a valuable surgical technique in head and neck surgery, providing optimal exposure, preservation of function, and cosmetically favorable outcomes for patients undergoing procedures involving the mandible, oral cavity, and neck (Roy et al., 2019).

7.4 Dissections

Once the incision has been made, subplatysma flaps are raised. The surgical field can extend to the inferior border superiorly, inferior border inferiorly, mastoid line posteriorly, and midline anteriorly. The neck fascia must be removed en bloc from the base of the skull to the pleural copula (Hamoir et al., 2014). The anatomical boundaries of the neck fascia are the base of the skull, which is marked by occipital vessels; prevertebral fascia covering the scalene muscle medially; anterior border of the trapezius muscle posteriorly; and transverse cervical vessels inferiorly (Roy et al., 2019).

7.4.1 Dissection of the Sternocleidomastoid Muscle

The dissection exposes levels II–IV. An incision is made at the posterior border of the SCM. The fascial layer is dissected from posterior to anterior until the muscle is completely exposed (Gavilán et al., 1993). The accessory nerve is identified as the SCM is dissected. Blunt dissection is used to complete the release of the SCM. The SCM is released from the clavicle by an incision on the anterior aspect of the clavicle and sternum. The SCM must be retracted superiorly. This should be followed by skeletonizing the EJV (Bocca et al., 1980).

7.4.2 Dissection of the Submandibular Triangle

The dissection of levels I–IV is at times indicated in oral and pharyngeal cancers, but dissection of level I is not necessary in laryngeal, hypopharyngeal, and thyroid gland cancers (Roy et al., 2019).

7.4.2.1 Levels IA and IB Dissection

The fascia is incised along the submandibular fossa parallel to the inferior border of the mandible. The submental and submandibular lymph nodes must be dissected from the mylohyoid muscle. The fascia of the mylohyoid muscle must also be dissected together with lymphatic material. Care must be taken to protect the marginal mandibular nerve (Gogna et al., 2019), and the use of intraoperative nerve monitoring must be considered to prevent injury to this nerve. The submandibular gland is dissected completely from its fascial covering and retracted superiorly. The fibrofatty tissue with the nodes is grasped and dissected off the submandibular fossa, preserving the gland (Gogna et al., 2019). The dissection is continued to the submental group. The submandibular and submental fibrofatty tissue is reflected inferiorly with the lymph nodes, then the fascia must be dissected from the digastric and stylohyoid muscles. The dissection is then carried posteriorly. The digastric and stylohyoid muscles are retracted superiorly so that the fascial sheath can be easily dissected from the inferior aspect of the digastric muscle and the upper jugular spaces (Gogna et al., 2019).

The dissection is carried out superior to the hypoglossal nerve, which must be identified. At this stage, several lingual veins should be ligated and divided, preserving the hypoglossal nerve. The fascia that covers the outer surface of the SCM and omohyoid muscle is dissected out, exposing the IJV. This vessel is gently skeletonized up to the level of the clavicle. An incision along the carotid sheath is made. The fascia is dissected from the IJV. The SCM is retracted anteriorly, while the omohyoid muscle is retracted inferiorly. The fibrofatty tissue with nodes is dissected in an anterior-medial direction. At the end of the procedure, the SCM is sutured into the clavicle and sternum. A drain is placed and the soft tissue closed (Gogna et al., 2019).

7.4.2.2 Complications of Functional Neck Dissections

Complication from FND occurred in 33.97% in a sample of 768 cases, with infection being the most common complication. A study by Chiesa-Estomba revealed that 40% of their series had complications from the FND procedure. The most common complication was spinal accessory nerve injury (10%) (Chiesa-Estomba et al., 2021). Table 7.2 summarizes the complications of FND in HNC.

Table 7.2 Complications of functional neck dissections (FND) in head and neck cancer

Complication	Description	References
Recurrence	Recurrence of the disease was 3% in patient treated with FND. The study by Minghua et al. did not find statistical difference in recurrence between modified FND (mFND) and FND.	Minghua et al., 2005
Nerve injury	The numbness of the skin over the neck is one of the complications FND. This numbness can be prevented by dissecting the nerves that supply the skin, thus protecting them from injury. While both transient and permanent injury accounted for 6.5% of the complications. Some studies have reported dysfunction of the shoulder from FND. This suggests that even if the integrity of the nerve is maintained, trauma from stretching the nerve can also cause injury. It is recommended that care should be taken when dissecting superior cervical chain.	Minghua et al., 2005
Infections	Some of the local complications include wound infection, seroma or hematoma, and dehiscence of the wound. The causes of these complications are multifactorial, affected by the choice of incision and surgical skills rather than FND.	Herranz et al., 2000
Chylous fistula	This complication can be avoided by delicate dissection of the thoracic duct, and surgeons are advised to repair the thoracic duct intraoperatively if it is severed. Application of pressure is not effective because of SCM.	Herranz et al., 2000
Hemorrhage	Hemorrhage is usually from the rupture of the carotid artery or internal jugular vein. This is very rare in FND as the vessels are covered by muscles.	Herranz et al., 2000

FND is a well-described surgical procedure, and its principles and philosophy are applied in other forms of neck dissections such as supra-omohyoid, selective neck dissection, and modified neck dissection. The development of modified FND suggests that there are clinicians who are determined to improve FND neck dissection and the quality of life of their patients (Herranz et al., 2000).

7.5 Minimally Invasive Neck Dissections

Technology and innovation have reduced morbidity and improved the cosmetic appearance of the neck through the use of minimally invasive techniques (Figure 7.9). Loco-regional neck dissection in head and neck oncology is paramount in improving both overall survival and disease-free survival (Nayak & Jayaprasad, 2017). Minimally invasive neck dissection (MIND) should not only be cosmetically pleasing, but it also needs to adhere to the principles of oncological surgery. This method provides access to the spaces in the neck using laparoscopic

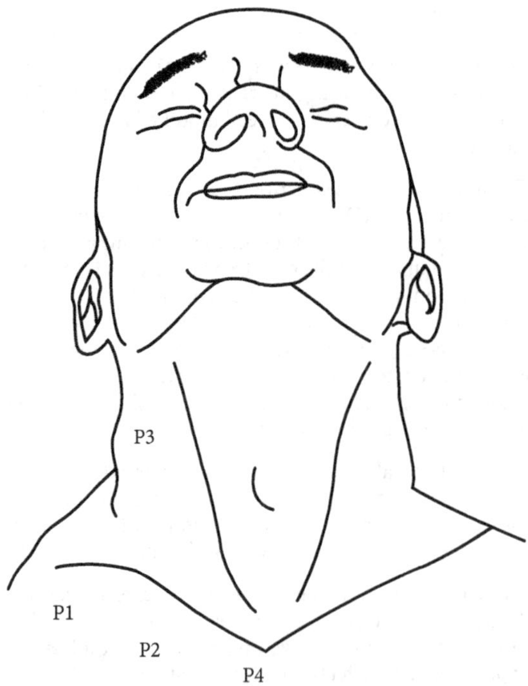

Figure 7.9 Minimally invasive neck dissection (MIND) technique. Primary port (P1) Working ports (P2 and P3) and assistant port (P4).
Figure adapted from Nayak & Jayaprasad, 2017.

endoscopes and/or robotic equipment. The procedure is performed under general anesthesia, with the patient in a supine position with the neck extended to expose the neck and the clavicle up to the nipple line (Nayak & Jayaprasad, 2017). The trocars and endoscopes are inserted 2–3 cm below the clavicle via a 2.5 cm incision. An airtight seal is necessary for placement of the trocars and endoscopes, and the instruments should triangulate for best access and visibility. The spaces are then insufflated with carbon dioxide at a pressure of 10 mm Hg. A skin flap in the subplatysmal plane is developed using laparoscopic instruments (Coyle et al., 2016; Nayak & Jayaprasad, 2017).

The plane is further developed after placing working ports medial to the first port (P2) and one near the posterior border of the SCM (P3). An assistant port is placed medial to the second working port as medially as possible (P4) (see Figure 7.9). This port is mainly used to retract the SCM. Planes are developed to expose the desired lymph node levels sufficiently. The extent of flap elevation is guided by surface landmarks that can be palpated externally, as well as by anatomical landmarks identified visually (Nayak & Jayaprasad, 2017). This technique and approach have successfully managed to expose and visualize lymph nodes from levels I through V in multiple observational studies in the management of an No neck in HNCs involving the oral cavity.

7.5.1 The Pros and Cons of Minimally Invasive Neck Dissections

The distinct advantages of MIND over open approaches, regardless of type of incision, is the absence of a scar on the anterior aspect of the neck and the shorter length of hospital stay postoperatively. The maximum length of hospital stay following MIND, in a paper published by Nayak et al., was 6 days, compared to the mean length of hospital stay of 14.55 days reported in an enhanced recovery after surgery (ERAS) study for head and neck surgery (Coyle et al., 2016; Nayak & Jayaprasad, 2017). The development of skin edema has also been reported to be less in the MIND group when compared with open neck dissection patients. The marginal mandibular and accessory nerves can be preserved successfully in this method. MIND has been tried and tested in numerous publications, many from India, in the management of an No neck in oral cavity malignancies. The use of MIND in this group proved to be successful and beneficial when measures such as access to levels I–V of the neck, neurovascular preservation, complete lymph node dissection, shorter hospital stay, and absence of a scar on the anterior neck are quantified (Nayak & Jayaprasad, 2017).

However, as with everything in life including surgery, MIND has its limits. The absence of the platysma muscle over anterior part of the neck at level I makes the skin over that area prone to injury due to the energy source, especially in lean patients. This may result in unintended perforation of the skin, which may need repair, which goes against the desired effect of MIND (i.e., the absence of a surgical scar in the neck area) (Coyle et al., 2016; Nayak & Jayaprasad, 2017). Proper selection of patients is necessary as this approach may be limited to patients with minor/smaller lymph nodes. The size of the lymph node is another limiting factor because the larger the nodes, the higher the risk of extranodal spread, thus placing the EJV at risk of injury (Coyle et al., 2016). These challenges make MIND limited to a select number of patients, especially in developing countries where patients present late with advanced disease and comorbidities. Furthermore, MIND does not negate the requirements of a surgeon to possess the necessary skills in open approaches should uncontrollable bleeding be encountered (Coyle et al., 2016). Like most technology, cost is a major limiting factor especially in the healthcare centers of developing countries. The equipment in itself and its maintenance, especially the ongoing need for consumables, is costly especially for already stretched healthcare budgets. Endoscopic skills acquisition, though costly, is achievable as many otolaryngologists and general surgeons nowadays are skilled in endoscopic surgery, including many in sub-Saharan Africa (Coyle et al., 2016; Nayak & Jayaprasad, 2017).

7.6 Nerve-Sparing Techniques

The main therapeutic dilemma in surgical management of head and neck oncology is damage to the nerves. Damage to these structures results in delayed surgical recovery, a negative impact on return to normal function, and poor quality of life for the affected patient (Kyriazis et al., 2022). In head and neck oncology, the nerves commonly encountered and impacting quality of life are the facial nerve in facial, parotid, and temporal bone surgery; the spinal accessory nerve in neck dissections; the recurrent laryngeal nerve in thyroid surgery; and the hypoglossal nerve in submandibular gland excision and suprahyoid surgery (Rob et al., 2010). Great lengths have been taken in the intraoperative preservation of these nerves because injury, whether intentional or unintentional, results in unsatisfactory outcomes. The number one preservation method to injury of these delicate structures is surgical planning and thorough knowledge of surgical anatomy. Surgical anatomy can be further enhanced by radiological anatomy for best evaluation of tumor position, its relation to other anatomical structures, and the best location of the nerves (Michl et al., 2016). Furthermore, intraoperative care of these structures leads to better postoperative outcomes. These intraoperative techniques range from limited use of electrocautery around the nerves, wet swab use throughout the procedure, less or no devascularization of the nerves, less or no pranging of the nerves, direct vision of the nerve at all times, the use of magnification, and nerve monitoring in the form of electromyography (EMG) (Kyriazis et al., 2022).

The history of intraoperative nerve monitoring (IONM) began in the 1898, when Dr. Fedor Krause of Berlin, Germany, used monopolar faradic stimulation during an acoustic nerve neurectomy to check the function of the facial nerve after performing a cochlear nerve section for uncontrollable tinnitus. Krause stimulated the facial nerve and observed contractions of the facial region, especially of the orbicularis oculi as well as the branches supplying the nose and the mouth (Rob et al., 2010). The popularity of its use grew through the years. The use of IONM has become standard in many institutions where it is used mainly as an identifying tool during careful dissection in the proximity of a nerve. Monitoring is conducted during the course of the surgical procedure (Michl et al., 2016). The surgeon uses a nerve stimulator probe to identify the nerve and differentiate it from other tissue. The probe is placed onto the nerve, thus closing a circuit and producing further visual or acoustic stimuli every time the nerve is touched. Such an application can be defined as intermittent or continuous. Most head and neck surgeons use intermittent stimulus to avoid nerve fatigue, which may lead to paresis (Kyriazis et al., 2022).

7.6.1 Facial Nerve Preservation

Facial nerve preservation is crucial in head and neck surgery. Damage to this structure leads to loss of function of the facial musculature. This loss may lead to incomplete eye closure, which places the eye at risk of exposure keratitis, and oral insufficiency (Yang et al., 2024). The current protocols in perifacial nerve surgery dictate that if the nerve is intact preoperatively it needs to be intact postoperatively (López et al., 2001). Facial nerve preservation has given rise to numerous debates in oncological surgery especially when there is nerve involvement, microscopically and macroscopically (Yang et al., 2024). To preserve or to sacrifice? The arguments seem to tilt toward preservation. Preservation comes with its own difficulties in large tumors, with or without involvement of the surrounding structures, especially in parotid surgery (López et al., 2001) where anatomical landmarks may be lost. The use of nerve monitoring has been popularized by these challenges. Several studies have demonstrated that facial nerve monitoring reduced the incidence and severity of facial nerve paralysis independently of the kind of surgery performed. The incidence of temporary facial paralysis was significantly lower in the monitored group (36%) than in the unmonitored group (70%) ($p = 0.013$). The rates of permanent deficit were 4% for the monitored group and 30% for the unmonitored group ($p = 0.025$). These results suggest that intraoperative facial nerve monitoring reduces the incidence of postoperative facial deficit. Monitoring is considered useful in surgeries where there is a higher risk of injury to the facial nerve (e.g., total parotidectomy, repeat interventions, or chronic inflammatory conditions) (López et al., 2001).

On the other hand, there are studies stating that IONM does not lead to less paresis after surgery. Thus, there is no clear recommendation on whether a head and neck surgeon should use IONM when performing surgeries on the parotid gland. As a result, 40% of otolaryngologists in United States do not currently routinely use IONM but rely rather on their surgical skills and knowledge of anatomical landmarks (Yang et al., 2024). A recent meta-analysis comparing parotidectomies with and without iIONM found the incidence of immediate postoperative facial nerve palsy following parotidectomy while using IONM to be significantly lower when compared with procedures without monitoring (Stankovic et al., 2020).

Recently, the development of IONM has been enhanced by the establishment of so-called continuous intraoperative neuromonitoring (cIONM) in clinical practice. This aims to provide real-time monitoring of the nerve status during the entire course of exposure and, perhaps more importantly, predict postoperative function. This is done either actively (acIONM) or passively (pcIONM) (Choi et al., 2024). During acIONM, the nerve is stimulated continuously during the whole procedure. This can be facilitated using either an electrode placed on or near the nerve, by transcranial nerve stimulation, or, in the case of vestibulocochlear monitoring, using acoustic stimuli at a given frequency (Hz). This development does not assist in nerve sparing for quality of life but has in other instances been mentioned in medicolegal scenarios when nerve damage occurs postoperatively (Yang et al., 2024). The nerve monitoring report provides a technological report of nerve status as opposed to the clinical presentation noted at the end of surgery. It further provides hope and promise of recovery when immediate postoperative paresis occurs. This technology is limited in its use by cost, availability, and training. However great its benefit, it has not replaced the knowledge of surgical landmarks in safely identifying and sparing the nerve (Choi et al., 2024).

7.6.2 Recurrent Laryngeal Nerve Preservation

Thyroid surgery carries the highest risk of recurrent laryngeal nerve (RLN) injuries. Emphasis on anatomical landmarks can never be replaced by nerve monitoring, but it can guide the surgeon in identifying the nerve and preserving it (Russell et al., 2024). RLN injury leads to vocal cord paresis or paralysis, which presents clinically as hoarseness and aspiration in patients whose contralateral vocal cord cannot compensate. It affects quality of life in unilateral injury; this quality of life worsens with bilateral loss, which may present as airway emergencies and death if not attended to in a timely manner (Choi et al., 2024). acIONM has been developed and used in thyroid surgery, and intermittent monitoring is still widely used. Like facial nerve monitoring, its use has resulted in less postoperative fallout than without its use. With that said, its use is not to date recommended as standard practice (Stankovic et al., 2020).

7.6.3 Accessory Nerve

The accessory nerve is often encountered in neck dissections during head and neck surgery. Historically it was dissected and sacrificed as part of comprehensive surgery in RNDs. Progress in surgical practices has seen a new age of minimalism, functional preservation, and quality of life after cancer while maintaining the principles of cancer management (Choi et al., 2024). The widely used MRND has led to a detailed description of accessory nerve preservation, with the nerve being the last structure to be sacrificed in a neck dissection. Accessory nerve damage leads to loss of shoulder function, loss of trapezius muscle function, and frozen shoulder syndrome. To date, its preservation is best achieved with good intraoperative surgical skills in identifying and preserving the nerve. Intraoperative monitoring is not used routinely in this regard (Russell et al., 2024).

7.6.4 Hypoglossal Nerve

Hypoglossal nerve injury results in loss of tongue musculature, which may result in feeding and articulating difficulties. Its preservation, as with the accessory nerve, depends on thorough knowledge of surgical anatomy. The nerve is often encountered in neck dissections, transhyoid surgery, and total laryngectomy (Choi et al., 2024). Monitoring this nerve mechanically is not standard practice for a head and neck surgeon. Preservation of neurovascular structures is essential for maintaining optimal functional outcomes in HNC surgery. Nerve-sparing techniques aim to identify and preserve critical nerves such as the facial nerve, recurrent laryngeal nerve, and hypoglossal nerve during tumor resection, reducing the risk of postoperative deficits such as facial paralysis and voice changes (Russell et al., 2024).

7.7 Intraoperative Neuromonitoring

Head and neck oncology surgery presents special difficulties due to the intricate anatomy and close proximity to critical neural structures. The use of IONM, which provides real-time feedback and improves surgical techniques, has expanded in recent years. The section examines the use of IONM in head and neck oncology surgery, highlighting its advantages, techniques, indications, and future prospects (Palacios-García et al., 2021). To reduce damage and enable early diagnosis of impending nerve injury, IONM allows for the continuous monitoring of neural integrity throughout surgery (Schneider et al., 2018). The ability to monitor neural function intraoperatively improves patient safety by reducing the risk of postoperative complications such as nerve paralysis, parenthesis, and dysphagia, and, in doing so, improving overall postsurgical outcomes (Zhu et al., 2021). IONM makes it easier to perform surgical procedures that spare nerves, allowing for the preservation of critical neural structures while ensuring effective tumor resection and functional preservation (Schneider et al., 2018).

Table 7.3 highlights some examples of IONM techniques. In head and neck oncology surgery, IONM has become an indispensable adjunct, especially for procedures like parotidectomy, neck dissection, thyroid surgery, and other procedures. During surgical intervention, this advanced approach continually monitors the integrity of nerves that are in danger of injury in an effort to preserve neurologic function (Schneider et al., 2018).

Table 7.3 Intraoperative neuromonitoring techniques in head and neck cancer

Techniques	Description
Electromyography (EMG)	EMG records the electrical activity in muscles in response to nerve stimulation. This technique provides valuable information regarding the integrity of the motor nerves and facilitates the identification and preservation of motor nerve function.
Somatosensory evoked potentials (SSEPs)	SSEPs help to preserve sensory nerve function and reduce the risk of sensor deficits by recording cortical responses to peripheral nerve stimulation, which allows for the assessment of the integrity of sensory pathways.
Auditory evoked potential (AEPs)	AEPs allow for the early detection of auditory nerve injury and the preservation of hearing function by evaluating the integrity of the auditory pathways during surgery involving the base of skull and associated structures.

Source: Schneider et al., 2018.

The facial nerve, which passes through the gland dividing it into superficial and deep lobes, is at risk of injury during a parotidectomy or in a transparotid approach for surgical access to the temporomandibular joint (TMJ) (Schneider et al., 2018). During parotid or transparotid surgery, IONM is essential for locating and protecting the facial nerve. Surgeons can modify their approaches to avoid nerve stress and lower the risk of facial paralysis or weakness after surgery by receiving real-time feedback on the nerve function (Schneider et al., 2018). Neck dissection involves the removal of lymph nodes at risk of metastases, and neck dissection is a routine treatment in head and neck oncology. The process entails a complex dissection close to vital structures, including the branches of the cervical plexus, marginal mandibular nerve, and the spinal accessory nerve (SAN) (Palacios-García et al., 2021). By mapping near routes and tracking nerve function during the dissection, IONM helps surgeons prevent unintentional nerve damage and the ensuing functional consequences, such as shoulder dysfunction (if the SAN is affected) or deformity on mouth opening, smiling, or grimacing (if the marginal mandibular nerve is affected) (Schneider et al., 2018). The recurrent laryngeal nerve (RLN) and the exterior branch of the superior laryngeal nerve (EBSLN), which are essential for vocal cord function, are at risk of injury after thyroidectomy, whether partial or complete (Zhu et al., 2021).

During thyroid surgery, IONM offers real-time feedback on vocal cord function, enabling surgeons to modify their strategy if any impairment to nerve integrity is found. Maintaining voice quality and swallowing function after surgery depends on RLN and EBSLN function preservation (Palacios-García et al., 2021). IONM can be helpful in various head and neck oncologic procedures involving nerves at risk, such laryngectomy, pharyngectomy, and mandibulectomy, in addition to parotid surgery, neck dissection, and thyroid surgery (Higuchi-Sanabria et al., 2014). Future developments in neuromonitoring technology, such as nerve stimulators, high-definition electrodes, and signal processing algorithms, should improve IONM sensitivity and specificity even more. Combining several neuromonitoring modalities, such as EMG, somatosensory evoked potentials (SSEPs), and auditory evoked potentials (AEPs), allows for more thorough evaluation of neural function and may enhance nerve localization and preservation precision. By incorporating patient-specific data into surgical planning, such as neurophysiological mapping and preoperative imaging, head and neck oncology surgeons may be able to optimize outcomes and reduce morbidity (Cozzi et al., 2023, 2021; Ling et al., 2020).

Intraoperative monitoring is a useful addition to head and neck real-time evaluation of neural function, increases surgical accuracy, and promotes patient safety. With the ongoing advancement in technology and comprehension of neurophysiology, IONM is expected to become more crucial in the treatment of head and neck oncology, ultimately improving patient outcomes (Ling et al., 2020; Schneider et al., 2018).

7.8 Laser Surgery in Head and Neck Oncology

The work of Albert Einstein on the principle of stimulated emission was the basis for the development of laser surgery. On May 16, 1960, at Hughes Malibu laboratories (Los Angeles, CA, USA), Maiman's solid-state pink ruby laser emitted mankind's first coherent light, with rays all the same wavelength and fully in phase. After its initial industrial applications, many other laser applications were developed in the medical field. In 1972, Strong and Jako reported the first application of the carbon dioxide (CO_2) laser in transoral surgery. Many applications were then developed in microsurgery for the resection of early-stage vocal cord cancer lesions (Hans et al., 2022). The second part of the 20th century was characterized by the development of fiberoptic, endoscopic, and robotic technologies.

The management of laryngeal cancer through partial/near total laryngectomy has evolved over the past centuries, from the use of open partial laryngeal surgery to transoral laryngeal microsurgery (TLM) and transoral robotic surgery (TORS) (Wang et al., 2021). (A hybrid of TLM and TORS is another modality that is gaining the attention of scientists and surgeons and gaining momentum over the years. At the rate at which technology is advancing, its availability may be present at time of publication.) The development of TLM was an important step in the history of conservative laryngeal surgery (Tan et al., 2024). Its main objective was to reduce both morbidity and mortality related to postoperative complications while maintaining adequate overall survival and recurrence-free survival. In its early days, it was mainly used for early glottic cancer, but it has hence progressed to utilization in advanced disease and salvage surgery (Wang et al., 2021).

7.8.1 Transoral Laryngeal Microsurgery in Laryngeal Cancer

In the early days of the technology, TLM was mainly indicated for early-stage glottic vocal fold cancers (Tis, T1, T2), and its limitations for resection included tumors with reduced vocal cord mobility, which could be due to cricoarytenoid joint involvement, cricoid cartilage involvement, and posterior paraglottic region involvement. This created a stringent selection criterion for patient selection. TLM became the gold standard for surgical treatment in early vocal cord cancer due to its benefits (Wang et al., 2021). It is associated with comparable or superior oncological outcomes that include high disease-free survival and high local or regional control rates and larynx preservation rates when compared to partial surgery and radiation therapy with and without chemotherapy. These parameters of measure (i.e., disease-free survival, local or regional control rates, and laryngeal preservation) have been used since the inception of laryngeal surgery for cancer and have stood the test of time in gauging improvements in overall survival (Meulemans et al., 2017). A large cohort series conducted by Ambrosch and Fazel reported 5-year local control and laryngeal preservation rates of patients treated with TLM for Tis–T2. Laryngeal carcinomas were higher than those who received ration therapy (RT) (Ambrosch, 2011). Furthermore, many other studies that followed proved better overall survival, disease-free survival, and preservation rates of TLM versus RT. There was better short- and long-term morbidity in the TLM group versus the partial laryngectomy and radiation groups in additional studies (Ambrosch, 2011; Hans et al., 2022).

The healthcare system costs of TLM treatment were significantly lower than those for partial laryngectomies or radiation therapy and resulted in the same if not better outcomes. Impact on morbidity and the lack of a need for a tracheostomy or feeding tube also added benefit to TLM use versus its counterparts in early glottic cancer (Brudasca et al., 2023). In this context, careful presurgical, clinical, and radiographic staging is paramount to determine whether the lesion will be amenable to TLM to achieve local and regional surgical control (Meulemans et al., 2017). These presurgical assessments are to date best discussed in a multidisciplinary team setting using radiology to carefully assess the tumor for better surgical planning. TLM is not a technique suited to all surgeons at all centers. It requires training of the entire surgical team and surgical unit and requires that the operating surgeon be trained equally in open laryngeal surgery and endoscopic approaches should a need arise (Wang et al., 2021).

The excellent results reported in the use of TLM are further advanced by using intraoperative frozen sections that require assessment by pathologists to clear the margins. This modality requires patience from the surgical team because it may require more time (Meulemans et al., 2017) and multiple and extensive resections, hence the need for a surgeon to be skilled both in open and endoscopic procedures. The success of TLM in early glottic cancer opened an avenue for its use in advanced disease (T3 and T4), with preserving organ function, avoiding chemoradiation effects, and preventing swallowing dysfunction as its end goals (Brudasca et al., 2023). In most instances, however, because TLM alone did not suffice in T3/T4 glottic cancer, many clinicians added postoperative radiation therapy to achieve results comparable to a total laryngectomy with or without radiation therapy. Poor voicing and aspiration post TLM for advanced lesions are often encountered in the early postoperative period but recover in most patients; with that said, many patients still opt for organ preservation despite these known challenges (Wang et al., 2021).

The increasing success of TLM in laryngeal cancer further challenged the progress of laryngeal cancer management for patients with recurrent disease. Recurrence after radiation therapy, depending on staging, often poses a challenge to the patient and surgeon on whether laryngeal preservation can be achieved safely (Wang et al., 2021). Previously, the gold standard for recurrent laryngeal cancer was open surgery, either partial or total laryngectomy, leading to aphonia, lifestyle challenges posed by the stoma, the high risk of pharyngeal fistulas, aspiration pneumonia, swallowing difficulty, and a prolonged hospital stay. The advent of TLM and its possibilities has changed the playing field for recurrent disease (Brudasca et al., 2023). Meulemans et al. reported that salvage TLM compared to open partial laryngeal surgery techniques as a treatment modality for radio-recurrent laryngeal cancer combined good oncological outcomes with the advantages of reduced complications. The study demonstrated better functional outcomes in terms of voice and swallowing and shortened hospital stays (Meulemans et al., 2017).

It unfortunately also demonstrated a trend toward inferior local controls even after repeated TLM when compared with open techniques. However, when combining all the data, TLM surgery alone in the salvage of radio-recurrent disease did not seem to negatively affect ultimate local control or overall survival because many other factors were at play. This approach is, however, best carried out in centers that are well experienced in salvage surgery (Meulemans et al., 2017). Previously radiated tissues pose a great challenge not only to open procedures but to endoscopic procedures, too. Healing is often delayed or slow. With manipulation of the larynx, the risk of aspiration in the immediate postoperative period poses a risk of pneumonia and may result in longer hospital stays. Laryngeal cancer is often a disease of smokers who may have poorer lung reserves that place them at higher risk of aspiration pneumonia. Therefore, preclinical workup and patient selection is important in this regard (Brudasca et al., 2023).

7.8.2 Transoral Laryngeal Microsurgery in Oropharyngeal Cancer

TLM resection of base tongue lesions offers significant advantages over open procedures especially from tumors that can be visualized using endoscopic technology. The first reported cases of TLM in tongue base lesions were conducted in 2003, and many others thereafter reported good results in both tumor control and postoperative morbidity. TLM resection spares a patient from transpharyngeal, transmandibular, and lip splitting approaches, which results in shorter hospital stays (Petruzzelli, 2009). TLM also has been expanded for use in the tonsil fossa and posterior pharyngeal wall. However, the advent of TORS has superseded TLM use because the laser used in TLM follows a straight line, thus making it challenging for difficult to reach places around corners. In resection of oropharyngeal lesions, without a doubt TORS is superior, but it is greatly disadvantaged by costs and a steep learning curve for the management team. Functional and oncology outcomes for patients treated with TLM for tongue base resection shows disease-specific survival compares favorably with chemoradiation. Swallowing and gastrostomy dependence were less common in the TLM group than in the chemoradiation group (Tan et al., 2024).

7.8.3 Transoral Laryngeal Microsurgery in Hypopharyngeal Cancer

Hypopharyngeal cancer lesions are often diagnosed at an advanced stage and carry a poor prognosis, which can be further worsened by histological type and patient factors. TLM in this population has been used in a small selection of patients (i.e., those with very early disease involving the piriform sinus). The rate of salvage total laryngectomy was 2%, and gastrostomy and tracheotomy use was reported at 4% (Petruzzelli, 2009). Other documented uses include accessible chemoradiation-recurrent disease. Further studies and its use in this regard are necessary to weigh benefits that will affect quality of life and improve survival (Luna-Ortiz, 2019).

7.8.4 Transoral Laryngeal Microsurgery in the Oral Cavity

Cancer of the oral cavity and oropharynx is the sixth leading cancer globally with an overall survival of 40–45%. Surgery has been performed using traditional scalpels, electrocautery, cryotherapy, and lasers. Laser surgery in the oral cavity has been in use since the 1960s. Its advantages included clean margins, decreased tissue damage, and decreased need for reconstruction in this area. With the assistance of a microscope, its precision has improved remarkably, too (Meulemans et al., 2017). Multiple studies have proved laser to be effective in both premalignant and malignant lesions of the oral cavity. However, there has been no conclusive evidence that outrightly makes it superior to other traditional methods in improving the local control rates and overall survival. Its use in oral cavity cancer resection results in minimal damage to the surrounding structures, reduction of acute inflammation reaction, and a decrease in fibroblast activity leading to reduced scarring. This results in less postoperative morbidity, a shorter time to oral intake, decreased dependency on tube feeding, and shorter hospital stays (Luna-Ortiz, 2019). The evolution of oncology surgery and advances in technology have led to the decision to perform increasingly less-invasive surgical procedures especially when the results of open surgery are comparable (Meulemans et al., 2017).

7.8.5 The Pros and Cons of Transoral Laryngeal Microsurgery

TLM is minimally invasive microsurgery that presents an oncologically sound approach for selected patients with malignant tumors while maintaining the desired outcomes in cancer management. It is a vital tool for the oncology surgeon and gives patients options for management of their disease (Hans et al., 2022). Numerous studies have documented its efficacy in reducing tissue damage, its increased precision with the use of a microscope, and its ability to reduce postoperative pain by reducing the inflammatory process that occurs with resections using other methods (Meulemans et al., 2017). It has been demonstrated to be the best technique in organ preservation in laryngeal malignancies and is a cornerstone in the evolution of oncology surgery. Many are living longer as technology and research advances. A cancer diagnosis, regardless of stage, poses a lifelong risk of recurrence or other cancerous lesions. The standard methods of management for recurrent disease have for the longest time been limited to radical surgery. TLM has become an alternative that not only resolves the disease but offers a better quality of life (Hans et al., 2022).

The use of laser is not without risk. Stringent efforts must be made to minimize the chance of damage. To this end, rigid safety protocols are applied whenever lasers are used surgically. These protocols differ from center to center and require training by all theater personnel (Hans et al., 2022). Technological advances and an increasing familiarity with lasers have made their use simpler and better; however, despite technological advantages, lasers, if used inappropriately, are dangerous and may result in inadvertent damage to the patient and/or the surgeon or theater staff. All theater staff must wear specialized eye protection, and the operator is only exempt if he or she is using the microscope as this confers eye protection (Meulemans et al., 2017). Laser-use warning signs must be visible inside and outside the theater where a laser is being used. All metal equipment used throughout the operation must be minimally or nonreflective. These measures are not without cost and the need for training time for personnel (Ahmed et al., 2010).

Transoral laser surgery demands the utilization of specially designed equipment, including endoscopes in which smoke-evacuating suction catheters are incorporated into the body of the endoscope and micro-manipulator units that, when attached to the microscope, allow precise maneuverability of the laser aiming beam, which in turn ensures accurate tissue resection under magnification (Hans et al., 2022). This apparatus has cost implications to a healthcare industry that is already tearing at the seams and struggling with affordability, especially in the lower-income countries. The oncological outcomes of TLM versus established techniques are more or less the same with the equipment available in most centers that treat HNCs (Meulemans et al., 2017). Acquiring this technology will no doubt be an added cost. Laser surgery utilizes high-energy light beams to precisely remove tumors in the head and neck region. This technique offers advantages such as minimal blood loss, precise tissue ablation, and preservation of adjacent structures, making it a valuable tool in the management of early-stage tumors and in cases where organ preservation is critical (Hans et al., 2022).

7.9 Transoral Robotic Surgery

TORS is a minimally invasive surgical technique applied in head and neck surgery for benign and malignant lesions (Yee, 2017). The most commonly used system is the DaVinci, marketed by Intuitive. In this system, the surgical team uses minimally invasive, robot-assisted technology to excise suspicious and histologically proven lesions via the oral cavity. The hardware in the da Vinci system allows surgeons to achieve excellent visualization of the tumor anatomy, and the operative instruments are controlled remotely within the visual field with excellent maneuverability. The operator remotely controls these instruments from a console across the operating room. The use of the "robot" eliminates tremor and allows movements in seven degrees of freedom, which would be impossible with the human wrist (Hamilton & Paleri, 2017).Several robotic systems will be available in the future, judging from the rate of advancement in technology and artificial intelligence (AI).

The TORS da Vinci technique is currently applicable for use in the oropharynx (tonsils, base of tongue, palate and parapharyngeal space), larynx and hypopharynx (supraglottis, glottis, piriform fossa, pharyngeal wall), and skull base (Yee, 2017). TORS has proved through progressive use and advancements in its technology to reduce morbidity and improve the accessibility of hard-to-reach lesions better than open approaches and transoral laser techniques (Nichols et al., 2019). With that said, not all patients are candidates for TORS (Yee, 2017). In 2009, the US Food and Drug Administration (FDA) approved the use of TORS for resection of benign and malignant tumors in otolaryngology procedures staged as T1 and T2 (very early and early, respectively) and for benign tongue base procedures. The contraindications for its use included patients with contraindications to anesthesia, locally advanced tumors that were unresectable, invasion into the mandible, advanced tongue base tumors requiring > 50% resection of the tongue, advanced pharyngeal tumors requiring > 50% resection of the posterior wall, and involvement of the vertebra (Yee, 2017).

In general, surgery is the primary treatment of cancers arising from the oral cavity, oropharynx, larynx, hypopharynx, and the skull base. It is often followed by radiation therapy and secondary treatment, with or without chemotherapy depending on the pathological staging (Yee, 2017). The current methods of approach to lesions arising from these sites include open excision en bloc, laser excision (piecemeal, minimally invasive surgery), endoscopic approaches, and robotic surgery in the form of TORS. Currently TORS is the method closest to the traditional surgical approaches to malignant lesions (i.e., en bloc resection with a margin), hence its preference over TLM. The application of TORS has expanded since its inception from resection of T1 and T2 oral cavity and oropharyngeal lesions to current applications in carcinoma of unknown primary (CUP) and recurrent disease (Hamilton & Paleri, 2017).

7.9.1 Transoral Robotic Surgery in Oropharyngeal Squamous Cell Carcinoma

Approximately 500,000 new cases of head and neck squamous cell carcinoma (HNSCC) are diagnosed each year making HNSCC the sixth most common cancer worldwide. The rate of HNSCC has been increasing recently secondary to an epidemic of human papillomavirus (HPV)-related oropharyngeal SCC (OPSCC) (Ferlay et al., 2010). The advent of OPSCC has demonstrated a shift in the demographics of the disease toward the younger population, with good functional status and less comorbidities. This population group prompted scientists and surgeons to revisit the management of OPSCC with the goal of organ preservation to achieve better treatment functionality and outcomes (Ferlay et al., 2010). The proportion of patients cured of HPV-positive OPSCC is higher than the HPV-negative OPSCC often described in the elderly and in smokers with or without concurrent alcohol intake. The management of OPSCC has relied on radiotherapy-based approaches. Older surgical approaches consist of techniques that required large incisions, such as mandibulotomies and division of the floor-of-mouth musculature. These techniques, though widely used, were not favored at most institutions because of the high morbidity and mortality shown in observational studies (Ferlay et al., 2010).

The addition of concurrent chemotherapy to radiotherapy has improved oncological outcomes and survival at the cost of markedly increased toxicity, with a treatment-related mortality risk of up to 3% (Nichols et al., 2019). Advances in radiation therapy further progressed to limit the side effects of radiation through the introduction of intensity-modulated radiation therapy (IMRT) but did not totally resolve the long-term effects of radiation (e.g., mucositis, esophageal webs, persistent xerostomia, and probable feeding tube dependency). The advent of minimally invasive surgery (TLM and TORS) placed surgery back on the management table of OPSCC (Nichols et al., 2019). In the United States, based on data from the National Cancer Database, the percentage of patients undergoing primary surgery for T1–T2 stage OPSCC increased from 56% (318 of 568) in 2004 to 82% (837 of 1021) in 2013, driven by patient preferences and assumptions of reduced toxicity or improved quality of life (Cracchiolo et al., 2016).

The ORATOR trial was an investigator-initiated, multicenter, international, open-label, parallel-group, phase II, randomized study. Patients with T1 or T2, N0–N2 (maximum nodal size ≤4 cm) OPSCC were randomly assigned to either radiotherapy with concurrent chemotherapy in node-positive patients (radiotherapy group), or to TORS plus neck dissection with adjuvant therapy depending on pathological findings (TORS plus neck dissection group) (Nichols et al., 2019). In the radiotherapy group, radiation was delivered using intensity-modulated radiotherapy techniques, including volumetric modulated arc therapy. In the TORS plus neck dissection group, a surgical robot was used to excise the primary tumor with 1 cm margins, with selective neck dissections done at the time of surgery or within 2 weeks. Adjuvant radiotherapy, to a total dose of 60 Gy in 30 fractions and starting within 6 weeks of surgery, was recommended for patients based on intermediate-risk pathological features (pT3 or pT4 disease, close resection margins [<2 mm], nodal disease, or lymph vascular invasion) (Hutcheson et al., 2016).

In situations with high-risk features (positive margins or extranodal extension), adjuvant chemoradiotherapy was given, and the radiation dose was increased to 64 Gy in 30 fractions. Follow-up occurred every 3 months for the first 2 years, and every 6 months thereafter until 5 years and included patient history and physical examination (all visits), adverse event monitoring (all visits), quality of life scoring (every 6 months), chest x-ray every 6 months except at 1 year when a CT of the neck and chest was completed, and an audiogram 1 year after treatment. The primary quality of life tool used was the MD Anderson Dysphagia Index (MDADI). The MDADI score ranges between 20 and 100, and a higher score represents better quality of life (Hutcheson et al., 2016).

The primary endpoint was a definitive comparison of the total score on the MDADI at 1 year. Prespecified secondary endpoints were overall survival, defined as time from randomization to death from any cause, and progression-free survival, defined as time from randomization to death or recurrence, whichever occurred first. TORS did not outrightly result in being superior to radiotherapy using the units of measure applied to the trial (Hutcheson et al., 2016). It did, however, open an avenue on research in HPV + OPSCC with regards to de-escalation approaches in the younger population through the use of surgery, TORS, and lower doses of postoperative radiation. At 1 year quality of life and feeding were reported to be better in the TORS and neck dissection approach group. In OPSCC, TORS offers an opportunity for excision of the hard-to-reach areas of the oropharynx with less morbidity. However, intraoperative bleeding is still a complication worth consideration (Hutcheson et al., 2016).

7.9.2 Transoral Robotic Surgery in Carcinoma of Unknown Primary

To this day, despite the advent of radiological advances in the form of fluorodeoxyglucose positron emission tomography (FDG-PET) scans, CUP persists, with the majority being attributed to OPSCC. According to the literature this group accounts for 2–5% of HNCs, a relatively small percentage in relation to all head and neck malignancies (Mehta et al., 2013). Management of these lesions includes fine needle or core biopsy of the involved lymph node, flexible endoscopy, assessment of all primary sites, and palpation of the tonsils plus base of tongue. If the primary site is not identified, then an FDG-PET scan is recommended, which increases rate of primary tumor identification by 44% (Hamilton & Paleri, 2017). If the PET scan demonstrates uptake only at the nodal site, then traditionally the patient undergoes an endoscopic assessment of the upper aerodigestive tract and bilateral tonsillectomies with random biopsies of the postnasal space and the base of tongue. Despite these rigorous attempts, a number of patients remained with an unknown primary site, thus posing a long-standing debate on neck dissection alone for an N1 node without extracapsular extension as compared to concurrent chemotherapy with total mucosal irradiation of the upper aerodigestive tract, which carries a substantial amount of adverse reactions (Hamilton & Paleri, 2017).

The advent of TORS came to the fore as another alternative mode in detecting the unknown primary. With TORS precise mucosectomies could be achieved, negating human errors in anatomical precision, reduction in hand tremor, and better visualization of the tongue base from the circumvallate papillae to the vallecula (Hamilton & Paleri, 2017). Mucosectomies can be carried out bilaterally using TORS up to the level of the tongue base musculature. This technique has demonstrated a primary detection rate averaged at 89% and spared radiation to the pharynx in 36% of patients (Hamilton & Paleri, 2017). A thorough analysis of the literature led the UK National Institute for Health and Care Excellence

(NICE) to recommend that if FDG PET-CT does not identify a primary site, then the next step should include tongue base mucosectomy if the facilities and expertise are available (Hamilton & Paleri, 2017). TORS mucosectomy has been demonstrated to be superior to endoscopic (pan endoscopy) approaches in obtaining tissue to identify the primary. Furthermore, when undertaken together with a neck dissection, it may act as primary treatment and limit the use of radiation therapy (Hamilton & Paleri, 2017)

7.9.3 Transoral Robotic Surgery in Recurrent Disease

TORS has been mainly applied to primary early-stage disease of the head and neck. Its success in this regard has prompted surgeons and scientists to further evaluate its use in residual or recurrent disease (White et al., 2013). This idea has been largely prompted by the younger patient population with HPV + OPSCC who present with residual disease that is amenable to surgical resection. Older techniques of surgical resection usually necessitate wide resection margins often in difficult-to-reach places, which further requires insertion of free flaps transorally, which can be achieved through the use of TORS (White et al., 2013). The technique is only feasible in selected patients, with trismus as a main contraindication. The main advantage of the TORS approach in recurrent/residual disease is avoidance of a mandibulotomy, with disruption of the floor of mouth, which can delay healing significantly in a previously radiated field. There is demonstrated success with the use of TORS in this patient population, the most notable being a retrospective multi-institutional case-control study of March 2003 through October 2011 conducted at four tertiary care institutions (White et al., 2013).

Sixty-four patients who underwent salvage TORS for recurrent oropharyngeal SCC were matched by tumor, node, and metastasis (TNM) stage to 64 patients who underwent open salvage resection. Patient demographics, operative data, and functional and oncologic outcomes were recorded and compared with a similarly TNM-matched patient group that underwent salvage surgical resection by traditional open surgical approaches (White et al., 2013). Patients treated with TORS were found to have a significantly lower incidence of tracheostomy use ($n = 14$ vs. $n = 50$; $P < .001$), feeding tube use ($n = 23$ vs. $n = 48$; $P < .001$), shorter overall hospital stays (3.8 days vs. 8.0 days; $P < .001$), decreased operative time (111 minutes vs. 350 minutes; $P < .001$), less blood loss (49 mL vs. 331 mL; $P < .001$), and significantly decreased incidence of positive margins ($n = 6$ vs. $n = 19$; $P = .007$). The 2-year recurrence-free survival rate was significantly higher in the TORS group than in the open approach group (74% and 43%, respectively) ($P = .01$) (White et al., 2013). The study demonstrated that TORS offers an alternative surgical approach to recurrent tumors of the oropharynx with acceptable oncologic outcomes and better functional outcomes than traditional open surgical approaches. This adds to the growing amount of clinical evidence to support the use of TORS in selected patients with recurrent oropharyngeal SCC as a feasible and oncological sound method of treatment (White et al., 2013).

7.9.4 The Pros and Cons of Transoral Robotic Surgery

The primary advantage of TORS is computerized mechanization that allows surgeons deeper access and better dissection of tumors that would otherwise be cumbersome or require extensive surgery to access. It further controls and negates the possible tremor that may be present in the human hand. It allows for cross-continental surgery and collaborations (Tan et al., 2024). The greatest of all benefits is to the patient: TORS results in a reduction of facial scarring from the lip spilt used in mandibulotomy and there is no large neck incision from base of tongue or pharyngeal approaches, no malocclusion or malunion of the mandible resulting in dysfunction, and no possibility of postoperative hardware extrusion from fixation techniques. TORS further results in decreased incidence of a tracheostomy, decreased nasogastric feed, more rapid swallowing rehabilitation, decreased blood loss, a shorter recovery period, and a faster return to normal activities (Hamilton & Paleri, 2017).

However, not all is bright and beautiful. The most limiting factor in robotic surgery is cost. The technology is expensive and not accessible to many centers globally. This cost is not only driven by the technology and the console itself but further ballooned by the cost of disposable and nondisposable robotic instruments, dedicated and delicate micro-instruments, and robotic supplies (Tan et al., 2024). It further requires infrastructure development or upgrades to accommodate the device, a cost that very few institutions can carry to accommodate a device that services a minimal portion of healthcare consumers (Hamilton & Paleri, 2017). The procedures conducted using TORS themselves are technically challenging, requiring training of the surgical services personnel from procurement, use, and nursing to cleaning and storage—a steep learning curve that may take time and redirect resources that are already stretched, especially in low-income countries (Tan et al., 2024). The TORS technology carries a further risk that echoes throughout many medical fields that are affected by AI: the loss of tactile sensation for the surgeon.

In addition, injury to the lips and teeth, mucosal injury from instrumentation, facial laceration, cervical spine injuries caused by robotic instrumentation, and ocular injuries also can occur. For now these are still manageable by the attending clinical team while the technology advances. Several robotic systems other than the da Vinci will be available in the future judging by the rate of advancement in technology and AI (Hamilton & Paleri, 2017).

TORS is a minimally invasive surgical technique that allows surgeons to access tumors in the oropharynx and larynx through the mouth using a robotic system. This approach offers improved visualization, maneuverability, and access to difficult-to-reach areas, leading to reduced morbidity and faster recovery compared to traditional open surgery (Tan et al., 2024). Technology is rapidly advancing to include more subsites and advanced disease. The greatest limit to this invention is cost, making its availability limited to developed countries involved in research. This dimension limits its use in multicenter trials and presents trials with limited numbers of patients. Reduction in cost may assist in advancing this technology for better precision in both diagnostic and therapeutic outcomes (Hamilton & Paleri, 2017).

7.9.5 Other Areas of Robotic Surgery Application in the Head and Neck

Technology has led to further innovation in the application of robotic surgery in the head and neck region. These areas include salivary gland surgery, thyroid surgery, and neck dissections. Robotic surgery for the salivary gland lesion is often conducted transorally, and access to the parapharyngeal space is accessible and often undertaken for pleomorphic adenomas, cysts, and schwannomas involving this area. The approach saves the patient from having an external scar. The transoral approach leads to better access of the parapharyngeal space for complete tumor resection. However, there have been multiple reports of tumor capsule rupture when using this technique, which may result in intraoperative tumor spillage. This complication is less common in open approaches. The majority of lesions that were operated using robot-assisted salivary gland excision were benign, with the majority being pleomorphic adenomas. The rate of tumor spillage was high, which poses a very high risk of recurrence (Hussain, 2022) and is a long-term complication that is often challenging to treat.

Robotic surgery also has gained its popularity in neck surgery due to its avoidance of a clearly visible external scar. Large studies in the literature describe the results of robot-assisted surgery for cervical lymph node surgery (i.e., neck dissections) and thyroid surgery. The surgical route of access is commonly taken via the modified facelift approach from the postauricular region. Sukato et al.'s metanalysis of 655 patients showed comparable results of robotic neck dissections using the da Vinci system compared to conventional neck dissection. The measured outcome was postoperative complications (i.e., postoperative bleeding, chyle leak/fistula formation, nerve injury, and wound infections). The number of dissected lymph nodes did not differ between the two approaches. However, the surgical time was longer in the traditional open approaches for modified RND despite the length of surgical experience. Patients were more satisfied with cosmetic outcome in the robot-assisted group (Sukato et al., 2019). Assessment of long-term oncologic outcomes is still ongoing.

Robot-assisted thyroid surgery is yet another avenue that is growing in popularity and improvement. An axillary approach can be used, which was established nearly 20 years ago. Its main purpose is to avoid a scar in the anterior aspect of the neck. Despite its good results, tumors > 5 cm, a body mass index of > 35 kg/m^2, and thyroid diseases such as Hashimoto thyroiditis or Graves disease are considered contraindications for robot-assisted thyroid surgery. To date, numerous meta-analyses have demonstrated excellent oncological outcomes with robot-assisted thyroid surgery. Robot-assisted surgery also demonstrated lower to equal rates of injury to the recurrent laryngeal nerve when compared to open approaches. However, the surgical time was much longer in robot-assisted thyroid surgery when compared to traditional open approaches (Holsinger & Chung, 2014).

Robot-assisted salivary gland and neck surgery offers cosmetic advantages due to the access route: an obvious scar can be avoided. Comparable results can be achieved to some extent with established endoscopic techniques. Although longer-term oncologic outcomes are already available for robotic thyroid surgery, for robot-assisted neck dissection, no final conclusions on the long-term impact on oncologic disease progression can be drawn at this point. Thus, an evaluation of the most important parameter for potential patient benefit, namely the impact on cure and survival, is still pending. In all areas of application, the use of robotic technology significantly prolongs the duration of surgery (Hussain, 2022).

7.10 Enhanced Recovery after Surgery Protocols

Enhanced recovery after surgery (ERAS) protocols have emerged as a valuable approach to optimizing perioperative care and improving postoperative outcomes in various surgical specialties, including HNC surgery (Nieminen et al., 2024). ERAS protocols are multidisciplinary, perioperative, evidence-based care pathways designed to minimize surgical stress, reduce complications, accelerate recovery, and enhance patient satisfaction (Kattar et al., 2023; Nieminen et al., 2024). While originally developed for colorectal surgery, ERAS principles have been adapted and implemented in HNC surgery to address the unique challenges and complexities of this patient population. These protocols incorporate strategies such as preoperative counseling, multimodal pain management, early mobilization, and nutritional support to minimize complications, shorten hospital stays, and improve overall outcomes in HNC patients undergoing surgery (Figure 7.10) (Nieminen et al., 2024).

Patients are provided with comprehensive information about their surgery, expected recovery, and strategies for postoperative pain management, nutrition, and mobility (Kattar et al., 2023). Nutritional assessment and supplementation are initiated preoperatively to optimize nutritional status and reduce the risk of postoperative complications. Smoking cessation programs are implemented preoperatively to reduce the risk of wound healing complications and respiratory complications (Fagan, 2021; Nieminen et al., 2024). Minimally invasive surgical approaches are utilized to reduce surgical trauma, minimize tissue damage, and expedite recovery whenever feasible (List et al., 2023). Regional anesthesia techniques, such as nerve blocks and local infiltration anesthesia, are used to reduce the need for systemic opioids and minimize postoperative pain. Fluid administration is guided by hemodynamic monitoring and individualized

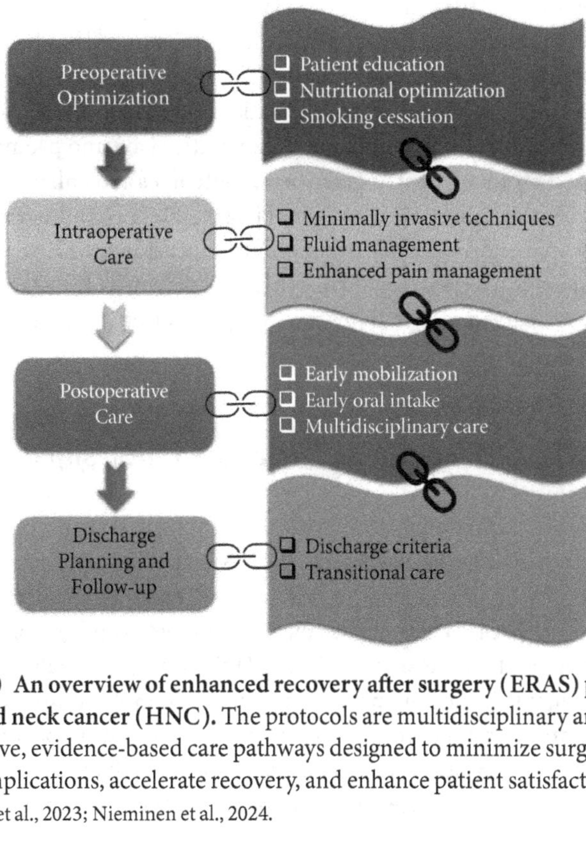

Figure 7.10 An overview of enhanced recovery after surgery (ERAS) protocols in head and neck cancer (HNC). The protocols are multidisciplinary and perioperative, evidence-based care pathways designed to minimize surgical stress, reduce complications, accelerate recovery, and enhance patient satisfaction
From Kattar et al., 2023; Nieminen et al., 2024.

goals to maintain adequate tissue perfusion while minimizing fluid overload and associated complications (Nieminen et al., 2024).

Patients are encouraged to resume oral intake as soon as possible after surgery to promote gastrointestinal function, prevent dehydration, and reduce the risk of ileus. Early mobilization and ambulation are encouraged to prevent complications such as venous thromboembolism, atelectasis, and pneumonia (List et al., 2023). A multimodal approach to pain management is employed, combining nonopioid analgesics, regional anesthesia techniques, and judicious use of opioids to minimize pain and opioid-related side effects. Criteria-based discharge protocols are utilized to facilitate early discharge and transition to home or rehabilitation facilities. Patients receive postoperative follow-up care, including monitoring for complications, wound care instructions, and rehabilitation services as needed (Nieminen et al., 2024). ERAS protocols involve collaboration among various healthcare providers, including surgeons, anesthesiologists, nurses, dietitians, physiotherapists, and other allied health professionals. This multidisciplinary approach ensures comprehensive perioperative care and coordination of services throughout the patient's surgical journey (Coyle et al., 2016; List et al., 2023).

The implementation of ERAS protocols in HNC surgery has been shown to result in several benefits, including reduced length of hospital stay, decreased postoperative complications, improved patient satisfaction, and cost savings (Nieminen et al., 2024). By optimizing perioperative care and promoting faster recovery, ERAS protocols contribute to better outcomes and enhanced quality of life for patients undergoing HNC surgery (Fagan, 2021; Nieminen et al., 2024). Ongoing research efforts aim to further refine and customize ERAS protocols to address the specific needs and challenges of HNC patients, ultimately improving the delivery of care and outcomes in this population (Kattar et al., 2023; Nieminen et al., 2024).

7.11 Telemedicine and Remote Surgical Support

Telemedicine platforms and remote surgical support systems have emerged as valuable tools in the management of HNC, facilitating access to specialized care, improving treatment coordination, and enhancing patient outcomes (Nieminen et al., 2024). They enable collaboration between surgeons, multidisciplinary teams, and remote experts during HNC surgeries (Mali, 2024). These technologies enable healthcare providers to deliver remote consultations, monitor patients' progress, and provide real-time guidance and support to surgeons performing complex procedures. These technologies facilitate real-time consultation, intraoperative guidance, and postoperative follow-up, enhancing access to specialized care and improving outcomes, particularly in underserved or remote areas (van de Weerd et al., 2023).

Telemedicine platforms allow HNC patients to consult with their healthcare providers remotely, eliminating the need for in-person visits and reducing travel burdens, particularly for patients residing in remote or underserved areas (Mali, 2024). Remote consultations enable healthcare providers to review imaging studies, discuss treatment options, and provide ongoing support and education to patients and their families throughout the cancer care continuum (Dhillon et al., 2022). Telemedicine also facilitates postoperative follow-up appointments, enabling healthcare providers to monitor patients' progress, assess treatment response, and address any concerns or complications without requiring patients to travel to the clinic (Mali, 2024). Telemedicine platforms can be used to facilitate preoperative consultations and multidisciplinary tumor board meetings, allowing surgeons, oncologists, radiologists, and other specialists to collaborate remotely and develop individualized treatment plans for HNC patients (da Silva et al., 2022). Virtual tumor board meetings enable healthcare providers to review patient cases, discuss treatment options, and make informed decisions regarding surgical approaches, adjuvant therapies, and patient management strategies (Dhillon et al., 2022).

Remote surgical support technologies, such as teleconferencing, video streaming, and tele mentoring, enable expert surgeons to provide real-time guidance and support to less-experienced surgeons performing complex HNC surgeries (Caputo et al., 2023). Remote surgical support allows expert surgeons to remotely visualize the surgical field, provide intraoperative feedback, and assist with decision-making, technique refinement, and troubleshooting during the procedure (Mali, 2024). Telemonitoring programs facilitate the transfer of surgical skills and expertise to less-experienced surgeons, promoting professional development and enhancing surgical proficiency in complex head and neck procedures (Dhillon et al., 2022). Telemedicine platforms can be used to deliver postoperative care and rehabilitation services to HNC patients, including speech therapy, swallow evaluations, and nutritional counseling (Mali, 2024). Remote monitoring technologies, such as wearable devices and telehealth applications, enable healthcare providers to remotely assess patients' functional status, monitor for complications, and provide timely interventions to optimize recovery and quality of life (Caputo et al., 2023).

While telemedicine and remote surgical support offer numerous benefits, there are also challenges and considerations to address, including technological limitations, privacy and security concerns, licensure and reimbursement issues, and disparities in access to technology and internet connectivity. Healthcare providers must ensure that telemedicine services comply with regulatory requirements, maintain patient confidentiality, and provide high-quality, equitable care to all patients, regardless of their geographic location or socioeconomic status (Dhillon et al., 2022). Thus, telemedicine and remote surgical support play an increasingly important role in the management of HNC, enabling healthcare providers to deliver high-quality, patient-centered care, improve treatment coordination, and optimize patient outcomes (Caputo et al., 2023). By harnessing the power of technology, telemedicine and remote surgical support have the potential to overcome geographic barriers, enhance access to specialized expertise, and revolutionize the delivery of care in head and neck oncology. Ongoing research and innovation in this field will continue to expand the capabilities of telemedicine and remote surgical support, further improving the delivery of care and outcomes for HNC patients (Mali, 2024)

7.12 Future Prospectives and Outlook

The future prospects and outlook of surgical innovations in HNCs are promising, with ongoing advancements poised to revolutionize the field and improve patient outcomes (Jayawickrama et al., 2024). Continued advancements in imaging modalities, including high-resolution magnetic resonance imaging, PET-CT, and intraoperative imaging techniques, will enable surgeons to better delineate tumor margins, identify critical structures, and tailor surgical approaches to individual patient anatomy (Mali, 2024). Integration of AI and machine learning algorithms into surgical planning and navigation systems holds promise for enhancing surgical precision, optimizing tumor resection, and minimizing damage to surrounding healthy tissues (Jayawickrama et al., 2024). Further development and refinement of minimally invasive surgical techniques, such as TORS, endoscopic approaches, and laser surgery, will enable more precise tumor resection with reduced morbidity and improved functional outcomes. Organ-sparing approaches, including partial laryngectomy, TLM, and supracricoid laryngectomy, will continue to gain prominence, allowing for preservation of critical functions such as speech, swallowing, and airway protection (Bhat et al., 2021; Jayawickrama et al., 2024).

Advancements in molecular profiling, genomic sequencing, and biomarker identification will enable more precise characterization of head and neck tumors, guiding personalized treatment strategies tailored to the unique genetic and molecular features of each patient's cancer (Jayawickrama et al., 2024). Targeted therapies, immunotherapies, and combination treatment approaches based on molecular profiling and tumor biology will revolutionize treatment paradigms, offering more effective and tailored therapeutic options for HNC patients (Mali, 2024). Innovations in tissue engineering, regenerative medicine, and 3D printing technology will enable more sophisticated and personalized approaches to reconstructive surgery, facilitating restoration of form and function following tumor resection (Han et al., 2024; Jayawickrama et al., 2024). Development of novel biomaterials, scaffolds, and bioengineered tissues will enhance the durability, biocompatibility, and aesthetic outcomes of reconstructive procedures, improving patient satisfaction and quality of life (Han et al., 2024). Expansion of telemedicine platforms, remote surgical support technologies, and virtual reality–based training programs will facilitate collaboration among multidisciplinary teams, enhance access to specialized expertise, and enable remote consultation and surgical mentoring for less-experienced surgeons (Jayawickrama et al., 2024).

Integration of telemedicine and remote surgical support into routine clinical practice will improve treatment coordination, optimize perioperative care, and enhance patient outcomes, particularly for patients residing in underserved or remote areas (Jayawickrama et al., 2024). The future of surgical innovations in HNCs is characterized by a convergence of technological advancements, personalized treatment approaches, and multidisciplinary collaboration (Mali, 2024). By harnessing the power of precision surgery, minimally invasive techniques, precision oncology, reconstructive surgery, and telemedicine, the field is poised to revolutionize the management of HNCs, offering new hope and improved outcomes for patients worldwide (Jayawickrama et al., 2024). Ongoing research, innovation, and collaboration among clinicians, researchers, industry partners, and patient advocates will be essential to realizing the full potential of surgical innovations in the years to come (Han et al., 2024).

7.13 Conclusion

Surgical innovations have transformed the landscape of HNC management, ushering in a new era of precision, minimally invasive, and function-preserving approaches to tumor resection and reconstruction (Ritter et al., 2024). From the advent of TORS to the integration of precision oncology and telemedicine technologies, the field has witnessed remarkable advancements that have revolutionized treatment paradigms, improved patient outcomes, and enhanced quality of life for individuals facing this complex and challenging disease (Kattar et al., 2023; Wojtera et al., 2024). The evolution of surgical techniques, guided by advancements in imaging, navigation, and intraoperative monitoring, has enabled surgeons to achieve more precise tumor resection while minimizing damage to surrounding healthy tissues. Minimally invasive approaches, including endoscopic and laser surgery, have reduced morbidity and expedited recovery, allowing patients to return to normal function more quickly (Fagan, 2021).

Moreover, the integration of precision oncology principles, including molecular profiling and targeted therapies, has facilitated personalized treatment strategies tailored to the unique genetic and molecular characteristics of each patient's cancer. This approach has led to improved treatment response rates, enhanced survival outcomes, and reduced treatment-related toxicities (Nieminen et al., 2024). In parallel, telemedicine and remote surgical support technologies have expanded access to specialized expertise, improved treatment coordination, and facilitated multidisciplinary collaboration, particularly for patients residing in remote or underserved areas (Jayawickrama et al., 2024). The future of surgical innovations in HNCs holds immense promise, with ongoing advancements poised to further optimize treatment outcomes, enhance patient satisfaction, and shape the standard of care (Mali, 2024). By harnessing the power of precision surgery, minimally invasive techniques, precision oncology, reconstructive surgery, and telemedicine, the field is poised to continue making significant strides in improving the lives of patients with HNC. The journey of conquering HNCs is earmarked by the relentless pursuit of better solutions through collective effort and dedication (Dhillon et al., 2022).

References

AGRAWAL, G., GUPTA, A., CHORARIA, A., TIWARI, S., & CHAUDHARY, V. 2018. Comparison of standard modified shrobingers incision versus transverse cervical incision for neck dissection: Our experience. *Otolaryngol Case Rep*, 6, 47–50.

AHMED, F., KINSHUCK, A. J., HARRISON, M., O'BRIEN, D., LANCASTER, J., ROLAND, N. J., JACKSON, S. R., & JONES, T. M. 2010. Laser safety in head and neck cancer surgery. *Eur Arch Oto-Rhino-Laryngol*, 267, 1779–84.

ALMANGUSH, A., MÄKITIE, A. A., TRIANTAFYLLOU, A., DE BREE, R., STROJAN, P., RINALDO, A., HERNANDEZ-PRERA, J. C., SUÁREZ, C., KOWALSKI, L. P., & FERLITO, A. 2020. Staging and grading of oral squamous cell carcinoma: An update. *Oral Oncol*, 107, 104799.

AMBROSCH, P. 2011. Functional organ preservation in laryngeal and hypopharyngeal cancer. GMS Curr Topics Otorhinolaryngol *Head Neck Surg*, 10, Doc02.

BHAT, G. R., HYOLE, R. G., & LI, J. 2021. Head and neck cancer: Current challenges and future perspectives. *Adv Cancer Res*, 152, 67–102.

BOCCA, E. 1975. Conservative neck dissection. *Laryngoscope*, 85, 1511–15.

BOCCA, E., & PIGNATARO, O. 1968. A conservation technique in radical neck dissection. *Plastic Reconstruct Surg*, 42, 607.

BOCCA, E., PIGNATARO, O., OLDINI, C., & CAPPA, C. 1984. Functional neck dissection: An evaluation and review of 843 cases. *Laryngoscope*, 94, 942–5.

BOCCA, E., PIGNATARO, O., & SASAKI, C. T. 1980. Functional neck dissection: A description of operative technique. *Arch Otolaryngol* 106, 524–7.

BRUDASCA, I., PHILOUZE, P., MORINIÈRE, S., LALLEMANT, B., VERGEZ, S., MALARD, O., ROUX, P.-E., ROSSELLO, N., PAYEN, C., & CÉRUSE, P. 2023. Transoral laser microsurgery versus robot-assisted surgery for squamous cell carcinoma of the tongue base (oncological and functional results): A retrospective GETTEC multicenter study. *J Clin Med*, 12, 4210.

CAPUTO, M. P., RODRIGUEZ, C. S., PADHYA, T. A., & MIFSUD, M. J. 2023. Telehealth interventions in head and neck cancer patients: A systematic review. *Cancer Nurs*, 46, E320–7.

CHIESA-ESTOMBA, C. M., SORIANO-REIXACH, M., THOMAS-ARRIZABALAGA, I., SISTIAGA-SUAREZ, J. A., GONZÁLEZ-GARCÍA, J. A., LARRUSCAIN, E., & ALTUNA, X. 2021. Complications after functional neck dissection in head and neck cancer patients: An observational, retrospective, single-centre study. *ORL*, 83, 372–80.

CHOI, J., DÍAZ-BAAMONDE, A., ROLDÁN, M. D. L. Á. S., PESCADOR, A. M., KIM, J.-S., TÉLLEZ, M. J., PARK, K. S., & DELETIS, V. 2024. Advancing intraoperative neurophysiological monitoring with human reflexes. *J Clin Neurol (Seoul, Korea)*, 20, 119.

COYLE, M., MAIN, B., HUGHES, C., CRAVEN, R., ALEXANDER, R., PORTER, G., & THOMAS, S. 2016. Enhanced recovery after surgery (ERAS) for head and neck oncology patients. *Clin Otolaryngol*, 41, 118–26.

COZZI, A. T., OTTAVI, A., LOZZA, P., MACCARI, A., BORLONI, R., NITRO, L., FELISATI, E. G., ALLIATA, A., MARTINO, B., CACIOPPO, G., FUCCILLO, M., ROSSO, C., PIPOLO, C., FELISATI, G., DE PASQUALE, L., & SAIBENE, A. M. 2023. Intraoperative neuromonitoring does not reduce the risk of temporary and definitive recurrent laryngeal nerve damage during thyroid surgery: A systematic review and meta-analysis of endoscopic findings from 73,325 nerves at risk. *J Personal Med*, 13, 1429.

CRACCHIOLO, J., BAXI, S., GANLY, I., PATEL, S., COHEN, M., & ROMAN, B. 2016. Increasing primary surgical treatment of T1 and T2 oropharyngeal squamous cell carcinoma and the treatment selection learning curve: National Cancer Data Base. *Int J Radiat Oncol Biol Physics*, 94, 872.

CRILE, G. 1906. Excision of cancer of the head and neck: With special reference to the plan of dissection based on one hundred and thirty-two operations. *JAMA*, 47, 1780–6.

DA SILVA, H. E. C., SANTOS, G. N. M., FERREIRA LEITE, A., MESQUITA, C. R. M., DE SOUZA FIGUEIREDO, P. T., MIRON STEFANI, C., & DE SANTOS MELO, N. 2022. The feasibility of telehealth in the monitoring of head and neck cancer patients: A systematic review on remote technology, user adherence, user satisfaction, and quality of life. *Support Care Cancer*, 30, 8391–404.

DHILLON, K., MANJI, J., TAPIA CÉSPEDES, M., PRASAD, J., KLEID, S., FLATMAN, S., NGUYEN, K., MCLEAN, T., & MAGAREY, M. 2022. Use of telemedicine consultations in head and neck cancer: Patient perceptions, acceptability and accessibility. *ANZ J Surg*, 92, 1415–22.

FAGAN, J. J. 2021. Africa: A window on challenges and opportunities for head and neck cancer. *Laryngoscope Invest Otolaryngol*, 6, 414–19.

FERLAY, J., SHIN, H. R., BRAY, F., FORMAN, D., MATHERS, C., & PARKIN, D. M. 2010. Estimates of worldwide burden of cancer in 2008: GLOBOCAN 2008. *Int J Cancer*, 127, 2893–917.

FERLITO, A., RINALDO, A., ROBBINS, K. T., & SILVER, C. E. 2006a. Neck dissection: Past, present and future? *J Laryngol Otol*, 120, 87–92.

FERLITO, A., RINALDO, A., SILVER, C. E., SHAH, J. P., SUÁREZ, C., MEDINA, J. E., KOWALSKI, L. P., JOHNSON, J. T., STROME, M., & RODRIGO, J. P. 2006b. Neck dissection: Then and now. *Auris Nasus Larynx*, 33, 365–74.

FERLITO, A., ROBBINS, K. T., SHAH, J. P., MEDINA, J. E., SILVER, C. E., AL-TAMIMI, S., FAGAN, J. J., PALERI, V., TAKES, R. P., & BRADFORD, C. R. 2011. Proposal for a rational classification of neck dissections. *Head Neck*, 33, 445–50.

GAVILÁN, J., HERRANZ, J., & MARTÍN, L. 2004. Functional neck dissection: The Latin approach. *Operat Techn Otolaryngol Head Neck Surg*, 15, 168–75.

GAVILÁN, J., MOÑUX, A., HERRANZ, J., & GAVILÁN, C. 1993. Functional neck dissection: Surgical technique. *Operat Techn Otolaryngol Head Neck Surg*, 4, 258–265.

GOGNA, S., KASHYAP, S., & GUPTA, N. 2019. Neck Cancer Resection and Dissection. In *StatPearls*. Treasure Island (FL): StatPearls Publishing. Available at: https://www.ncbi.nlm.nih.gov/books/NBK536998/.

HAMILTON, D., & PALERI, V. 2017. Role of transoral robotic surgery in current head and neck practice. *Surgeon*, 15, 147–54.

HAMOIR, M., SCHMITZ, S., & GREGOIRE, V. 2014. The role of neck dissection in squamous cell carcinoma of the head and neck. *Curr Treat Opt Oncol*, 15, 611–24.

HAN, P., LI, F., ZHANG, Y., GAO, L., ZHANG, G., GUO, Q., ZHU, Y., & SU, Q. 2024. B-ultrasound or CT-guided 3D-printing individualized non-coplanar template brachytherapy for the treatment of locally uncontrolled recurrent head and neck squamous cell carcinoma. *Adv Dermatol Allergol Postępy Dermatol*, 41, 41–8.

HANS, S., BAUDOUIN, R., CIRCIU, M. P., COUINEAU, F., LISAN, Q., CREVIER-BUCHMAN, L., & LECHIEN, J. R. 2022. Laryngeal cancer surgery: History and current indications of transoral laser microsurgery and transoral robotic surgery. *J Clin Med*, 11, 5769.

HARISH, K. 2005. Neck dissections: Radical to conservative. *World J Surg Oncol*, 3(1), 21.

HERRANZ, J., SARANDESES, A., FERNÁNDEZ, M. F., BARRO, C. V., VIDAL, J. M., & GAVILÁN, J. 2000. Complications after total laryngectomy in nonradiated laryngeal and hypopharyngeal carcinomas. *Otolaryngol Head Neck Surg*, 122, 892–8.

HIGUCHI-SANABRIA, R., PERNICE, W. M., VEVEA, J. D., ALESSI WOLKEN, D. M., BOLDOGH, I. R., & PON, L. A. 2014. Role of asymmetric cell division in lifespan control in Saccharomyces cerevisiae. *FEMS Yeast Res* 14, 1133–46.

HOLSINGER, F. C., & CHUNG, W. Y. 2014. Robotic thyroidectomy. *Otolaryngol Clin North Am*, 47, 373–378.

HUSSAIN, T. 2022. Patient benefit and quality of life after robot-assisted head and neck surgery. *Laryngorhinootologie*, 101, S160–85.

HUTCHESON, K. A., BARROW, M. P., LISEC, A., BARRINGER, D. A., GRIES, K., & LEWIN, J. S. 2016. What is a clinically relevant difference in MDADI scores between groups of head and neck cancer patients? *Laryngoscope*, 126, 1108–13.

JAYAWICKRAMA, S. M., RANAWEERA, P. M., PRADEEP, R. G. G. R., JAYASINGHE, Y. A., SENEVIRATHNA, K., HILMI, A. J., RAJAPAKSE, R. M. G., KANMODI, K. K., & JAYASINGHE, R. D. 2024. Developments and future prospects of personalized medicine in head and neck squamous cell carcinoma diagnoses and treatments. *Cancer Rep*, 7, e2045.

KARNATZ, N., MÖLLMANN, H. L., WILKAT, M., PARVIZ, A., & RANA, M. 2022. Advances and innovations in ablative head and neck oncologic surgery using mixed reality technologies in personalized medicine. *J Clin Med*, 11, 4767.

KATTAR, N., WANG, S. X., TROJAN, J. D., BALLARD, C. R., MCCOUL, E. D., & MOORE, B. A. 2023. Enhanced recovery after surgery protocols for head and neck cancer: Systematic review and meta-analysis. *Otolaryngol Head Neck Surg*, 168, 593–601.

KERAWALA, C. J., & HELIOTOS, M. 2009. Prevention of complications in neck dissection. *Head Neck Oncol*, 1, 1–6.

KYRIAZIS, I., SPINOS, T., TSATURYAN, A., KALLIDONIS, P., STOLZENBURG, J. U., & LIATSIKOS, E. 2022. Different nerve-sparing techniques during radical prostatectomy and their impact on functional outcomes. *Cancers*, 14, 1601.

LASARIDIS, N., DALABIRAS, S., & KARAKASSIS, D. 1994. Modification of the Conley incision for neck dissection. *J Oral Maxillofac Surg*, 52(10), 1046–9.

LASSALETTA, L., GARCÍA-PALLARÉS, M., MORERA, E., SALINAS, S., BERNÁLDEZ, R., PATRÓN, M., & GAVILÁN, J. 2002. Functional neck dissection for the clinically negative neck: effectiveness and controversies. *Ann Otol Rhinol Laryngol*, 111, 169–73.

LING, Y., ZHAO, J., ZHAO, Y., LI, K., WANG, Y., & KANG, H. 2020. Role of intraoperative neuromonitoring of recurrent laryngeal nerve in thyroid and parathyroid surgery. *J Int Med Res*, 48, 0300060520952646.

LIST, M. A., KNACKSTEDT, M., LIU, L., KASABALI, A., MANSOUR, J., PANG, J., ASARKAR, A. A., & NATHAN, C.-A. 2023. Enhanced recovery after surgery, current, and future considerations in head and neck cancer. *Laryngoscope Invest Otolaryngol*, 8, 1240–56.

LÓPEZ, M., QUER, M., LEÓN, X., ORÚS, C., RECHER, K., & VERGÉS, J. 2001. [Usefulness of facial nerve monitoring during parotidectomy]. *Acta Otorrinolaringol Esp*, 52, 418–21.

LUNA-ORTIZ, K. 2019. Tumors of the oral cavity: CO2 laser management. *Medicina Oral, Patología Oral y Cirugía Bucal*, 24, e84–8.

MALI, S. B. 2024. Role of telemedicine in head neck cancer. *Oral Oncol*, 151, 106746.

MASTRONICOLA, R., LE ROUX, P., CASSE, A., CORTESE, S., BEULQUE, E., PERNA, M., & DOLIVET, G. 2023. Current approaches to salvage surgery for head and neck cancer: A comprehensive review. *Cancers*, 15, 2625.

MEDINA, J. E. 1989. *A Rational Classification of Neck Dissections*. Los Angeles: Sage.

MEHTA, V., JOHNSON, P., TASSLER, A., KIM, S., FERRIS, R. L., NANCE, M., JOHNSON, J. T., & DUVVURI, U. 2013. A new paradigm for the diagnosis and management of unknown primary tumors of the head and neck: A role for transoral robotic surgery. *Laryngoscope*, 123, 146–51.

MEULEMANS, J., DELAERE, P., NUYTS, S., CLEMENT, P. M., HERMANS, R., & VANDER POORTEN, V. 2017. Salvage transoral laser microsurgery for radiorecurrent laryngeal cancer: Indications, limits, and outcomes. *Curr Otorhinolaryngol Rep*, 5, 83–91.

MICHL, U., TENNSTEDT, P., FELDMEIER, L., MANDEL, P., OH, S. J., AHYAI, S., BUDÄUS, L., CHUN, F. K. H., HAESE, A., HEINZER, H., SALOMON, G., SCHLOMM, T., STEUBER, T., HULAND, H., GRAEFEN, M., & TILKI, D. 2016. Nerve-sparing surgery technique, not the preservation of the neurovascular bundles, leads to improved long-term continence rates after radical prostatectomy. *Eur Urol*, 69, 584–9.

MINGHUA, G., ZHIYUAN, G., ZHUN, J., & HAN, C. 2005. Modified functional neck dissection: A useful technique for oral cancers. *Oral Oncology*, 41, 978–83.

MURCHITE, S. A., GOWTHAM, T., KADIYAL, A. M., GAIKWAD, V. V., & TIWARI, A. 2021. Guidelines for safe and optimum neck dissection: A review article. *Int Surg J*, 8, 1394–401.

NAYAK, S. P., & JAYAPRASAD, K. 2017. Minimally invasive neck dissection (MIND) using standard laparoscopic equipment: A preliminary report and description of technique. *Indian J Surg Oncol*, 8, 217–21.

NICHOLS, A. C., THEURER, J., PRISMAN, E., READ, N., BERTHELET, E., TRAN, E., FUNG, K., DE ALMEIDA, J. R., BAYLEY, A., & GOLDSTEIN, D. P. 2019. Radiotherapy versus transoral robotic surgery and neck dissection for oropharyngeal squamous cell carcinoma (ORATOR): An open-label, phase 2, randomised trial. *Lancet Oncol*, 20, 1349–59.

NIEMINEN, T., TAPIOVAARA, L., BÄCK, L., LINDFORD, A., LASSUS, P., LEHTONEN, L., MÄKITIE, A., & KESKI-SÄNTTI, H. 2024. Enhanced recovery after surgery (ERAS) protocol improves patient outcomes in free flap surgery for head and neck cancer. *Eur Arch Oto-Rhino-Laryngol*, 281, 907–14.

ODATE, T., KAWAI, M., IIO, K., FUNAYAMA, S., FUTAMATA, H., & TAKEDA, S. 2012. Anatomy of the levator claviculae, with an overview and a literature survey. *Anat Sci Int*, 87, 203–11.

ORHAN, K. S., DEMIREL, T., BASLO, B., ORHAN, E. K., YÜCEL, E. A., GÜLDIKEN, Y., & DEĞER, K. 2007. Spinal accessory nerve function after neck dissections. *J Laryngol Otol*, 121(1), 44–8.

OSBORNE, J. E., CLAYTON, M., & FENWICK, J. D. 1987. The Leeds modified Weber-Fergusson incision. *J Laryngol Otol*, 101(5), 465–6.

PALACIOS-GARCÍA, J. M., VIZCARRA-MELGAR, J., & SÁNCHEZ-GÓMEZ, S. 2021. Intraoperative spinal accessory nerve monitoring in neck dissections. *Eur Arch Otorhinolaryngol*, 278(9), 3579–81.

PETRUZZELLI, G. J. 2009. Transoral laser microsurgery: Applications in head and neck oncology. *Exp Rev Med Devices*, 6, 599–602.

RAGOS, V., TSIAMBAS, E., MARTIS, K., KITSAKOS, A., FOTIADES, P. P., ASPROUDIS, I., STAMATELOPOULOS, A., & MARTIS, C. 2016. Impact of the functional neck dissection in maxillofacial surgical oncology: its role in robotic-based surgery era. *J BU ON*, 21, 516–19.

RITTER, A., LEVYN, H., & SHAH, J. 2024. Recent advances in head and neck surgical oncology. *J Surg Oncol*, 129, 32–9.

ROB, L., HALASKA, M., & ROBOVA, H. 2010. Nerve-sparing and individually tailored surgery for cervical cancer. *Lancet Oncol*, 11, 292–301.

ROBBINS, K. T., CLAYMAN, G., LEVINE, P. A., MEDINA, J., SESSIONS, R., SHAHA, A., SOM, P., & WOLF, G. T. 2002. Neck dissection classification update: Revisions proposed by the American Head and Neck Society and the American Academy of Otolaryngology–Head and Neck Surgery. *Arch Otolaryngol Head Neck Surg*, 128, 751–8.

ROY, S., SHETTY, V., SHERIGAR, V., HEGDE, P., & PRASAD, R. 2019. Evaluation of four incisions used for radical neck dissection: A comparative study. *Asian Pac J Cancer Prev*, 20, 575–80.

RUSSELL, M. D., ABDELHAMID AHMED, A. H., FENG, Z., SHONKA JR, D. C., KARCIOGLU, A. S., IWATA, A. J., KYRIAZIDIS, N., SIDDIQUI, S. H., ATHNI, T. S., PARK, J. C., WIRTH, L. J., ZAFEREO, M. E., & RANDOLPH, G. W. 2024. Recovery of recurrent laryngeal nerve function with neoadjuvant treatment: Neural characterization. *Laryngoscope*, 134(7), 3415–19.

SCHNEIDER, R., RANDOLPH, G. W., DIONIGI, G., WU, C.-W., BARCZYNSKI, M., CHIANG, F.-Y., AL-QUARYSHI, Z., ANGELOS, P., BRAUCKHOFF, K., CERNEA, C. R., CHAPLIN, J., CHEETHAM, J., DAVIES, L., GORETZKI, P. E., HARTL, D., KAMANI, D., KANDIL, E., KYRIAZIDIS, N., LIDDY, W., ORLOFF, L., SCHARPF, J., SERPELL, J., SHIN, J. J., SINCLAIR, C. F., SINGER, M. C., SNYDER, S. K., TOLLEY, N. S., VAN SLYCKE, S., VOLPI, E., WITTERICK, I., WONG, R. J., WOODSON, G., ZAFEREO, M., & DRALLE, H. 2018. International neural monitoring study group guideline 2018 part I: Staging bilateral thyroid surgery with monitoring loss of signal. *Laryngoscope*, 128, S1–17.

STANKOVIC, P., WITTLINGER, J., GEORGIEW, R., DOMINAS, N., HOCH, S., & WILHELM, T. 2020. Continuous intraoperative neuromonitoring (cIONM) in head and neck surgery-a review. *Hno*, 68, 86–92.

SUKATO, D. C., BALLARD, D. P., ABRAMOWITZ, J. M., ROSENFELD, R. M., & MLOT, S. 2019. Robotic versus conventional neck dissection: A systematic review and meta-analysis. *Laryngoscope*, 129, 1587–96.

TAN, W., BUI, R., RANASINGHE, V. J., COBLENS, O., & SHABANI, S. 2024. Transoral robotic surgery for oropharyngeal and hypopharyngeal squamous cell carcinoma. *Cureus*, 16, e57186.

VAN DE WEERD, C., EBBERS, T., SMILDE, D. E. M., VAN TOL-GEERDINK, J. J., TAKES, R. P., VAN DEN BROEK, G. B., HERMENS, R. P. M. G., & KOOL, R. B. 2023. Evaluation of a remote monitoring app in head and neck cancer follow-up care. *Cancer Med*, 12, 15552–66.

WANG, C.-C., LIN, W.-J., LIU, Y.-C., CHEN, C.-C., WU, S.-H., LIU, S.-A., & LIANG, K.-L. 2021. Transoral robotic surgery for pharyngeal and laryngeal cancers: A prospective medium-term study. *J Clin Med*, 10, 967.

WHITE, H., FORD, S., BUSH, B., HOLSINGER, F. C., MOORE, E., GHANEM, T., CARROLL, W., ROSENTHAL, E., & MAGNUSON, J. S. 2013. Salvage surgery for recurrent cancers of the oropharynx comparing TORS with standard open surgical approaches. *JAMA Otolaryngol Head Neck Surg*, 139, 773–8.

WOJTERA, B., SZEWCZYK, M., PIEŃKOWSKI, P., & GOLUSIŃSKI, W. 2024. Artificial intelligence in head and neck surgery: Potential applications and future perspectives. *J Surg Oncol*, 129, 1051–5.

YANG, B., XIE, P., XU, Y., YANG, X., REN, J., LIU, T., JIANG, Y., & HUA, Q. 2024. [Facial nerve protection in surgery for rare tumors of the internal auditory canal]. *Lin chuang er bi yan hou tou jing wai ke za zhi/J Clin Otorhinolaryngol Head Neck Surg*, 38, 400–404, 410.

YEE, S. 2017. Transoral robotic surgery. *AORN J*, 105, 73–84.

ZHU, Y., GAO, D. S., LIN, J., WANG, Y., & YU, L. 2021. Intraoperative neuromonitoring in thyroid and parathyroid surgery. *J Laparoendosc Adv Surg Techn*, 31, 18–23.

8

Radiation Therapy Advancements in Head and Neck Cancer

Lloyd Mabonga, Thulo Molefi, Abidemi Paul Kappo, Stylianos Makrogkikas, Georgios Lolas, and Zodwa Dlamini

8.1 Introduction

Head and neck cancer (HNC) refers to a group of malignancies that develop in the tissues of the head and neck region, which includes the oral cavity, pharynx, larynx, nasal cavity, paranasal sinuses, salivary glands, and thyroid gland (Zhang et al., 2023). These cancers can arise from various cell types, including squamous cells, which line the mucosal surfaces of these areas. HNC is among the most common cancers worldwide, accounting for a significant portion of cancer cases globally. The prevalence varies across different regions, with higher rates typically seen in areas where tobacco and alcohol consumption are common (Alfouzan, 2021; Runnels et al., 2023). Several factors increase the risk of developing HNC, including tobacco use (smoking or chewing), excessive alcohol consumption, human papillomavirus (HPV) infection (particularly HPV16 and HPV18), poor oral hygiene, occupational exposure to certain chemicals or dust, chronic irritation or inflammation of the oral cavity or throat, family history of HNC, areca or betel nut (*Areca catechu*) quid chewing (common in some Asian countries), and virus infection (associated with nasopharyngeal carcinoma) (Anderson et al., 2021; Runnels et al., 2023; Zhang et al., 2023). Early detection is crucial for successful treatment, which may involve surgery, radiation therapy (RT), chemotherapy, targeted therapy, or a combination of these approaches to provide comprehensive care tailored to the individual's needs (Anderson et al., 2021).

RT plays a pivotal role in the multidisciplinary management of HNC, offering effective tumor control while preserving organ function and quality of life (Runnels et al., 2023; Zhang et al., 2023). Over the years, significant advancements in RT techniques and technologies have revolutionized the treatment landscape, providing clinicians with innovative tools to optimize treatment outcomes and minimize treatment-related toxicities (Koka et al., 2022). The recent advancements in RT for HNC highlight the evolution from conventional techniques to modern approaches such as intensity-modulated RT (IMRT), image-guided RT (IGRT), and stereotactic RT (SRT) (Runnels et al., 2023; Zhang et al., 2023). By leveraging these advancements, radiation oncologists can tailor treatment plans to individual patient characteristics, delivering precise radiation doses to tumor targets while sparing surrounding healthy tissues (Alfouzan, 2021; Yeh, 2010). This chapter sets the stage for exploring the critical advancements in RT and their impact on improving outcomes in HNC treatment in Africa.

8.2 Traditional Radiation Therapy Techniques

"Traditional RT techniques" refer to the methods of delivering radiation to cancerous or diseased tissues using external beam RT (EBRT) (Maitre et al., 2022). Traditional RT techniques have evolved and have been instrumental in the treatment of various cancers and continue to play a crucial role in cancer care. They are often used alone or in combination with surgery and/or chemotherapy in managing HNC (Zhang et al., 2023). The choice of technique depends on various factors, including the tumor's location and size, the disease's stage, and the patient's overall health and treatment goals. Over the years, HNC was treated with conventional two-dimensional (2D) techniques that included simple field arrangements, such as parallel-opposed portals with or without a matching low anterior neck field or antero-lateral wedge pair based on 2D fluoroscopic imaging, with little emphasis on normal tissue shielding (Ratko et al., 2014).

2D RT (2D-RT) involves the delivery of radiation beams based on a simple, 2D representation of the patient's anatomy, typically using x-rays. The treatment plan for 2D-RT is based on anatomical landmarks and measurements obtained from plain x-ray images of glands (Kearney et al., 2020). In this case, radiation beams are directed at the tumor from various angles to maximize dose delivery to the target while minimizing exposure to adjacent normal tissues. Treatment fields are shaped using physical collimators or blocks to shield critical structures from radiation exposure (Ratko et al., 2014). While 2D-RT is relatively simple and cost-effective, it cannot precisely conform the radiation dose to the shape of the tumor, leading to higher doses to surrounding healthy tissues and increased risk of radiation-related toxicities. Hence, measures have been taken to address these limitations. In the *opposed fields* technique, radiation beams are directed at the tumor from opposite sides of the patient's head and neck. This technique ensures adequate tumor coverage while minimizing radiation exposure to critical structures such as the spinal cord and salivary glands (Kearney et al., 2020).

In the *anterior-posterior (AP) fields* technique, radiation beams are delivered from the anterior and posterior directions, targeting the tumor from the front and back of the patient. The AP fields technique allows for effective dose delivery to the tumor while sparing critical structures in the anterior and posterior neck regions (Muzaffar et al., 2021). In *compensator-based* techniques, physical compensators or bolus materials are used to modulate the radiation beam intensity and compensate for tissue thickness and density variations within the treatment field (Kearney et al., 2020). The compensators are customized to match the patient's anatomy and tumor shape, helping to ensure more uniform dose distribution and improved target coverage (Nangia et al., 2006). In the same context, *fractionated* RT emerged as a standard approach used in treating HNC. Fractionated RT involves delivering radiation in multiple smaller doses, or fractions, over some time. This fractionation schedule effectively destroys cancer cells while minimizing damage to surrounding healthy tissues (Anderson et al., 2021).

Fractionated RT takes advantage of the fact that cancer cells are generally less capable of repairing radiation-induced damage compared to normal cells. By delivering radiation in smaller doses over several sessions, normal tissues have time to repair themselves between treatments, thus reducing the risk of radiation-related side effects (Anderson et al., 2021; Moon et al., 2024). By delivering radiation in multiple smaller doses over several weeks, fractionation allows for the effective destruction of cancer cells while minimizing damage to surrounding healthy tissues, thereby improving treatment outcomes and quality of life for patients. It enables greater precision in targeting the tumor while sparing adjacent critical structures and minimizing toxicity (Anderson et al., 2021). Thus, fractionated RT became a standard and practical traditional approach to treating HNC (Anderson et al., 2021; Moon et al., 2024).

Brachytherapy is another type of traditional RT that has been used over the years. While primarily used for certain types of cancers (such as prostate, cervical, and gynecological cancers), brachytherapy is a traditional RT technique in HNC treatment (Makarewicz et al., 2024). It involves placing radioactive sources directly into or near the tumor, allowing for the delivery of high-dose radiation to the target area while minimizing exposure to surrounding healthy tissues (Bhalavat et al., 2020). Brachytherapy can be delivered using temporary or permanent implants. Temporary implants involve the placement of radioactive sources into the tumor for a specific period before removal, while permanent implants involve leaving the radioactive sources in place indefinitely (Meyer et al., 2010). In *intracavitary* brachytherapy, radioactive sources are placed within natural body cavities such as the mouth or throat to deliver radiation directly to the tumor. In *interstitial* brachytherapy, radioactive sources are placed directly into the tumor tissue using needles or catheters inserted through the skin (Lapeyre et al., 2013). Brachytherapy is not typically a first-line treatment for HNC; however, it can be used in specific situations, particularly for superficial or recurrent tumors (Makarewicz et al., 2024).

Brachytherapy represents a valuable therapeutic modality for the treatment of HNC due to its ability to provide a targeted and efficient approach to cancer therapy, offering various advantages such as precise targeting of tumors, delivery of high radiation doses to the tumor site, and minimized exposure of adjacent healthy tissues (Lapeyre et al., 2013; Makarewicz et al., 2024). Nonetheless, the utilization of brachytherapy is accompanied by inherent risks and potential complications, notably radiation-induced side effects like mucositis, dysphagia (difficulty swallowing), xerostomia (dry mouth), and tissue fibrosis (Makarewicz et al., 2024). Such risks contribute significantly to morbidity (Chambers et al., 2004) and give rise to adverse effects such as dry mouth, sticky saliva, swallowing difficulties, and subcutaneous fibrosis. These adverse effects collectively exert a profound impact on the health-related quality of life (QOL) of long-term survivors (Ge et al., 2020; Scott-Brown et al., 2010).

Traditional RT techniques continue to be used in specific clinical scenarios, particularly in resource-constrained settings in Africa or for palliative care purposes where the emphasis is on alleviating symptoms rather than aiming for a cure (Gupta et al., 2020; Muzaffar et al., 2021; Rahim et al., 2020). However, more advanced RT techniques, such as 3D conformal RT (3D-CRT) and intensity-modulated RT (IMRT), have emerged to address the limitations of the traditional methods (Gupta et al., 2020; Muzaffar et al., 2021). They offer additional benefits in terms of precision and reduced treatment duration and are preferred for optimizing treatment outcomes and minimizing treatment-related side effects (Anderson et al., 2021). Thus, RT techniques continue to evolve and are progressively supplemented or replaced by more advanced approaches to improve precision and minimize damage to surrounding healthy tissues (Das et al., 2023; Zhang et al., 2023).

8.3 Advancements in Radiation Delivery

Advanced radiation delivery techniques have revolutionized the treatment of HNC by offering improved dose conformity and sparing critical structures, thus potentially reducing treatment-related toxicities (Zhang et al., 2023). They utilize sophisticated technology and precise treatment planning to deliver radiation more accurately and precisely. Advanced radiation delivery techniques represent significant advancements in radiation oncology, offering improved precision in treating HNC (Kearney et al., 2020). The techniques contribute to better outcomes and enhanced quality of life for patients undergoing RT for HNC by reducing treatment-related toxicities and improving tumor control (Zhang et al., 2023). The most common advanced RT techniques used in HNC include 3D-CRT, IMRT, volumetric modulated arc therapy (VMAT), fractionated RT, and brachytherapy (Maitre et al., 2022; Zhang et al., 2023).

8.3.1 Three-Dimensional Conformal Radiation Therapy

3D-CRT is an advanced technique used to treat HNC. It uses advanced imaging techniques, such as computed tomography (CT) scans, to precisely map the tumor's size, shape, location, and surrounding critical structures (Gupta et al., 2020; Tomizawa et al., 2024). Radiation beams in 3D-CRT are shaped and aimed from different angles to conform to the tumor's shape while minimizing radiation exposure to nearby healthy tissues (Sachan et al., 2022). Unlike traditional two-dimensional techniques, 3D-CRT incorporates detailed three-dimensional imaging of the patient's anatomy to target the tumor while sparing adjacent healthy tissues precisely (Gupta et al., 2020; Tomizawa et al., 2024). 3D-CRT operational procedures begin with the acquisition of high-resolution imaging studies such as CT, magnetic resonance imaging (MRI), or positron emission tomography (PET) scans to visualize the tumor and surrounding anatomy in three dimensions (Gupta et al., 2020). The obtained imaging studies provide detailed information about the tumor's size, shape, and location, as well as the proximity of critical structures such as the spinal cord, salivary glands, and major blood vessels. According to Gupta and co-workers (2020), treatment planning software is used to precisely delineate the target volume (gross tumor volume or GTV) and to define critical structures to be spared from radiation exposure (organs at risk or OAR) (Tomizawa et al., 2024).

Once the imaging data and treatment planning are obtained, radiation oncologists design customized treatment fields and beam arrangements to deliver radiation to the tumor while minimizing dose to surrounding healthy tissues (Gupta et al., 2020; Tomizawa et al., 2024). Multiple radiation beams from different angles converge on the tumor target, ensuring that the radiation dose conforms closely to the shape and size of the tumor while sparing adjacent critical structures (Gupta et al., 2020). The beam intensity modulation is adjusted to optimize dose distribution and achieve uniform target volume coverage while minimizing dose to OARs. This may involve the use of physical blocks, multileaf collimators (MLCs), or dynamic techniques such as IMRT (Tomizawa et al., 2024). Once the treatment plan is finalized, patients undergo treatment sessions, typically delivered daily over several weeks. Patients lie on a treatment table in a precisely reproducible position during treatment, and radiation beams are delivered according to the planned treatment fields and beam arrangements (Gupta et al., 2020; Tomizawa et al., 2024).

Image guidance techniques such as cone-beam CT (CBCT) or kilovoltage (kV) imaging are used to verify patient positioning and ensure accurate delivery of radiation. 3D-CRT allows more precise tumor targeting, minimizing the risk of underdosing the tumor or irradiating adjacent healthy tissues (Gupta et al., 2020). 3D-CRT can help reduce treatment-related side effects such as xerostomia, dysphagia, and radiation-induced toxicity to the skin and mucosa by sparing critical structures from unnecessary radiation exposure (Tomizawa et al., 2024). It improves local tumor control rates and overall treatment outcomes in HNC patients by optimizing dose distribution and target coverage. Thus, 3D-CRT represents a significant advancement in the treatment of HNC, allowing for more precise tumor targeting while minimizing radiation-related toxicity to adjacent healthy tissues (Gupta et al., 2020). Incorporating detailed imaging and advanced treatment planning techniques helps optimize treatment outcomes and improve the quality of life for patients undergoing RT for HNC (Gupta et al., 2020; Tomizawa et al., 2024).

8.3.2 Intensity-Modulated Radiation Therapy

IMRT is an advanced form of EBRT that allows for more precise targeting of radiation beams. It uses computer-controlled linear accelerators to deliver radiation at varying intensities and angles, adjusting the radiation dose to conform to the tumor's shape while sparing nearby healthy tissues (Gutiontov et al., 2016; Mackeprang et al., 2024). IMRT delivers highly conformal doses of radiation, reducing side effects while improving treatment outcomes. It allows for exact radiation delivery to the tumor while minimizing exposure to surrounding critical structures, such as the salivary glands, spinal cord, and swallowing muscles (Bhide et al., 2012). It delivers highly conformal radiation doses to the tumor by modulating the intensity of radiation beams across multiple beam angles and from various directions (Gutiontov et al., 2016; Marta et al., 2014).

Unlike conventional radiation techniques, which use fixed radiation beam shapes and intensities, IMRT employs computer-controlled dynamic MLCs or other beam-shaping devices to adjust the intensity of radiation beams continuously throughout each treatment session (Mackeprang et al., 2024; Marta et al., 2014). The modulation allows for varying radiation doses within each treatment field, sculpting the dose distribution to match the shape and size of the tumor while sparing nearby critical structures. By modulating the intensity of radiation beams and delivering them from multiple angles, IMRT can sculpt the radiation dose to conform to the tumor's shape while sparing nearby critical structures

(Gutiontov et al., 2016; Marta et al., 2014). IMRT enables clinicians to deliver higher doses of radiation to the tumor while minimizing the risk of damage to healthy tissues, reducing treatment-related toxicities such as xerostomia, dysphagia, and radiation-induced mucositis (Mackeprang et al., 2024).

IMRT treatment planning begins with detailed imaging studies such as CT, MRI, or PET scans to visualize the tumor and surrounding anatomy in three dimensions (Nath et al., 2009). Radiation oncologists use specialized treatment planning software to delineate the target volume (GTV) and identify critical structures to be spared from radiation exposure, such as the spinal cord, salivary glands, and major blood vessels (Nutting et al., 2011). The treatment planning software then optimizes the intensity of radiation beams to achieve uniform dose distribution within the target volume while minimizing the dose to adjacent healthy tissues. The optimization process considers the complex geometry of the tumor and surrounding anatomy, as well as dose constraints for critical structures (Nutting et al., 2011). Patients lie on a table in a reproducible position during treatment sessions, and radiation beams are delivered according to the optimized treatment plan. IMRT treatments are typically delivered over several weeks, with daily sessions lasting a few minutes each. Image guidance techniques such as CBCT or kV imaging may be used to verify patient positioning and ensure accurate radiation delivery (Mackeprang et al., 2024; Nath et al., 2009).

IMRT allows for highly conformal dose delivery to the tumor, reducing the risk of underdosing the tumor or irradiating adjacent healthy tissues. By sparing critical structures from unnecessary radiation exposure, it helps minimize treatment-related side effects such as xerostomia, dysphagia, and radiation-induced toxicity to the skin and mucosa (Mackeprang et al., 2024; Nath et al., 2009). IMRT can improve local tumor control rates and overall treatment outcomes in HNC patients by optimizing dose distribution and minimizing toxicity. Thus, IMRT represents a significant advancement in the treatment of HNC, offering improved dose conformity, reduced toxicity, and enhanced treatment outcomes compared to conventional radiation techniques (Nath et al., 2009). By incorporating advanced treatment planning and delivery techniques, IMRT helps optimize treatment efficacy and quality of life for patients undergoing RT for HNC (Mackeprang et al., 2024).

8.3.3 Volumetric Modulated Arc Therapy

VMAT is an advanced form of RT that combines IMRT elements with dynamic arc therapy. VMAT optimizes radiation delivery by dynamically adjusting the radiation beams' shape, intensity, and speed as the treatment machine rotates around the patient (Patodi et al., 2024; Toya et al., 2020). It delivers highly conformal radiation doses to the tumor while minimizing radiation exposure to surrounding healthy tissues, making it an effective treatment option for HNC. Compared to IMRT, the dynamic modulation of VMAT allows for faster treatment delivery and improved dose conformity as the treatment machine continuously adjusts the radiation intensity and shape of the beam as it rotates around the patient, sparing critical structures and reducing treatment-related toxicities (Buciuman & Marcu, 2022a, 2022b; Patodi et al., 2024).

VMAT delivers radiation using a rotating gantry that continuously adjusts the radiation beams' shape, intensity, and speed as they arc around the patient. The dynamic modulation allows for precise dose delivery to the tumor from multiple angles while minimizing dose to nearby critical structures (Bertholet et al., 2022). VMAT, like IMRT, utilizes computer-controlled dynamic MLCs or other beam-shaping devices to modulate the intensity of radiation beams throughout each treatment session (Buciuman & Marcu, 2022). Its treatment planning begins with detailed imaging studies such as CT, MRI, or PET scans to visualize the tumor and surrounding anatomy in three dimensions (Bertholet et al., 2022; Toya et al., 2020). Radiation oncologists use specialized treatment planning software to delineate the target volume (GTV) and define critical structures to be spared from radiation exposure. The treatment planning software optimizes the intensity and trajectory of radiation beams to achieve highly conformal dose distribution within the target volume while minimizing the dose to adjacent healthy tissues. The optimization process considers the complex geometry of the tumor and surrounding anatomy, as well as dose constraints for critical structures (Buciuman & Marcu, 2022a, 2022b; Toya et al., 2020).

During treatment sessions, the radiation machine rotates around the patient lying on a treatment table, delivering radiation beams according to the optimized treatment plan. VMAT treatments are typically delivered over several weeks, with daily sessions lasting a few minutes each (Buciuman & Marcu, 2022a, 2022b; Patodi et al., 2024). Image guidance techniques such as CBCT or kV imaging are used to verify patient positioning and ensure accurate delivery of radiation. VMAT allows for highly conformal dose delivery to the tumor from multiple angles, reducing the risk of underdosing or irradiating adjacent healthy tissues (Buciuman & Marcu, 2022a, 2022b; Toya et al., 2020). VMAT treatments are delivered more efficiently than conventional radiation techniques, with shorter treatment times and fewer treatment sessions required. By sparing critical structures from unnecessary radiation exposure, VMAT can help minimize treatment-related side effects such as xerostomia, dysphagia, and radiation-induced toxicity to the skin and mucosa (Patodi et al., 2024).

VMAT can improve local tumor control rates and overall treatment outcomes in HNC patients by optimizing dose distribution and minimizing toxicity. Thus it represents a significant advancement in the treatment of HNC, offering improved dose conformity, treatment efficiency, and reduced toxicity compared to conventional radiation techniques (Buciuman & Marcu, 2022a; Toya et al., 2020). VMAT helps to optimize treatment efficacy and quality of life for patients undergoing RT for HNC by incorporating dynamic arc therapy with intensity modulation (Patodi et al., 2024).

8.3.4 Image-Guided Radiation Therapy

IGRT plays a crucial role in the treatment of head and neck tumors by facilitating accurate tumor localization and precise treatment delivery while minimizing irradiation of healthy tissues. It combines advanced imaging techniques such as CT scans or CBCT with precise radiation delivery to ensure accurate tumor targeting and alignment during treatment (Kearney et al., 2020). IGRT allows clinicians to visualize the tumor and surrounding critical structures in real time before each treatment session, enabling precise adjustments to the treatment plan to account for any changes in tumor size, shape, or position. By accurately targeting the tumor while minimizing exposure to nearby healthy tissues, IGRT helps to reduce the risk of treatment-related toxicities and improve treatment outcomes (Mireştean et al., 2023). IGRT utilizes advanced imaging technologies to precisely locate the tumor and surrounding critical structures immediately before or during each radiation treatment session. This allows for accurate tumor targeting while minimizing radiation exposure to healthy tissues (Kearney et al., 2020). IGRT utilizes advanced imaging technologies, such as CBCT or onboard imaging systems, to acquire high-resolution images of the patient's anatomy immediately before or during each radiation treatment session. The real-time images provide detailed information about the position, size, and shape of the tumor, as well as the surrounding critical structures (Mireştean et al., 2023). CBCT is a specialized form of CT imaging that uses a cone-shaped x-ray beam and a flat-panel detector to generate high-resolution 3D images of the patient's anatomy (Kearney et al., 2020; Mireştean et al., 2023).

In IGRT, CBCT is typically integrated into the RT treatment machine, allowing for the acquisition of images immediately before or during each treatment session. Figure 8.1 illustrates how CBCT works in the context of IGRT, from patient setup to treatment delivery (Fernández-Rodríguez et al., 2022). The CBCT images are aligned with the reference images from the treatment planning CT scan to allow clinicians to compare the position of the tumor and critical structures in real time and make necessary adjustments to the treatment plan (Kearney et al., 2020; Mireştean et al., 2023). By comparing the acquired images to the reference images, IGRT allows clinicians to precisely localize the tumor and ensure that the radiation beams are accurately targeted to the intended

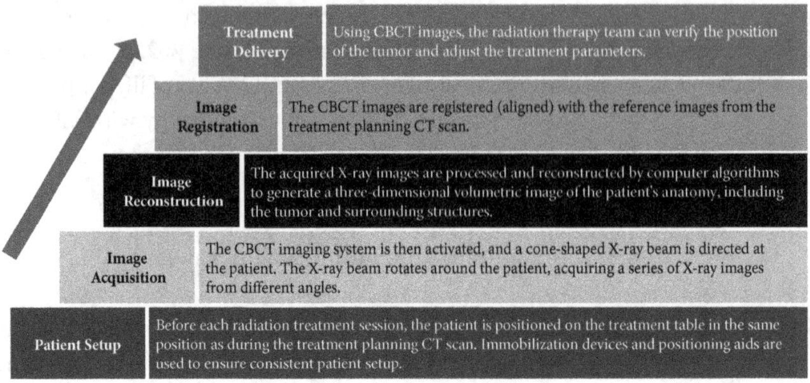

Figure 8.1 How cone-beam computed tomography (CBCT) works in image-guided radiation therapy (IGRT), from patient set-up to treatment delivery. CBCT provides detailed, real-time imaging of the patient's anatomy, allowing for precise tumor localization and accurate radiation delivery during each treatment session.

treatment area. This is particularly important in HNC, where tumors may be located near critical structures such as the spinal cord, salivary glands, and swallowing muscles (Kearney et al., 2020). Based on the information from the CBCT images, the RT team can verify the position of the tumor and adjust the treatment parameters, such as the beam angles or patient positioning, to ensure accurate delivery of radiation to the target while sparing nearby healthy tissues (Mireştean et al., 2023).

CBCT provides detailed, real-time imaging of the patient's anatomy, allowing for precise tumor localization and accurate radiation delivery during each treatment session. This helps to minimize setup errors and intra-fraction motion, improving the effectiveness of RT and reducing the risk of damage to surrounding critical structures (Kearney et al., 2020). IGRT helps to identify and correct any setup errors or changes in the position of the tumor that may occur between treatment sessions or during treatment delivery. For example, if the tumor has shifted slightly due to patient movement or changes in anatomy, IGRT allows clinicians to make real-time adjustments to the treatment plan to ensure accurate radiation delivery (Kearney et al., 2020; Mireştean et al., 2023).

Radiation oncologists can optimize treatment parameters such as beam angles, field size, and dose distribution to maximize the dose to the tumor while sparing nearby healthy tissues based on the information provided by IGRT (Kearney et al., 2020; Mireştean et al., 2023). This personalized approach helps to minimize the risk of treatment-related toxicities, such as xerostomia, dysphagia, and radiation-induced mucositis. In addition to facilitating accurate treatment delivery, IGRT also allows clinicians to monitor the response of the tumor to RT throughout treatment. Radiation oncologists can adapt the treatment plan as needed to optimize tumor control while minimizing toxicity by assessing tumor size and shape changes on serial imaging studies (Kearney et al., 2020). Thus, IGRT enables precise targeting of head and neck tumors while minimizing irradiation of healthy tissues, leading to improved treatment outcomes and reduced side effects for patients undergoing RT. It enhances the effectiveness and safety of RT for HNC by providing real-time imaging and continuous treatment process monitoring (Fernández-Rodríguez et al., 2022; Mireştean et al., 2023).

"Onboard imaging systems" refer to integrated devices built directly into the RT treatment machine, allowing for imaging immediately before or during treatment delivery. These systems may include CBCT and other imaging modalities such as kV x-ray imaging or ultrasound (Nath et al., 2009). Onboard imaging systems offer real-time, integrated workflow and high-quality imaging benefits. Imaging can be performed immediately before or during treatment delivery, allowing for real-time tumor position verification and adjustment of treatment parameters as needed. The imaging system is seamlessly integrated into the treatment machine, streamlining the workflow and minimizing treatment delays (Mireştean et al., 2023). Onboard imaging systems typically provide high-resolution images, allowing for accurate localization of the tumor and precise delivery of radiation. Thus, onboard imaging systems enhance the accuracy and precision of RT delivery, improving treatment outcomes and reducing toxicity for patients undergoing IGRT for HNC treatment (Fernández-Rodríguez et al., 2022).

8.3.5 Stereotactic Body Radiation Therapy

SBRT or stereotactic radiosurgery (SRS) delivers high doses of radiation to the tumor in a few treatment sessions, typically 1–5 sessions, using precise targeting and immobilization techniques to ablate or destroy the tumor cells while sparing nearby healthy tissues (Wang et al., 2024). This highly conformal and ablative approach suits small, well-defined, or recurrent head and neck tumors (Kodani et al., 2011; Nath et al., 2009). SBRT offers excellent tumor control by minimizing radiation exposure, resulting in reduced treatment-related toxicities and the subsequent improvement of patients' quality of life. While these techniques are more commonly associated with treating small, well-defined tumors in other parts of the body, they are increasingly being utilized in managing HNC, particularly for certain cases (Nath et al., 2009). The use of SBRT in Africa faces several challenges from limited access to technology, shortage of skilled personnel, and financial constraints to lack of awareness and education (Kodani et al., 2011). The challenges present opportunities for collaboration and partnerships, capacity building, technology adaptation, research, and clinical trials to improve the region's cancer care. Hence, the acquisition of SBRT technologies remains crucial to improving cancer care and outcomes for African patients (Baliga et al., 2017).

SBRT can treat small, early-stage tumors in the head and neck region. These tumors may include early-stage or recurrent cancers of the larynx, nasopharynx, oropharynx, or other sites within the head and neck area (Mutsaers et al., 2024). SBRT delivers highly precise and focused radiation beams to the tumor while minimizing radiation exposure to surrounding healthy tissues. This is achieved through advanced imaging techniques and specialized treatment planning, allowing for accurate tumor targeting with submillimeter precision (Nath et al., 2009). SBRT typically involves shorter treatment courses compared to conventional RT, with fewer treatment sessions required. This is advantageous for patients with early-stage tumors who may benefit from a more convenient and condensed treatment schedule. By delivering high doses of radiation with precise targeting, SBRT aims to maximize tumor control while minimizing damage to nearby critical structures. This can help reduce the risk of treatment-related side effects, such as xerostomia, dysphagia, and radiation-induced mucositis (Mutsaers et al., 2024).

SBRT is also used in the management of HNC patients with oligometastatic disease, where the cancer has spread to a limited number of distant sites, such as the lungs or lymph nodes (Mutsaers et al., 2024). It is employed to treat localized recurrences or residual disease following surgery or conventional RT in the head and neck region, including recurrent tumors in the neck or primary site that are not amenable to surgical resection (Mohamad et al., 2023). SBRT's ablative approach mainly benefits patients with limited treatment options (Mohamad et al., 2023). SBRT treatment plans are tailored to the individual patient's anatomy and tumor characteristics, allowing for personalized treatment that optimizes tumor control while minimizing toxicity. This individualized approach may involve advanced imaging techniques, such as CT or MRI scans, to accurately delineate the target and nearby critical structures (Nath et al., 2009; Wang et al., 2024). Thus, SBRT is increasingly being integrated into the multidisciplinary management of HNC to optimize treatment outcomes and enhance patient care. SBRT in Africa can improve cancer care and outcomes for patients in the region and simultaneously leverage opportunities for collaboration in addressing the challenges (Nath et al., 2009).

8.4 Proton Therapy

Proton therapy is an advanced form of RT that uses protons rather than photons to deliver radiation to the tumor (Baliga et al., 2017). While proton therapy is most associated with the treatment of tumors in the body, it can also be utilized in the management of HNC. Proton therapy offers superior dose distribution and sparing of healthy tissues compared to conventional photon-based RT, particularly in cases where the tumor is located near critical structures. By precisely targeting the tumor while minimizing radiation exposure to surrounding normal tissues, proton therapy can reduce the risk of treatment-related toxicities and improve long-term outcomes for patients with HNC (Kodani et al., 2011; Nath et al., 2009). Proton therapy takes advantage of the unique physical properties of protons, which deposit most of their radiation dose at the tumor site while minimizing radiation exposure to surrounding healthy tissues. Unlike conventional photon-based RT, which delivers radiation along the entire path of the beam, proton therapy allows for precise modulation of the radiation dose depth, known as the *Bragg peak*, resulting in reduced dose to normal tissues beyond the tumor (Mohamad et al., 2023).

Proton therapy may be considered for patients with head and neck cancers, particularly those with tumors located close to critical structures such as the spinal cord, brainstem, or optic nerves, where sparing healthy tissue is paramount. It may also be suitable for patients with recurrent or unresectable tumors who have previously received RT because proton therapy can provide a highly conformal dose distribution while minimizing the risk of re-irradiation injury to surrounding normal tissues (Nath et al., 2009). Proton therapy treatment planning begins with detailed imaging studies, such as CT, MRI, or PET scans, to precisely delineate the tumor and surrounding anatomy. Treatment planning software optimizes the radiation dose distribution to ensure adequate tumor coverage while sparing critical structures. Proton therapy treatments are typically delivered over several weeks, with daily sessions lasting a few minutes each. Patients undergo treatment while lying on a treatment table, and proton beams are delivered according to the optimized treatment plan. Proton therapy allows for exact tumor targeting, minimizing radiation exposure to surrounding healthy tissues and reducing the risk of treatment-related side effects (Mohamad et al., 2023).

By sparing critical structures from unnecessary radiation exposure, proton therapy can help minimize acute and late radiation-related side effects such as xerostomia, dysphagia, and radiation-induced toxicity to the skin and mucosa. It offers the potential for improved tumor control rates and overall treatment outcomes in selected patients with HNC, particularly those with tumors located near critical structures where sparing healthy tissue is crucial. Thus, proton therapy represents a valuable treatment option for HNC patients in Africa, offering enhanced precision and reduced toxicity compared to conventional RT. While unsuitable for all patients or tumor types, proton therapy plays an important role in the multidisciplinary management of HNC, providing many individuals an effective and well-tolerated treatment option (Mutsaers et al., 2024).

8.5 Adaptive Radiation Therapy

Adaptive RT (ART) holds significant promise in treating HNC due to its complex anatomy and the potential for anatomical changes during treatment (Castelli et al., 2023; Guberina et al., 2024). The technique allows radiation oncologists to adapt treatment delivery to account for tumor and normal tissue anatomy variations, ensuring optimal tumor targeting while minimizing radiation exposure to surrounding healthy tissues, as shown in Figure 8.2 (Gan et al., 2024). ART manages anatomical changes, tumor regression, response assessment, OAR sparing

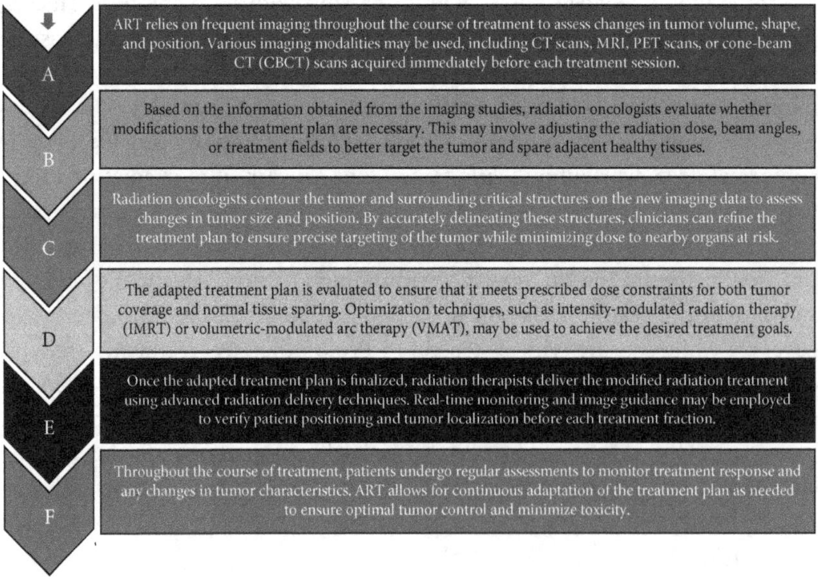

Figure 8.2 Overview of adaptive radiation therapy (ART) procedure. The procedure allows the adaptation of treatment delivery that accounts for variations in tumor and normal tissue anatomy, ensuring optimal tumor targeting while minimizing radiation exposure to surrounding healthy tissues.
A, imaging for adaptation; B, treatment plan modification; C, contouring and targeting; D, plan evaluation and optimization; E, treatment delivery; and F, ongoing assessment.

and reducing toxicity, and it provides adaptive planning strategies, real-time monitoring and feedback, and personalized treatment approaches (Perrier et al., 2024). Head and neck tumors can exhibit significant changes in size, shape, and position throughout RT due to factors such as tumor regression, tumor growth, organ motion, or changes in patient anatomy (e.g., weight loss or tumor shrinkage). By adapting treatment plans based on changes in tumor anatomy, ART can enhance tumor targeting and improve local control rates (Guberina et al., 2024).

ART allows for the adaptation of treatment plans to accommodate these variations, ensuring that the radiation dose is accurately delivered to the target while minimizing irradiation of nearby critical structures (Castelli et al., 2023; Perrier et al., 2024). It enables clinicians to monitor tumor response to treatment and adjust RT plans accordingly. As tumors regress or shrink in response to radiation, adaptive replanning ensures that the remaining tumor volume continues to receive an adequate radiation dose while sparing healthy tissues. The proximity of critical structures such as the spinal cord, salivary glands, swallowing muscles, and the oral cavity poses a challenge in head and neck RT (Castelli et al., 2023; Gan et al., 2024). ART allows for the optimization of treatment plans to minimize radiation dose to these structures, reducing the risk of treatment-related toxicities such as xerostomia, dysphagia, and mucositis (Guberina et al., 2024).

ART employs various planning strategies to dynamically adjust radiation treatment plans based on changes in tumor anatomy, response, or patient characteristics. Table 8.1 highlights the adaptive planning strategies commonly employed in HNC treatment using ART. The adaptive planning strategies enable personalized and precise radiation delivery, ensuring optimal tumor coverage while minimizing radiation exposure to surrounding healthy tissues and reducing treatment-related toxicity. (Guberina et al., 2024; Perrier et al., 2024). Advanced radiation delivery techniques, such as IMRT or VMAT, can achieve conformal dose distributions and minimize dose to OARs. ART involves real-time treatment delivery and patient response monitoring using imaging modalities such as CBCT or MRI (Gan et al., 2024). This allows for timely adjustments to the treatment plan based on changes in tumor anatomy or patient positioning, thus ensuring accurate and precise radiation delivery. By incorporating real-time imaging and plan adaptation, ART enhances treatment precision and accuracy, improving patient outcomes (Guberina et al., 2024).

ART allows a personalized treatment approach tailored to the patient's anatomy and tumor characteristics. It optimizes treatment outcomes and improves patient care by continuously adapting treatment plans based on evolving clinical parameters (Perrier et al., 2024). Thus, ART represents a sophisticated approach to radiation treatment planning and delivery, offering personalized and dynamic adjustments to optimize treatment outcomes in cancer patients (Castelli et al., 2023). It represents a valuable tool in managing HNC by accommodating anatomical changes, optimizing target coverage,

Table 8.1 Adaptive planning strategies commonly employed in head and neck cancer treatment using adaptive radiation therapy (RT)

Strategy	Remarks	References
Anatomy-based adaptation	Regular imaging studies, such as computed tomography (CT) scans or cone-beam CT (CBCT), are used to assess changes in tumor volume, shape, and position throughout the course of treatment. Adaptation of treatment plans involves modifying radiation beam angles, adjusting treatment margins, or altering dose distributions to account for changes in tumor anatomy and ensure optimal tumor coverage.	Guberina et al., 2024
Dose escalation or de-escalation	ART allows for dose escalation (increasing radiation dose) or de-escalation (reducing radiation dose) based on observed changes in tumor response or surrounding normal tissue toxicity. Dose adjustments may be made to target areas of residual disease or areas at high risk of recurrence while sparing critical structures from excessive radiation exposure.	Perrier et al., 2024
Organs-at-risk (OAR) sparing	ART enables real-time adaptation of treatment plans to minimize radiation exposure to critical structures such as the spinal cord, salivary glands, and major blood vessels. Modifications to treatment plans may involve reducing radiation dose to OARs experiencing increased toxicity or shifting radiation beams to avoid critical structures that have shifted position.	Guberina et al., 2024
Margin reduction	As treatment progresses, ART allows for the reduction of treatment margins around the tumor target volume based on observed tumor shrinkage or changes in tumor position. Margin reduction helps to minimize radiation exposure to surrounding healthy tissues while maintaining adequate tumor coverage.	Guberina et al., 2024

Table 8.1 Continued

Strategy	Remarks	References
Replanning based on functional imaging	Functional imaging modalities such as positron emission tomography (PET) scans or magnetic resonance imaging (MRI) may be used to assess treatment response and guide adaptive planning strategies. Replanning based on functional imaging allows for the adaptation of treatment plans to target areas of persistent metabolic activity or identify regions of treatment resistance.	Perrier et al., 2024
Hybrid ART techniques	Hybrid ART techniques combine multiple imaging modalities or treatment delivery methods to optimize treatment planning and delivery. Examples include integrating MRI-guided RT(MRgRT) with daily adaptive planning or combining intensity-modulated RT (IMRT) with proton therapy for precise dose delivery.	Gan et al., 2024
Multidisciplinary collaboration	ART requires close collaboration among radiation oncologists, medical physicists, dosimetrists, and radiation therapists to assess imaging data, develop adaptive strategies, and effectively implement treatment adjustments. Multidisciplinary meetings are convened regularly to review patient progress, discuss adaptive planning strategies, and make informed decisions regarding treatment modifications.	Gan et al., 2024

sparing critical structures, and reducing treatment-related toxicities (Gan et al., 2024). ART allows for better sparing of nearby healthy tissues, reducing the risk of radiation-related side effects and enhancing the quality of life for patients with HNC by providing a dynamic and personalized approach to RT (Castelli et al., 2023; Guberina et al., 2024).

8.6 Biologically Integrated Radiation Therapy

Biologically integrated RT (BIRT) has emerged as a promising strategy to address HNC by tailoring treatment regimens based on the unique biological characteristics of individual tumors (Eberly et al., 2024). It is a relatively new approach in radiation oncology that aims to tailor radiation doses based on the individual's biology, including the tumor's characteristics and the patient's genetic makeup (McDonald et al., 2024). The BIRT technique recognizes that tumors within the same anatomical site can exhibit considerable heterogeneity in biological behaviors, such as proliferation rates, oxygenation levels, and sensitivity to radiation (Nutting, 2016). It seeks to optimize treatment outcomes by delivering radiation doses tailored to the specific biology of each tumor. BIRT addresses key biological factors such as hypoxia, proliferation, and radioresistance to optimize treatment outcomes of HNC (McDonald et al., 2024; Runnels et al., 2023). Hypoxia, or low oxygen levels within tumors, is a well-known factor that contributes to radioresistance. Tumor cells in hypoxic regions are less susceptible to radiation-induced DNA damage and therefore more likely to survive treatment (McDonald et al., 2024; Nutting, 2016).

BIRT utilizes advanced imaging techniques such as PET-CT or MRI to identify hypoxic regions within head and neck tumors. Identifying hypoxic regions allows radiation oncologists to apply *dose-painting* strategies, which involve selectively boosting radiation doses to hypoxic areas while sparing surrounding healthy tissues (Eberly et al., 2024). The spatially targeted approach aims to overcome the radioresistance associated with hypoxia and improve local tumor control. By delivering higher radiation doses to these resistant regions, BIRT aims to improve local tumor control. In some cases, adjunctive therapies may address tumor hypoxia (Nutting, 2016; Runnels et al., 2023). BIRT may utilize oxygenation modifiers to enhance tumor oxygenation and sensitize hypoxic cells to radiation. For instance, hyperbaric oxygen therapy or hypoxia-activated prodrugs can enhance tumor oxygenation and sensitize hypoxic cells to radiation thereby increasing the effectiveness of radiotherapy against head and neck tumors. These oxygenating agents can be integrated into treatment regimens to augment the effectiveness of RT in hypoxic tumors (Eberly et al., 2024; Runnels et al., 2023).

Head and neck tumors often exhibit high proliferation rates, making them sensitive to RT due to their increased susceptibility to DNA damage. BIRT techniques account for tumor proliferation dynamics through radiobiological modeling and fractionation schemes (Nutting, 2016; Runnels et al., 2023). With radiobiological modeling, BIRT incorporates mathematical models that predict tumor response to radiation based on proliferation rates and other biological parameters. It employs radiobiological models that consider tumor proliferation dynamics. These models guide treatment planning by optimizing radiation doses to maximize tumor control while minimizing normal tissue toxicity (Eberly et al., 2024; Runnels et al., 2023). However, with fractionation schemes, BIRT utilizes altered fractionation schedules, such as accelerated fractionation or hyperfractionation, to exploit differences in tumor proliferation rates

(Runnels et al., 2023). The schedules aim to deliver higher biologically effective doses to rapidly proliferating tumors while minimizing the risk of late radiation-induced toxicity. By delivering radiation in a more intensive or fractionated manner, BIRT aims to increase the sensitivity of rapidly proliferating tumor cells to radiation-induced DNA damage (McDonald et al., 2024; Runnels et al., 2023).

Head and neck tumor cells can develop mechanisms of radioresistance that render them less susceptible to the cytotoxic effects of radiation. BIRT techniques address radioresistance through various approaches that include molecular profiling and radiosensitization strategies (Eberly et al., 2024). It incorporates molecular profiling techniques to identify genetic mutations or biomarkers associated with radioresistance in head and neck tumors. Clinicians can tailor treatment strategies to target specific resistance mechanisms, such as DNA repair pathways or anti-apoptotic signaling pathways, by characterizing the molecular landscape of tumors (Runnels et al., 2023). BIRT combines RT with radiosensitizing agents, such as targeted therapies or chemotherapy, to enhance tumor cell killing and overcome radioresistance. According to Eberly and co-workers, such combination approaches aim to disrupt key cellular pathways involved in radioresistance, thereby improving treatment outcomes (Eberly et al., 2024). Thus, BIRT holds promise for improving the efficacy and precision of RT in HNC treatment while minimizing adverse effects on surrounding healthy tissues by tailoring treatment regimens to individual tumor characteristics (McDonald et al., 2024; Runnels et al., 2023).

In this context, dose-painting and radiobiological optimization stand out as innovative techniques that offer the potential for improved outcomes in HNC management. Dose-painting, a concept rooted in the principles of radiobiology and advanced imaging, involves the delivery of heterogeneous radiation doses within the tumor volume (Eberly et al., 2024). Unlike conventional uniform dose distribution, dose-painting allows for the selective escalation of radiation to regions of high tumor burden while sparing surrounding healthy tissues. The spatially tailored approach is particularly advantageous in HNC, where tumors often exhibit heterogeneous biological characteristics and varying degrees of radiation sensitivity (Runnels et al., 2023). Dose-painting aims to enhance local control rates and reduce treatment-related toxicities by targeting aggressive tumor subvolumes while minimizing radiation exposure to critical structures (McDonald et al., 2024). Radiobiological optimization represents another integral component of BIRT, wherein treatment planning is guided by mathematical models that account for the complex interplay between radiation dose, tumor biology, and normal tissue response (Eberly et al., 2024). It seeks to maximize therapeutic efficacy while minimizing the risk of radiation-induced complications by integrating radiobiological parameters such as tumor clonogen density, cell proliferation rates, and tissue repair kinetics into treatment planning algorithms

(Runnels et al., 2023). Radiobiological optimization enables the customization of radiation doses based on tumor-specific biological factors, thereby optimizing the therapeutic ratio and improving clinical outcomes (McDonald et al., 2024).

BIRT holds significant promise because it addresses the complex anatomy and diverse biological behaviors of tumors in HNC. It is integrated into managing HNC through a precision medicine approach, radiation sensitivity prediction, dose escalation and de-escalation, ART, radiosensitization strategies, functional imaging guidance, and biomarker-driven decision-making (Eberly et al., 2024). The technique employs precision medicine principles to personalize treatment strategies. By analyzing the genetic and molecular profile of the tumor, clinicians can identify specific vulnerabilities or biomarkers that can guide radiation dose selection and treatment response prediction (Eberly et al., 2024; McDonald et al., 2024). Specific genetic mutations or molecular features can influence a tumor's sensitivity to radiation. BIRT utilizes these factors to predict how tumors respond to RT, allowing for optimized dose delivery. This approach helps spare normal tissues while maximizing tumor control (Eberly et al., 2024). Unlike traditional RT, which often delivers a uniform dose to the entire tumor volume, dose escalation to particularly resistant areas is applied within the tumor or dose de-escalation to spare sensitive structures like critical organs or tissues. Thus, BIRT aims to improve treatment outcomes while minimizing toxicity (McDonald et al., 2024; Runnels et al., 2023).

BIRT frequently incorporates ART, where treatment plans are modified in real-time based on changes in tumor size, shape, or response during treatment. ART allows clinicians to adapt radiation doses to evolving tumor characteristics, thus enhancing treatment precision and efficacy (Runnels et al., 2023). BIRT also involves combining RT with other treatment modalities, such as chemotherapy or targeted therapies, to enhance tumor response. By exploiting synergistic interactions between radiation and systemic agents, BIRT can achieve superior tumor control while potentially reducing radiation doses and associated toxicities (McDonald et al., 2024). BIRT often utilizes advanced imaging techniques like PET-CT or MRI to assess tumor biology, metabolism, and perfusion. Functional imaging provides valuable insights into tumor behavior and response to treatment, enabling more accurate target delineation and dose optimization (Eberly et al., 2024). BIRT incorporates biomarkers into treatment decision-making processes, allowing clinicians to stratify patients based on their molecular profiles and select the most appropriate treatment strategies (Runnels et al., 2023). Biomarker-driven approaches enable tailored treatments that address the specific biological characteristics of each patient's tumor (McDonald et al., 2024).

Thus, BIRT offers a promising avenue for improving outcomes in HNC, especially in resource-limited settings like Africa. By leveraging personalized treatment approaches based on the individual's biology, managing HNC through a precision medicine approach will help transform HNC treatment in Africa as a region (Eberly et al., 2024). BIRT represents a paradigm shift toward personalized and biologically driven RT, offering new avenues for enhancing treatment's precision, efficacy, and safety in this challenging disease setting. It aims to achieve better tumor control while minimizing treatment-related toxicities by optimizing radiation doses and treatment strategies according to tumor characteristics and patient factors (Eberly et al., 2024; McDonald et al., 2024).

8.7 Immunotherapy and Radiation Synergy

The emerging role of immunotherapy in combination with RT for HNC represents a significant advancement in the treatment landscape, offering new avenues to improve therapeutic outcomes and patient survival (Runnels et al., 2023). Immunotherapy harnesses the body's immune system to recognize and destroy cancer cells, while RT exerts its cytotoxic effects through DNA damage and tumor cell death. Combined, these modalities can complement each other's mechanisms of action and enhance antitumor immune responses (Qian & Schoenfeld, 2021). RT has been shown to improve the immunogenicity of tumors by inducing immunogenic cell death, releasing tumor antigens, and modulating the tumor microenvironment to favor immune cell infiltration and activation (Rajeev-Kumar & Pitroda, 2023). Conversely, immunotherapy potentiates the antitumor immune response by overcoming immune suppression and promoting immune cell–mediated tumor killing. Together, these modalities can amplify the immune system's ability to recognize and eliminate cancer cells, leading to more robust and durable responses (Mireştean et al., 2020).

Combining immunotherapy with RT can improve HNC's local and systemic disease control (Qian & Schoenfeld, 2021). While RT targets the primary tumor and locoregional disease, immunotherapy can activate systemic immune responses that target distant metastases and micrometastatic disease. The dual approach leads to a more comprehensive eradication of cancer cells throughout the body, reducing the risk of recurrence and distant metastasis (Runnels et al., 2023). HNCs often exhibit intrinsic and acquired resistance to both RT and immunotherapy. However, combining these modalities can help overcome resistance through complementary mechanisms of action (Rajeev-Kumar & Pitroda, 2023). For example, RT can sensitize tumor cells to immunotherapy by upregulating the expression of tumor-associated antigens and immune checkpoint molecules (Qian & Schoenfeld, 2021). Conversely, immunotherapy can enhance the efficacy of RT by promoting immune-mediated tumor cell killing and abscopal effects, where radiation-induced antitumor immune responses extend beyond the irradiated site (Mireştean et al., 2020).

Combining immunotherapy and RT opens opportunities for treatment personalization and the identification of predictive biomarkers (Qian & Schoenfeld, 2021). By analyzing the tumor immune microenvironment and molecular profiles, clinicians can identify patients most likely to benefit from combination therapy and tailor treatment strategies accordingly (Runnels et al., 2023). Biomarkers such as programmed death-ligand 1 (PD-L1) expression, tumor mutational burden, and immune cell infiltration may help guide patient selection and treatment response prediction (Mireştean et al., 2020). Preclinical and clinical studies investigating the synergistic effects of RT and immunotherapy agents—remarkably immune checkpoint inhibitors (ICIs)—have provided compelling evidence for the potential of combination therapy in enhancing antitumor immune responses and improving treatment outcomes in HNC (Rajeev-Kumar & Pitroda, 2023). The studies have demonstrated that combining immunotherapy and RT can improve tumor control and survival outcomes compared to either modality alone (Mireştean et al., 2020; Runnels et al., 2023). The intricate relationship between radiation-induced immune responses and the tumor microenvironment lays the foundation for innovative treatment strategies that leverage the immune system's power to combat cancer (Qian & Schoenfeld, 2021). Research efforts are ongoing to optimize combination regimens, identify predictive biomarkers, and expand the applicability of combination therapy to additional cancer types and patient populations (Runnels et al., 2023).

In the same context, preclinical studies have consistently demonstrated synergistic antitumor effects when combining RT with ICIs such as anti–cytotoxic T-lymphocyte-associated protein 4 (CTLA-4) and anti–programmed cell death protein 1 (PD-1)/PD-L1 antibodies (Rajeev-Kumar & Pitroda, 2023). These studies demonstrate that RT can enhance the immunogenicity of tumors by promoting the release of tumor antigens and upregulating the expression of immune checkpoint molecules, making tumors more susceptible to immune-mediated destruction (Mireştean et al., 2020). Preclinical models observed that RT can induce systemic antitumor immune responses, leading to regression of distant metastases outside the irradiated field, a phenomenon known as the *abscopal effect.* ICIs can potentiate this effect by overcoming immune suppression and enhancing immune cell infiltration and activation within tumors (Runnels et al., 2023).

Clinical trials evaluating the combination of immunotherapy and RT in HNC have shown promising results, leading to regulatory approvals and ongoing research efforts. Studies in melanoma, non-small cell lung cancer (NSCLC), HNC, and various other cancers have shown enhanced local disease management and survival rates through the utilization of a combined approach involving RT and ICIs (Qian & Schoenfeld, 2021). For example, in HNC, the phase III KEYNOTE-048 trial showed that the addition of pembrolizumab, an anti–PD-1 antibody, to standard platinum-based chemotherapy and RT led to significantly improved overall survival compared to chemotherapy and RT alone (Mireştean et al., 2020; Rajeev-Kumar & Pitroda, 2023). Combination therapy with radiation and ICIs is associated with higher response rates and prolonged responses compared to either modality alone. This is particularly evident in patients with metastatic disease or locally advanced tumors where conventional therapies have limited efficacy. While the combination of RT and ICIs has shown promising efficacy, it is also essential to consider the safety and tolerability of treatment (Rajeev-Kumar & Pitroda, 2023; Runnels et al., 2023).

Nonetheless, combination therapy has been well-tolerated in most clinical studies, with manageable side effects such as fatigue, skin reactions, and immune-related adverse events. Careful monitoring and managing adverse events are essential to ensure patient safety (Qian & Schoenfeld, 2021). Future directions include exploring novel immunotherapy agents, optimizing treatment schedules and sequencing, and identifying rational combination strategies with other treatment modalities such as chemotherapy and targeted therapy (Rajeev-Kumar & Pitroda, 2023). Additionally, efforts to elucidate synergistic mechanisms between immunotherapy and RT will inform the development of more effective combination regimens and improve patient outcomes (Mireştean et al., 2020). Thus, the emerging role of immunotherapy in combination with RT holds great promise for improving outcomes in HNC, especially in resource-disadvantaged regions like Africa. By harnessing these modalities' complementary mechanisms of action, clinicians can achieve enhanced tumor control, overcome resistance, and improve patient survival (Rajeev-Kumar & Pitroda, 2023). Further research efforts will continue to refine treatment approaches and identify optimal combination strategies, ultimately benefiting patients with this challenging disease (Qian & Schoenfeld, 2021; Runnels et al., 2023).

8.8 Future Directions and Challenges

Research efforts in RT for HNC are ongoing, and they encompass a broad range of areas including technological advancements, treatment optimization strategies, and novel combination approaches. The efforts aim to improve treatment outcomes, reduce treatment-related toxicities, and enhance patient quality of life (Eberly et al., 2024). Proton therapy offers the potential for more precise dose delivery and reduced radiation exposure to surrounding healthy tissues compared to conventional photon-based RT. Ongoing research is evaluating the role of proton therapy in HNC to determine its efficacy in improving tumor control and reducing treatment-related toxicities (Moon et al., 2024). SBRT delivers high doses of radiation to tumors with exquisite precision, typically in a limited number of fractions. Studies investigating the role of SBRT in managing HNC, particularly in the re-irradiation setting or for treating oligometastatic disease, are under way (Tomizawa et al., 2024). Research exploring the potential benefits of ART in HNC, including improved target coverage and sparing of critical structures, is currently being explored (Makarewicz et al., 2024). Research focusing on refining BIRT techniques, incorporating advanced imaging modalities, biomarker-driven treatment strategies, and molecular profiling to optimize treatment outcomes in HNC is being fostered (McDonald et al., 2024). Combining RT with immunotherapy agents, such as ICIs, is an area of active investigation. Currently, clinical trials evaluate novel combination regimens, treatment sequencing, and predictive biomarkers to maximize the synergistic effects of radiation and immunotherapy in HNC (Qian & Schoenfeld, 2021).

Researchers are investigating and identifying predictive biomarkers to guide treatment selection, predict treatment response, and inform personalized treatment strategies in HNC. Biomarkers such as PD-L1 expression, tumor mutational burden, and immune cell infiltration are being studied to optimize patient selection for immunotherapy and other targeted treatments (Runnels et al., 2023). In addition to tumor-directed therapies, future research efforts are focused on improving supportive care measures and addressing the long-term sequelae of treatment in HNC survivors. This includes interventions to manage treatment-related toxicities, preserve functional outcomes, and enhance patient quality of life (Makarewicz et al., 2024). Future research efforts in RT for HNC focus on advancing treatment techniques, optimizing therapeutic strategies, and integrating emerging treatment modalities to improve patient outcomes and quality of life. Continued collaboration among multidisciplinary teams, investment in translational research, and participation in clinical trials will drive future advancements in the field (Runnels et al., 2023).

Despite significant advancements in RT for HNC, several challenges persist, spanning optimization of treatment outcomes and management of treatment-related toxicities and addressing disparities in access to advanced radiation technologies. Achieving optimal locoregional control remains challenging, particularly in locally advanced or recurrent diseases (Makarewicz et al., 2024). Strategies to improve tumor response rates and minimize disease recurrence are needed. While advancements have been made in improving survival rates with multimodal treatments, further efforts are required to enhance long-term survival outcomes, especially in patients with aggressive or metastatic disease. Some tumors develop resistance to RT over time, leading to treatment failure (Runnels et al., 2023). Understanding resistance mechanisms and developing targeted therapies to overcome resistance are essential for improving treatment outcomes (Moon et al., 2024). RT can cause acute toxicities such as mucositis, xerostomia, dysphagia, and dermatitis, which can significantly impact patient quality of life and treatment adherence. Effective management strategies, including supportive care measures and symptom control, are needed to alleviate treatment-related toxicities (Makarewicz et al., 2024).

Long-term toxicities, such as radiation-induced fibrosis, dysphagia, and xerostomia, can persist for years after treatment completion and affect functional outcomes and patient well-being. Strategies for mitigating late effects and preserving organ function are essential for improving long-term quality of life (Moon et al., 2024). Access to advanced radiation technologies, such as proton therapy or SBRT, may be limited in specific geographic regions like Africa, leading to disparities in treatment options and outcomes. Cost considerations, insurance coverage, and financial constraints may hinder accessing advanced radiation technologies, particularly for underserved or uninsured patients (Moon et al., 2024). Disparities in healthcare infrastructure and resources can impact access to specialized radiation oncology services, including comprehensive cancer centers and academic medical centers, where advanced radiation technologies are often available. Addressing these challenges requires a multifaceted approach involving collaboration among healthcare providers, policymakers, patient advocacy groups, and community stakeholders (Makarewicz et al., 2024).

Continued research efforts to develop novel treatment strategies, biomarker-driven therapies, and targeted radiation techniques to improve treatment outcomes and minimize toxicities remain crucial objectives in HNC management. Patient education initiatives to raise awareness about treatment options, side effects, supportive care measures, and efforts to reduce stigma and improve health literacy are paramount (Moon et al., 2024). Advocacy for policies that promote equitable access to advanced radiation technologies, expand insurance coverage for cancer treatment, and address social determinants of health that contribute to disparities in care need to be addressed. Implementing multidisciplinary care models that integrate radiation oncology, medical oncology, surgery, and supportive care services to optimize treatment planning, delivery, and survivorship care remains a priority in the future (Makarewicz et al., 2024). Initiatives to foster engagement with community organizations, patient advocacy groups, and local healthcare providers to identify and address barriers to care, improve access to screening and early detection programs, and promote health equity initiatives remain vital in HNC management. By addressing these challenges collaboratively and proactively, it is possible to improve the quality of RT for HNC patients and ensure that all individuals have access to high-quality, equitable cancer care (Makarewicz et al., 2024).

8.9 Conclusion

The advancements in RT for HNC represent a transformative evolution in managing this complex and challenging disease. From technological innovations to treatment optimization strategies and novel combination approaches, RT has significantly improved treatment outcomes, enhanced patient quality of life, and expanded therapeutic options for individuals diagnosed with HNC (Makarewicz et al., 2024). Integrating advanced radiation delivery techniques, such as proton therapy and SBRT, has enabled more precise and targeted treatment delivery, reducing radiation exposure to surrounding healthy tissues and minimizing treatment-related toxicities (McDonald et al., 2024). BIRT approaches have further personalized treatment regimens based on tumor biology, thereby optimizing radiation doses to maximize tumor control while minimizing adverse effects. Combining RT with immunotherapy agents, particularly ICIs, has emerged as a promising strategy to enhance antitumor immune responses, overcome treatment resistance, and improve treatment outcomes (Eberly et al., 2024). Ongoing research efforts continue to refine treatment approaches, identify predictive biomarkers, and address remaining challenges, including optimizing treatment outcomes, managing treatment-related toxicities, and addressing disparities in access to advanced radiation technologies (Makarewicz et al., 2024). Moving forward, collaboration among multidisciplinary teams, investment in translational research, and participation in clinical trials will be essential to drive further advancements in RT for HNC. By leveraging cutting-edge technologies, implementing evidence-based treatment strategies, and advocating for equitable access to care, we can improve patient outcomes, enhance survivorship, and work toward eradicating HNC (Eberly et al., 2024).

References

ALFOUZAN, A. F. 2021. Radiation therapy in head and neck cancer. *Saudi Med J*, 42(3), 247–54.

ANDERSON, G., EBADI, M., VO, K., NOVAK, J., GOVINDARAJAN, A., & AMINI, A. 2021. An updated review on head and neck cancer treatment with radiation therapy. *Cancers (Basel)*, 13(19), 4912.

BALIGA, S., KABARRITI, R., OHRI, N., HAYNES-LEWIS, H., YAPARPALVI, R., KALNICKI, S., & GARG, M. K. 2017. Stereotactic body radiotherapy for recurrent head and neck cancer: A critical review. *Head Neck*, 39(3), 595–601.

BERTHOLET, J., MACKEPRANG, P. H., MUELLER, S., GUYER, G., LOEBNER, H. A., WYSS, Y., FREI, D., VOLKEN, W., ELICIN, O., AEBERSOLD, D. M., FIX, M. K., & MANSER, P. 2022. Organ-at-risk sparing with dynamic trajectory radiotherapy for head and neck cancer: comparison with volumetric arc therapy on a publicly available library of cases. *Radiat Oncol*, 17(1), 122.

BHALAVAT, R., BUDRUKKAR, A., LASKAR, S. G., SHARMA, D., MUKHERJI, A., CHANDRA, M., MAHANTSHETTY, U., PAREEK, V., BAUSKAR, P., & SARAF, S. 2020. Brachytherapy in head and neck malignancies: Indian Brachytherapy Society (IBS) recommendations and guidelines. *J Contemp Brachytherapy*, 12(5), 501–11.

BHIDE, S. A., GULLIFORD, S., SCHICK, U., MIAH, A., ZAIDI, S., NEWBOLD, K., NUTTING, C. M., & HARRINGTON, K. J. 2012. Dose-response analysis of acute oral mucositis and pharyngeal dysphagia in patients receiving induction chemotherapy followed by concomitant chemo-IMRT for head and neck cancer. *Radiother Oncol*, 103(1), 88–91.

BUCIUMAN, N., & MARCU, L. G. 2022a. Adaptive radiotherapy in head and neck cancer using volumetric modulated arc therapy. *J Pers Med*, 12(5), 668.

BUCIUMAN, N., & MARCU, L. G. 2022b. Is there a dosimetric advantage of volumetric modulated arc therapy over intensity modulated radiotherapy in head and neck cancer? *Eur Arch Otorhinolaryngol*, 279(11), 5311–21.

CASTELLI, J., THARIAT, J., BENEZERY, K., HASBINI, A., GERY, B., BERGER, A., LIEM, X., GUIHARD, S., CHAPET, S., THUREAU, S., AUBERDIAC, P., POMMIER, P., RUFFIER, A., PERRIER, L., DEVILLERS, A., CAMPILLO-GIMENEZ, B., & DE CREVOISIER, R. 2023. Weekly adaptive radiotherapy vs standard intensity-modulated radiotherapy for improving salivary function in patients with head and neck cancer: A phase 3 randomized clinical trial. *JAMA Oncol*, 9(8), 1056–64.

CHAMBERS, M. S., GARDEN, A. S., KIES, M. S., & MARTIN, J. W. 2004. Radiation-induced xerostomia in patients with head and neck cancer: Pathogenesis, impact on quality of life and management. *Head Neck*, 26(9), 797–807.

DAS, S. M., ROY, N., SINGH, D., SARDAR, P. K., & DAS, S. 2023. A comparative prospective study between conventional chemo-radiotherapy and pure accelerated radiotherapy with concurrent chemotherapy for the treatment of locally advanced head and neck cancer. *Cureus*, 15(7), e42206.

EBERLY, H. W., SCISCENT, B. Y., LORENZ, F. J., RETTIG, E. M., & GOYAL, N. 2024. Current and emerging diagnostic, prognostic, and predictive biomarkers in head and neck cancer. *Biomedicines*, 12(2), 415.

FERNÁNDEZ-RODRÍGUEZ, L. J., ARENS-BENITES, M. A., & MALDONADO-PIJOAN, X. 2022. Image-guided radiation therapy for squamous cell cancer of the head and neck in a specialized Peruvian public hospital. *Cureus*, 14(2), e22569.

GAN, Y., LANGENDIJK, J. A., OLDEHINKEL, E., LIN, Z., BOTH, S., & BROUWER, C. L. 2024. Optimal timing of re-planning for head and neck adaptive radiotherapy. Radiother Oncol, 194, 110145.

GE, X., LIAO, Z., YUAN, J., MAO, D., LI, Y., YU, E., WANG, X., & DING, Z. 2020. Radiotherapy-related quality of life in patients with head and neck cancers: A meta-analysis. *Support Care Cancer*, 28(6), 2701–12.

GUBERINA, M., GUBERINA, N., HOFFMANN, C., GOGISHVILI, A., FREISLEBEN, F., HERZ, A., HLOUSCHEK, J., GAULER, T., LANG, S., STÄHR, K., HÖING, B., PÖTTGEN, C., INDENKÄMPEN, F., SANTIAGO, A., KHOUYA, A., MATTHEIS, S., & STUSCHKE, M. 2024. Prospects for online adaptive radiation therapy (ART) for head and neck cancer. *Radiat Oncol*, 19(1), 4.

#GUPTA, T., SINHA, S., GHOSH-LASKAR, S., BUDRUKKAR, A., MUMMUDI, N., SWAIN, M., PHURAILATPAM, R., PRABHASH, K., & AGARWAL, J. P. 2020. Intensity-modulated radiation therapy versus three-dimensional conformal radiotherapy in head and neck squamous cell carcinoma: Long-term and mature outcomes of a prospective randomized trial. *Radiat Oncol*, 15(1), 218.

GUTIONTOV, S. I., SHIN, E. J., LOK, B., LEE, N. Y., & CABANILLAS, R. 2016. Intensity-modulated radiotherapy for head and neck surgeons. *Head Neck*, 38 (Suppl 1), E2368–73.

KEARNEY, M., COFFEY, M., & LEONG, A. 2020. A review of image guided radiation therapy in head and neck cancer from 2009–2010: Best practice recommendations for RTTs in the clinic. *Tech Innov Patient Support Radiat Oncol*, 14, 43–50.

KODANI, N., YAMAZAKI, H., TSUBOKURA, T., SHIOMI, H., KOBAYASHI, K., NISHIMURA, T., AIBE, N., IKENO, H., & NISHIMURA, T. 2011. Stereotactic body radiation therapy for head and neck tumor: Disease control and morbidity outcomes. *J Radiat Res*, 52(1), 24–31.

KOKA, K., VERMA, A., DWARAKANATH, B. S., & PAPINENI, R. V. L. 2022. Technological advancements in external beam radiation therapy (EBRT): An indispensable tool for cancer treatment. *Cancer Manag Res*, 14, 1421–9.

LAPEYRE, M., COCHE-DEQUÉANT, B., MOREIRA, J. F., LE BOURHIS, J., & PEIFFERT, D. 2013. Curiethérapie des cancers des voies aérodigestives supérieures [Brachytherapy for head and neck cancers]. *Cancer Radiother*, 17(2), 130–5.

MACKEPRANG, P. H., BRYJOVA, K., HEUSEL, A. E., HENZEN, D., SCRICCIOLO, M., & ELICIN, O. 2024. EORTC Head & Neck Young Investigators Group. Consideration of image guidance in patterns of failure analyses of intensity-modulated radiotherapy for head and neck cancer: A systematic review. *Radiat Oncol*, 19(1), 30.

MAITRE, P., KRISHNATRY, R., CHOPRA, S., GONDHOWIARDJO, S., LIKONDA, B. M., HUSSAIN, Q. M., ZUBIZARRETA, E. H., & AGARWAL, J. P. 2022. Modern radiotherapy technology: Obstacles and opportunities to access in low- and middle-income countries. *JCO Glob Oncol*, 8, e2100376.

MAKAREWICZ, J., KAŹMIERCZAK-SIEDLECKA, K., SOBOCKI, B. K., DOBRUCKI, I. T., KALINOWSKI, L., & STACHOWSKA, E. 2024. Anti-cancer management of head and neck cancers and oral microbiome: What can we clinically obtain? *Front Cell Infect Microbiol*, 14, 1329057.

MARTA, G. N., SILVA, V., DE ANDRADE CARVALHO, H., DE ARRUDA, F. F., HANNA, S. A., GADIA, R., DA SILVA, J. L., CORREA, S. F., VITA ABREU, C. E., & RIERA, R. 2014. Intensity-modulated radiation therapy for head and neck cancer: systematic review and meta-analysis. *Radiother Oncol*, 110(1), 9–15.

MCDONALD, B. A., DAL BELLO, R., FULLER, C. D., & BALERMPAS, P. 2024. The use of MR-guided radiation therapy for head and neck cancer and recommended reporting guidance. *Semin Radiat Oncol*, 34(1), 69–83.

MEYER, J. E., BROCKS, C., MAUNE, S., STRNAD, V., WERNER, J. A., WOLLENBERG, B., & KOVÁCS, G. 2010. Brachytherapie für die Behandlung von Kopf-Hals-Karzinomen [Brachytherapy for the treatment of head and neck cancer]. *HNO*, 58(9), 947–58.

MIREŞTEAN, C. C., CRIŞAN, A., BUZEA, C., IANCU, R. I., & IANCU, D. T. 2020. Synergies radiotherapy-immunotherapy in head and neck cancers: A new concept for radiotherapy target volumes – "immunological dose painting." *Medicina* (Kaunas), 57(1), 6.

MIREŞTEAN, C. C., IANCU, R. I., & IANCU, D. P. T. 2023. Image guided radiotherapy (IGRT) and delta (Δ) radiomics: An urgent alliance for the front line of the war against head and neck cancers. *Diagnostics* (Basel), 13(12), 2045.

MOHAMAD, I., KARAM, I., EL-SEHEMY, A., ABU-GHEIDA, I., AL-IBRAHEEM, A., AL-ASSAF, H., ALDEHAIM, M., ALGHAMDI, M., ALOTAIN, I., ASHOUR, M., BUSHEHRI, A., ELHADDAD, M., & HOSNI, A. 2023. The evolving role of stereotactic body radiation therapy for head and neck cancer: Where do we stand? *Cancers* (Basel), 15(20), 5010.

MOON, D. H., AVKSHTOL, V., VO, D., AHN, C., SUMER, B., DAY, A. T., TILLMAN, B., MYERS, L., TRUELSON, J., & SHER, D. J. 2024. HYPORT: Phase 1 study of 3-week hypofractionated postoperative radiation therapy for head and neck squamous cell carcinoma. *Int J Radiat Oncol Biol Phys*, 118(1), 157–64.

MUTSAERS, A., ABUGHARIB, A., POON, I., LOBLAW, J., BAYLEY, A., ZHANG, L., CHIN, L., GALAPIN, M., ERLER, D., SAHGAL, A., HIGGINS, K., ENEPEKIDES, D., ESKANDER, A., & KARAM, I. 2024. Stereotactic body radiotherapy for distant metastases to the head and neck. *Support Care Cancer*, 32(4), 230.

MUZAFFAR, J., BARI, S., KIRTANE, K., & CHUNG, C. H. 2021. Recent advances and future directions in clinical management of head and neck squamous cell carcinoma. *Cancers* (Basel), 13(2), 338.

NANGIA, S., CHUFAL, K. S., ARIVAZHAGAN, V., SRINIVAS, P., TYAGI, A., & GHOSH, D. 2006. Compensator-based intensity-modulated radiotherapy in head and neck cancer: Our experience in achieving dosimetric parameters and their clinical correlation. *Clin Oncol (R Coll Radiol)*, 18(6), 485–92.

NATH, S. K., SIMPSON, D. R., ROSE, B. S., & SANDHU, A. P. 2009. Recent advances in image-guided radiotherapy for head and neck carcinoma. *J Oncol*, 2009, 752135.

NUTTING, C. 2016. Radiotherapy in head and neck cancer management: United Kingdom National Multidisciplinary Guidelines. *J Laryngol Otol*, 130(S2), S66–7.

NUTTING, C. M., MORDEN, J. P., HARRINGTON, K. J., URBANO, T. G., BHIDE, S. A., CLARK, C., MILES, E. A., MIAH, A. B., NEWBOLD, K., TANAY, M., ADAB, F., JEFFERIES, S. J., SCRASE, C., YAP, B. K., A'HERN, R. P., SYDENHAM, M. A., EMSON, M., & HALL, E.; PARSPORT TRIAL MANAGEMENT GROUP. 2011. Parotid-sparing intensity modulated versus conventional radiotherapy in head and neck cancer (PARSPORT): A phase 3 multicentre randomised controlled trial. *Lancet Oncol*, 12(2), 127–36.

PATODI, V., SONI, T. P., SINGH, D. K., PATNI, N., JAKHOTIA, N., CHITTAPPURATH, V., KUYYANANGADAN, R., JENNY, A., KANNIYAPPAN, E., GUPTA, A. K., GUPTA, T. C., SINGHAL, H., NATRAJAN, T., & KATHER, F. S. 2024. Dosimetric comparison of O-ring versus conventional C-arm linear accelerator for volumetric modulated arc therapy (VMAT) of head and neck cancer and carcinoma cervix patients. *Radiat Prot Dosimetry*, 200(6), 538–43.

PERRIER, L., BALUSSON, F., MORELLE, M., CASTELLI, J., THARIAT, J., BENEZERY, K., HASBINI, A., GERY, B., BERGER, A., LIEM, X., GUIHARD, S., CHAPET, S., THUREAU, S., AUBERDIAC, P., POMMIER, P., RUFFIER, A., DEVILLERS, A., OGER, E., CAMPILLO-GIMENEZ, B., & DE CREVOISIER, R. 2024. Cost-effectiveness of weekly adaptive radiotherapy versus standard IMRT in head and neck cancer alongside the ARTIX trial. *Radiother Oncol*, 193, 110116.

QIAN, J. M., & SCHOENFELD, J. D. 2021. Radiotherapy and immunotherapy for head and neck cancer: Current evidence and challenges. *Front Oncol*, 10, 608772.

RAHIM, S., KORTE, J., HARDCASTLE, N., HEGARTY, S., KRON, T., & EVERITT, S. 2020. Upright radiation therapy: A historical reflection and opportunities for future applications. *Front Oncol*, 10, 213.

RAJEEV-KUMAR, G., & PITRODA, S. P. 2023. Synergizing radiotherapy and immunotherapy: Current challenges and strategies for optimization. *Neoplasia*, 36, 100867.

RATKO, T. A., DOUGLAS, G. W., DE SOUZA, J. A., BELINSON, S. E., & ARONSON, N. 2014. Radiotherapy treatments for head and neck cancer update [Internet]. Rockville (MD): Agency for Healthcare Research and Quality (US); Report No, 15-EHC001-EF. https://www.ncbi.nlm.nih.gov/books/NBK269010/

RUNNELS, J., BLOOM, J. R., HSIEH, K., DICKSTEIN, D. R., SHI, Y., JONES, B. M., LEHRER, E. J., & BAKST, R. L. 2023. Combining radiotherapy and immunotherapy in head and neck cancer. *Biomedicines*, 11(8), 2097.

SACHAN, A., GUPTA, S., & SINGH, N. 2022. Correlation of 3DCRT and open field treatment techniques in advanced head and neck cancer patients treated by chemoradiation. *J Biomed Phys Eng*, 12(1), 83–90.

SCOTT-BROWN, M., MIAH, A., HARRINGTON, K., & NUTTING, C. 2010. Evidence-based review: Quality of life following head and neck intensity-modulated radiotherapy. *Radiother Oncol*, 97, 249–57.

TOMIZAWA, K., MOTEGI, A., OYOSHI, H., FUJISAWA, T., ZENDA, S., ZHOU, Y., NAKAMURA, M., HIRATA, H., HOJO, H., KAGEYAMA, S. I., HIROTAKI, K., MATSUURA, K., & AKIMOTO, T. 2024. Accelerated three-dimensional conformal radiotherapy for early-stage glottic cancer in reducing dose to the internal carotid artery and pharyngeal constrictor muscles. *Head Neck*, 46(2), 239–48.

TOYA, R., SAITO, T., YAMAGUCHI, K., MATSUYAMA, T., WATAKABE, T., MATSUMOTO, T., YOSHIDA, R., HIROSUE, A., MURAKAMI, D., ORITA, Y., NAKAYAMA, H., & OYA,

N. 2020. Hypofractionated palliative volumetric modulated arc radiotherapy with the Radiation Oncology Study Group 8502 "QUAD shot" regimen for incurable head and neck cancer. *Radiat Oncol*, 15(1), 123.

WANG, H., YANG, J., LEE, A., PHAN, J., LIM, T. Y., FULLER, C. D., HAN, E. Y., RHEE, D. J., SALZILLO, T., ZHAO, Y., CHOPRA, N., PHAM, M., CASTILLO, P., SOBREMONTE, A., MORENO, A. C., REDDY, J. P., ROSENTHAL, D., GARDEN, A. S., & WANG, X. 2024. MR-guided stereotactic radiation therapy for head and neck cancers. *Clin Transl Radiat Oncol*, 46, 100760.

YEH, S. A. 2010. Radiotherapy for head and neck cancer. *Semin Plast Surg*, 24(2), 127–36.

ZHANG, S., ZENG, N., YANG, J., HE, J., ZHU, F., LIAO, W., XIONG, M., & LI, Y. 2023. Advancements of radiotherapy for recurrent head and neck cancer in modern era. *Radiat Oncol*, 18(1), 166.

9
Multidisciplinary Approaches in Head and Neck Cancer

Talent Chipiti, Thifhelimbilu Emmanuel Luvhengo, Batsirai Mabvakure, and Zodwa Dlamini

9.1 Introduction

Head and neck cancer (HNC) is a term used to describe a diverse set of cancerous tumors that develop in various locations throughout the head and neck, including the oral cavity, pharynx, larynx, paranasal sinuses, and nasal cavity. Due to their distinct clinical attributes, histological subtypes, and prognostic outcomes, these tumors necessitate a thorough and multidisciplinary management strategy (Ferlay et al., 2020). Despite advancements in cancer care, HNC remains a significant global health challenge, exerting a substantial burden of morbidity and mortality worldwide. These cancers can have significant impacts on speech, swallowing, and overall quality of life, presenting a considerable burden on affected individuals (Sung et al., 2021). Globally, HNC accounts for a significant burden of cancer morbidity and mortality, with an estimated incidence of > 947,000 new cases and approximately 482,000 deaths annually (Bray et al., 2018; Sung et al., 2021).

In Africa, HNC constitutes a considerable public health concern, reflecting the continent's diverse population, socioeconomic disparities, and varying levels of healthcare access. Although comprehensive epidemiological data on head and neck cancer in Africa are limited, studies suggest that the incidence rates vary across different regions of the continent. Notably, factors such as tobacco and alcohol consumption, human papillomavirus (HPV) infection, dietary habits, and exposure to environmental carcinogens contribute to the burden of HNC in Africa (O'Sullivan et al., 2016). The multifactorial nature of HNC incidence and mortality rates in Africa emphasizes the importance of comprehensive and multidimensional approaches to disease prevention, early detection, and treatment. Efforts to address the complex interplay of genetic, environmental, and socioeconomic determinants are crucial for reducing the burden of HNC and improving outcomes for affected individuals and communities across the continent.

As illustrated in Table 9.1, the incidence and mortality rates of HNC in South Africa vary across different population groups and geographical regions. The top 15 countries reported in Table 9.1 all have age-standardized incidence rates (ASIR) > 6, going up to the highest of around 13 ASIR for France La Reunion. The mortality rate was mostly below 4 ASIR except in a few countries, with the highest mortality rate reported in the Namibian population, which was > 6 ASIR. In countries like Kenya, Cameroon, Uganda, and Namibia the incidence rate is almost equal to the mortality rate, which calls for better action to ensure better outcomes (Global Cancer Observatory, 2022).

The reported cancers include lip, oral cavity, oropharynx, nasopharynx, hypopharynx, and larynx cancers, which are often referred to as HNCs. The statistics on the incidence and mortality rates from the top 15 African countries with the highest incidences are provided in Table 9.1. The ASIR or mortality rate is a weighted average of the age-specific mortality rates per 100,000 persons, where

Table 9.1 Age-standardized incidence rate (world) per 100,000, incidence and mortality, both sexes (2022)

ASIR (world) per 100,000		
Country	**Incidence rate**	**Mortality rate**
France la Reunion	13.2	4.6
Namibia	11.1	6.3
Tunisia	8.6	4.7
Gabon	7.8	4.0
Botswana	7.6	4.0
Angola	7.4	4.3
Kenya	7.1	4.8
Morocco	7.0	4.3
Algeria	6.9	4.0
Uganda	6.8	5.3
South Africa	6.7	2.8
Libya	6.5	4.2
Mauritius	6.3	3.6
Cameroon	6.1	4.8
Cape Verde	6.0	3.2

the weights are the proportions of persons in the corresponding age groups of the World Health Organization's (WHO) standard population.

In South Africa, HNC remains a significant health challenge, with substantial morbidity and mortality rates. According to recent statistics, HNC ranks among the top 10 most prevalent cancers in South Africa, accounting for a notable proportion of cancer-related deaths in the country (South African National Cancer Registry, 2021). The incidence and mortality rates of HNC in South Africa vary across different population groups and geographical regions, underscoring the complex interplay of genetic, environmental, and socioeconomic factors influencing disease outcomes (Mendenhall et al., 2019). In a comprehensive review of HNCs in Africa, Seedat et al. (2023) documented a 12% prevalence. In Africa, there is a noticeable variation in national HNC mortality rates, as measured by ASIR per 100,000 population. The rates vary between African nations, with Tunisia (8.7), Uganda (7.2), South Africa (7.0), and Namibia having the highest rate (12), followed by Morocco (7.7), Kenya (7.8), Gabon (8.5), Cameroon (7.6), Botswana (8.0), Angola (8.3), and Algeria (7.1). The remaining African countries have ASIRs of > 7, and Sierra Leone has the lowest with 0.04. Age-specific mortality attributable to HNC increases from the fifth decade onward, reaching peak mortality in those older than 90 years, both sexes included (Statssa, 2008).

Understanding the epidemiology, risk factors, and healthcare disparities associated with HNC is crucial for implementing effective prevention, early detection, and treatment strategies in Africa, particularly in regions with limited resources and access to healthcare services. The multidisciplinary approach to HNC management involves collaboration among various healthcare professionals, including surgeons, medical oncologists, radiation oncologists, pathologists, radiologists, speech therapists, dietitians, and social workers, as highlighted in Figure 9.1. This comprehensive team-based approach allows for individualized treatment planning tailored to each patient's unique clinical presentation, disease stage, comorbidities, and treatment goals (Jin et al., 2021).

The significance of a multidisciplinary approach in HNC care is underscored by its impact on treatment decision-making, treatment adherence, and patient outcomes. Multidisciplinary team (MDT) meetings facilitate interdisciplinary discussions where treatment options are deliberated, consensus is reached, and personalized treatment plans are formulated based on evidence-based guidelines and expert consensus (Nutting et al., 2011). Furthermore, MDT meetings provide opportunities for clinical trial enrollment, supportive care interventions, and psychosocial support, thereby addressing the holistic needs of HNC patients throughout their cancer journey (Licitra et al., 2016).

Studies have demonstrated the superiority of multidisciplinary care in improving treatment outcomes and survival rates for patients with HNC.

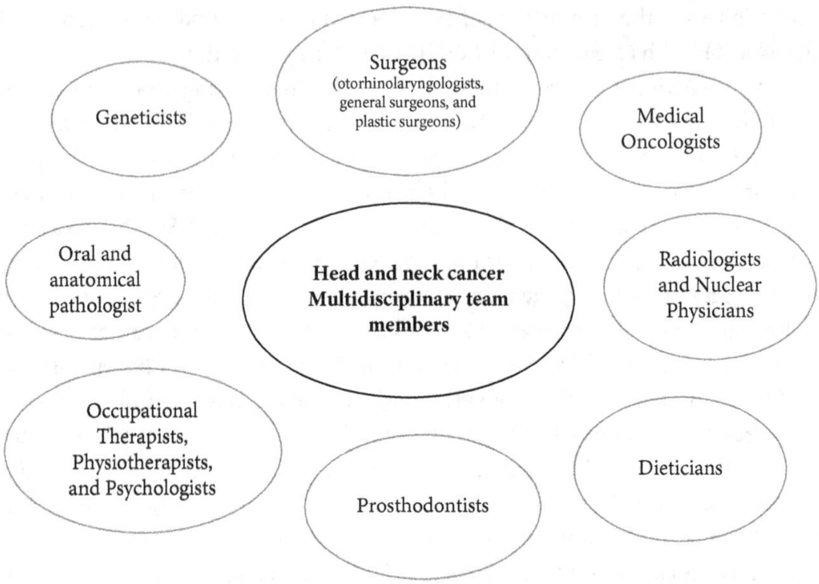

Figure 9.1 Integration of multidisciplinary efforts in head and neck cancer (HNC) care. Healthcare professionals from different disciplines work together to provide holistic care for patients with HNC. It highlights the collaborative nature of multidisciplinary efforts, emphasizing the importance of communication and coordination among team members. The inclusion of external factors underscores the need to consider various aspects of patient care, including individual preferences and available resources.

A systematic review by Porceddu et al. (2011) found that MDT-based care was associated with improved locoregional control, disease-free survival, and overall survival compared to non-MDT care. Additionally, MDT involvement has been shown to reduce treatment delays, minimize treatment-related toxicities, and enhance patient satisfaction and quality of life (Murphy et al., 2016).

9.2 Multidisciplinary Team Member Roles

9.2.1 Surgeons

Surgical expertise is integral to the multidisciplinary approach in managing HNCs, with otorhinolaryngologists (ENT surgeons), general surgeons, and plastic surgeons forming vital members of the team. These specialists are crucial in performing a range of surgeries aimed at both curing and palliating HNCs. Curative surgeries are primarily employed for oral cavity cancers and locally advanced tumors, including laryngeal carcinoma, and focus on complete tumor removal and disease control (Loewen et al., 2021). Noteworthy advancements in surgical techniques, such as function-preserving surgery and robotic-assisted procedures, have revolutionized treatment paradigms, emphasizing organ preservation and improved functional outcomes. Additionally, palliative surgeries play a crucial role in alleviating symptoms like airway obstruction or swallowing difficulties, thereby enhancing patients' quality of life (Colevas et al., 2021; Loewen et al., 2021; Luryi et al., 2016).

Function-preserving surgery, a hallmark of modern HNC management, aims to maximize functional outcomes while achieving oncological control, thereby preserving vital structures like speech and swallowing apparatus. This approach has significantly improved patients' postoperative quality of life and functional outcomes compared to traditional radical surgeries. Moreover, robotic-assisted surgery has emerged as a promising modality, offering enhanced precision, dexterity, and visualization particularly in complex anatomical regions like the oropharynx and larynx. Robotic platforms facilitate minimally invasive procedures with reduced morbidity, shorter hospital stays, and faster recovery, thereby optimizing patient outcomes (Genden et al., 2016; Haughey et al., 2011; Loewen et al., 2021).

Palliative surgeries address symptomatic relief in advanced or metastatic HNCs, focusing on mitigating airway compromise, dysphagia, or pain. These procedures, including tracheostomies or feeding tube placements, aim to enhance patients' comfort and overall well-being, particularly in cases where curative treatment modalities may not be feasible or appropriate. By alleviating distressing symptoms and improving functional status, palliative surgeries play a crucial role in optimizing patients' end-of-life care and ensuring dignity in terminal illness (Colevas et al., 2021; Luryi et al., 2016).

9.2.2 Medical Oncologists

Medical oncologists play pivotal roles in the multidisciplinary management of HNC, overseeing chemotherapy, immunotherapy, and targeted therapy modalities. Their responsibilities encompass comprehensive assessment, strategic planning, administration, and close monitoring of chemotherapy regimens tailored to individual patient needs. Chemotherapy represents a cornerstone in the treatment of locally advanced HNC, aiming to achieve tumor control and improve patient outcomes (Colevas et al., 2021). However, the unpredictable nature of tumor responses and the frequent occurrence of side effects, such as bone marrow suppression, cardiotoxicity, and mucositis, necessitate vigilant monitoring and supportive care interventions (Argiris, Li, et al., 2019).

In recent years, immunotherapy has emerged as a promising therapeutic avenue in HNC treatment, revolutionizing the treatment landscape. Medical oncologists oversee the incorporation of immunotherapeutic agents such as immune checkpoint inhibitors into treatment protocols, harnessing the patient's immune system to target and eradicate cancer cells. Immunotherapy holds particular promise in patients with recurrent or metastatic disease, offering durable responses and improved survival outcomes (Ferris et al., 2018). Additionally, precision medicine approaches, including targeted therapies directed against specific molecular alterations, have revolutionized treatment paradigms, offering personalized treatment options and improved therapeutic efficacy (Cohen, Bell, et al., 2019).

Furthermore, medical oncologists are at the forefront of integrating novel treatment modalities into clinical practice, including *oncolytic virotherapy*, which has shown promising results as an adjuvant therapy in HNC management. Oncolytic viruses selectively replicate within tumor cells, inducing tumor cell lysis and stimulating antitumor immune responses, thereby enhancing treatment efficacy (Russell et al., 2018). When used synergistically with immunotherapy, oncolytic virotherapy holds immense potential in augmenting treatment responses and overcoming therapeutic resistance (Rutkowski et al., 2015).

In summary, medical oncologists play instrumental roles in orchestrating multimodal treatment strategies for HNC patients, ensuring optimal therapeutic outcomes and improved quality of life. Their expertise in chemotherapy administration, immunotherapy integration, and adoption of precision medicine approaches underscores their indispensable contributions to the multidisciplinary care team.

9.2.3 Radiologists and Nuclear Physicians

Radiologists and nuclear physicians are integral members of the MDT involved in the diagnosis and management of HNCs, employing advanced imaging techniques to facilitate accurate staging and treatment planning. Utilizing modalities such as ultrasound and computed tomography (CT) scans, they play a pivotal role in the initial assessment of patients, providing detailed anatomical information and identifying primary tumors, lymph node involvement, and potential metastatic spread. Moreover, their expertise in interpreting imaging results enables the detection of subtle abnormalities, including invasion of cranial nerves and adjacent structures, which are crucial for determining the extent of disease and formulating appropriate treatment strategies (Ogura et al., 2017).

In recent years, significant advancements in nuclear medicine have further revolutionized the diagnostic approach to HNCs, with positron emission tomography (PET) imaging emerging as a valuable tool for tumor detection, staging, and monitoring treatment response. Combined PET/CT and PET/magnetic resonance imaging (PET/MRI) modalities offer enhanced sensitivity and specificity, providing comprehensive anatomical and functional information to guide clinical decision-making (Marcus et al., 2018). Additionally, molecular imaging techniques utilizing radiotracers targeted to specific biomarkers enable the characterization of tumor biology and aid in the identification of potential therapeutic targets, paving the way for personalized treatment approaches (Paidpally et al., 2017).

Furthermore, the role of radiologists and nuclear physicians extends beyond diagnostic imaging to include image-guided interventions and treatment planning. They collaborate closely with other members of the MDT to ensure accurate delineation of target volumes and critical structures during radiation therapy planning, thus optimizing treatment delivery and minimizing radiation-related toxicity (Chen et al., 2019). Moreover, their expertise in functional imaging modalities, such as diffusion-weighted imaging and dynamic contrast-enhanced MRI, enables the assessment of treatment response and the early detection of recurrent disease, facilitating timely interventions and improving patient outcomes (Jentsch et al., 2015).

In summary, radiologists and nuclear physicians play indispensable roles in the comprehensive management of HNCs, leveraging advanced imaging technologies to facilitate early diagnosis, precise staging, and individualized treatment planning. Their contributions are instrumental in improving patient care and outcomes, underscoring the importance of multidisciplinary collaboration in tackling this complex disease.

9.2.4 Dieticians

Dieticians play a crucial role in the comprehensive care of patients with HNC, addressing the complex nutritional challenges associated with the disease and its treatment. Their primary responsibility involves assessing the nutritional status of patients and developing individualized pre-treatment nutrition plans tailored to their specific needs. Given that HNCs frequently impair chewing and swallowing functions, leading to malnutrition, dieticians are instrumental in identifying and addressing these issues to optimize patients' nutritional intake and overall health (Isenring et al., 2017).

One of the key interventions recommended by dieticians is the placement of feeding gastrostomy tubes, either percutaneously or through open surgery, particularly for severely malnourished patients or those with significant swallowing difficulties. This proactive approach ensures adequate nutritional delivery during prehabilitation and facilitates optimal treatment tolerance and recovery (Kam et al., 2019). Moreover, dieticians collaborate closely with other members of the MDT to integrate nutrition support strategies into the overall treatment plan, particularly for patients undergoing surgery, radiotherapy, or chemotherapy for HNC (Zhang et al., 2020).

Furthermore, recent advances in the management of HNC have emphasized the importance of function-preserving treatments and the modulation of radiotherapy to minimize treatment-related complications, such as dysphagia. Dieticians play a vital role in these efforts by providing ongoing nutritional guidance and support to mitigate the impact of treatment on swallowing function and overall quality of life (Chasen et al., 2018).

Dietitians are a crucial part of the MDT responsible for caring for patients with HNC. They provide invaluable knowledge and support in nutritional assessment, intervention, and management throughout the treatment process to proactively address malnutrition and swallowing issues. This valuable contribution significantly enhances patient outcomes and overall quality of life.

9.2.5 Occupational Therapists, Physiotherapists, and Psychologists

HNC patients often face a variety of physical and emotional challenges during their treatment journey. To ensure comprehensive care, a team of healthcare professionals work together to support these patients. Among these vital team members are occupational therapists, physiotherapists, and psychologists. These experts play a crucial role in addressing the physical and psychosocial needs of patients, making their journey through treatment smoother and more manageable. By providing specialized care, these healthcare professionals help patients regain their quality of life and achieve the best possible outcomes.

Occupational therapists and physiotherapists are primarily responsible for assessing the functional status of patients and implementing physical prehabilitation programs aimed at improving functional outcomes and quality of life. This may include prescribing swallowing exercises to mitigate dysphagia, which is a common issue among HNC patients, even in the absence of physical obstruction. These exercises help maintain or improve swallowing function and prevent complications arising from treatment-induced sarcopenia and dysphagia (Zopf et al., 2020).

Furthermore, occupational therapists and physiotherapists play a crucial role in addressing treatment-related impairments, such as weakness and mobility limitations, which may result from surgery, radiotherapy, or chemotherapy. By providing personalized rehabilitation plans and ongoing support, they help patients regain independence in daily activities and optimize their overall functional capacity (Cnossen et al., 2019).

Psychologists are essential members of the MDT, offering psychological support and counseling to patients and their families throughout the cancer journey. The diagnosis and treatment of HNC can have profound psychological impacts, often triggering feelings of anxiety, depression, and distress. Psychologists provide a safe and supportive environment for patients to express their emotions, cope with treatment-related challenges, and develop effective coping strategies (Verdonck-de Leeuw et al., 2019). Occupational therapists, physiotherapists, and psychologists all play complementary roles in meeting the physical and emotional requirements of patients with HNC, resulting in more comprehensive treatment and better patient outcomes.

9.2.6 Geneticists

Geneticists are key members of the MDT for managing patients with HNC because of their competence in analyzing genetic alterations linked with these malignancies. With recent advances in genomic technology, geneticists play a vital role in the diagnosis, risk classification, and development of targeted therapeutic methods for head and neck malignancies. HNCs can be viral-induced (e.g., human papillomavirus [HPV]-positive or HPV-negative). As well, there are different subtypes of the HNC groups, and a complete diagnosis through genetic analysis can make these distinctions to develop an effective treatment and management plan.

One of the primary responsibilities of geneticists is to conduct comprehensive genetic analyses to identify specific genetic alterations present in tumors. These analyses help to characterize the molecular profile of individual tumors, which can provide valuable insights into their behavior, prognosis, and response to treatment (Chung et al., 2019). Furthermore, geneticists play a key role in risk stratification, where they assess the inherited genetic predisposition of patients to develop HNCs. By identifying germline mutations associated with increased cancer susceptibility, geneticists can offer genetic counseling and implement appropriate surveillance strategies for at-risk individuals and their families (Ghadimi et al., 2020).

Moreover, geneticists are instrumental in guiding personalized treatment approaches based on the genetic profile of tumors. They collaborate closely with other members of the MDT to interpret genetic analysis results and recommend targeted therapies tailored to the specific molecular alterations present in individual tumors. This personalized approach to treatment holds promise for improving treatment efficacy and minimizing adverse effects (Marur et al., 2017).

In summary, geneticists play a vital role in the MDT for HNC care by conducting genetic analyses, risk assessment, and guiding personalized treatment strategies based on the molecular characteristics of tumors. Their contributions contribute to more precise and effective management of patients with HNC.

9.3 Current Treatment Interventions for Head and Neck Cancers

Surgical interventions play a critical role in the comprehensive management of HNC, encompassing various techniques, innovations, and strategies aimed at achieving optimal oncologic outcomes while preserving essential functions and maximizing the quality of life for patients. Below are detailed accounts of surgical techniques, innovations, and rehabilitation/reconstruction approaches in HNC care.

9.3.1 Surgical Techniques and Innovations

9.3.1.1 Transoral Robotic Surgery

Transoral robotic surgery (TORS), as described by Burton et al. (2015), represents a significant advancement in minimally invasive surgical techniques for HNC. This approach allows for precise resection of tumors located in challenging anatomical sites within the oropharynx, larynx, and hypopharynx using robot-assisted instrumentation (Genden & O'Malley, 2016). By accessing tumors through the mouth, TORS offers several advantages, including avoidance of external neck incisions, reduced trauma to surrounding tissues, and improved postoperative functional outcomes (Gorphe et al., 2019). With TORS, surgeons can perform complex procedures without the need for traditional open neck incisions, minimizing scarring and potential complications associated with extensive neck dissection. TORS facilitates the preservation of critical anatomical structures involved in swallowing, speech, and other vital functions, leading to improved functional outcomes and quality of life for HNC patients (Weinstein et al., 2012). TORS enables diagnostic biopsies with minimal excision of the tongue base, particularly beneficial in patients with cancer of unknown primary (CUP), allowing for accurate tumor identification and subsequent treatment planning. Studies have reported comparable disease control rates between TORS and conventional surgical approaches, highlighting the efficacy and oncological outcomes of this innovative technique (Burton et al., 2015).

9.3.1.2 Surgical Rehabilitation and Reconstruction in Head and Neck Cancer Care

Surgical resection of HNC often necessitates reconstruction to restore form and function, particularly in cases involving extensive tissue loss or functional impairment (Chow et al., 2020; Momeni et al., 2020). Microvascular free tissue transfer techniques, such as free flap reconstruction, are commonly employed to reconstruct defects following tumor resection. These techniques involve transferring vascularized tissue from distant donor sites to reconstruct complex defects in the head and neck region, restoring both aesthetic appearance and functional integrity (Dholam et al., 2013). In addition to restoring anatomical structures, surgical rehabilitation encompasses multidisciplinary efforts aimed at optimizing functional outcomes, including speech therapy, swallow rehabilitation, and dental rehabilitation. These interventions aim to address functional deficits resulting from surgery and improve patients' overall quality of life (Carnaby et al., 2020).

Incorporating these surgical techniques and rehabilitation strategies into comprehensive treatment plans requires multidisciplinary collaboration among surgeons, oncologists, rehabilitation specialists, and allied healthcare professionals. By leveraging innovative surgical approaches and rehabilitative interventions, clinicians can enhance the outcomes and quality of life for patients undergoing treatment for HNC (Burton et al., 2015; Chow et al., 2020).

9.3.2 Radiation Therapy

Radiation oncologists are integral members of the MDT involved in managing patients with HNC, given the frequent use of radiotherapy in treatment protocols. Radiotherapy serves both curative and palliative purposes in HNC, either alone for early-stage cancer or in combination with chemotherapy for locally advanced disease. The addition of chemotherapy to radiotherapy aims at radiosensitization, enhancing its effectiveness (Jethwa & Johung, 2020). Furthermore, adjuvant radiotherapy may be employed following surgical resection for locally advanced tumors or those with lymph node metastasis and extranodal extension to reduce recurrence risk. Palliative radiotherapy is often necessary for pain relief or hemostasis. However, radiotherapy in the head and neck region frequently leads to acute and chronic complications, including mucositis, dysphagia, xerostomia, and osteoradionecrosis (Alfonzan et al., 2021; Gupta & Paul, 2021). Hence, the role of a radiation oncologist encompasses not only delivering effective radiotherapy but also minimizing treatment-related side effects through various strategies and techniques. These include utilizing advanced imaging techniques such as 3D imaging to delineate tumor volumes and adjacent tissues accurately, planning conformal radiotherapy with techniques like intensity-modulated radiation therapy (IMRT) and volumetric modulated arc radiotherapy (VMAT) to target tumors while sparing normal tissues, and implementing fractionation methods like hyperfractionation and accelerated radiotherapy to optimize treatment outcomes. Additionally, adaptive radiotherapy is employed to adjust for anatomical changes during treatment, and proton radiotherapy may be utilized when critical structures are in close proximity to the tumor (Blanchard & Blanchard, 2019). However, it is crucial to recognize that toxicity from radiation, both acute and chronic, is higher when combined with chemotherapy, leading to adverse effects such as mucositis, dermatitis, trismus, and dysphagia.

Overall, radiation oncologists play a vital role in the comprehensive management of HNC, focusing on delivering effective treatment while minimizing treatment-related toxicities. Recent studies, such as Alfonzan et al. (2021) in the *Saudi Medical Journal*, have emphasized advancements in radiotherapy techniques and their impact on HNC treatment outcomes, further highlighting the importance of radiation oncologists in the multidisciplinary care of these patients. Additionally, recent reviews and clinical trials, such as those by Gupta et al. (2016) and Zafereo et al. (2020), provide valuable insights into emerging strategies and advancements in radiation therapy for HNC management, contributing to ongoing improvements in patient care and outcomes. Recent research by Alfonzan (2021) underscores the importance of such multidisciplinary approaches in the management of HNC, highlighting the necessity for ongoing advancements in treatment strategies to address the unique challenges posed by this complex disease (Alfonzan, 2021).

9.3.3 Systemic Treatments

HNC management involves a range of treatment modalities aimed at improving patient outcomes and quality of life. In recent years, noteworthy progress has been made in the development of chemotherapy, targeted therapy, immunotherapy, and the exploration of novel treatment approaches through clinical trials. These advancements have the potential to benefit patients and improve their overall well-being greatly.

9.3.3.1 Chemotherapy and Targeted Therapy

Chemotherapy is still an essential form of systemic treatment for advanced or recurrent HNC. It can be used as a standalone treatment or in combination with other treatment options. Platinum-based regimens, like cisplatin or carboplatin, are typically used along with agents such as 5-fluorouracil (5-FU) or taxanes (Vermorken et al., 2008). The treatment of HNC has been revolutionized by targeted therapies that exploit specific molecular pathways involved in tumor growth and progression.

In the past few years, targeted therapies have become a promising option for managing HNC. These treatments aim to target specific molecular pathways involved in the growth and progression of tumors. They have the potential to be more effective and cause fewer side effects compared to traditional chemotherapy (Argiris et al., 2008). Cetuximab, a monoclonal antibody targeting epidermal growth factor receptor (EGFR), has shown effectiveness with chemo or radiation for metastatic disease. (Vermorken et al., 2008).

9.3.3.2 Immunotherapy Approaches

The introduction of immunotherapy has brought a significant transformation in the treatment landscape for HNC. Immune checkpoint inhibitors, including pembrolizumab and nivolumab, have demonstrated noteworthy clinical benefits in patients who are experiencing recurrent or metastatic disease and have shown no response to platinum-based chemotherapy. These advancements have opened up new avenues for cancer treatment and can prove to be a significant milestone in the field of oncology (Cohen, Soulières, et al., 2019; Ferris et al., 2016). These agents stimulate the immune system to recognize and eliminate tumor cells, resulting in long-lasting responses and better survival rates for some patients.

In addition to immune checkpoint inhibitors, clinical trials are investigating other immunotherapy approaches, such as cancer vaccines and adoptive cell therapies, to enhance antitumor immune responses and overcome treatment resistance (Schumacher & Schreiber, 2015). New strategies are being developed to improve outcomes in HNC patients. Personalized medicine is key, tailoring treatment to a patient's unique needs. Other promising approaches include targeted therapies, immunotherapies, and novel surgical techniques. These innovations offer hope for better management and treatment of this devastating disease (Cohen, Soulières, et al., 2019).

9.3.4 Clinical Trials and Emerging Therapies

Clinical trials are a critical component in the development of HNC treatments. These trials evaluate new therapeutic approaches, identify new treatment paradigms, and help to advance the field. Several ongoing trials are currently investigating the efficacy and safety of combination therapies, novel targeted agents, and immunotherapy-based regimens in various disease settings (Argiris et al., 2019). New cancer therapies like epigenetic modifiers, DNA damage repair inhibitors, and tumor-agnostic treatments offer hope for patients with refractory disease. These treatments improve outcomes by targeting cancer cells with specific genetic mutations, leading to more effective and personalized cancer treatments in the future.

9.3.5 Supportive Care

Supportive care plays a crucial role in the comprehensive management of HNC, encompassing various interventions aimed at alleviating symptoms, optimizing nutritional status, and improving functional outcomes. Three key aspects of supportive care in HNC include palliative care, nutritional support, and speech and swallowing rehabilitation:

Palliative care focuses on enhancing the quality of life and addressing the physical, psychological, and spiritual needs of patients with advanced or incurable HNC. Palliative interventions aim to manage symptoms such as pain, dysphagia, dyspnea, and psychological distress through a multidisciplinary approach involving physicians, nurses, social workers, and psychologists (Ferrell et al., 2016). Advanced symptom management strategies, including opioid analgesia, corticosteroids, and supportive medications, are utilized to improve symptom control and overall well-being in HNC patients receiving palliative care (Lacouture et al., 2021).

Nutritional support is essential in HNC patients to prevent malnutrition, maintain body weight, and optimize treatment outcomes. Dieticians play a significant role in assessing nutritional status, implementing dietary modifications, and providing enteral or parenteral nutrition support, when necessary, particularly in patients with dysphagia or severe weight loss (Corry et al., 2022). Strategies such as the use of high-protein, high-calorie supplements; swallowing exercises; and dietary counseling help mitigate the impact of dysphagia and ensure adequate nutritional intake during and after treatment (Kulbersh et al., 2020).

Speech and swallowing rehabilitation are integral components of supportive care in HNC, aimed at restoring functional abilities and improving quality of life. Speech-language pathologists (SLPs) work closely with patients to assess swallowing function, provide therapeutic exercises, and implement swallowing strategies to address dysphagia and improve oral intake (Govender et al., 2020). Additionally, SLPs offer voice therapy to manage voice changes resulting from surgery, radiation therapy, or tumor-related complications, helping patients regain vocal function and communication skills (Hutcheson et al., 2019).

Supportive care therapies such as palliative care, nutritional assistance, and speech and swallowing therapy are essential components of the complete management of patients with HNC. These treatments play critical roles in meeting patients' complex requirements throughout the illness trajectory, from diagnosis to survivorship or end-of-life care.

9.4 Integration of Multidisciplinary Efforts

9.4.1 Team-Based Care Models

Collaboration among healthcare professionals is a vital aspect of managing HNC (HNC). Team-based care models facilitate this collaboration by bringing together a range of experts to address the complex needs of patients. MDTs comprised of surgeons, medical oncologists, radiation oncologists, pathologists, radiologists, speech therapists, dietitians, and social workers work together to develop personalized treatment plans for each patient. These plans are tailored to the patient's clinical presentation and preferences, and this approach to care has been globally recognized as effective in managing HNC (Nutting et al., 2011; Rutherford et al., 2017). In countries like South Africa, where the burden of HNC is high, team-based care models improve treatment outcomes, reduce delays, and enhance patient satisfaction (Ogunleye et al., 2019). In South Africa, MDTs are critical in providing comprehensive and coordinated care for HNC patients across diverse healthcare settings, including academic centers and rural hospitals (Sayed et al., 2019). The team-based care models underscore the significance of communication, coordination, and shared decision-making among healthcare professionals to enhance treatment outcomes and patient satisfaction. The success of these models hinges on the collaboration of various healthcare professionals, including physicians, nurses, and other stakeholders. The models ensure that healthcare professionals work together to provide optimal care to patients. The benefits of these models include augmented patient satisfaction, decreased healthcare costs, and improved health outcomes.

9.4.2 Tumor Boards and Case Conferences

The hospital tumor board is a vital forum for multidisciplinary collaboration in cancer care. It brings together physicians from various specialties to review complex cancer cases to improve the quality of care and provide educational opportunities. By incorporating diverse perspectives from medical oncologists, surgical oncologists, radiation oncologists, pathologists, radiologists, and others, the board ensures that all relevant factors are considered when making decisions. This collaborative approach promotes patient-centered care that integrates a range of treatment options and expertise (American Society of Clinical Oncology, 2017).

For more than five decades, tumor boards have served as a vital platform for medical professionals from diverse fields to collaborate and discuss the best possible treatment options for patients. Initially, these boards held physical meetings, but now virtual tumor boards have become increasingly popular. In addition, *mini-tumor boards* cater to cases that require a subset of specialists, while *molecular tumor boards* rely on genetic cancer cell profiling to make personalized treatment decisions. In general, a multidisciplinary tumor board (MTB) comprises a "core team" of healthcare professionals such as oncologists, surgeons, pathologists, and radiotherapists who are specialized in the type of cancer being discussed. The "non-core team" may include additional members such as palliative care physicians, medical students, psychologists, and physicians in training, as shown in Figure 9.2. Tumor boards provide a platform for personalized treatment plans that incorporate the latest medical advancements (Berardi et al., 2020).

For patients with HNC, tumor boards and case conferences are vital components of comprehensive care. They offer a valuable platform for the entire medical team to examine individual cases, deliberate on diagnostic results, consider treatment alternatives, and devise personalized management strategies grounded in the most current evidence and expert agreement (Naidoo et al., 2018). Tumor boards are a valuable resource in African settings where access to specialized expertise may be limited. They promote knowledge exchange, capacity building, and quality assurance, as illustrated in Figure 9.3. In South Africa, tumor boards are increasingly recognized as platforms for fostering collaboration, promoting best practices, and addressing disparities in access to care among diverse patient populations (Fagan, Mubuuke, et al., 2016; Sayed et al., 2020). By leveraging multidisciplinary expertise, tumor boards play a vital role in optimizing treatment decision-making and improving clinical outcomes in HNC patients.

Tumor boards and case conferences are meetings where healthcare professionals from various disciplines come together to discuss treatment options for patients with HNC based on evidence-based guidelines, expert consensus, and individual patient factors (Nutting et al., 2011). These forums provide an opportunity for experts to share their knowledge, review diagnostic studies, and formulate personalized management plans for patients. In Africa, tumor boards and case conferences have become an essential part of HNC care, promoting collaboration among specialists and encouraging best practices in treatment decision-making (Fagan, Mubuuke, et al., 2016).

The main goal of tumor conferences in HNC care is to create tailored treatment plans based on individual patients' specific needs and circumstances, using evidence-based methods. By employing a multidisciplinary approach, all available treatment options are evaluated and optimized to achieve the most

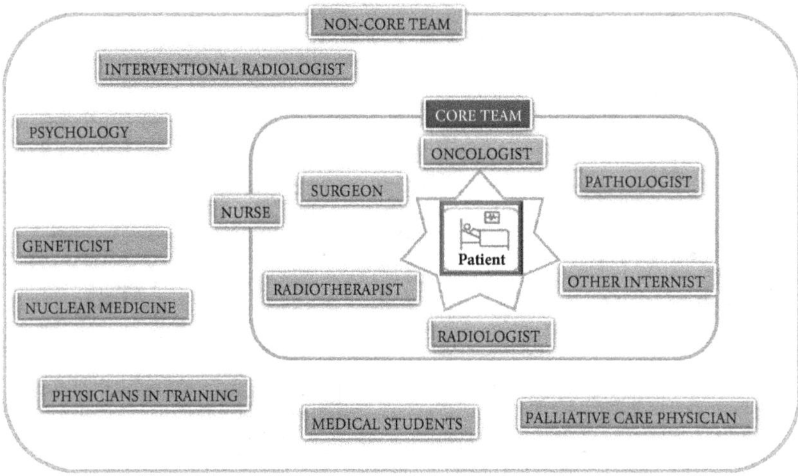

Figure 9.2 Further classification of tumor board. A multidisciplinary tumor board (MTB) typically consists of a "core team" of specialists, including oncologists, surgeons with various specialties, pathologists, radiotherapists, and other experts depending on the type of cancer being discussed (such as breast, head and neck, gastrointestinal, or genitourinary). The MTB welcomes other members who are not part of the "core team," such as psychologists, medical students, nursing staff specialists, research nurses, coordinators, and palliative care physicians. In some countries, nurses are included in the core team rather than the non-core team and play a critical role in influencing treatment decisions (Berardi et al., 2020). Tumor board meetings provide a vital forum for healthcare professionals to exchange ideas and insights on innovative cancer treatment options and research findings. By facilitating ongoing professional growth and knowledge-sharing, these meetings help advance cancer care standards not only within the hospital but also across the broader medical community. The tumor board serves as a key catalyst for fostering interdisciplinary collaboration, promoting professional development, and driving quality improvement initiatives (NCCN, 2021).

favorable outcomes, including surgery, radiation therapy, chemotherapy, immunotherapy, and targeted therapy (Lamb et al., 2011).

Furthermore, tumor conferences facilitate communication and coordination among team members, promoting seamless transitions of care and continuity throughout the patient's cancer journey. They also provide opportunities for education, professional development, and quality assurance within healthcare institutions.

Numerous studies have shown how tumor boards can improve patient outcomes, treatment decision-making, adherence to clinical guidelines, and overall quality of cancer care. For example, Lamb et al. conducted a study that

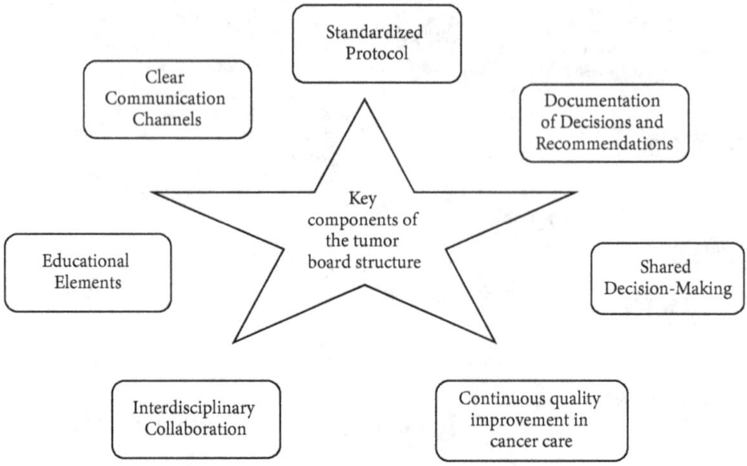

Figure 9.3 Head and neck tumor board key components. Tumor boards are designed to facilitate interdisciplinary collaboration, shared decision-making, and continuous quality improvement in cancer care. Key components of the tumor board structure include the establishment of clear communication channels, the use of standardized protocols for case presentation and discussion, and the documentation of decisions and recommendations made during the meetings. Additionally, tumor boards may include educational elements to promote ongoing professional development for team members. Overall, the organizational structure of tumor boards is crucial for improving the quality of cancer care and ensuring that patients receive the best possible treatment.

demonstrated the significant influence of multidisciplinary tumor conferences on treatment recommendations and management plans for HNC patients (Lamb et al., 2011). Additionally, a study by Liu et al. highlighted the role of tumor boards in enhancing treatment consensus and optimizing outcomes in HNC care (Liu et al., 2020).

Tumor conferences play a crucial role in the multidisciplinary management of patients with HNC. They help in carrying out a comprehensive evaluation, collaborative decision-making, and personalized treatment planning. They are an important part of providing high-quality cancer care, which ensures that patients receive the most effective and coordinated therapeutic interventions.

9.4.3 Patient-Centered Approach to Treatment Planning

When it comes to treating HNC, it is crucial to adopt a patient-centered approach that factors in each patient's distinct preferences and needs. This global effort to boost patient engagement and empowerment takes many forms, including educational resources, decision-making tools, and supportive care services that aim to address the physical, emotional, and psychosocial aspects of HNC care (Ganzer et al., 2015). In the African context, cultural beliefs, socioeconomic factors, and healthcare access barriers exert a significant influence on patients' treatment decisions and adherence to therapy. Meanwhile, the global paradigm shift toward patient-centered care underscores the importance of shared decision-making, informed consent, and psychosocial support as essential components of the cancer care continuum (Langendijk et al., 2010). In Africa, patient-centered care initiatives such as patient navigation programs and survivorship clinics are emerging to improve patient outcomes and quality of life (Moreno & Fagan, 2018). In South Africa, various programs and efforts are aimed at improving patient engagement, empowering patients as active participants in their care, and enhancing health outcomes. These include patient navigation programs, survivorship clinics, and community outreach initiatives (Mao et al., 2018). By prioritizing the values, preferences, and quality of life of patients, a patient-centered approach promotes trust, satisfaction with treatment, and holistic well-being in HNC survivors.

9.5 Future Directions

Despite significant advancements in the treatment of HNC, the overall outcomes for patients remain suboptimal. Traditional prognostic tools such as the tumor-node-metastasis (TNM) staging system, which categorizes tumors based on tumor size, lymph node involvement, and metastasis, often fail to accurately predict patient outcomes. This discrepancy highlights the need for more precise and personalized approaches to HNC management, emphasizing the importance of precision oncology. The TNM staging system, while valuable for providing a general overview of disease extent, may not fully capture the heterogeneity of HNC. Patients with tumors classified under the same TNM stage may exhibit vastly different responses to treatment and overall survival rates. This variability underscores the limitations of relying solely on conventional staging systems to guide treatment decisions and prognostication (Kong et al., 2016).

Precision oncology offers a promising solution to address these challenges by integrating comprehensive molecular profiling of tumors with targeted therapeutic interventions tailored to the specific genetic alterations driving tumor growth. By analyzing the genomic landscape of individual tumors, clinicians can identify actionable mutations or molecular biomarkers that may inform treatment selection and predict treatment response more accurately. Furthermore, precision oncology allows for the identification of novel therapeutic targets and the development of innovative treatment strategies, such as targeted therapies and immunotherapies. These therapies aim to selectively target cancer cells while sparing normal tissues, thereby minimizing treatment-related toxicities and improving therapeutic efficacy (Machiels et al., 2015).

Incorporating precision medicine approaches into HNC care requires collaboration among MDTs, including medical oncologists, radiation oncologists, surgical oncologists, pathologists, and geneticists. Together, these experts can utilize advanced molecular profiling techniques, such as next-generation sequencing, to identify actionable genomic alterations and translate these findings into personalized treatment plans tailored to each patient's unique tumor biology (Lheureux et al., 2020).

As the field of oncology continues to evolve, several promising avenues are emerging for the future of HNC care, with a particular emphasis on genomics, pharmacogenomics, and robotic surgery.

Genomic research has revolutionized our understanding of HNC biology and treatment response. By elucidating the intricate molecular mechanisms underlying tumor initiation, progression, and metastasis, genomic studies have identified novel therapeutic targets and prognostic biomarkers. Next-generation sequencing technologies enable comprehensive profiling of tumor genomes, transcriptomes, and epigenomes, facilitating personalized treatment approaches based on the specific molecular alterations driving tumor growth (Lheureux et al., 2020).

Pharmacogenomics holds immense promise in optimizing therapeutic outcomes and minimizing treatment-related toxicities in HNC patients. By analyzing genetic variations in drug metabolism pathways and drug targets, pharmacogenomic testing can identify individuals at risk of adverse drug reactions or poor treatment responses. Tailoring treatment regimens based on patients' genetic profiles allows for personalized drug selection, dosage adjustments, and treatment modifications, ultimately enhancing treatment efficacy and safety (Chong & Jänne, 2020).

Robot-assisted surgery has emerged as a minimally invasive alternative to traditional open surgical approaches for HNC resection. With enhanced dexterity, precision, and visualization capabilities, robotic surgical systems enable surgeons to perform complex procedures with greater accuracy and control while minimizing trauma to surrounding healthy tissues. Robotic surgery offers several potential benefits for HNC patients, including reduced blood loss, shorter hospital stays, faster recovery times, and improved functional outcomes (O'Malley Jr et al., 2020).

To implement these advances in clinical practice, oncologists, surgeons, geneticists, pharmacologists, and bioinformaticians must work together. Using genetic insights, pharmacogenomic tactics, and robotic surgical procedures, doctors may provide more accurate, personalized, and effective care to HNC patients, thereby enhancing treatment results and quality of life.

To summarize, the continued poor results in HNC treatment, along with the limits of standard prognostic techniques, highlight the crucial need for precision oncology methods. Precision medicine has the potential to revolutionize HNC treatment paradigms by using molecular profiling and tailored medicines to provide patients with better results and a higher quality of life.

9.6 Limitations and Challenges

The implementation of a multidisciplinary approach for cancer patient care has demonstrated benefits, primarily through collaborative decision-making in diagnostic and therapeutic settings. Yet certain elements of this approach may impede its use in clinical practice, particularly in resource-constrained environments. As a result, these prospective challenges remain a subject of noteworthy apprehension and ongoing discussion (Berardi et al., 2020).

Effective communication among MDT members is crucial for collaborative decision-making and coordinated patient care. However, communication breakdowns, inadequate information sharing, and differences in professional terminology can hinder effective teamwork and compromise patient safety. Limited access to specialized equipment, facilities, and support services can impede the delivery of comprehensive care within MDTs (Ward et al., 2021). Resource constraints may include inadequate staffing, funding shortages, and logistical challenges, particularly in resource-limited healthcare settings. Unclear delineation of roles and responsibilities among MDT members can lead to confusion, duplication of efforts, and conflicts within the team. Role ambiguity may arise from overlapping scopes of practice, hierarchical structures, and variations in professional training and expertise. Institutional culture and leadership support significantly influence the functioning of MDTs (Ward et al., 2021). Resistance to change, hierarchical structures, and competing priorities within healthcare organizations may hinder the adoption of multidisciplinary approaches and collaborative practices. Despite the benefits of MDT collaboration, achieving truly patient-centered care remains a challenge. Factors such as patient preferences, cultural beliefs, and socioeconomic disparities may influence treatment decisions and patient engagement in the decision-making process (Mehanna et al., 2016; Ward et al., 2021).

9.6.1 Remedies and Strategies

Implementing structured communication protocols, interdisciplinary meetings, and electronic health record systems can facilitate information exchange and improve communication among MDT members. Clear documentation of treatment plans and regular team debriefings can also enhance coordination and collaboration. Adequate resource allocation, including staffing, funding, and infrastructure, is essential for supporting MDTs and ensuring access to comprehensive HNC care. Healthcare organizations should prioritize investments in multidisciplinary cancer centers and supportive services to address resource constraints (Ferris, Nikitakis, et al., 2021).

Clarifying roles and responsibilities through job descriptions, training programs, and interprofessional education can mitigate role ambiguity and promote effective teamwork within MDTs. Professional development opportunities and ongoing training in collaborative practice skills are essential for enhancing interprofessional collaboration. Healthcare leaders should foster a culture of collaboration, teamwork, and innovation within organizations to support MDT integration. Creating interdisciplinary care pathways, establishing governance structures, and incentivizing collaborative behavior can promote organizational buy-in and sustainability (Mehanna et al., 2016).

Incorporating patient perspectives, preferences, and values into treatment decision-making processes is essential for achieving patient-centered care. Shared decision-making approaches, patient education materials, and culturally sensitive communication strategies can empower patients to actively participate in their care and treatment planning. By addressing these limitations and implementing strategies to enhance multidisciplinary collaboration, healthcare organizations can optimize HNC care delivery, improve patient outcomes, and enhance the overall quality of care (Bossi & Loewen, 2021).

9.7 Conclusion

MDT meetings are becoming increasingly essential in the management of HNCs. These meetings offer a collaborative platform for healthcare professionals to share their expertise and insights to optimize patient care. The forums not only foster knowledge sharing and awareness but also alleviate anxiety among participants. Despite their endorsement in various guidelines, there is still no consensus on evaluation methodologies, making it challenging to determine the impact of MTBs on cancer survival. Therefore, it is crucial to establish robust methods for determining the effectiveness of MTBs in improving patient outcomes, reinforcing their role as a cornerstone in the comprehensive care of HNC patients.

MDTs and oncologic functional units play a crucial role in enhancing the quality of cancer care. By integrating various departments and professionals involved in the treatment of specific cancers, MDTs ensure comprehensive and continuous support for patients throughout the entire care continuum, from diagnosis to treatment and follow-up. Patients highly value this collaborative approach because it ensures a holistic and personalized approach to their care. Within an MDT, different members contribute to close management of symptoms and both acute and long-term side effects, as well as provide essential nutritional support, psychosocial reinforcement, and individualized follow-up care. The specialized care provided by MDTs leads to improved treatment adherence and tolerance, a reduction in long-term side effects, enhanced quality of life, and, ultimately, better treatment outcomes and survival rates for patients with HNC.

Expanding further, numerous studies have demonstrated the significant benefits of MDTs in oncology care. For instance, research by Taylor et al. (2019) highlights how the integration of MDTs results in more timely diagnosis, appropriate treatment planning, and better coordination of care, ultimately leading to improved patient outcomes. Similarly, a study by Maguire et al. (2020) underscores the positive impact of MDTs on treatment adherence, patient satisfaction, and overall survival rates among HNC patients. Furthermore, the multidisciplinary approach ensures that patients receive comprehensive support, addressing not only their medical needs but also their psychosocial and nutritional requirements, as emphasized by studies such as that by Taylor et al. (2010). By providing specialized care tailored to the individual needs of patients, MDTs contribute significantly to enhancing the overall quality of cancer care and optimizing treatment outcomes.

Additionally, the seamless coordination and collaboration facilitated by MDTs enable the timely identification and management of treatment-related complications, thereby minimizing the burden of side effects and improving patients' overall well-being. Moreover, the ongoing monitoring and follow-up provided by MDTs ensure that patients receive continued support and guidance throughout their cancer journey, promoting adherence to treatment plans and facilitating timely interventions when necessary. Overall, the integration of specialized MDTs in HNC care represents a cornerstone in delivering patient-centered, evidence-based care that maximizes treatment efficacy and enhances patients' quality of life.

References

ALFONZAN, A. 2021. Multidisciplinary approach in the management of head and neck cancer. *Saudi Medical Journal*, 42(3), 247–54.

AMERICAN SOCIETY OF CLINICAL ONCOLOGY. 2017. Cancer.Net: Understanding the tumor board. Available at: https://www.cancer.org/search.html?q=tumor+boards

ARGIRIS, A., KARAMOUZIS, M. V., RABEN, D., & FERRIS, R. L. 2008. Head and neck cancer. *Lancet*, 371(9625), 1695–709.

ARGIRIS, A., LI, S., GHEBREMICHAEL, M., EGLOFF, A. M., WANG, L., FORASTIERE, A. A., BURTNESS, B., & MEHRA, R. 2014. Prognostic significance of human papillomavirus in recurrent or metastatic head and neck cancer: An analysis of Eastern Cooperative Oncology Group trials. *Ann Oncol*, 25(7), 1410–16.

ARGIRIS, A., LI, S., SAVVIDES, P., OHR, J. P., GILBERT, J., LEVINE, M. A., CHAKRAVARTI, A., HAIGENTZ, M. JR, SABA, N. F., IKPEAZU, C. V., SCHNEIDER, C. J., PINTO, H. A., FORASTIERE, A. A., & BURTNESS, B. 2019. Phase III randomized trial of chemotherapy with or without bevacizumab in patients with recurrent or metastatic head and neck cancer. *J Clin Oncol*, 37(34), 3266–74. doi:10.1200/JCO.19.00555

BERARDI, R., MORGESE, F., RINALDI, S., TORNIAI, M., MENTRASTI, G., SCORTICHINI, L., & GIAMPIERI, R. 2020. Benefits and limitations of a multidisciplinary approach in cancer patient management. *Cancer Manage Res*, 12, 9363–74.

BLANCHARD, P., & BLANCHARD, P. 2019. Role of radiation therapy in the treatment of head and neck cancer. *Exp Rev Anticancer Ther*, 19(4), 327–33.

BOSSI, P., & LOEWEN, I. J. S. 2021. Head and neck cancer: toward precision medicine. *Front Oncol*, 11, 690226.

BRAY, F., FERLAY, J., SOERJOMATARAM, I., SIEGEL, R. L., TORRE, L. A., & JEMAL, A. 2018. Global cancer statistics 2018: GLOBOCAN estimates of incidence and mortality worldwide for 36 cancers in 185 countries. *CA: Cancer J Clin*, 68(6), 394–424.

BURTON, A. M., PATEL, M. R., & CANNADY, S. B. 2015. Robotic-assisted surgery in the head and neck. *Cancer Control*, 22(3), 331–4.

CARNABY, G., HARENBERG, L., CRARY, M., & MCWEENEY, L. 2020. Early speech and swallowing therapy in patients with head and neck cancer: A controlled study. *Arch Physical Med Rehabil*, 101(7), 1131–8.

CHASEN, M. R., BHARGAVA, R., AMSELLEM, M., CARVALHO, C., CHEN, J., DEWALD, L., & SEHGAL, M. 2018. Dysphagia management in head and neck cancer: ASCO guideline. *J Clin Oncol*, 36(24), 2421–49.

CHEN, A. M., FELIX, C., WANG, P. C., HSU, S., BASEHART, V., GARST, J., BERON, P., WONG, D., ROSOVE, M. H., RAO, S., MELANSON, H., KIM, E., PALMER, D., QI, L., KELLY, K., STEINBERG, M. L., KUPELIAN, P. A., & DALY, M. E. 2019. Reduced-dose radiation therapy for HPV-associated oropharyngeal carcinoma (NRG Oncology HN002). *JNCI*, 111(5), 477–85.

CHOW, L. Q. M., HEAD, T., CHAJUT, A., KLAMPATSA, A., MAHAL, B. A., & CASTIGLIONI, M. 2020. Microvascular reconstruction of the head and neck. *J Clin Oncol*, 38(15_suppl), e17599.

CHUNG, C. H., GUTHRIE, V. B., MASICA, D. L., TOKHEIM, C., KANG, H., RICHMON, J., & SLEBOS, R. J. 2019. Genomic alterations in head and neck squamous cell carcinoma determined by cancer gene-targeted sequencing. *Ann Oncol*, 30(4), 608–17.

CNOSSEN, I. C., VAN UDEN-KRAAN, C. F., EERENSTEIN, S. E., JANSEN, F., WITTE, B. I., LACKO, M., HARDILLO, J. A., HONINGS, J., HALMOS, G. B., GOEDHART-SCHWANDT, N. L., DE BREE, R., LEEMANS, C. R., & VERDONCK-DE LEEUW, I. M. 2019. An online self-care education program to support patients after total laryngectomy: Feasibility and satisfaction. *Support Care Cancer*, 27(2), 559–67.

COHEN, E. E., BELL, R. B., BIFULCO, C. B., BURTNESS, B., GILLISON, M. L., HARRINGTON, K. J., LE, Q. T., LEE, N. Y., LEIDNER, R., LEWIS, R. L., LICITRA, L., MEHANNA, H., MELL, L. K., RABEN, A., SIKORA, A. G., UPPALURI, R., WHITWORTH, F., ZANDBERG, D. P., & FERRIS, R. L. 2019. The Society for Immunotherapy of Cancer consensus statement on immunotherapy for the treatment of squamous cell carcinoma of the head and neck (HNSCC). *J ImmunoThera Cancer*, 7(1), 1–26.

COHEN, E. E. W., SOULIÈRES, D., & LE TOURNEAU, C. 2019. Pembrolizumab versus methotrexate, docetaxel, or cetuximab for recurrent or metastatic head-and-neck squamous cell carcinoma (KEYNOTE-040), a randomised, open-label, phase 3 study. *Lancet*, 393(10167), 156–67.

COLEVAS, A. D., YOM, S. S., PFISTER, D. G., SPENCER, S., ADELSTEIN, D., ADKINS, D., BRIZEL, D. M., BURTNESS, B., BUSSE, P. M., CAUDELL, J. J., CMELAK, A. J., EISELE, D. W., FENTON, M., FOOTE, R. L., GILBERT, J., GILLISON, M. L., HADDAD, R. I., HICKS, W. L., HITCHCOCK, Y. J., JIMENO, A., LEIZMAN, D., MAGHAMI, E., MELL, L. K., MITTAL, B. B., PINTO, H. A., RIDGE, J. A., ROCCO, J., RODRIGUEZ, C. P., SHAH, J. P., WEBER, R. S., WITEK, M., WORDEN, F., ZHEN, W., BURNS, J. L., & DARLOW, S. D. 2021. NCCN Guidelines Insights: Head and neck cancers, version 3.2021. *J Nat Comp Cancer Netw*, 19(6), 550–61.

CORRY, J., NG, W. T., MA, S. J., SINGH, A. K., DE GRAEFF, P., & OOSTING, S. F. 2022. Disadvantaged subgroups within the global head and neck cancer population: How can we optimize care?. *Am Soc Clin Oncol Educ Book*, 42, 501–10.

DHOLAM, K. P., PUSALKAR, H. A., YADAV, P. S., QUAZI, G. A., & SOMANI, P. P. 2013. Implant-retained dental rehabilitation in head and neck cancer patients: an assessment of success and failure. *Implant Dent*, 22(6), 604–9. doi:10.1097/ID.0b013e3182a4d7bc.

FAGAN, J. J., MUBUUKE, A. G., & MWANDA, W. O. 2016. Tumour board: An essential component of multidisciplinary cancer care. *East Afr Med J*, 93(1 Suppl), S3–S4.

FERLAY, J., ERVIK, M., LAM, F., COLOMBET, M., MERY, L., PIÑEROS, M., ZNAOR, A., SOERJOMATARAM, I., & BRAY, F. 2020. Global cancer observatory: Cancer today. Lyon, France: International Agency for Research on Cancer. Available at: https://gco.iarc.fr/today.

FERRELL, B. R., TEMEL, J. S., TEMIN, S., ALESI, E. R., BALBONI, T. A., BASCH, E. M., FIRN, J. I., PAICE, J. A., PEPPERCORN, J. M., PHILLIPS, T., STOVALL, E. L., ZIMMERMANN, C., & SMITH, T. J. 2016. Integration of palliative care into standard oncology care: American Society of Clinical Oncology Clinical Practice Guideline Update. *J Clin Oncol*, 35(6), 96–112.

FERRIS, R. L., BLUMENSCHEIN JR, G., FAYETTE, J., GUIGAY, J., COLEVAS, A. D., LICITRA, L., HARRINGTON, K., KASPER, S., VOKES, E. E., EVEN, C., WORDEN, F., SABA, N. F., IGLESIAS DOCAMPO, L. C., HADDAD, R., RORDORF, T., KIYOTA, N., TAHARA, M., MONGA, M., LYNCH, M., GEESE, W. J., KOPIT, J., SHAW, J. W., & GILLISON, M. L. 2016. Nivolumab for recurrent squamous-cell carcinoma of the head and neck. *N Engl J Med*, 375(19), 1856–67.

FERRIS, R. L., NIKITAKIS, N., EGLOFF, A. M., & MULVEY, C. 2021. The multidisciplinary management of head and neck cancer: present and future considerations. *J Nat Comp Cancer Netw*, 19(1), 12–20.

GENDEN, E. M., & O'MALLEY JR, B. W. 2016. Transoral robotic surgery for the management of head and neck cancer: A preliminary experience. *Head Neck*, 38(S1), E417–23.

GENDEN, E. M., O'MALLEY JR, B. W., & WEINSTEIN, G. S. 2016. Transoral robotic surgery: Role in the management of upper aerodigestive tract tumors. *Head Neck*, 38(2), 184–93.

GHADIMI, M., JOHANSEN, P., STEENHOLDT, C., MERL, M., LASSMANN, S., NIELSEN, D. L., & HORAK, I. D. 2020. Danish national guidelines for treatment of squamous cell carcinoma of the head and neck. *Acta Oncologica*, 59(4), 395–402.

GLOBAL CANCER OBSERVATORY. 2022. Cancer Today. https://gco.iarc.fr/today/en/data viz/bars?mode=population&cancers=1_3_4_5_14&multiple_cancers=1&group_populati ons=0&multiple_populations=1&types=0_1&populations

GORPHE, P., BEDDOK, A., HERBORT, M., HANS, S., FERNANDEZ, J., HARTL, D. M., & JANOT, F. 2019. Transoral robotic surgery in head and neck cancer: What we learned from over 500 procedures. *Eur Arch Oto-Rhino-Laryngol*, 276(3), 813–19.

GOVENDER, R., SMITH, C. H., TAYLOR, S. A., SIVASUBRAMANIAM, R., GREEN, S., WILLIS, C., & JONES, T. M. 2020. The role of speech therapy in managing disordered swallowing (dysphagia) in adults with head and neck cancer: A systematic review. *Cancer Treat Rev*, 85, 101994.

GUPTA, B., JOHNSON, N. W., & KUMAR, N. 2016. Global epidemiology of head and neck cancers: A continuing challenge. *Oncology*, 91(1), 13–23. doi:10.1159/000446117

HAUGHEY, B. H., HINNI, M. L., SALASSA, J. R., HAYDEN, R. E., GRANT, D. G., RICH, J. T., MILOV, S., LEWIS, J. S. Jr, & KRISHNA, M. 2011. Transoral laser microsurgery as primary treatment for advanced-stage oropharyngeal cancer: A United States multicenter study. *Head Neck*, 33(12), 1683–94.

HUTCHESON, K. A., BARRINGER, D. A., ROSENTHAL, D. I., MAY, A. H., ROBERTS, D. B., & LEWIN, J. S. 2019. Swallowing outcomes after radiotherapy for laryngeal carcinoma. *Arch Otolaryngol Head Neck Surg*, 135(9), 929–35.

ISENRING, E., ELIA, M., KISS, N., BAUER, J., & CAPRA, S. 2017. The evidence of improved nutritional outcomes in cancer patients using multidisciplinary team interventions: A systematic review. *Eur J Clin Nutr*, 71(3), 332–41.

JENTSCH, C., BEUTHIEN-BAUMANN, B., TROOST, E. G., & SHAKIRIN, G. 2015. Validation of functional imaging as a biomarker for radiation treatment response. *Br J Radiol*, 88(1051), 20150014. doi:10.1259/bjr.20150014

JIN, Y., AHMAD, S., RITTER, A., BUSS, M., HEROLD-MENDE, C., DYCKHOFF, G. 2021. Multidisciplinary team meetings for head and neck cancer in Germany: A systematic literature review. *BMC Cancer*, 21, 609.

KAM, A. W., KEAT, C. S., AZLAN, A. H., HAFIZAH, N., & LEONG, W. L. 2019. Nutritional support for patients undergoing radiotherapy for head and neck cancer: A systematic review. *Malaysian J Nutr*, 25(2), 239–54.

KONG, C. S., NARASIMHAN, B., CAO, H., KWOK, S., ERICKSON, J. P., KOONG, A., & PARSA, A. T. 2016. The relationship between human papillomavirus status and other molecular prognostic markers in head and neck squamous cell carcinomas. *Int J Radiat Oncol Biol Physics*, 96(2), 379–86.

KULBERSH, B. D., ROSENTHAL, E. L., & MCGREW, B. M. 2020. Impact of swallowing therapy on aspiration rate following treatment for head and neck cancer. *Dysphagia*, 35(5), 812–18.

LACOUTURE, M. E., SIBAUD, V., GERBER, P. A., VAN DEN HURK, C., FERNÁNDEZ-PEÑAS, P., SANTINI, D., & STÄNDER, S. 2021. Management of dermatologic adverse events to immune checkpoint inhibitors: Recommendations from an expert panel of dermatologists and oncologists. *J Clin Oncol*, 39(8), 851–63.

LAMB, B. W., BROWN, K. F., NAGPAL, K., VINCENT, C., GREEN, J. S., & SEVDALIS, N. 2011. Quality of care management decisions by multidisciplinary cancer teams: A systematic review. *Ann Surg Oncol*,18(8), 2116–25.

LANGENDIJK, J. A., FERLITO, A., TAKES, R. P., RODRIGO, J. P., SUÁREZ, C., STROJAN, P., HAIGENTZ, M. JR, & RINALDO, A. 2010. Postoperative strategies after primary surgery for squamous cell carcinoma of the head and neck. *Oral Oncol*, 46(8), 577–85.

LHEUREUX, S., DENOYELLE, C., OHASHI, P. S., & DE BONO, J. S. 2020. MARCH: A precision medicine platform for patients with recurrent or metastatic head and neck cancer. *Exp Rev Precision Med Drug Develop*, 5(2), 99–110.

LICITRA, L., KEILHOLZ, U., TAHARA, M., LIN, J. C., CHOMETTE, P., CERUSE, P., HARRINGTON, K., & MESIA, R. 2016. Evaluation of the benefit and use of multidisciplinary teams in the treatment of head and neck cancer. *Oral Oncol*, 59, 73–9.

LIU, J. C., KAPLON, A., BLACKMAN, E., MIYAMOTO, C., SAVIOR, D., & RAGIN, C. 2020. The impact of the multidisciplinary tumor board on head and neck cancer outcomes. *Laryngoscope*, 130(4), 946–50. doi:10.1002/lary.28066

LOEWEN, D., D'AGUILLO, C., NGUYEN, D., & HARRIS, J. 2021. The role of multidisciplinary teams in the management of head and neck cancer: A scoping review. *J Otolaryngol Head Neck Surg*, 50(1), 2.

LURYI, A. L., CHEN, M. M., MEHRA, S., ROMAN, S. A., & SOSA, J. A. 2016. Judicious opioid use in head and neck cancer patients undergoing surgery. *Head Neck*, 38(6), 846–51.

MACHIELS, J. P. H., HADDAD, R. I., FAYETTE, J., LICITRA, L. F., TAHARA, M., VERMORKEN, J. B., CLEMENT, P. M., GAULER, T., CUPISSOL, D., GRAU, J. J., GUIGAY, J., CAPONIGRO, F., DE CASTRO, G. JR, DE SOUZA VIANA, L., KEILHOLZ, U., DEL CAMPO, J. M., CONG, X. J., EHRNROOTH, E., COHEN, E. E.; LUX-H&N 1 INVESTIGATORS. 2015. Afatinib versus methotrexate as second-line treatment in patients with recurrent or metastatic squamous-cell carcinoma of the head and neck progressing on or after platinum-based therapy (LUX-Head & Neck 1), an open-label, randomised phase 3 trial. *Lancet Oncol*, 16(5), 583–94.

MAGUIRE, E., THOMPSON, L., TONIGAN, S. 2020. Multidisciplinary team care in head and neck cancer: The otolaryngologist's perspective. *Curr Oncol Rep*, 22, 51.

MAO, J. J., PALMER, S. C., & DESAI, K. 2018. Development of a model of integrative oncology care for patients with head and neck cancer. *J Altern Complement Med*. 24(3), 252–9.

MARCUS, C., CIARALLO, A., TAHARI, A. K., & SUBRAMANIAM, R. M. 2018. PET/CT in the management of head and neck cancers: Current perspectives and emerging applications. *J Nucl Med*, 59(5), 716–24.

MARUR, S., LI, S., CMELAK, A. J., GILLISON, M. L., ZHAO, W. J., FERRIS, R. L., WESTRA, W. H., GILBERT, J., BAUMAN, J. E., WAGNER, L. I., TREVARTHEN, D. R., BALKRISHNA, J., MURPHY, B. A., AGRAWAL, N., COLEVAS, A. D., CHUNG, C. H., BURTNESS, B. A. 2017. E1308: Phase II trial of induction chemotherapy followed by reduced-dose radiation and weekly cetuximab in patients with HPV-associated resectable squamous cell carcinoma of the oropharynx—ECOG-ACRIN Cancer Research Group. *J Clin Oncol*, 35(5), 490–7.

MEHANNA, H., EVANS, M., BEASLEY, M., CHATTERJEE, S., DILKES, M., HOMER, J., O'HARA, J., ROBINSON, M., SHAW, R., & SLOAN, P. 2016. Oropharyngeal cancer: United Kingdom National Multidisciplinary Guidelines. *J Laryngol Otology*, 130(S2), S90–S96.

MENDENHALL, W. M., WERNING, J. W., PFISTER, D. G., MALYAPA, R. S., & ROBBINS, K. T. 2019. *Essentials of Head and Neck Oncology*. New York: Springer.

MOMENI, A., PATEL, P. N., KATTAN, A., & BHADKAMKAR, M. A. 2020. Management of head and neck reconstruction. *Surg Clin*, 100(1), 157–76.

MURPHY, C. T., GALLOWAY, T. J., HANDORF, E. A., EGLESTON, B. L., WANG, L. S., MEHRA, R., FLIEDER, D. B., & RIDGE, J. A. 2016. Survival impact of increasing time to treatment initiation for patients with head and neck cancer in the United States. *J Clin Oncol*, 34(2), 169–78.

NAIDOO, Y., SINGH, B., KRIEGLER, S., et al. 2018. Multidisciplinary management of head and neck cancer in South Africa: The importance of partnerships and collaboration. *S Afr Med J*, 108(9), 729–33.

NUTTING, C., HORLOCK, N., A'HERN, R., & DEARNALEY, D. P. 2011. Intensity-modulated radiotherapy in head and neck cancers: Early experience of a UK regional centre. *Br J Radiol*, 84(1004), 358–63.

OGUNLEYE, T., ROBINSON, M., ALABI, B. 2019. Implementation of multidisciplinary team meetings in diagnostic and treatment services of head and neck cancer patients in a semi-urban Nigerian setting. *Pan Afr Med J*, 33:56.

OGURA, I., SAITO, M., & KIYOTA, N. 2017. PET imaging for head and neck cancers: Current status and future directions. *Oncol Lett*, 14(1), 5–11.

O'MALLEY JR, B. W., WEINSTEIN, G. S., SNYDERMAN, C. H., & HOCKSTEIN, N. G. 2020. Robotic surgery for head and neck cancer: A review of current clinical outcomes. *Future Oncol*, 16(17), 1205–19.

O'SULLIVAN, B., HUANG, S. H., SU, J., GARDEN, A. S., STURGIS, E. M., DAHLSTROM, K., LEE, N., RIAZ, N., PEI, X., KOYFMAN, S. A., ADELSTEIN, D., BURKEY, B. B., FRIBORG, J., KRISTENSEN, C. A., GOTHELF, A. B., HOEBERS, F., KREMER, B., SPEEL, E. J., BOWLES, D. W., RABEN, D., KARAM, S. D., YU, E., & XU, W. 2016. Development and validation of a staging system for HPV-related oropharyngeal cancer by the International

Collaboration on Oropharyngeal cancer Network for Staging (ICON-S), a multicentre cohort study. *Lancet Oncol*, 17(4), 440–51.

PAIDPALLY, V., CHIRINDEL, A., LAM, S., AGRAWAL, N., QUON, H., & SUBRAMANIAM, R. M. 2017. FDG-PET/CT imaging biomarkers in head and neck squamous cell carcinoma. *Imaging Med*, 9(4), 119–33.

PORCEDDU, S. V., PRYOR, D. I., BURMEISTER, E., BURMEISTER, B. H., POULSEN, M. G., FOOTE, M. C., PANIZZA, B., COMAN, S., MCFARLANE, D., & COMAN, W. 2011. Results of a prospective study of positron emission tomography-directed management of residual nodal abnormalities in node-positive head and neck cancer after definitive radiotherapy with or without systemic therapy. *Head Neck*, 33(12), 1675–82.

RUSSELL, S. J., BABOVIC-VUKSANOVIC, D., & BEXON, A. 2018. Oncolytic viruses: Cancer therapy with targeted virotherapy. *Nat Rev Drug Discov*, 17(9), 673–92.

RUTHERFORD, M., STEVENS, T. M., ZAMMIT-MAEMPEL, I., & HARTLEY, A. 2017. Development of a multidisciplinary team meeting model for head and neck cancer patients in a district general hospital: A review of current practice. *Int J Oral Maxillofac Surg*, 46(6), 715–21.

RUTKOWSKI, M. R., STEPHEN, T. L., SVORONOS, N., ALLEGREZZA, M. J., TESONE, A. J., PERALES-PUCHALT, A., BRENCICOVA, E., ESCOVAR-FADUL, X., NGUYEN, J. M., CADUNGOG, M. G., ZHANG, R., SALATINO, M., TCHOU, J., RABINOVICH, G. A., & CONEJO-GARCIA, J. R. 2015. Microbially driven TLR5-dependent signaling governs distal malignant progression through tumor-promoting inflammation. *Cancer Cell*, 27(1), 27–40.

SAYED, S. I., ESTERHUIZEN, T. M., SWANEPOEL, A. C. 2019. Management of head and neck cancer: A South African perspective. *S Afr Med J*. 109(7), 501–5.

SAYED, S. I., LIN, J., KRIEGLER, S. 2020. Factors influencing treatment decisions in head and neck cancer: perspectives from South African radiation oncologists. *S Afr Med J*, 110(1), 65–71.

SCHUMACHER, T. N., & SCHREIBER, R. D. 2015. Neoantigens in cancer immunotherapy. *Science*, 3486230, 69–74.

SEEDAT, J., COUTTS, K., & VLOK, E. 2023. Epidemiology and demographics of head and neck cancer in Africa: A scoping review. *Afr J Prim Health Care Fam Med*, 15(1), e1–e13. doi:10.4102/phcfm.v15i1.3749. PMID: 37526561; PMCID: PMC11022662.

SOUTH AFRICAN NATIONAL CANCER REGISTRY. 2021. Cancer in South Africa 2021. National Cancer Registry, National Health Laboratory Service. Available at: http://www.nioh.ac.za/assets/files/NCR/Cancer%20in%20SA%202021.pdf

STATSSA. 2008. Cancer in South Africa, 2008–2019. Available at: www.statssa.gov.za/publications/03-08-00/03-08-002023.pdf [Accessed May 16, 2024.]

SUNG, H., FERLAY, J., SIEGEL, R. L., LAVERSANNE, M., SOERJOMATARAM, I., JEMAL, A., & BRAY, F. 2021. Global cancer statistics 2020: GLOBOCAN estimates of incidence and mortality worldwide for 36 cancers in 185 countries. *CA: Cancer J*, 71(3), 209–49.

TAYLOR, C., MUNRO, A. J., GLYNNE-JONES, R., GRIFFITH, C., TREVATT, P., RICHARDS, M., & RAMIREZ, A. J. 2010. Multidisciplinary team working in cancer: What is the evidence? *BMJ*, 340, c951. doi:10.1136/bmj.c951

TAYLOR, C., SHEWBRIDGE, A., HARRIS, J., et al. 2019. Benefits of multidisciplinary teamwork in the management of breast cancer. *Breast Cancer (Dove Med Press)*, 11, 435–48.

VERDONCK-DE LEEUW, I. M., JANSEN, F., BRAKENHOFF, R. H., LANGENDIJK, J. A., TAKES, R. P., TERHAARD, C. H. J., BAATENBURG DE JONG, R. J., SMIT, J. H., & LEEMANS, C. R. 2019. Advancing interdisciplinary research in head and neck cancer through a multicenter longitudinal prospective cohort study: The NETherlands QUality of life and BIomedical Cohort (NET-QUBIC) data warehouse and biobank. *BMC Cancer*, 19(1), 765. doi:10.1186/s12885-019-5866-z. Erratum in: BMC Cancer. 2019 Oct 22;19(1):982. doi:10.1186/s12885-019-6223-y.

VERMORKEN, J. B., MESIA, R., RIVERA, F., REMENAR, E., KAWECKI, A., ROTTEY, S., ERFAN, J., ZABOLOTNYY, D., KIENZER, H. R., CUPISSOL, D., & PEYRADE, F. 2008. Platinum-based chemotherapy plus cetuximab in head and neck cancer. *N Engl J Med*, 359(11), 1116–27.

WARD, M. C., REDDY, C. A., ADELSTEIN, D. J., & KOYFMAN, S. A. 2021. Multidisciplinary management of locally advanced head and neck cancer. *Semin Radiat Oncol*, 31(1), 32–40.

WEINSTEIN, G. S., O'MALLEY, B. W. JR, MAGNUSON, J. S., CARROLL, W. R., OLSEN, K. D., DAIO, L., MOORE, E. J., & HOLSINGER, F. C. 2012. Transoral robotic surgery: A multicenter study to assess feasibility, safety, and surgical margins. *Laryngoscope*, 122(8), 1701–7.

ZAFEREO, M., YU, J., ONAKOYA, P. A., ASWANI, J., BAIDOO, K., BOGALE, M., CAIRNCROSS, L., CORDES, S., DANIEL, A., DIOM, E., MAURICE, M. E., MOHAMMED, G. M., BIADGELIGN, M. G., KONÉ, F. I., ITIERE, A., KOCH, W., KONNEY, A., KUNDIONA, I., MACHARIA, C., MASHAMBA, V., MOORE, M. G., MUGABO, R. M., NOAH, P., OMUTSANI, M., ORLOFF, L. A., OTITI, J., RANDOLPH, G. W., SEBELIK, M., TODSEN, T., TWIER, K., & FAGAN, J. J. 2020. African Head and Neck Society Clinical Practice guidelines for thyroid nodules and cancer in developing countries and limited resource settings. *Head Neck*, 42(8), 1746–56. doi:10.1002/hed.26094

ZHANG, Z., LI, Y., YAN, L., LUO, X., TAO, L., & ZHU, S. 2020. Role of a clinical dietician in patients with head and neck cancer treated with radiotherapy. *Support Care Cancer*, 28(6), 2921–6.

ZOPF, D. A., HOLLENBEAK, C. S., MULLADY, D. K., & GANGNON, R. E. 2020. Determinants of long-term swallowing outcomes following chemoradiotherapy for head and neck cancer. *Otolaryngol Head Neck Surg*, 163(5), 989–95.

10

Health Systems and Organization of Head and Neck Cancer Care

Nkhensani Chauke-Malinga, Lloyd Mabonga Talent Chipiti, Mohammed Alaouna, Kenneth Segwapa, Thendo Netshiongolwe, Alexis Koskan, and Zodwa Dlamini

10.1 Introduction

The integration of a well-coordinated health system to deliver optimal head and neck cancer (HNC) care outcomes involves a multifaceted approach. Health systems encompass all the organizations, institutions, resources, and people whose primary purpose is to improve health (Solanki et al., 2024). They consist of various components, including service delivery, health workforce, health information systems, access to essential medicines, financing, and leadership/governance (Kutzin & Sparkes, 2016). These systems operate at multiple levels, from local clinics to national health ministries, aiming to provide equitable, efficient, and quality healthcare services to populations (Malakoane et al., 2020). The organization and delivery of HNC care vary significantly across different health systems and is influenced by factors such as healthcare infrastructure, resource allocation, policy frameworks, and the availability of specialized care facilities (Matolengwe et al., 2024). Moreso, the implementation of multidisciplinary teams (MDTs) is central to HNC care. MDTs facilitate comprehensive care planning and delivery, ensuring that patients receive tailored and holistic treatment plans. This team-based approach enhances clinical decision-making and improves patient outcomes by integrating various expertise and perspectives (Matolengwe et al., 2024; Solanki et al., 2024).

The South African health system is a complex and multifaceted entity, characterized by a dual structure of public and private sectors (Solanki et al., 2024). As a result of racial segregation in the apartheid era, South Africa has a deeply ingrained history of healthcare inequality. This is reflected by disparities in health status and access to healthcare between the different ethnic groups in South Africa, as well as for patients with HNC (de Villiers, 2021; Maphumulo & Bhengu, 2019). The two-tier system is characterized by an inequitable distribution of national healthcare resources, with some parts of the country's public healthcare system providing suboptimal care for patients with HNC (Solanki et al., 2024). South Africa has an estimated population of between 60.9 and 62 million, and an annual population growth rate of 0.8%, which is equivalent to 0.75% of the total world population (Worldometer, 2024). The median age is 27.6 years, and life expectancy is 63 years old (Kruger & Shongwe, 2004; Pillay & Siyothula, 2008). Sixty percent of the population is younger than 25 years, and < 9% are older than 60 (Gómez-Olivé et al., 2018).

South Africa has a diverse population with the ethnic distribution consisting of 81.4% black, 7.3% white, 8.2% colored (mixed race), and 2.7% Indian (Yamoah et al., 2022). Significant health disparities exist among these ethnic groups. The black African population has diverse cultures, defined by language, religion, political beliefs, coupled with high internal and international migration (Roy et al., 2022). A large proportion of the population is economically dependent on 30% of the population. Migration from rural to urban areas over the past 40 years from former homelands and other rural areas to the nine major metropolitan areas has been significant (Collinson et al., 2007). The reasons for this migration have been social, economic, and political, with the intention of obtaining access to better amenities and living conditions. However, a large portion of South Africa still lives in inadequate informal housing (Zulu & Perry, 2021). This migration to cities has implications for healthcare because it places pressure on already strained tertiary services in urban areas. This tapestry is an important consideration when providing cancer care because cultural beliefs and practices impact patients' understanding of and approach to the disease (Roy et al., 2022).

South Africa is an upper-middle-income country and is one of the most well-developed and robust economies in Africa. It is the economic powerhouse of the continent and the only country in Africa that is a member of G20 (Dlamini & Ngalawa, 2021). According to the World Bank, South Africa is considered a newly industrialized country (World Bank, 2024). It ranks 34th in the world in terms of its economy, with a gross domestic product (GDP) of US$351.4 billion in 2020, which translates to around US$6,287 per capita, which is quite high by African standards (Olayungbo & Iqbal, 2021). However, according to Statistics South Africa (2024), South Africa has a very high unemployment rate, standing at approximately 33% in the third quarter of 2024, which is indeed a significant concern (Visagie & Posel, 2013). Youth unemployment remains particularly high, with 43.4% of individuals ages 15–34 unemployed. This demographic challenge highlights the ongoing struggle to integrate young people into the workforce effectively (Statistics South Africa, 2024).

The high unemployment rate, particularly among youth, underscores structural issues within the South African economy that need to be addressed through comprehensive strategies focusing on both demand and supply sides of the labor market (Paver et al., 2020). It is generally agreed that being employed enhances physical and mental well-being and is a significant social predictor of health because most individuals rely on jobs to provide for their daily needs, including healthcare (Doku et al., 2019; Thern et al., 2017). People without employment are less likely to have access to healthcare and have a greater probability of becoming ill (Silver et al., 2022). Additionally, South Africa's high rates of unemployment are directly linked to poverty, a predictor of untreated or late-stage diagnosis for HNCs. One US study links poverty to HNC, describing how the poor have increased exposure to risk factors such as poor nutrition, environmental carcinogens, and human papillomavirus (HPV) infection (Hoffman et al., 1998). Similar results were reported in India, where poverty was identified as a cause of delayed presentation and, hence, more advanced stages of the disease at presentation and less access to treatment for HNC (Hoffman et al., 1998).

Sub-Saharan Africa has a severe shortage of health workers, with < 2.3 health workers working per 10,000 inhabitants (Masis et al., 2021). South Africa also has a shortage of healthcare workers and an uneven distribution of medical expertise, causing some institutions to be overwhelmed due to insufficient financial and human resources (Aluttis et al., 2014). The lack of healthcare workers in South Africa is aggravated by the emigration of health professionals to affluent countries, including Australia, Canada, New Zealand, the United Kingdom, and the United States (Masis et al., 2021). This career-driven migration creates a challenge in managing patients with HNC. Ayoub and Pulijala reported that although oral cancer is the sixth most common cancer among men in South Africa, there is a severe shortage of professionals trained in otolaryngorhinology and maxillofacial surgery (Ayoub & Pulijala, 2019). The high burden imposed on healthcare by HIV/AIDS, tuberculosis, maternal and child health, noncommunicable diseases, and trauma competes with the care that can be provided to HNC patients (Delobelle et al., 2011; Mhlanga & Garidzirai, 2020).

HNC is a critical public health issue within South Africa, representing a substantial portion of the country's cancer burden (Solanki et al., 2024). The prevalence of HNC is influenced by a variety of risk factors prevalent in the population, such as tobacco use, alcohol consumption, and HPV infection (Roy et al., 2022). The epidemiology of HNC in South Africa reflects both global trends and region-specific risk profiles, necessitating targeted public health interventions. Early detection and timely treatment of HNC are essential for improving patient outcomes (Solanki et al., 2024). However, in the South African context, these are often hindered by late presentations, limited access to specialized care, and socioeconomic barriers (Nash et al., 2024). The disparity between the public and private healthcare sectors further exacerbates these challenges, leading to inequitable health outcomes across different population groups (Nash et al., 2024; Solanki et al., 2024).

Addressing the burden of HNC in South Africa requires a multifaceted approach, one that include enhancing public health campaigns aimed at early detection, expanding HPV vaccination programs, and improving the overall healthcare infrastructure (Nash et al., 2024; Solanki et al., 2024). Moreover, policy interventions and increased funding are crucial to bridging the gap between the public and private sectors, ensuring that all South Africans have access to quality care for HNC (Solanki et al., 2024). In this context, understanding the dynamics of the South African healthcare system and its impact on the management of HNC is vital for developing effective strategies to combat this disease and improve health outcomes for the population (Nash et al., 2024; Roy et al., 2022). This chapter conducts a comprehensive examination of the organization and structure of health systems dedicated to managing HNC. It explores the intricate multidisciplinary approaches employed within these health systems to address the diverse facets of care for affected individuals. The chapter delves into the challenges faced in organizing and delivering effective HNC care, offering insights into the complexities inherent in the healthcare landscape. Moreover, it identifies opportunities for improvement, presenting a nuanced discussion on potential strategies to enhance the overall organization and delivery of care for individuals facing HNC.

10.2 South African Healthcare System

The South African health system is a dual structure composed of public and private sectors, each with its own organizational framework, resources, and service delivery mechanisms (Malakoane et al., 2020; Matolengwe et al., 2024). This system aims to provide comprehensive health services to a diverse population but faces significant challenges in terms of equity, accessibility, and quality of care (Solanki et al., 2024). Public healthcare in South Africa was restructured in 1994, after the end of apartheid, as the country made a new effort to address disparities in healthcare linked to race and class (McLaren et al., 2014). The goal of the government was to move the nation slowly toward a more centralized healthcare system by creating a two-tier healthcare structure with a large public sector and a smaller, high-quality private sector (Younger, 2016). The tiers differ in that there is a maldistribution of resources between the private and public sectors. Elite and middle-class populations predominantly use private healthcare, which provides them with a high standard of care (Nash et al., 2024).

The public healthcare sector serves approximately 84% of the South African population but is burdened by resource limitations, infrastructural deficiencies, and high patient loads; it primarily caters to lower-income individuals who do not have access to private health insurance (Matolengwe et al., 2024; Solanki et al., 2024). It is funded by the government through general taxation and is characterized by a tiered system of healthcare delivery. The cornerstone of the public health system, primary healthcare (PHC) services are delivered through a network of clinics and community health centers (Nash et al., 2024). These facilities provide essential health services, including preventive care, maternal and child health, immunizations, and basic medical treatments. PHC aims to be the first point of contact for patients, emphasizing accessibility and community-based care (Malakoane et al., 2020; Solanki et al., 2024). The public sector is characterized as having lower health expenditures and, consequently, fewer resources (Matolengwe et al., 2024). This underfunding, coupled with an inequitable distribution of resources, has resulted in inadequate access to quality healthcare (M'bouaffou et al., 2022; Rensburg, 2021). The public healthcare system is also under immense strain due to poor economic growth, increased unemployment, urbanization, the influx of health and economic migrants from member states of the Southern African Development Community (SADC), and poor management (Mhlanga & Garidzirai, 2020; Singh, 2021).

Conversely, the private healthcare sector accounts for the remaining 16% and offers more immediate and higher-quality access to specialized care, benefiting as it does from better resources and advanced medical technologies (M'bouaffou et al., 2022). According to the World Health Organization (WHO) report, South Africa spends a larger percentage (41.8%) of its overall health expenditure on voluntary private health insurance as compared to other nations, even though it only caters to 16% of the population (WHO, 2019). The Organization for Economic Cooperation and Development (OECD) reports an average of 6.3% of GDP expenditure on healthcare worldwide (OECD, 2021). However, it is important to note that this figure reflects spending in OECD member countries, which represent only about 16% of the global population. Despite catering to a relatively small portion of the global population, the high expenditure underscores significant investments in healthcare within these developed nations (World Bank, 2021). This discrepancy highlights disparities in healthcare funding and access between OECD countries and the rest of the world (Schneider et al., 2021).

Private health insurance is individually funded, although taxpayers younger than 65 years can claim medical tax credit for contributions to medical schemes. This suggests that, despite the high total cost of healthcare, the government still subsidizes individuals covered by private healthcare insurance (Schneider et al., 2021). However, this sector remains accessible primarily to the affluent minority with health insurance coverage, leaving a significant portion of the population reliant on the underresourced public sector (Mhlanga & Garidzirai, 2020). In the public sector, diagnostic and treatment delays are common due to resource constraints. Advanced cases often present late, limiting treatment options and reducing survival rates (Singh, 2021). The private sector, with its better resources, offers more timely and effective treatment, but this is not a viable option for the majority of the population (Solanki et al., 2024). This disparity creates a dual system in which patient and institutional health outcomes are closely tied to socioeconomic status (Singh, 2021). Table 10.1 is an overview summary of patient and institutional outcomes in South African public health and private institutions. The disparities between private and public health institutions in South Africa highlight significant inequities in access to quality healthcare (Schneider et al., 2021; Solanki et al., 2024). To improve patient and institutional outcomes across the board, it is essential to address these disparities through policy reforms, increased funding for public health, and initiatives aimed at improving efficiency and care quality in public hospitals. This could involve public–private partnerships, better resource allocation, and investment in healthcare infrastructure and workforce development in public institutions (Schneider et al., 2021).

The national Minister of Health (MoH) oversees establishing national health policy and has the authority to define and establish the parameters of this policy in national legislation. The MoH also has the power to ensure that all levels of the healthcare system adhere to these policies (van den Heever, 2016). Policy coordination occurs through a National Health Council (NHC) that is made up of provincial Members of the Executive Council (provincial ministers) who are responsible for health and of relevant departmental heads (Mhlanga & Garidzirai, 2020). Nine provinces and local governments (8 metropolitan, 44 district, and 226 local municipalities) are devolved tiers of government with their own powers to make legislation, raise funds, and execute programs (shown in Figure 10.1) (van den Heever, 2016).

The Council for Medical Schemes (CMS), an ostensibly independent statutory organization, regulates medical schemes, which are a significant component of the health system. The CMS reports to the MoH. It is also accountable for the prudential regulation of schemes and their overall conduct (van den Heever, 2016). As of March 31, 2022, the CMS regulates 72 medical schemes, 27 administrators (including self-administered schemes), 44 managed care organizations (including schemes providing their own managed care services to members), 2,156 broker organizations, and 7,530 individual brokers. The role of the CMS is to ensure that these entities utilizing the MSA and its regulations protect the interests of all 8.95 million scheme beneficiaries (Council for Medical Schemes [CMS], 2024).

Table 10.1 A comparison of patient and institutional outcomes between South African public and private health institutions

	Public health institutions	Private health institutions
	Patient outcomes	
Quality of care	Public health institutions often struggle with limited resources, resulting in longer wait times, overcrowded facilities, and shortages of medical supplies and staff. The quality of care can vary significantly depending on the location and the specific facility, with rural areas often facing more severe challenges.	Generally, private health institutions in South Africa offer higher quality care compared to public facilities. This is attributed to better funding, more advanced medical technology, and lower patient-to-doctor ratios. Private hospitals tend to have shorter wait times for treatments and procedures, which contributes to higher patient satisfaction and better health outcomes.
Patient satisfaction	Patient satisfaction in public hospitals is generally lower due to the aforementioned issues. However, these institutions are crucial for providing care to the majority of South Africans who cannot afford private healthcare.	Surveys indicate that patient satisfaction is typically higher in private institutions. This is largely due to more personalized care, better amenities, and more efficient service delivery.
Health outcomes	Public institutions face challenges in managing and treating chronic diseases effectively, partly due to resource constraints and high patient loads. This often leads to poorer health outcomes compared to private institutions.	Outcomes for treatments such as surgeries and chronic disease management are generally better in private institutions. This is because these institutions often have better-equipped facilities and more specialized healthcare professionals
	Institutional outcomes	
Efficiency	Public hospitals often face inefficiencies due to bureaucratic constraints, limited funding, and high patient volumes. This impacts the overall effectiveness of service delivery and patient care.	Private hospitals generally operate more efficiently due to better management practices and more significant financial resources. They can invest in state-of-the-art technology and infrastructure, which contributes to better overall performance.

Table 10.1 Continued

	Public health institutions	**Private health institutions**
Financial stability	Public health institutions are heavily reliant on government funding, which can be insufficient to meet the growing healthcare demands. This leads to resource shortages and impacts the quality of care provided.	Private health institutions often have better financial stability, allowing for continuous improvements and investments in healthcare delivery. However, they rely heavily on medical aid schemes and out-of-pocket payments from patients.
Workforce	Public hospitals face challenges in retaining skilled healthcare professionals due to lower salaries and difficult working conditions. This can lead to high turnover rates and staffing shortages, further affecting institutional outcomes.	The workforce in private institutions often includes highly skilled professionals who are attracted by better working conditions and higher salaries. This contributes to better service delivery and institutional performance.

Source: Department of Health, 2017.

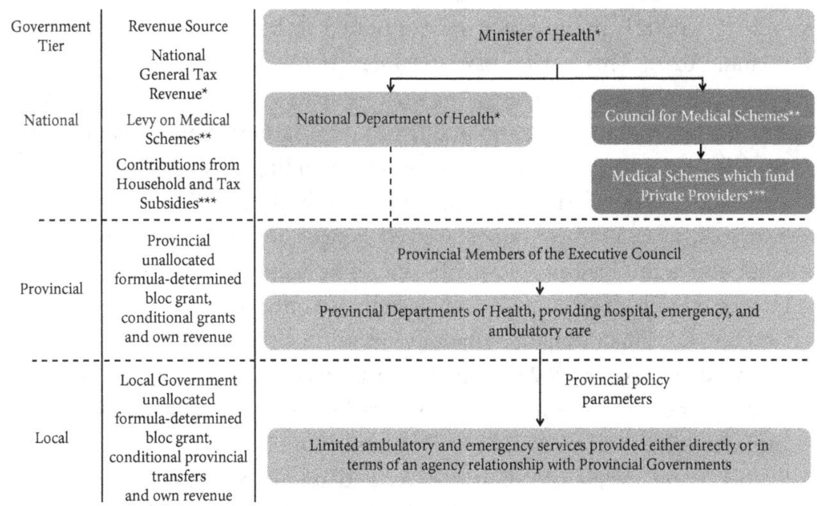

Figure 10.1 Organization and structure of the South African healthcare system. The system is a complex and dual-structured entity with distinct public and private sectors. While the public sector strives to provide essential health services to the majority of the population, it faces significant challenges related to funding, resources, and accessibility. The private sector, though better resourced, is accessible primarily to those who can afford private health insurance. Addressing these challenges requires coordinated efforts from the government, healthcare providers, and the community to ensure a sustainable and inclusive healthcare system. Asterisks indicate which revenue source matches a national function.

10.2.1 South Africa's Healthcare System Expenditure

The South African health system expenditure is divided among various sectors and services, reflecting the allocation of resources to meet the diverse healthcare needs of the population. The healthcare system is divided into two parts (Solanki et al., 2024). As of 2021, South Africa's overall health system expenditure amounted to approximately 8.3% of GDP. Of this total expenditure, around 48% was accounted for by the public sector, while medical schemes constituted about 41% of the total health spending (Africa Health Exhibition, 2020; Knoema, 2023; World Bank, 2024). The healthcare expenditure in South Africa as a percentage of GDP has shown significant fluctuations from 2000 to 2021 (Figure 10.2). In the early 2000s, the health expenditure was around 7% of GDP. This figure saw a gradual increase over the years, reflecting the country's efforts to improve healthcare infrastructure and access (Knoema, 2023). By 2010, health expenditure had risen to approximately 8% of GDP. This increase was partly driven by the government's initiatives to tackle major public health challenges, including the HIV/AIDS epidemic and tuberculosis (World Bank, 2021).

The introduction of more comprehensive health programs and improved healthcare services contributed to this upward trend. In the subsequent decade, from 2011 to 2021, the expenditure continued to hover around 8% of GDP (Knoema, 2023). This period saw sustained investments in both the public and private health sectors. The public sector's focus was on expanding primary healthcare, hospital services, and public health programs (Solanki et al., 2024). Meanwhile, the private sector saw increased spending on specialized medical services and advanced treatment facilities (Nash et al., 2024). Despite these investments, the healthcare system faced challenges such as resource constraints, unequal access to services, and inefficiencies in healthcare delivery (Knoema, 2023; World Bank, 2024). By 2021, the health expenditure remained significant, at 8.3% of GDP, illustrating the ongoing commitment to addressing the nation's health needs (Knoema, 2023). These data underscore the dynamic nature of healthcare funding in South Africa, driven by both public health needs and economic factors (Solanki et al., 2024; World Bank, 2021).

The focus on hospitals, primary care, and public health programs in the public sector as shown in the National Treasury 2024 Budget Review breakdown of 2024/2025 (Figure 10.3) ensures a comprehensive approach to healthcare delivery (Maphumulo et al., 2019; Solanki et al., 2024). The private sector complements this with specialized services and pharmaceuticals, while donor and nongovernmental organization (NGO) funding supports critical health initiatives like HIV/AIDS and tuberculosis programs (CMS, 2024; Knoema, 2023). The distribution reflects the dual nature of South Africa's health system whose public and private sectors cater to different segments of the population.

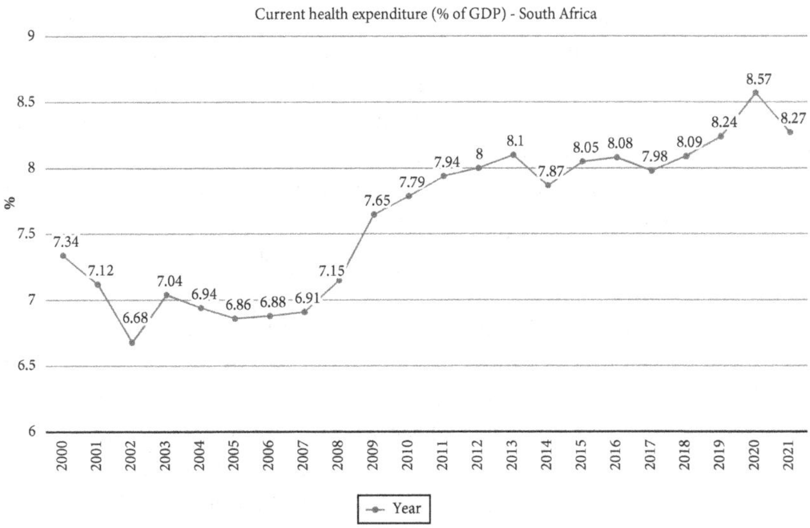

Figure 10.2 South African healthcare system expenditure (% of GDP) from 2000 to 2021. The healthcare expenditure in South Africa, as a percentage of GDP, has shown significant fluctuations from 2000 to 2021. The gradual increase over the years reflects the country's efforts to improve healthcare infrastructure and access.

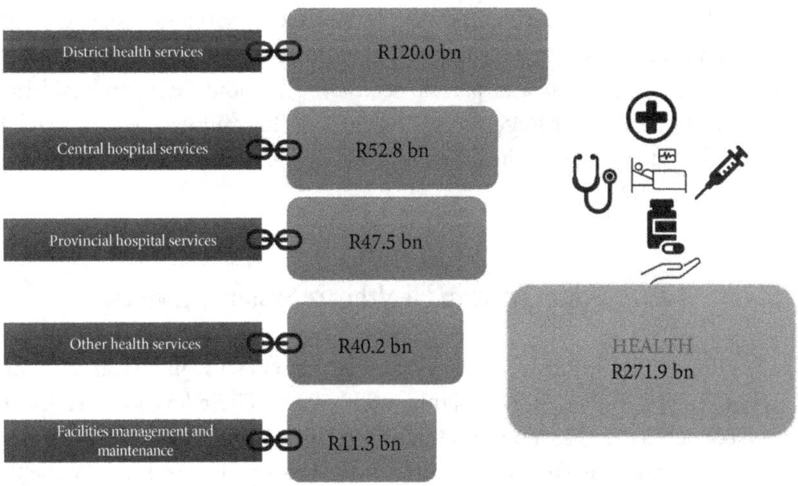

Figure 10.3 South African healthcare system 2024–2025 budget review allocation. The focus on hospitals, primary care, and public health programs in the public sector ensures a comprehensive approach to healthcare delivery (National Treasury, 2024 Budget Review).

The medical schemes system provides cover mainly to income earners for families with breadwinners above the tax threshold (taxpayers), totaling 8.8 million beneficiaries (members and dependents) or 16.3% of the general population (CMS, 2024; Knoema, 2023). The remaining 45.2 million (83.7%) are effectively covered by public services without user charges. (In practice, every citizen is covered in one way or another, most often by both for-profit and public healthcare systems, but, unlike in regions where the influence of nonfinancial barriers is negligible, public services cover the large majority of cases; see Knoema, 2023; World Bank, 2024.)

On the other hand, the 5.5 million being served by public hospitals are left without coverage because a means test for public sector services makes them technically uninsured (these figures were estimated through extrapolation from a Ministerial Task Team (2005) report on South Africa's National Health Insurance [NHI] (van den Heever, 2016). Primary care is free for all, irrespective of patient participation in a medical scheme or their income. Both systems together achieve a high level of financial risk protection, with low rates of out-of-pocket (OOP) payment—only about 7.1% of total expenditure (or under 1% of GDP) (Solanki et al., 2024). Two-thirds of this expenditure (mainly in the form of medicine, pharmacy, and practitioner expenses by medical schemes beneficiaries) accounts for most of the total OOP expenditures, not burdening the poor (Nash et al., 2024). Nonetheless, an increasing number of people use private ambulatory care within the public sector services (Solanki et al., 2024). Table 10.2 provides a structured breakdown of how health expenditure is allocated for the public and private sectors in the South African healthcare system (National Cancer Registry [NCR], 2020). This multifaceted approach is essential for addressing the healthcare needs of the South African population (Solanki et al., 2024).

10.2.2 South African Healthcare System Services

The South African healthcare system comprises primary, secondary, and tertiary levels of service (Keller, 2024; Solanki et al., 2024). These levels of healthcare can be conceptualized as a pyramid, with less specialized care at the bottom of the pyramid and more specialized treatment at the top (Figure 10.4). While the top of the pyramid is just as significant and important as the bottom of the pyramid, it is very important to realize that the bottom of the pyramid resonates with most South Africa's disadvantaged population (Hunter et al., 2024). If the foundation of the structure is not secure, then the whole system is faced with disparities and challenges in offering specialized patient care (Ramlagan et al., 2024; Solanki et al., 2024). A well-functioning health system matches all patients

Table 10.2 South Africa's Health care system expenditure breakdown

Sectors	Percentage	Description
Hospitals	40%	Includes tertiary, secondary, and district hospitals Expenditures cover inpatient care, specialized treatments, and hospital-based services
Primary health care	25%	Encompasses clinics and community health services Focuses on preventive care, outpatient services, and basic medical care
Administration and management	10%	Salaries and operational costs for administrative functions Management of healthcare facilities and public health initiatives
Public health programs	15%	Programs such as immunization, maternal and child health, and disease prevention Funding for public health campaigns and community outreach
Capital expenditure	10%	Investment in infrastructure, new healthcare facilities, and equipment Upgrading existing facilities and purchasing advanced medical technology
Private hospitals	35%	Private inpatient and outpatient hospital services Includes costs for specialized treatments and elective surgeries
Specialist services	25%	Specialist consultations and diagnostic services Includes advanced medical imaging, laboratory tests, and specialist care
General practitioner services	15%	Primary care services provided by general practitioners Routine check-ups, minor procedures, and initial medical consultations
Pharmaceuticals	15%	Medication, vaccines, and other pharmaceutical products Both prescription and over-the-counter drugs
Medical schemes administration	10%	Management and operational costs of medical aid schemes Includes administrative expenses and claim processing

Source: National Cancer Registry (NCR), 2020.

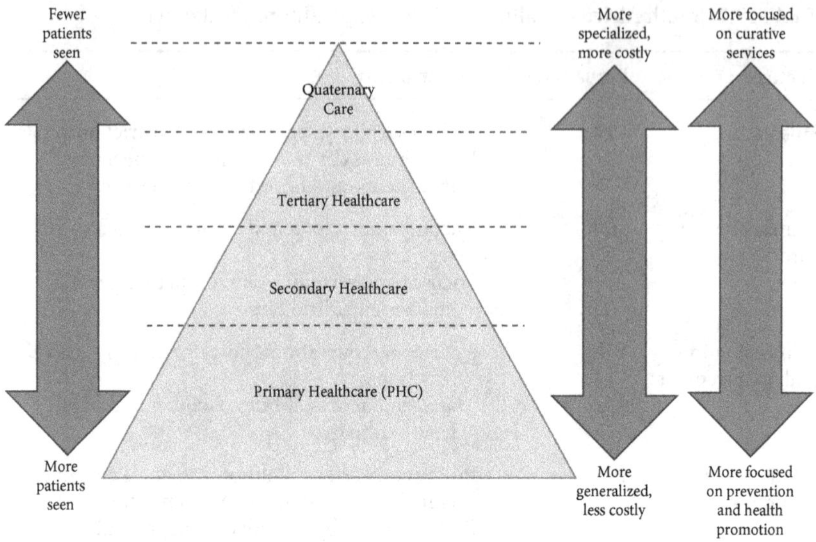

Figure 10.4 Illustration of South African healthcare system services. The levels of healthcare services are conceptualized as a pyramid going from less specialized at the bottom to more specialized healthcare at the top of the pyramid. In a well-functioning healthcare system, patients are matched with the right level of care.

equally with the right level of care without discrimination, so that all those who need the more costly services can have access to them (Keller, 2024).

Government-funded health services are structured to prioritize primary care as the initial point of contact for patients (Solanki et al., 2024). If necessary, patients can then be sent to higher levels of care that offer more specialized services (Ramlagan et al., 2024). Primary care services encompass clinics, mobile clinics, and district hospitals. Accessing higher levels of specialized care is contingent upon receiving referrals (Nash et al., 2024). Figure 10.5 displays the referral pathways that exist throughout government health services. Patients requiring more specialized care are referred from primary healthcare facilities to secondary and tertiary hospitals (Zulu & Perry, 2021). Secondary hospitals offer more complex care, including specialized medical, surgical, and diagnostic services. Tertiary hospitals, mostly located in urban centers, provide highly specialized and advanced medical care, including oncology services necessary for HNC treatment (Matolengwe et al., 2024). However, these facilities are often overwhelmed, resulting in long waiting times and limited access to timely and effective care (Zulu & Perry, 2021).

Rural and periurban areas are particularly disadvantaged, with patients frequently required to travel long distances to access specialized services. Some

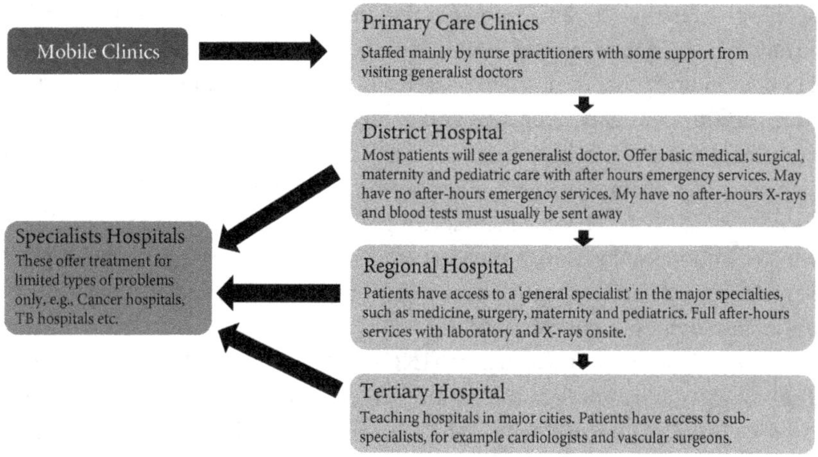

Figure 10.5 Facilities and referral pathways in the South African healthcare system. Referral pathways in the South African healthcare system are structured to ensure that patients receive the appropriate level of care at the right time. The system is designed to facilitate a smooth transition of patients from primary healthcare (PHC) facilities to secondary and tertiary care, ensuring comprehensive management of their health needs.

hospitals offer quaternary care, which involves even more specialized and advanced medical treatment and procedures, often linked to academic and research institutions (Matolengwe et al., 2024; Ramlagan et al., 2024). The public healthcare system is managed at both the provincial and national levels. Provincial health departments are responsible for the delivery of healthcare services within their regions, including the management of hospitals, clinics, and health programs (Keller, 2024; Zulu and Perry, 2021). The National Department of Health provides overarching policies, standards, and funding allocations to ensure uniformity and address national health priorities (Matolengwe et al., 2024).

10.3 Prevalence of Head and Neck Cancer in Africa

In a scoping review on HNCs in Africa, Seedat et al. (2023) reported that HNC prevalence in Africa varies significantly across the continent and is generally lower compared to more developed regions of the world. However, there are notable hotspots within Africa, particularly in southern and eastern Africa, where incidence rates can be quite high (Okerosi et al., 2023). For example, regions in southern Africa and parts of eastern Africa report higher age-standardized incidence rates (ASIR) for HNC, sometimes exceeding 13.1 cases per 100,000 people (Melariri et al., 2023). In contrast, northern and central Africa tend to have lower incidence rates of HNC, often below 6.2 cases per 100,000 people. The data indicate that the burden of HNC in Africa is not uniformly distributed, with certain areas experiencing significantly higher rates. For example, HNC prevalence ranges from Nigeria, at 27%, to Tunisia at 12%, South Africa at 12%, Tunisia at 12%, Morocco at 8%, Algeria at 7%, Sudan at 7%, and Uganda at 4% (Seedat et al., 2023). These percentages highlight the total population residing in selected countries that have a high prevalence of HNC. Nigeria has the highest prevalence, followed by South Africa and Morocco with Uganda having the least prevalence of these eight countries.

The incidence and prevalence of HNCs in Africa are likely to increase with public awareness, improved access, and screening (Solanki et al., 2024). This is largely a result of improvements in healthcare and a decline in overall mortality rates. The upward trend in the number of elderly individuals also leads to an increase in HNC incidences (Seedat et al., 2023). While more than half of the HNC cases were cancers of the oral cavity or larynx, pharyngeal cancer accounted for the remaining half (Melariri et al., 2023). Globally, the highest ASIRs for HNC are found in northern and eastern Europe and parts of Asia, where incidence rates can exceed 20 cases per 100,000 people. In North America, the incidence rates are generally lower, with most regions reporting rates below 13.1 cases per 100,000 people (Okerosi et al., 2023). The discrepancies in HNC prevalence between Africa and other regions can be attributed to several factors, including differences in risk factors like tobacco and alcohol use, HPV infection rates, and access to healthcare services for early detection and treatment (Solanki et al., 2024). Additionally, the lack of comprehensive cancer registries and diagnostic infrastructure in many African countries poses challenges in accurately assessing and managing the true burden of HNC on the continent (Keller, 2024; Zulu & Perry, 2021).

10.4 Overview of Head and Neck Cancer in South Africa

HNCs are relatively common in South Africa compared to other regions on the continent. This high prevalence is attributed to various risk factors prevalent in the population, including tobacco use, alcohol consumption, and HPV infections (Zwane et al., 2018). When assessed in terms of the proportion of HNCs to all other cancers, tobacco-related HNCs were unusually high in South African “colored” and “black” populations. Seventy percent of those diagnosed with HNC are black people (Zwane et al., 2018). The high rates of smoking and alcohol consumption in the country significantly contribute to the incidence of these cancers (Matolengwe et al., 2024). A growing body of evidence suggests that HPV, particularly HPV16, is an important etiological factor for oropharyngeal cancers in South Africa. The rise in HPV-related HNC cases mirrors trends observed in developed countries (Okerosi et al., 2023). Socioeconomic disparities also play a crucial role, with lower-income populations having higher exposure to risk factors and less access to early detection and treatment services. This disparity leads to more advanced disease at the time of diagnosis and poorer outcomes (Matolengwe et al., 2024).

Within South Africa, the prevalence of HNC is not uniform, with some regions reporting higher incidence rates. Southern African regions, including parts of South Africa, have some of the highest incidence rates of HNC on the continent. This regional variance is influenced by differing lifestyles, healthcare access, and public health policies (Ramlagan et al., 2024). Compared to other parts of the world, South Africa has a higher prevalence of HNC than most regions in Africa but lower than hotspots in northern and eastern Europe and parts of Asia (Solanki et al., 2024). In these global hotspots, the ASIRs for HNC can exceed 20 cases per 100,000 people, while in South Africa, it varies significantly but can reach similarly high rates in certain regions (Matolengwe et al., 2024). Figure 10.6 illustrates the number of histologically diagnosed HNC patients in 2020 according to the NCR.

The incidence of HNC in South Africa reflects global trends, where males typically exhibit higher rates of these cancers compared to females (Okerosi et al., 2023; Solanki et al., 2024). Several factors contribute to this disparity, including higher rates of tobacco and alcohol use among males, as well as occupational exposures and HPV infections, as highlighted earlier (Okerosi et al., 2023). Males in South Africa generally have a higher incidence of HNC compared to females for oral and laryngeal cancer (Zwane et al., 2018). There is reportedly increasing oropharyngeal cancer incidences in both genders, particularly linked to HPV, with a notable rise in females due to changes in sexual behaviors and HPV prevalence (Seedat et al., 2023). This is consistent with global patterns, where lifestyle factors such as smoking and heavy alcohol consumption are more prevalent among men. While females have a lower incidence of HNC, the rate is still significant and often linked to factors such as HPV infections, particularly in cancers of the oropharynx (Keller, 2024; Maphumulo et al., 2019).

The frequency of histologically diagnosed HNC cases in South Africa revealed a significant burden of this disease in the population, with new cases reported annually (Matolengwe et al., 2024). HNC diagnosis primarily involves histopathological examination following biopsies of suspected lesions. The availability of diagnostic resources varies, often impacting the timely and accurate diagnosis of HNC (Mhlanga & Garidzirai, 2020). Treatment modalities in South Africa include surgery, radiation therapy, and chemotherapy, similar to global standards; however, access to these treatments can be inconsistent across

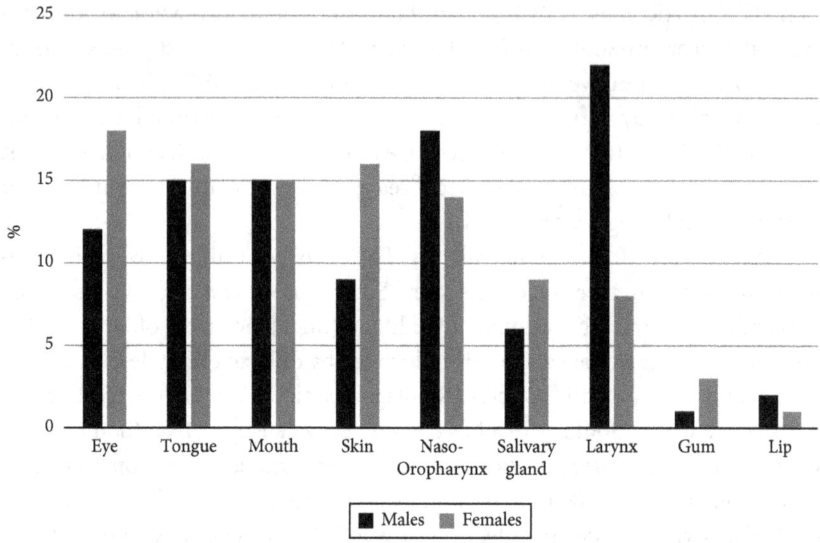

Figure 10.6 Histologically diagnosed head and neck cancer (HNC) patients in 2020 according to the National Cancer Registry. Laryngeal cancer is the most common type of HNC cancer. Although not all skin cancer cancers are located in the head and neck region, 89.9% of skin tumors have a preponderance of the head and neck region. Eye cancers occur mostly in women > 40, while gum cancers occur in females > 80 years.

different regions (Maphumulo et al., 2019). The WHO has noted the significant burden of HNCs in South Africa and highlights the need for improved healthcare infrastructure to manage this growing concern (WHO, 2024).

10.5 Background of Head and Neck Cancer Centers

HNC centers in South Africa are integral parts of the country's healthcare infrastructure, aiming to provide specialized care and treatment for patients suffering from various forms of cancer within the head and neck region (Fagan et al., 2021; Seedat et al., 2023). Table 10.3 summarizes the major HNC centers in South Africa as published by the NCR (2020). These centers are typically located within major public hospitals and private healthcare institutions, reflecting the dual nature of South Africa's healthcare system (Seedat et al., 2023). They also give an accurate picture of the national resources and health services available in South Africa for HNC treatment (Dalvie, 2019). Both public and private HNC centers in South Africa utilize MDTs comprising oncologists,

Table 10.3 Head and neck cancer centers in South Africa

HNC center	Description	Location
	Public healthcare sector	
Chris Hani Baragwanath Academic Hospital	One of the largest hospitals in the world and serves as a major referral center for HNC cases. It is affiliated with the University of the Witwatersrand and provides comprehensive cancer care, including surgery, chemotherapy, and radiation therapy.	Johannesburg
Groote Schuur Hospital	It is known for its advanced medical services and is affiliated with the University of Cape Town. The hospital has a dedicated oncology department that handles a significant number of HNC cases, offering multidisciplinary treatment options.	Cape Town
Steve Biko Academic Hospital	The hospital is another key facility for cancer treatment, including HNCs. It is affiliated with the University of Pretoria and offers specialized care through a team of oncologists, surgeons, and other healthcare professionals.	Pretoria
	Private healthcare sector	
Netcare Cancer Care	The Netcare group centers provide advanced oncological services, including for HNCs. They offer state-of-the-art technology and personalized care plans for patients.	Spread across South Africa
Life Healthcare	This private healthcare group includes several hospitals with oncology units that specialize in HNC treatment. These centers provide a range of services from diagnostic imaging to advanced surgical procedures and radiation therapy.	Spread across South Africa
Mediclinic Southern Africa	Mediclinic is a major private healthcare provider with facilities that offer comprehensive cancer care. They focus on a multidisciplinary approach to treat HNCs, incorporating the latest treatment modalities and technologies.	Spread across South Africa

Source: National Cancer Registry (NCR), 2020.

surgeons, radiologists, pathologists, and allied healthcare professionals to provide holistic care (Fagan et al., 2021). These centers are equipped with advanced diagnostic tools like positron emission tomography/computed tomography (PET/CT) scanners, magnetic resonance imaging (MRI), and molecular diagnostic facilities (Melariri et al., 2023; Seedat et al., 2023). They offer treatment options that include minimally invasive surgeries, targeted radiotherapy, and chemotherapy. Moreso, the centers are affiliated with leading universities and research institutions, contributing to ongoing research in oncology and providing training for medical students and professionals (Fagan et al., 2021; Seedat et al., 2023).

Despite the presence of advanced HNC centers, South Africa faces several challenges, including resource constraints, geographic disparities, and cost barriers (Melariri et al., 2023; Seedat et al., 2023). Public hospitals often face shortages of medical staff and resources, impacting the quality and accessibility of care (Fagan et al., 2021). There is a significant disparity in the availability of specialized cancer care between urban and rural areas. High costs in the private sector can be prohibitive for many patients, while public sector services, though more affordable, may struggle with capacity issues (Seedat et al., 2023). However, initiatives to improve cancer care infrastructure and ongoing research efforts provide opportunities to enhance the quality and accessibility of HNC treatment in the country (Fagan et al., 2021). While significant strides have been made in offering advanced treatment options, ongoing efforts are needed to address resource limitations and ensure equitable access to care across the country (Melariri et al., 2023). Collaboration between public and private sectors, along with continued investment in healthcare infrastructure and professional training, will be key to improving outcomes for patients with HNCs in South Africa (Starzyńska et al., 2022).

10.6 Importance of Organizational Structures in the Management of Head and Neck Cancer

Organizational structures are considered the skeleton of the healthcare system, and subsequent decision-making processes for any department or service can affect the overall quality of care provided (Passchier et al., 2024). To effectively analyze and improve the current status of HNC care in South Africa, it is important to understand the various organizational structures in existence (Passchier et al., 2024). This assessment identifies the types of HNC services present in South Africa and elucidates their decision-making processes and budgets, providing information that is critical to evaluate, improve, and develop organizational structures for better HNC management services (Coutts et al., 2022). Prioritizing organizational structures and decision-making processes is indispensable in the provision of quality care. With vast improvements in preventive, diagnostic, and therapeutic modalities, the complexity and specialization of healthcare practices have multiplied, and organizational structure often influences important patient outcomes (Passchier et al., 2024). It is a natural step in clinical and health services research to attempt to understand which organizational structures are better than others and for what reasons. This is a stepping stone to understanding the best possible practice for patients and how it can be facilitated (Nasa et al., 2021).

10.6.1 Referral System and Organizational Structures of Head and Neck Cancer Units

The majority of patients at state care facilities gain access to services via the casualty/emergency department, either presenting complications or being referred from a primary healthcare facility (Nash et al., 2024). Patients with a known diagnosis and referred by a medical practitioner access a specific department directly, usually the department of surgery in the case of HNC (Zulu & Perry, 2021). Patients with minor symptoms and no diagnosis often experience significant delays before investigation or examination by an appropriate specialist due to insufficient resources, lack of prioritization, and inherent backlogs in the state health sector (Maphumulo & Bhengu, 2019). Although early cancer patients may be recognized and treated more effectively, referral delays and ambiguous symptomatology can lead to advancing HNC (Matolengwe et al., 2024). There is no shortage of therapeutic options for problems such as airway obstruction for patients in need of emergency care, and they are addressed swiftly. However, the final outcomes may vary (Maphumulo & Bhengu, 2019). Budgetary constraints and/or a lack of qualified staff may make the complex HNC surgery necessary to preserve form and function impractical; in these cases, palliative surgery or the best available medical therapy may be chosen (Becker et al., 2012). State care falls within the jurisdiction of the public health sector. State cancer centers manage patients' cancer care in their entirety. Typical management methods include a combination of surgery, radiotherapy, or chemotherapy. A team of specialists generally provides treatment (Matolengwe et al., 2024; Nash et al., 2024).

10.6.2 State Care Facilities

Presently, a referral system unique to oncology suggests that some of the larger centers of excellence ought to serve as regional oncology units offering a wide range of oncology services (Fagan et al., 2021). For most people, this would maximize access to the finest available cancer care. Specialist maxillofacial and head and neck surgeons' roles within this framework for integrated oncology services must be clarified and refined. This is part of a larger national health scheme/plan. A survey of the present services offered in a particular region is under way, and a minimal dataset regarding the composition and operation of hospitals offering oncology care has been developed (Ramutumbu et al., 2023). In recent years, cancer treatment has been decentralized to rural and underserved regions where the majority of the population lives. This is in recognition of the fact that all South African citizens have the right to access the same level and quality of healthcare. This move was an attempt to rectify the inequity of the past, where racial and social inequality often determined access to care (Fagan et al., 2021). This initiative was facilitated by an increase in funding from the central government for oncology services and the introduction of a global health funding project by the Department of Health, specializing in oncology services (Maphumulo & Bhengu, 2019).

Patients from metropolitan populations have traditionally been referred to large academic centers that house head and neck oncology services in major cities (Seedat et al., 2023). This was linked to the finest possible medical treatment in the area, but the way these services were integrated into the entire oncology framework was frequently subpar, and patients either lost track of their care or were directed back to adjacent state hospitals or clinics for radiotherapy (Melariri et al., 2023). Curative services for people diagnosed with cancer are mainly situated in academic settings and consist of medical/pediatric oncology, clinical hematology, radiation oncology, and specialized surgical services through a MDT. Infrastructure and capacity to treat adults with cancer are variable throughout the country (Fagan et al., 2021). For example, screening for cervical cancer and treatment of precancerous cells as well as education and awareness initiatives occur at a primary healthcare level and vary in terms of coverage and quality of care (Melariri et al., 2023; Seedat et al., 2023).

Many tertiary specialist units are grossly understaffed and poorly equipped and are thus unable to provide holistic care for the majority of patients (Maphumulo & Bhengu, 2019). To understand the current situation regarding cancer treatment centers, researchers audited some facilities to ascertain a baseline of service delivery (Fagan et al., 2021). This baseline informs the interventions required to strengthen current services, and work has commenced on addressing such needs. It is of concern that pediatric oncology services are limited in the provinces of Northern Cape, Northwest, Mpumalanga, Limpopo, and KwaZulu Natal (Zwane et al., 2018). Noting the existing situation in South Africa, the National Cancer Strategic Framework (NCSF) organization will prioritize health systems gaps related to equitable access to diagnostics and treatments. Table 10.4 is a summary of the current facilities that offer oncological services in South Africa.

Table 10.4 Current facilities that offer oncological services in the South Africa

Province	Hospital	Clinical oncology and hematology permanent staff	Pediatric oncology and hematology permanent staff	Radiation equipment	Surgical equipment	Pharmacy
Free State	National and Universitas Annex	4	1	Sufficient	Sufficient	Sufficient
Gauteng	CMJAH	9	4	Insufficient, outdated, poor maintenance	Sufficient	Good
Gauteng	CHBAH	Medical: 0 Haema: 3 Radiation: N/A	3	N/A	Good	Sufficient
Gauteng	George Mukhar	Unknown	1	Refer to SBAH	Refer to SBAH	Insufficient
Gauteng	Nelson Mandela Children's Hospital	Under construction	Under construction	N/A	Under Construction	Under construction
Gauteng	SBAH	Clinical: 5 Haema: 2	3	Sufficient but poor maintenance	Sufficient	Good
KZN	Addington	Clinical: 0 Haema: 1	2	Nonoperational	Sufficient	Sufficient
KZN	IALCH	0	0	Nonoperational	Sufficient	Sufficient
KZN	Greys	4	1	Sufficient for adult service only	Sufficient	Sufficient

(*continued*)

Table 10.4 Continued

Province	Hospital	Clinical oncology and hematology permanent staff	Pediatric oncology and hematology permanent staff	Radiation equipment	Surgical equipment	Pharmacy
KZN	Ngwelezana	2 part-time. Service rendered by public–private partnership	Service rendered by public–private partnership	Service rendered by public–private partnership	Service rendered by public–private partnership	Service rendered by public–private partnership
Northwest	Klerksdorp	2	0	Sufficient	Sufficient	Sufficient
Mpumalanga	Mbombela	0	0	Insufficient	Insufficient	Insufficient
Northern Cape	Kimberley	2	1	Not available	Insufficient	Sufficient
Eastern Cape	Frere	2	1	Sufficient	Sufficient	Sufficient
Eastern Cape	Livingston	2	1	Sufficient	Insufficient	Excellent
Eastern Cape	Nelson Mandela Central Hospital	Under construction	Under construction	Under construction	Under construction	Under construction
Limpopo	Polokwane	2	1	Insufficient	Insufficient	Insufficient
Western Cape	George	Service rendered by public–private partnership	Service rendered by public–private partnership	Service rendered by public–private partnership	Service rendered by public–private partnership	Service rendered by public–private partnership
Western Cape	Groote Schuur Hospital	9 + 12 Supernumerary	3 (Red Cross)	Sufficient	Sufficient	Good
Western Cape	Tygerberg	6	2	Sufficient	Sufficient	Sufficient

Source: National cancer strategic framework 2017–2023; Department of Health, 2017.

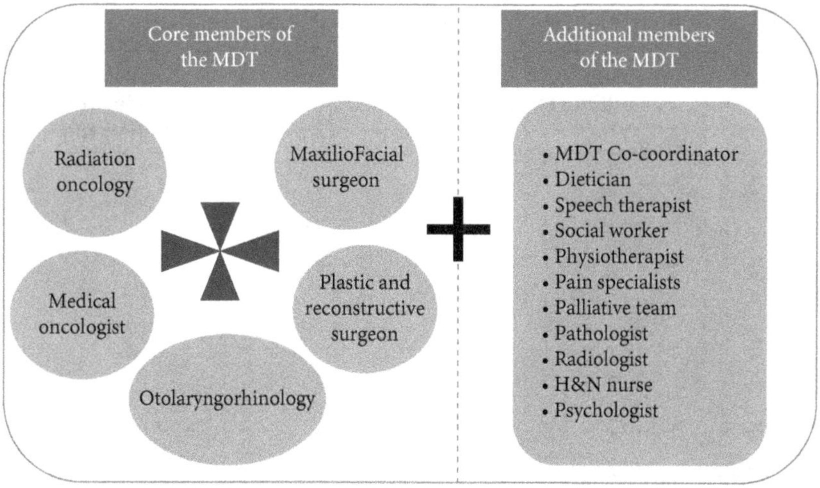

Figure 10.7 A summary of all multidisciplinary team members consisting of core members and additional team members. Head and neck cancer (HNC) presents a complex clinical challenge that necessitates a multidisciplinary approach for effective management and treatment.

10.6.3 Structure and Roles of Staff

HNC presents a complex clinical challenge that necessitates a multidisciplinary approach for effective management and treatment (Maphumulo & Bhengu, 2019). The South African healthcare system, comprising both public and private sectors, employs various strategies to integrate multiple disciplines in addressing HNC (Figure 10.7) (Malakoane et al., 2020; Matolengwe et al., 2024). This approach ensures comprehensive patient care, combining the expertise of various specialists to improve treatment outcomes and patient quality of life (Zulu & Perry, 2021). The interdisciplinary HNC team works together, but, in cases of advanced malignancy, the intensive care unit team plays a crucial role in the patient's postoperative care and is therefore an essential part of the management group (Melariri et al., 2023; Seedat et al., 2023). Apart from the core medical team stated above, the finance team and digital data systems representatives should ideally join the team to obtain a clear prospective costing of all interventions discussed and to correctly capture data for analytics later (Shellenberger & Weber, 2018).

10.7 Private Care Facilities

A few head and neck oncology surgeons have private hospital operating rights; however, it is difficult to distinguish between private and public health sector

Table 10.5 Number of private healthcare facilities per province

Province	Population (in millions)	GDP per province in US$ (2022)	Number of hospitals	Number of hospitals per 100K people
Gauteng	14.55	134,682	127	1
Western Cape	6.21	56,286	55	1
KwaZulu Natal	5.46	64,696	37	1
Eastern Cape	2.58	30,903	19	1
Free State	2.52	20,041	16	1
Northwest	1.22	26,903	11	1
Mpumalanga	1.37	32,598	10	1
Northern Cape	435.29	9,069	8	1
Limpopo	777.46	31,348	3	~1

Source: South African Health Review, 2020.

patient outcomes (Melariri et al., 2023; Seedat et al., 2023). Table 10.5 is a summary of the number of private healthcare facilities per province in South Africa (South African Health Review, 2020). Specialist physician care mainly occurs in rooms with or without day-clinic facilities. Medical and radiation oncologists share in the treatment of HNC (Matolengwe et al., 2024). South African medical oncology is also a small subspecialty with few practitioners; therefore, only a few medical oncologists specialize in head and neck oncology to treat patients undergoing systemic therapy (Malakoane et al., 2020; Matolengwe et al., 2024). A few private institutions have radiation therapy facilities, and participation in clinical trials through collaborative groups is increasing (Melariri et al., 2023). In a study involving private oncologists treating patients with HNC in Pretoria, 47% of the patients received radiation therapy as definitive treatment, 10% received adjuvant therapy, and 7% received palliative treatment. The remaining patients were referred to public institutions for treatment (Seedat et al., 2023).

10.8 Limitations and Challenges

The dual nature of the South African healthcare system creates a fragmented environment where public and private sectors operate independently, leading to inefficiencies and disparities in care (Solanki et al., 2024). The unequal distribution of resources between the public and private sectors exacerbates health disparities. The public healthcare sector in South Africa is severely underfunded, resulting in significant resource constraints (Nash et al., 2024). Public hospitals often lack the necessary equipment, medication, and trained personnel to provide comprehensive care for HNC patients (Malakoane et al., 2020). Coordination between these sectors is limited, thus hindering comprehensive and cohesive healthcare delivery. Limited financial resources lead to shortages of essential medical supplies, outdated equipment, and insufficient infrastructure, all of which impede the delivery of effective healthcare services, including those for HNC. Investments in health infrastructure and human resources are crucial to address these gaps (Malakoane et al., 2020; Matolengwe et al., 2024).

There is a critical shortage of healthcare professionals in the public sector. The imbalance between the number of patients and the available healthcare providers results in overworked staff and burnout, further diminishing the quality of care (Keller, 2024). The scarcity of specialists, particularly in oncology, exacerbates this issue, delaying diagnosis and treatment for HNC patients (Ramlagan et al., 2024). Increasing the number of trained specialists in the public sector and improving working conditions to retain these professionals are vital steps. Incentive programs and continued professional development opportunities can help achieve this goal. Specialized healthcare services, including oncology care for HNC, are predominantly concentrated in urban areas (Solanki et al., 2024). Figure 10.8 is a summary of the limitations in the South African healthcare system regarding the treatment of HNC.

Patients in rural and periurban regions face significant barriers to accessing these services, including long travel distances, transportation costs, and time away from work and family (Keller, 2024). This geographic disparity leads to delayed diagnoses and poorer outcomes for rural populations. Rural health facilities often lack the necessary infrastructure to provide comprehensive care. This includes inadequate diagnostic tools, limited surgical facilities, and insufficient follow-up care options (Ramlagan et al., 2024). Consequently, patients from these areas must travel to urban centers for specialized treatment, further exacerbating access issues. Financial constraints and lack of health insurance limit access to private healthcare services (Malakoane et al., 2020; Matolengwe et al., 2024). A significant portion of the South African population lacks health insurance, limiting their access to the private healthcare sector, which offers better resourced and more timely care. The out-of-pocket expenses for medical consultations, treatments, and travel can be prohibitive, particularly for low-income individuals and leads to delayed or foregone care (Keller, 2024).

South Africa's NHI aims to provide universal health coverage and improve access to quality care for all South Africans. While policies such as the NHI aim to

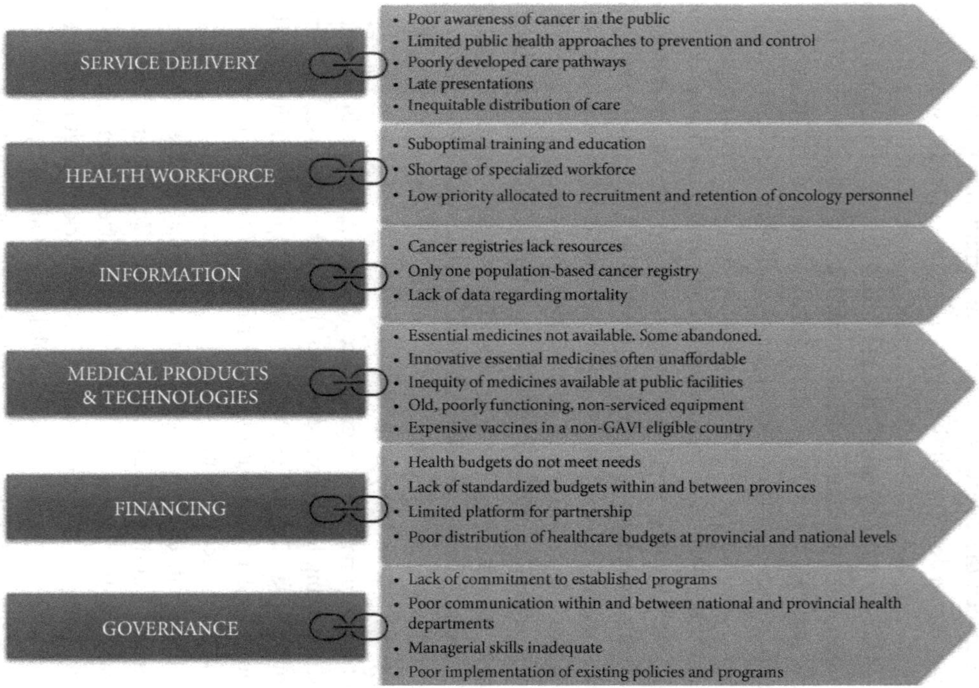

Figure 10.8 A summary of the limitations in the South African healthcare system regarding the treatment of head and neck cancer (HNC). Addressing these challenges requires a multifaceted approach that includes increased funding, improved healthcare infrastructure, enhanced training and recruitment of specialized healthcare professionals, and greater public awareness. Effective policy and governance reforms are also essential to ensure equitable access to high-quality cancer care for all South Africans.

improve access to healthcare, their implementation faces significant challenges (Solanki et al., 2024). Bureaucratic delays, resistance from vested interests, and logistical complexities impede the effective rollout of these policies (Malakoane et al., 2020; Matolengwe et al., 2024). Strengthening the public healthcare system and expanding health insurance coverage through initiatives like the NHI could mitigate these barriers and promote more equitable access to care (Keller, 2024). Successful implementation of the NHI could significantly enhance access to specialized services, including those for HNC, by redistributing resources and reducing the disparity between public and private healthcare sectors. Hence, ensuring that the NHI can bridge the gap between public and private healthcare remains a daunting task (Malakoane et al., 2020; Matolengwe et al., 2024).

Cultural stigma and misinformation surrounding cancer can lead to delays in seeking medical help (Ramlagan et al., 2024). Patients may resort to traditional or alternative remedies instead of seeking conventional medical treatment. Social stigma associated with conditions like HPV can also deter individuals from seeking timely care (Malakoane et al., 2020). Language and cultural differences between healthcare providers and patients can hinder effective communication, impacting the quality of care (Matolengwe et al., 2024). Misunderstandings and lack of culturally sensitive care can result in misdiagnoses, noncompliance with treatment plans, and overall poorer health outcomes (Ramlagan et al., 2024). Thus, the South African healthcare system faces numerous limitations and challenges in providing effective and equitable care for HNC (Seedat et al., 2023). Addressing these issues requires substantial investment in the public health sector, strategic policy implementation, and enhanced coordination between public and private health services (Matolengwe et al., 2024).

There is a lack of awareness and education about the risk factors, early symptoms, and importance of early detection of HNC (Okerosi et al., 2023). This is particularly prevalent in lower socioeconomic groups who may not have access to health education resources (Malakoane et al., 2020; Matolengwe et al., 2024). Public health campaigns are often underfunded and may not reach all segments of the population effectively. Effective public health campaigns focused on reducing tobacco and alcohol use and promoting HPV vaccination are critical (Hunter et al., 2024). HPV-related HNC is a growing concern. The introduction of HPV vaccination programs has the potential to reduce the incidence of these cancers significantly (Okerosi et al., 2023). However, widespread implementation and uptake of these programs are necessary to see a population-level impact, which requires coordinated public health efforts and sufficient funding (Malakoane et al., 2020).

These campaigns must be well-funded and tailored to reach diverse population groups, particularly those in underserved areas (Okerosi et al., 2023). Rural areas face significant barriers to accessing specialized care. Improving access to specialized care, particularly in rural areas, along with targeted public health campaigns and education initiatives, are crucial steps toward mitigating the burden of HNC in South Africa (Fagan et al., 2021). Improving transportation infrastructure and developing decentralized care models, such as telemedicine, could help bridge this gap (Seedat et al., 2023). Ensuring that rural health facilities are adequately equipped and staffed is also essential. Overcoming these challenges will involve a concerted effort from the government, healthcare providers, and the community to ensure that all South Africans receive the quality care they need and deserve (Malakoane et al., 2020; Matolengwe et al., 2024).

10.9 Conclusion

The South African healthcare system, characterized by its dual public and private sectors, faces significant challenges in providing equitable access to specialized and effective care for HNC. The public sector, serving the majority of the population, struggles with resource constraints, infrastructural deficiencies, and high patient loads, leading to delays in diagnosis and treatment. Conversely, the private sector, although well-resourced, remains accessible primarily to those with health insurance, thus exacerbating health disparities based on socioeconomic status. Addressing the disparities in access to specialized care necessitates comprehensive policy interventions, increased investment in the public health sector, and strategic investments in infrastructure and human resources. HNC represents a substantial public health issue in South Africa. Early detection and timely treatment are crucial for improving patient outcomes, yet these are often hindered by the limitations of the public health system. Efforts to promote HPV vaccination and reduce risk factors are essential but require adequate funding and strategic implementation to be effective. Enhancing public health campaigns and expanding health insurance coverage through initiatives like the NHI are crucial steps toward reducing health disparities and improving outcomes for HNC patients.

The proposed NHI scheme holds promise for providing more equitable access to quality care by redistributing resources and integrating the public and private health systems. Additionally, improving transportation infrastructure, decentralizing care models, and strengthening rural health facilities are critical steps toward ensuring that all South Africans, regardless of their location or socioeconomic status, can access the specialized care they need. Training and retaining more specialists within the public sector, along with improving working conditions, are vital for enhancing the quality of care for HNC patients. Continued professional development and incentive programs can help achieve this goal. While significant challenges remain, strategic investments, policy reforms, and coordinated efforts across all sectors of the healthcare system are essential for improving the management and treatment of HNC in South Africa. By addressing these issues, the country can move toward a more equitable healthcare system that provides comprehensive and effective care for all its citizens. Achieving these goals will require coordinated efforts from the government, healthcare providers, and the broader community to ensure that all South Africans have access to the care they need.

References

AFRICA HEALTH EXHIBITION. 2020. Industry insights: South Africa healthcare market overview. https://prod65.africahealthexhibition.com/content/dam/Informa/africahealthexhibition/en/2020/pdf/AFH19_Industry_Insights-SA_MARKET_REPORT.pdf

ALUTTIS, C., BISHAW, T., & FRANK, M. 2014. The workforce for health in a globalized context: Global shortages and international migration. *Glob Health Action*, 7(1), 23640. https://doi.org/10.3402/gha.v7.23640

AYOUB, A. & PULIJALA, Y. 2019. The application of virtual reality and augmented reality in oral and maxillofacial surgery. *BMC Oral Health*.

BECKER, J., DELL, A., JENKINS, L., & SAYED, R. 2012. Reasons why patients with primary health care problems access a secondary hospital emergency centre. *South African Medical Journal*, 102(10), 800–1.

COLLINSON, M., TOLLMAN, S., & KAHN, K. 2007. Migration, settlement change and health in post-apartheid South Africa: Triangulating health and demographic surveillance with national census data. *Scand J Public Health*, 69, 77–84.

COUNCIL FOR MEDICAL SCHEMES (CMS). 2024. Annual performance plan for 2023/24. https://www.medicalschemes.co.za/cms-annual-report-2023-24/

COUTTS, K. A., SEEDAT, J., & VLOK, E. 2022. The management of head and neck cancer in Africa: What lessons can be learned from African literature? *S Afr J Oncol*, 6(0), a204.

DALVIE, S. 2019. Head and neck cancer in Africa. *S Afr J Oncol*, 3(0), a67.

DE VILLIERS, K. 2021. Bridging the health inequality gap: An examination of South Africa's social innovation in health landscape. *Infect Dis Poverty* 10, 19.

DELOBELLE, P., RAWLINSON, J. L., NTULI, S., MALATSI, I., DECOCK, R., & DEPOORTER, A.-M. 2011. Job satisfaction and turnover intent of primary healthcare nurses in rural South Africa: A questionnaire survey. *J Adv Nurs*, 67(2), 371–83.

DEPARTMENT OF HEALTH. 2017. National Cancer Strategic Framework 2017–2023. Pretoria: Department of Health. Available at: http://www.health.gov.za/national_cancer_framework.pdf [Accessed June 30, 2024.]

DLAMINI, L. P., & NGALAWA, H. 2021. Macroprudential policy and house prices in an estimated dynamic stochastic general equilibrium model for South Africa. *Australian Economic Papers: Wiley Blackwell*, 61(2), 304–36.

DOKU, D. T., ACACIO-CLARO, P. J., KOIVUSILTA, L., & RIMPELÄ, A. 2019. Health and socioeconomic circumstances over three generations as predictors of youth unemployment trajectories. *Eur J Public Health*, 29(3), 517–23.

FAGAN, J. J., NORONHA, V., & GRABOYES, E. M. 2021. Making the best of limited resources: Improving outcomes in head and neck cancer. *American Society of Clinical Oncology educational book. American Society of Clinical Oncology. Annual Meeting*, 41, 1–11. https://doi.org/10.1200/EDBK_320923

GÓMEZ-OLIVÉ, F. X., MONTANA, L., WAGNER, R. G., KABUDULA, C. W., ROHR, J. K., KAHN, K., BÄRNIGHAUSEN, T., COLLINSON, M., CANNING, D., GAZIANO, T., SALOMON, J. A., PAYNE, C. F., WADE, A., TOLLMAN, S. M., & BERKMAN, L. 2018. Cohort profile: Health and ageing in Africa: A longitudinal study of an INDEPTH community in South Africa (HAALSI). *Int J Epidemiol*, 47(3), 689–90j.

HOFFMAN, H. T., FUNK, G. F., ROBINSON, R. A., & MENCK, H. R. 1998. The National Cancer Data Base report on cancer of the head and neck. *Arch Otolaryngol Head Neck Surg*, 124(9), 951–62.

HUNTER, M., PETERS, S., KHUMALO, N., & DAVIES, M. A. 2024. Analysis of patient flow and barriers to timely discharge from general medical wards at a tertiary academic hospital in Cape Town, South Africa. *BMC Health Serv Res*, 24(1), 287.

KELLER, M. M. 2024. National Health Insurance interprofessional practice implementation in hand rehabilitation service delivery in South Africa. *S Afr J Physiother*, 80(1), 1969.

KNOEMA. 2023. South Africa Health expenditure as a share of GDP, 1960–2023. Retrieved from Knoema. https://knoema.com/atlas/South-Africa/Health-expenditure-per-capita

KRUGER, A., & SHONGWE, S. 2004. Temperature trends in South Africa: 1960–2003. *Int J Climatol*, 24(15), 1929–45.

KUTZIN, J., & SPARKES, S. P. 2016. Health systems strengthening, universal health coverage, health security and resilience. *Bull WHO*, 94(1), 2.

MALAKOANE, B., HEUNIS, J. C., CHIKOBVU, P., et al., 2020. Public health system challenges in the free state, South Africa: A situation appraisal to inform health system strengthening. *BMC Health Serv Res*, 20(1), 1–14.

MAPHUMULO, W. T., & BHENGU, B. R. 2019. Challenges of quality improvement in the healthcare of South Africa post-apartheid: A critical review. *Curationis*, 42(1), e1–e9.

MASIS, L., GICHAGA, A., ZERAYACOB, T., LU, C., & PERRY, H. B. 2021. Community health workers at the dawn of a new era: 4. Programme financing. *Health Res Policy Syst*, 19(Suppl 3), 107.

MATOLENGWE, A., MURRAY, D., & OKAFOR, U. B. 2024. The challenges of implementing a health referral system in South Africa: A qualitative study. *Risk Manag Healthc Policy*, 17, 855–64.

M'BOUAFFOU, F., BUCH, É., OLORUNJU, S., & THSEHLA, E. 2022. Perceived knowledge of scheme members and their satisfaction with their medical schemes: A cross-sectional study in South Africa. *BMC Public Health*, 22(1), 1700.

MCLAREN, Z. M., ARDINGTON, C., & LEIBBRANDT, M. 2014. Distance decay and persistent health care disparities in South Africa. *BMC Health Serv Res*, 14, 541.

MELARIRI, H., ELS, T., OYEDELE, O., SUTTLE, T. K., BERMOSKY, K. T., DE FREITAS, A., MURTAZA, A., MOOSAJEE, M., & MELARIRI, P. E. 2023. Prevalence of locoregional recurrence and survival post-treatment of head and neck cancers in Africa: A systematic review and meta-analysis. *EClinicalMedicine*, 59, 101964.

MHLANGA, D., & GARIDZIRAI, R. 2020. The influence of racial differences in the demand for healthcare in South Africa: A case of public healthcare. *Int J Environ Res Public Health*, 17(14), 5043.

MINISTERIAL TASK TEAM ON SOCIAL HEALTH INSURANCE REFORM. 2005. Social health insurance options: Financial and fiscal impact assessment. Discussion Document. June 2005. https://www.gov.za/sites/default/files/nationalhealthinsurance.pdf

NASA, P., JAIN, R., & JUNEJA, D. 2021. Delphi methodology in healthcare research: How to decide its appropriateness. *World J Methodol*, 11(4), 116–29.

NASH, J., ROSS, A. J., NAIDOO, M., RAS, T., BRITS, H., & MATHEW, S. 2024. Health budget cuts will be paid for by the most vulnerable. *S Afr Fam Pract 2004*, 66(1), e1–e2.

NATIONAL CANCER REGISTRY (NCR). 2020. NCR Annual Reports. https://www.nicd.ac.za/centres/national-cancer-registry/

NATIONAL TREASURY 2024 BUDGET REVIEW. 2024. reasury.gov.za/documents/National%20Budget/2024/review/Chapter%206.pdf

OECD. 2021. Health Spending. OECD Health Statistics. https://www.oecd.org/content/dam/oecd/en/publications/reports/2024/12/latest-health-spending-trends_7332c460/df0bb1ba-en.pdf

OKEROSI, S., MOKOH, L. W., RUBAGUMYA, F., NIYIBIZI, B. A., NKYA, A., VAN LOON, K., BUCKLE, G., BENT, S., HA, P., FAGAN, J. J., NG, D., ASWANI, J., & XU, M. J. 2023. Human papillomavirus-associated head and neck malignancies in sub-Saharan Africa: A systematic review. *JCO Glob Oncol*, 9, e2200259.

OLAYUNGBO, D. O., & IQBAL, B. A. 2021. An empirical analysis of African trade blocs effects on the global economy: New evidence from the gravity model. *Future Business Journal*, 7, 45.

PASSCHIER, E., BECK, A. C. C., STUIVER, M. M., RETÈL, V. P., NAVRAN, A., VAN HARTEN, W. H., VAN DEN BREKEL, M. W. M., & VAN DER MOLEN, L. 2024. Dutch Head, Neck Society: Organization of head and neck cancer rehabilitation care: A national survey among healthcare professionals in Dutch head and neck cancer centers. *Eur Arch Otorhinolaryngol*, 281(5), 2575–85.

PAVER, R., DE WITTE, H., ROTHMANN, S., VAN DEN BROECK, A., & BLONK, R. W. B. 2020. The implementation and evaluation of the South African adaptation of the JOBS program. *Front Psychol*, 11, 1418.

PILLAY, A., & SIYOTHULA, E. -T. B. 2008. The training institutions of Black African clinical psychologists registered with the HPCSA in 2006. *S Afr J Psychol*, 38(4), 725–35.

RAMLAGAN, S., SEWPAUL, R., SHEAN, Y., SCHMIDT, T., NORTH, A., & REDDY, S. P. 2024. Psychological distress among South African healthcare workers during the COVID-19 pandemic. *Curationis*, 47(1), e1–e12.

RAMUTUMBU, N. J., RAMATHUBA, D. U., & MAPUTLE, M. S. 2023. Barriers to accessing oncology services for effective cancer care in the public health institutions in Limpopo Province, South Africa: A qualitative study. *Nurs Rep (Pavia, Italy)*, 13(3), 956–68.

RENSBURG, R. 2021. Healthcare in South Africa: How inequity is contributing to inefficiency, University of the Witwatersrand. The Conversation AFRICA, July 6, 2021. https://www.wits.ac.za/news/latest-news/opinion/2021/2021-07/healthcare-in-south-africa-how-inequity-is-contributing-to-inefficienc

ROY, K., HIMELFARB, A., KARRAH, K., PORTERFIELD, L., PAREMOER, L., SERAG, H., & LEE, W. C. 2022. The social, behavioral, and ethical modalities of COVID-19 on HIV care in South Africa: A systematic review. *Int J Environ Res Public Health*, 19(15), 9766.

SCHNEIDER, M. T., CHANG, A. Y., CHAPIN, A., CHEN, C. S., CROSBY, S. W., HARLE, A. C., TSAKALOS, G., ZLAVOG, B. S., & DIELEMAN, J. L. 2021. Health expenditures by services and providers for 195 countries, 2000–2017. *BMJ Global Health* 6, e005799.

SEEDAT, J., COUTTS, K., & VLOK, E. 2023. Epidemiology and demographics of head and neck cancer in Africa: A scoping review. *Afr J Prim Health Care Fam Med*, 15(1), e1–e13.

SHELLENBERGER, T. D., & WEBER, R. S. 2018. Multidisciplinary team planning for patients with head and neck cancer. *Oral Maxillofac Surg Clin North Am*, 30(4), 435–44.

SILVER, S. R., LI, J., & QUAY, B. 2022. Employment status, unemployment duration, and health-related metrics among US adults of prime working age: Behavioral risk factor surveillance system, 2018–2019. *Am J Indust Med*, 65(1), 59–71.

SINGH, G. K. 2021. Trends and social inequalities in maternal mortality in the United States, 1969–2018. *Int J Matern Child Health AIDS*, 10(1), 29–42.

SOLANKI, G., WILKINSON, T., MYBURGH, N. G., CORNELL, J. E., & BRIJLAL, V. 2024. South African healthcare reforms towards universal healthcare: Where to next? *S Afr Med J*, 114(3), e1571.

SOUTH AFRICAN HEALTH REVIEW. 2020. Health Systems Trust. https://www.hst.org.za/publications/Pages/SAHR2020.aspx

STARZYŃSKA, A., SOBOCKI, B. K., & ALTERIO, D. 2022. Current challenges in head and neck cancer management. *Cancers*, 14(2), 358.

STATISTICS SOUTH AFRICA. 2024. Quarterly labour force survey, Q1 2024. Available at: https://www.statssa.gov.za [Accessed June 27, 2024.]

THERN, E., MUNTER, J. D., HEMMINGSSON, T., & RASMUSSEN, F. 2017. Long-term effects of youth unemployment on mental health: Does an economic crisis affect mental health? *J Epidemiol Commun Health*, 71(4), 344–9.

VAN DEN HEEVER, A. M. 2016. South Africa's universal health coverage reforms in the post-apartheid period. *Health Policy*, 120(12), 1420–8.

VISAGIE, J., & POSEL, D. 2013. A reconsideration of what and who is middle class in South Africa. *Development Southern Africa*, 30(2), 149–67.

WORLD BANK. 2021. World development indicators: Health expenditure, total (% of GDP). https://data.worldbank.org/indicator/SH.XPD.CHEX.GD.ZS

WORLD BANK. 2024. Population data. World Bank Data. https://data.worldbank.org/indicator/SP.POP.TOTL

WORLD HEALTH ORGANIZATION. 2019. Global health expenditure database. https://apps.who.int/nha/database

WORLDOMETER. 2024. Available at: https://www.worldometers.info/world-population/ [Accessed June 27, 2024.]

YAMOAH, K., LEE, K. M., AWASTHI, S., ALBA, P. R., PEREZ, C., ANGLIN-FOOTE, T. R., ROBISON, B., GAO, A., DUVALL, S. L., KATSOULAKIS, E., WONG, Y. N., MARKT, S. C., ROSE, B. S., BURRI, R., WANG, C., ABOIRALOR, O., FINK, A. K., NICKOLS, N. G., LYNCH, J. A., & GARRAWAY, I. P. 2022. Racial and ethnic disparities in prostate cancer outcomes in the veterans' affairs healthcare system. *JAMA Netw Open*, 5, e2144027.

YOUNGER, D. S. 2016. Health care in South Africa. *Neurol Clin*, 34(4), 1127–36.

ZULU, J. M., & PERRY, H. B. 2021 Community health workers at the dawn of a new era. *Health Res Policy Syst*, 19(Suppl 3), 130.

ZWANE, N. B., MOHANGI, G. U., & SHANGASE, S. L. 2018. Head and neck cancers among HIV-positive patients: A five-year retrospective study from a Johannesburg hospital, South Africa. *S Afr Dental J*, 73(3), 121–6.

SECTION IV

SURVIVORSHIP, QUALITY OF LIFE, AND HOLISTIC CARE

11

Survivorship and Quality of Life in Head and Neck Cancer

Thabiso Victor Miya, Langanani Mbodi, Alexandre Kokoua, Emmanuel Konan, and Zodwa Dlamini

11.1 Introduction

11.1.1 Definition of Terms

Individuals who survive head and neck cancers (HNCs) are faced with lifetime challenges related to the disease process, complications of therapy, and adjustment to activities of daily living, workplace, and participation in communities. These problems could be emotional, physical, or a combination and the onset may vary depending on many factors (Ringash et al., 2018). The terms "survivorship care" and "palliative care" have been previously utilized interchangeably and even confused by both patients and caregivers. There is a need to clarify the nature of care described because patients may have both misunderstandings and different expectations (Geerse et al., 2018).

11.1.1.1 Survivorship

Survivorship care is often used to define the phase of care following completion of treatment. However, the phrase may also be applied to those living with the active disease (Hoffman et al., 2006). The definition by the National Cancer Institute extends from the period of diagnosis throughout life (Figure 11.1). It also includes all the support structures that the patient has (family, friends, caregivers, etc.) who are affected by the survivorship (Khan et al., 2012). In the modern day, although acknowledging that *survivorship* begins during the period of diagnosis, *survivorship care* is defined as the period after primary treatment. Survivorship in cancer in general is still not well understood, and there is no concrete agreement on its definition and scope in HNCs as well (Kean et al., 2021).

11.1.1.2 Palliative Care

To some, including patients and family, the concept of palliative care (PC) is confused with the end-of-life, terminal stage of the disease even though many

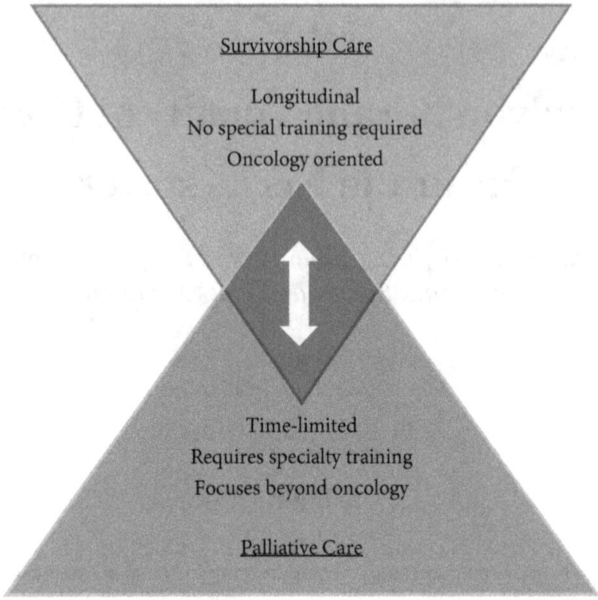

Figure 11.1 A comparison between survivorship care and palliative care appears to show an opposite, inverted picture of each other. However, they have the same goals of improving patient well-being and patient-centered care and they require interdisciplinary and multiprofessional collaboration.

patients have not reached the end of life (Zhi & Smith, 2015). By definition, it is care that focuses on symptom control and ameliorating quality of life (QOL), and it involves both patients and their support structure (Figure 11.1). This care is begun early in the stage of the disease and can be offered concurrently with chemotherapy or radiotherapy for HNCs. However, few patients receive PC services, especially in Africa and low- and middle-income countries (LMICs) (Ferrell et al., 2017).

HNC disrupts nutrition, emotional communication, feeding, respiratory, and comfort mechanisms. Physical effects include scarring, deformity, and a stoma for neck breathing (Chen et al., 2022b). HNC survivors confront two recovery challenges: systematic and locoregional. Pretreatment intervention, linkage, and education are crucial for setting realistic survivor expectations and functioning baselines. These routines impact the HNC survivor's experience from the outset (Jacobson, 2018; Malloy & Pou, 2017). The phrase "survivorship experience" refers to the broad idea that compiles the specifics of a cancer patient's complex post-diagnosis reality into a composite narrative that spans the course of the patient's life in all of its acute, protracted, and permanent phases (Kraus, 2016). It includes the accompanying life-altering events linked to shifting symptoms, functional difficulties, and effects on interpersonal relationships, finances, legal matters, and way of life (Nightingale et al., 2016). With the use of tradeoffs between treatment-related morbidity and survival advantages, patients are becoming increasingly involved in medical choices regarding oncological treatments. A patient's QOL, needs, preferences, and availability of caregivers are all elements that should be considered at the same time (Salvestrini et al., 2022). Windon et al. (2019) examined the viewpoints and preferences of patients with HNC in a recent paper (Windon et al., 2019). Preferences for "cure of disease," "survival as long as possible," and "trusting in healthcare providers" were most commonly expressed. All patients shared the fear of recurrence, and, compared to other HNC subgroups, laryngeal cancer patients gave speech difficulties far more thought (Bonomo et al., 2020; Windon et al., 2019). As such, this chapter focuses on the long-term management of patients who have survived HNC after primary therapy is completed. It delves into the mental, physical, and social dimensions of survivorship and includes approaches to facilitate the general QOL for individuals who have received medical treatment as well as rehabilitation and supporting care.

11.2 Survivorship in Head and Neck Cancer

The 2005 seminal publication, *From Cancer Patient to Cancer Survivor: Lost in Translation*, was the first to discuss the idea of survivorship care (National Research Council, 2006). In this publication, the authors outlined the necessity of a patients' survivorship care plan as well as (1) increased awareness of the functional, psychological, and medical impact of cancer and its treatments; (2) defined quality healthcare for survivors of cancer and identified strategies to acquire it; and (3) the necessity for policies to guarantee survivors' access to psychosocial services, health insurance, and fair employment practices to improve their QOL.

Since then, a large number of organizations have documented the late impact of cancer and therapy (both psychological and physical) and, even more important, have looked at the efficacy of various interventions to address them. Well-established programs are available for patients with colorectal cancer (Meyerhardt et al., 2013), breast cancer (American Society of Clinical Oncology, 1997; Khatcheressian et al., 2006; Runowicz et al., 2016; Smith et al., 1999), prostate cancer (Resnick et al., 2015; Skolarus et al., 2014), and malignancies associated with childhood, adolescence, and early adulthood (American Academy of Pediatrics, 2009; Ginsberg et al., 2006; Landier et al., 2004; Rosenberg-Yunger et al., 2013). Likewise, there has been interest in creating programs specifically for patients with HNC. This is partially because HNC patients are becoming more common survivors—they currently make up 3% of all cancer survivors (Miller et al., 2016). All HNC patients had the following overall survival (OS) rate over 5 years: 52.7% in 1982–1986, 58.6% in 1997–2001, and 65.9% in 2002–2006 ($p < 0.0001$). This observed increase in OS is probably partly because of advancements in therapeutic and diagnostic modalities, including systemic treatment standardization, intensity-modulated radiation therapy (IMRT), and improved surgical methods. These modalities include positron emission tomography-computed tomography (PET-CT) and CT/magnetic resonance imaging (CT/MRI). Additionally, the increased prevalence of oropharyngeal malignancies linked to HPV is a contributing factor (Chaturvedi et al., 2011; Gillison et al., 2015). Numerous organizations, including the American Cancer Society (ACS) (Cohen et al., 2016), the Cancer Council Australia (CCA) (2016), and the specialty organizations of the United Kingdom (Paleri & Roland, 2016), have reviewed published guidelines and literature detailing survivorship care in response to the increasing number of HNC survivors and the expanding body of research describing their condition.

11.2.1 Survivorship in Head and Neck Cancer Patients in Low- and Middle-Income Countries

A Pakistan study reported that, in HNCs, the prevalence of high resilience is most apparent in small families where the welfare of the rest of the family is the least prioritized over the ill patient. Several factors, such as formal education and the position and role of the patient in the family, impact this decision. These survivors still require resilience-building interventions to help them adapt and cope (Zahid et al., 2021). A retrospective study by Milas et al. (2022) supported that the implementation of a survivorship program is essential and helps patients identify and manage post-treatment sequelae (Milas et al., 2022). Survivorship objectives and strategies should be designed to extend beyond offering what may be perceived as PC and must encompass all aspects of survivorship (Garton et al., 2023).

11.2.2 Head and Neck Cancer Survivorship in Africa

HNC patients in Africa may have lower survival rates and a higher risk of recurrence since there are fewer diagnostic and therapeutic options available (Okoturo et al., 2020). In addition to these variables, patients with HNC in Africa have a higher likelihood of experiencing socioeconomic hardship, higher degrees of poverty, and detrimental sociocultural characteristics such as lower educational attainment (Nielsen-Scott et al., 2022). To comprehend the impact of local recurrence and patients' survival following therapy in this region, as well as to emphasize the need for clinical care, consistent prevalence figures from Africa are essential (Melariri et al., 2023).

HNCs (excluding eye and brain cancers) are difficult to manage in Côte d'Ivoire. Public care is concentrated in the country's five teaching hospitals. People are poorly trained in screening for precancerous lesions and early-stage lesions, and traditional therapy is still strongly embedded in their habits. These issues are responsible for frequent delays in consultation at early stages. Even when the diagnosis is made early (which represents a tiny percentage of patients), the use of traditional medicine therapy is still almost constant. Recent studies published in Ouagadougou and Dakar suggest a reversal in the sex ratio compared with the classic worldwide trend. In fact, in these countries, it seems that women are more affected by cancers of the oral cavity without any associated alcohol and/or tobacco abuse.

The survival rate for HNCs is closely related to the stage of diagnosis, the level of development of the patient's country, and access to primary healthcare. Reported survival rates are still very low in studies conducted by head and neck specialists, at around 9% at 5 years. In Côte d'Ivoire, cancers are diagnosed at relatively late stages, which explains the low survival rate, and palliative treatment is often the only option available. The situation sometimes deteriorates following unilateral surgical management carried out without any multidisciplinary consultation. Instead of improving the situation, the procedure becomes harmful and complicates subsequent management.

The recent advent of radiotherapy (2018) has undoubtedly improved the prognosis for HNCs, but the costs associated with radiotherapy and palliative care, which are not yet covered by the National Health Insurance Fund (CNAM), limit access for many patients. Large cancerous tumor resections are associated with a significant deterioration in patients' QOL, with compromised physiological functions (swallowing, chewing, phonation, etc.). Reconstructions of these large tissue losses, carried out using flaps, are not yet accessible to all patients, partly because of the lack of physicians qualified to do so and partly because of the cost, which remains high for patients.

In Côte d'Ivoire, reduced QOL is exacerbated by poor access to opioids for pain and the lack of policy, strategy, and guidelines for palliative care. Since 2013, however, due to political will, morphine powder has been added to the national list of essential medicines and palliative care providers and caregivers are trained in the psychology of patients and families and the management of painful symptoms.

Much progress is needed to improve the QOL of patients with HNCs. Efforts should focus on

- Early diagnosis, by educating patients to seek help when they experience even trivial signs, especially if risk factors are present.
- The systematic implementation of multidisciplinary consultation meetings for cancer management.
- Partial or total coverage by CNAM.
- Toughening laws against the use of tobacco in public and increasing the tobacco tax.
- Encouraging systematic multidisciplinary consensus meetings (MCM) for care.
- Training health workers in flap reconstruction techniques.

It is worth noting that QOL in cancer patients generally depends on multiple factors and may differ depending on whether such a patient is hospitalized or receiving care through outpatient facilities. These multiple factors and their effects are discussed in Table 11.1.

11.3 Unmet Needs of Survivorship among Head and Neck Cancer Patients and Their Caregivers

Unmet needs of survivors are widespread and were found in more than half of individuals with general cancer (McDowell et al., 2010). If these unmet requirements (Figure 11.2) are not addressed, they may have a detrimental impact on a patient's psychological health, QOL, and capacity to carry out everyday activities (So et al., 2014). The unique characteristics of unmet needs in HNC patients—a population that had been mainly ignored in earlier research in this field—have been the subject of recent research (Armes et al., 2009).

There are numerous validated instruments to evaluate survivability or unmet supportive care needs in patients with cancer; however, a thorough analysis of these tools is outside the purview of this chapter (see Carlson et al., 2012). The Cancer Survivors' Unmet Needs (CaSUN) instrument, a measure of patient-reported supportive care requirements for cancer survivors, is one such tool. It was created by a woman, and most cancer survivors on whom it was tested were female (Hodgkinson et al., 2007). The CaSUN examined unmet needs for survivorship in five domains: information (3 items), relationships (3 items), QOL (2 items), comprehensive cancer care (6 items), and existential survivorship (14 items). Respondents are asked to classify each item in the CaSUN into one of three categories: need is unmet, have need but it is met, or no need or not applicable. For partners or caregivers of cancer survivors, the Cancer Survivors' Partners Unmet Needs (CaSPUN) is a self-reported companion tool to the CaSUN (Hodgkinson et al., 2007).

Table 11.1 Determining association between health-related quality of life (QOL) and sociodemographic and clinical characteristics

Outpatient treatment cancer patients			**Hospitalized cancer patients**		
Factors	**Type/ Specifications**	**Level of QOL**	**Factors**	**Type/ Specifications**	**Level of QOL**
Age	Older age	Low	Age	Older age	Low
Education	Primary & middle	High	Education	Graduation & above	High
	Up to senior secondary	High			
	Graduation & above	High			
Type of treatment	Palliative care	Low	Type of treatment	Palliative care	Low
	Hormone therapy	High		Surgery	Low
	Others (clinical follow-up)	High		Combination therapy	Low
				Maintenance therapy	Low
				On diagnostic workup	Low
				Others (clinical follow-up)	Low
Line of treatment	Third line	Low	Line of treatment	Second line	Low
Response to treatment	Progressive	Low	Response to treatment	Progressive	Low
Adverse effect	Without adverse effect	High	Adverse effect	Without adverse effect	High
			Type of hospital	Semi-private	High
Area of residence	Slum	Low			
Cancer stage	Stage IV	Low			

Source: Dixit et al., 2024.

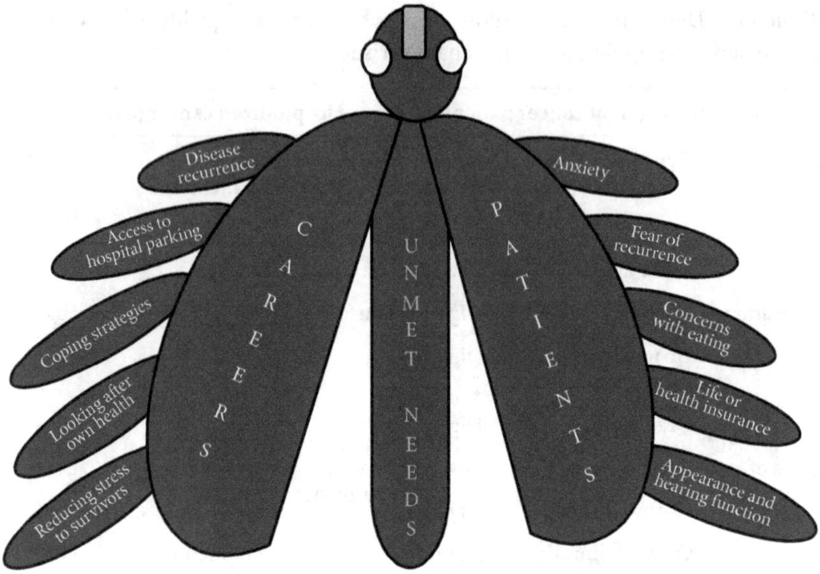

Figure 11.2 The illustration of the butterfly effect in the needs and strategies that need to be addressed to keep head and neck cancer (HNC) survivors in a better position to support themselves. If HCP survivorship is to take off, comparing it with a butterfly, there must be equal attention paid to the needs of both carergivers and patients. If one wing is neglected, the butterfly won't be able to fly.

Utilizing the CaSUN, a cross-sectional study of 158 HNC survivors was carried out at the Princess Margaret Cancer Center (Hodgkinson et al., 2007). Out of the 158 patients sampled, 96 (61%) had at least one unmet need, and 6 had a very high number of requirements (items 31–35 out of 35). There were an average of six unmet needs for each patient. Among individuals who had finished active treatment, "I need help to manage my concerns about the cancer coming back" was the most often expressed unmet need. "I need more easily accessible hospital parking," "I need assistance getting life and/or travel insurance because of my cancer," "I need up-to-date information," and "I need to know that all of my doctors communicate with one another to coordinate my care" were most often mentioned. Patients with higher numbers of unmet demands were highly likely to be younger, closer to the period of their cancer treatment, and to have experienced a worse QOL (List et al., 1996; Rosenthal et al., 2007) in the multivariable analysis (Giuliani et al., 2016).

Of the 158 participants in the aforementioned study, 44 partners finished the CaSPUN. With the use of 35 need items—six of which are positive change items—and one open-ended question, the CaSPUN evaluates and identifies the needs that partners have experienced in the past month. Four partners had a relatively high number of needs (31–35 out of 35 available items), and 29 of the 44 partners who took part in this element of the research reported having at least one unmet need. "I need help to manage my concerns about cancer coming back," "I need more accessible hospital parking," and "I need help to cope with others not acknowledging the impact that having a partner experience cancer has had on my own life" were the most commonly expressed unmet needs among the partners of HNC patients. There was a statistically significant correlation between the amount of unfulfilled wants in patients and their relationships (Giuliani et al., 2017).

A study that used the Supportive Care Needs Survey (SF34) found that 68% of 127 HNC patients had unmet needs (McElduff et al., 2004), thus supporting the findings from these investigations. Most of the unmet demands that were most frequently stated belonged to the psychological realm. They included melancholy, worries about friends and family, uncertainties about the future, and dread of cancer returning (Henry et al., 2014). Using the Partners and Caregiver Supportive Care Needs Survey (Girgis et al., 2011), Balfe and colleagues conducted a study with 197 caregivers of HNC survivors. They found that the most frequently mentioned unmet need was controlling anxieties about cancer recurrence (Balfe et al., 2016b). These striking statistics highlight important unmet requirements and can help direct the creation of survivor programs for HNC patients and their caregivers or partners. Additional approaches to address these demands might be necessary, particularly in smaller cancer centers (Ringash et al., 2018).

11.4 Issues Frequently Faced by Head and Neck Cancer Patients and Recommended Solutions

The crucial time after active treatment ends is known as "post-treatment survival," and it is usually split into two stages: permanent and extended. Survivors may experience a range of survival issues during this phase, including exhaustion, pain, poor body image and malfunction, anxiety about the disease coming back, disturbed sleep, and reluctance to go back to work. Furthermore, cancer survivors might have diminished psychological, social, and physical functioning, which could leave them in need of supporting care (Chen et al., 2022a; Emery et al., 2022; Hill et al., 2020; Tsatsou et al., 2021). Survivors of HNC frequently have serious long-term toxicity, delayed onset of symptoms, increased chance of developing a second primary cancer, and other medical conditions. Oral cancer patients experience greater degrees of suffering and unmet medical, psychological, and social demands compared to those with other cancer types. It is widely known that severe psychosocial morbidities, which include anxiety, depression, problems with social isolation, deficits in body image, and decreased well-being, can persist or even worsen over time in the face of treatment. Patients with oral cancer may experience significant obstacles, such as difficulties speaking and eating, adjustments to their work schedules, limitations on their ability to interact with others, and uncertainty about their prognosis. These issues are covered in various QOL instruments' content (Deshpande & Ghooi, 2017; Doss et al., 2017; Kumar et al., 2017; Wang et al., 2018). Following reconstructive procedures, oral cancer patients experience a variety of psychological and social difficulties, including facial deformity, various symptoms, and a lack of social support (Chen et al., 2022b). Patients' self-concept and body image may suffer as a result of facial deformity (Rhoten et al., 2013), which can make social interactions uncomfortable and challenging (Rifkin et al., 2018). The biggest risk factors for psychosocial maladjustment are low socioeconomic level, stage III or IV cancer, excruciating pain, increased social eating disorders, speech issues, and decreased sexuality. Social support is provided by giving someone within a social network the material and psychological resources to assist them in dealing with stress. Identifying groups at high risk for maladjustment and creating suitable interventions can be aided by knowledge of postoperative psychosocial adjustment modifications and the factors that influence them (Chen et al., 2019, 2022b; Dewa et al., 2018; Giuliani et al., 2019).

11.4.1 Chronic Pain

As many as 45% of individuals receiving treatment for HNC may experience chronic pain (Cramer et al., 2018; Terkawi et al., 2017). Among HNC survivors, this may have a significant impact on function and QOL. Patients with HNC do not have a clear, standardized method for evaluating chronic pain. Validated QOL or Likert scales or tools can be utilized as a supplement to measure the extent of disability a patient experiences more accurately as a result of their pain (Ojo et al., 2012). More than 20% of chronic pain sufferers fit the requirements for a major depressive episode (Cramer et al., 2018). In this case, patients should be assessed for depression symptoms and referred appropriately. Pain can be a sign of recurrent disease, even though it is most frequently linked to therapeutic side effects. Pain is the initial symptom that up to 70% of individuals with recurrent cancer may experience (Smit et al., 2001). When there is chronic post-treatment pain, an extensive evaluation of the upper aerodigestive tract is necessary, especially if there is lancinating focal pain that spreads to the mandible or unilateral ear (Goyal et al., 2022).

Although there are differing definitions in the literature, pain that lasts >3 months after the acute phase of treatment is widely regarded to be chronic pain, as long as the immediate effects of therapy have subsided (Dowell et al.,

2016). Opioids will be used continuously by 13–50% of patients receiving HNC-directed therapy to cure them. Pre-treatment opioid usage, alcohol addictions, nicotine dependency, and the use of induction chemotherapy or trimodal therapy are all linked to chronic opioid use and abuse post-treatment (Cramer et al., 2018; McDermott et al., 2019; Silver et al., 2019; Smith et al., 2019). Moreover, persistent opioid usage during cancer therapy is linked to anxiety and depression. Patients with oral cavity carcinoma have a worse disease-free survival rate when they use opioids on a chronic basis (Pang et al., 2017).

Patients (especially those in high-risk groups) need to undergo screening for chronic opioid use and addiction 3 months after treatment ends, given the current opioid crisis. Alternatives to opioids that are effective in treating chronic pain include nonsteroidal anti-inflammatory medications and acetaminophen. Neuromodulators, including gabapentin, have also shown promise in treating chronic cancer-related pain (Bar Ad, 2010) and acute treatment-associated pain during HNC therapy (Bar Ad et al., 2010; Sanders & Dawes, 2016).

Patients who continue to experience concerns about chronic opioid use or pain that does not improve with non-opioid therapy should be referred to a multidisciplinary pain management team or palliative care team. These specialist teams can integrate medication, physical therapy, psychotherapy, and nontraditional resources. They often handle chronic pain more holistically. In some situations, these diverse treatment approaches may help lower opioid dependence, costs, and pain-related morbidity (Binczak et al., 2014; Katz et al., 2015).

11.4.2 Musculoskeletal Restrictions and Physical Therapy

Following HNC-directed therapy, functional musculoskeletal restrictions are somewhat common but frequently go unreported and untreated. The ensuing impairment may cause HNC survivors' QOL and means of subsistence to significantly decline. Only a small percentage of HNC multidisciplinary teams regularly recommend patients to physical therapy (Robinson et al., 2018). The most prevalent musculoskeletal problems are trismus, which can be seen in as many as half of patients receiving radiation therapy to the pterygoid musculature/temporomandibular joint region, and shoulder dysfunction, which can be found in as many as 70% of patients undergoing neck dissection (Dijkstra et al., 2001; Weber et al., 2010). Reduced neck range of motion is another common post-treatment occurrence. In addition to regular post-treatment visits, baseline evaluations of shoulder, neck, and temporomandibular joint mobility should be carried out by HNC physicians as part of a thorough physical examination before therapy (Goyal et al., 2022).

There have been conflicting reports on the frequency of shoulder dysfunction following neck dissection, and it appears to be related to the degree of surgery. More than 90% of patients undergoing radical neck dissection and 23% of patients undergoing modified radical neck dissection had impaired abduction, according to a meta-analysis (Gane et al., 2017). A handheld goniometer and the standard Medical Research Council 0–5 scale can be used to objectively test a range of motion and shoulder strength, but this might not be feasible in a surgical clinic (Fan et al., 2010; Jepsen et al., 2004). To measure disability and determine the necessity for rehabilitation, several patient-directed questionnaires about shoulder function following neck dissection were devised (Goldstein et al., 2014). According to Goldstein et al. (2014), the only patient-reported outcome measure that particularly addresses shoulder function in patients who underwent neck dissection is the Neck Dissection Impairment Index (Goldstein et al., 2014).

Based on the available medical research, the efficacy of physiotherapy is not entirely clear when shoulder dysfunction, whether subjective or objective, is detected. McGarvey et al. (2011) pointed out that although physical therapy is well-tolerated by patients, little data support its efficacy in treating shoulder dysfunction following neck dissection (McGarvey et al., 2011). In follow-up research published by the same group, patients who underwent neck dissection were prospectively assigned to either a control group or a 12-week shoulder strength program. At 3 months following surgery, they discovered that the group receiving physical therapy had significantly improved shoulder abduction (McGarvey et al., 2015).

Transverse myelitis post-HNC treatment is extremely rare (<1% at 54 Gy with traditional fractionation) thanks to improvements in radiation therapy (Kirkpatrick et al., 2010). On the other hand, L'Hermitte's sign, which is defined as electric shock sensations down the spinal cord and into the limbs following neck flexion, may manifest as a minor form of spinal cord poisoning. In the past, rates of HNC treated with conformal, field-based radiation treatment have been reported to range from 3% to 13% (Ésik et al., 2003). Interestingly, an increased incidence of L'Hermitte's sign of between 15% and 29% was reported in research focused on intensity-modulated radiation therapy for thoracic and head and neck cancers. L'Hermitte's sign usually appears in the first few months after radiation therapy and rarely persists for >6 months (Pak et al., 2012). Patients with this illness continue to receive conservative treatment, which includes corticosteroids, hyperbaric oxygen, and soft neck collars (Gemici, 2010). Patients with HNC frequently experience trismus, also known as a restricted mouth opening. People who have trismus frequently have trouble doing everyday tasks including eating, drinking, laughing, and kissing. Their quality of life is negatively impacted by these challenges. Narrow inclusion criteria, a single tumor localization, a single treatment technique, short sample sizes, and varying trismus cutoff points have resulted in a wide range of trismus prevalence (from 5% to 65%) and trismus-related variables (van der Geer et al., 2018). Research indicates that between 25% and 40% of individuals with oral cavity or oropharyngeal primary tumors experience trismus after treatment. Risk factors for this condition include the tumor's initial stage, the necessity for reconstruction, chemotherapy, and radiation treatment (Pauli et al., 2013; van der Geer et al., 2019). Exercise therapy is effective in improving trismus, according to three recent systematic reviews, and early commencement and compliance led to better results. In comparing the TheraBite device to forced opening (1.1), tongue blades (1.5), or microcurrent therapy (0.3), the device considerably increased mouth opening (effect size of 2.6 in one evaluation). However, in the majority of cases, restoration to normal (>35 mm) levels was not possible (Dijkstra et al., 2004; Kamstra et al., 2017; Scherpenhuizen et al., 2015).

11.4.3 Lymphedema

Increased lymphatic load and a requirement for drainage beyond the lymphatic system's transit capability lead to lymphedema. In HNC, lymphedema develops secondary to lymphatic disruption brought on by the tumor load or cancer treatment (chemotherapy, radiation, or surgery) (Deng et al., 2011; Smith & Lewin, 2010). Insufficient drainage causes lymphatic fluid to build up in interstitial spaces and soft tissues, which can cause fibrosis and inflammation. This will show up as a large amount of dense soft tissue edema that might be internal (tongue, pharynx, and larynx) or external (facial and neck). Aesthetic deformities, shoulder and neck dysfunction, visual disturbance, dysphagia, dysphonia, and breathing difficulties are among the possible symptoms (Cohen et al., 2016). Occasionally, lymphedema may become severe enough to need a tracheotomy. With recorded rates ranging from 12% to 90%, the reported incidence of lymphedema differs and is probably linked to cancer stage, site, severity, and mix of treatment (Deng et al., 2011; Ridner et al., 2016).

Numerous studies have shown how lymphedema affects HNC survivors' QOL (Klernäs et al., 2018; Murphy & Gilbert, 2009; Penner, 2009; Poulsen et al., 2008). It is crucial to diagnose and treat it early because of its functional and psychosocial effects. A physical examination using precise measures and flexible fiberoptic laryngoscopy to detect internal lymphedema can be used to objectively identify head and neck lymphedema (Smith & Lewin, 2010). Although the Foldi lymphedema rating scale was designed with extremity lymphedema in mind, it is capable of supporting a qualitative grading system (Smith & Lewin, 2010). The University of Texas M. D. Anderson Cancer Center Head and Neck

Lymphedema Rating Scale was developed to solve this constraint. It was derived from the Foldi lymphedema rating scale, which uses a straightforward 5-point rating system to capture subtle presentations of HNC lymphedema (Smith & Lewin, 2010). Ameliorating lymphatic drainage with compressive bandages and manual massage is part of the treatment for lymphedema. To enhance lymphatic flow, manual lymphatic drainage (MLD) uses mild circular massage. Complete decongestive therapy (CDT) is the "gold standard" for management; it is administered by licensed lymphedema therapists and incorporates MLD, physical activity, skincare, and compressive bandages. For the first 2–4 weeks of this therapy, intense, nearly daily outpatient sessions are common. After that, patients or caregivers might be able to offer adequate and efficacious home care if regular clinic visits are not practicable (Yao et al., 2020). Exercises include swallowing exercises and range-of-motion exercises for the arms, shoulders, neck, and face. Although some institutions advocate applying compressive bandages before and after MLD, the bandages are typically used following MLD (Smith & Lewin, 2010). Patients with HNC can effectively manage their lymphedema using these therapies (Smith et al., 2015).

11.4.4 Dysphonia and Dysphagia

Patients with HNC frequently have symptoms associated with impaired voice, speech, and swallowing abilities, which lowers their QOL. Speech and swallowing difficulties might be induced by the cancer's inherent course or by the side effects of treatment, including radiation, surgery, or chemotherapy and radiation therapy (Wall et al., 2013). Mastication, deglutition, and nutritional maintenance may be adversely affected by anatomic changes, dentition loss, mucositis, trismus, post-treatment lymphedema, xerostomia, fibrosis, and neuropathy, among other factors (Gillespie et al., 2004; Lin et al., 2002). Swallowing disturbance symptoms are prevalent in HNC patients. The prevalence of aspiration pneumonia, dysphagia, and stricture was 8.7%, 10.2%, and 45.3%, respectively, in one epidemiology and results (SEER)-based investigation. According to the site (lower in the oral cavity), the stage (greater with more extensive malignancies), and the treatment modality (greater in patients receiving nonsurgical or various treatment modalities), the extent of these signs and symptoms varied (Hutcheson et al., 2019). According to other research, up to 84% of patients may experience aspiration, and almost half of patients have poor QOL as a result of dysphagia. Chemotherapy added as a radiosensitizer may make these symptoms even worse (Maurer et al., 2011).

Enhancements in QOL may result from cooperative multidisciplinary efforts focused on the patient's capacity to maintain and restore functional swallowing and speech (Clarke et al., 2016). Speech-language pathologist (SLP) professionals can assist in determining baseline swallowing and speech abnormalities and offer patients counseling and education to help them comprehend the consequences of their illness and how it affects their ability to speak and swallow (Pauloski et al., 2000). By evaluating baseline function, patients may be screened for chronic dysfunction to identify those who might need extra support for phonatory rehabilitation (e.g., non-laryngeal speech) or dietary demands (e.g., gastrostomy tube). SLP practitioners may instruct and promote preventive swallowing exercises in patients undergoing radiation or chemotherapy to enhance post-treatment functional results (Carnaby-Mann et al., 2012; Kotz et al., 2012). Swallowing exercises that support oral intake throughout treatment are linked to improved long-term swallowing outcomes and decreased reliance on gastric tubes in these individuals (Hutcheson et al., 2013). Along with speech and voice production issues, patients with HNC may present with reduced intelligibility, loss of natural speech, or low voice quality. Speech therapy can undoubtedly enhance the intelligibility and quality of speech (Langmore, 2001). Using an electrolarynx, esophageal speech therapy, or tracheoesophageal puncture, SLP practitioners can also assist in determining the best methods for speech rehabilitation and restoration in individuals with alaryngeal disorders. Therefore, as part of their assessment and treatment planning, patients with HNC should be referred to SLP specialists as soon as possible. SLPs can monitor functional outcomes linked to speech and swallowing to track patients' ongoing survivorship treatment. Tools for assessing symptoms-driven swallowing, such as videostroboscopy, fiberoptic endoscopic examination of swallowing, and modified barium swallow study, offer valuable information for creating focused therapies, such as teaching compensatory movements and swallowing exercises when necessary (Clarke et al., 2016). A long-term assessment of cranial nerve function, swallowing, and speech is recommended because radiation therapy patients may develop late toxicities (Goyal et al., 2022).

11.4.5 Hearing Loss

The effects of HNC therapy on auditory function can be significant. Radiation and surgery can both significantly impact the auditory system in cases of cancer affecting the nasopharynx, skull base, ear, and paranasal sinuses. Conductive hearing loss (CHL) will follow surgical resection of the tympanic membrane, middle ear space, or external auditory canal (EAC). Similar to this, surgery performed on the paranasal sinuses, nasal cavity, and/or base of the skull may result in trauma, edema, or Eustachian tube dysfunction, which might cause CHL from serous otitis media (Goyal et al., 2022).

Both CHL and sensorineural hearing loss (SNHL) may result from radiation therapy administered to the head and neck. Radiation alterations to the Eustachian tube system may result in CHL. In addition, external toxicity to the ear or EAC may cause ossicular necrosis, otitis externa, or EAC stenosis (Bhandare et al., 2007; Nader & Gidley, 2019). Anywhere in the auditory pathway from the brainstem to the cochlea, radiation to the inner ear might also result in sudden hearing loss. Research has shown that the frequency of ototoxicity is related to radiation dosage and method, age of the patient, and chemotherapy plus radiation. A higher incidence of irreversible ototoxicity may be linked to radiation doses to the cochlea of > 40–45 Gy according to some studies, while other studies have reported cases of SNHL at radiation doses as low as 20–25 Gy (Bhandare et al., 2007; Hitchcock et al., 2009; McDowell et al., 2018; Strojan et al., 2017; Zuur et al., 2009). Additionally, reports of ototoxicity encompassing a spectrum of radiation treatments vary from 0% to 43% (Strojan et al., 2017; Wakisaka et al., 2011; Zuur et al., 2009).

Chemotherapy, especially platinum-based drugs (mostly carboplatin, oxaliplatin, and cisplatin), can have a significant impact on the inner ear and cause tinnitus and high-frequency SNHL (Nader & Gidley, 2019). Patients who receive a total dose of > 100 mg/m^2 of cisplatin run the risk of suffering from high-frequency SNHL since these medications have cumulative dose-dependent effects (Cohen et al., 2016). Chemotherapy-related ototoxic symptoms might manifest as vestibular dysfunction (dizziness, imbalance, or vertigo), cochlear dysfunction (tinnitus, hearing loss, or hyperacusis), or as a mix of both (Cianfrone et al., 2011). It was estimated that 40% of chemotherapy patients experience tinnitus, which is described as a subjective impression of sound without an external source. Tinnitus can have a substantial detrimental influence on psychological status and QOL (Dille et al., 2013). Psychological symptoms as well as difficulties with driving, bicycling, and other activities can be brought on by vestibular symptoms, which can also result in a decline in QOL (Sun et al., 2014). As many as 18% of individuals who had cisplatin therapy may suffer progressive hearing loss due to cochleotoxicity, which can manifest either suddenly or slowly (Frisina et al., 2016). If hearing loss develops during treatment, another chemotherapy regimen might be considered (Goyal et al., 2022).

Although not yet standard of care, chemoprotective drugs have been researched (Nader & Gidley, 2019). The location and source of ototoxicity determine how it should be managed. While losses resulting from fibrosis, scarring, or Eustachian tube dysfunction might need surgical methods to relieve the specific obstruction, CHL secondary to edema typically resolves over time. While serous otitis media might also go away with time, patients who have had persistent CHL for 3–6 months might find that having a simple myringotomy or tympanostomy tube placed is beneficial (Nader & Gidley, 2019). Unfortunately, there is no proven treatment for SNHL, and hyperbaric oxygen therapy and high-dose steroid administration have had conflicting effects. According to the American Academy of Audiology, patients receiving platinum-based chemotherapy need to have pure tone audiometry performed a few months after the chemotherapy is finished. Patients should then continue to be monitored for at least 2 years while receiving concurrent radiation therapy because hearing loss may worsen over time. Additionally, utilization of hearing amplification (hearing aids) is essential for post-treatment SNHL rehabilitation (Strojan et al., 2017). Cochlear implantation is successful for patients with significant bilateral SNHL, and there is no difference in their prognosis from those who did not receive previous chemotherapy or radiation (Nader & Gidley, 2019; Strojan et al., 2017).

11.4.6 Psychosocial Problems

Psychosocial function can be severely impacted by HNC diagnosis and therapy. Following therapy, extremely apparent and socially significant changes are frequently observed because HNC occurs in places that are both cosmetically and functionally critical (Fingeret et al., 2012; Graboyes et al., 2019). Visible deformity, a compromised smile, dysphagia, dysphonia, and fear of recurrence can all contribute to significant psychological morbidity, such as anxiety, sadness, and body image issues (Fingeret et al., 2013; Graboyes et al., 2019; Henry et al., 2019; Rieke et al., 2017; Wu et al., 2016).

11.4.6.1 Body Image Disturbance

Body image disturbance (BID) is a multifaceted condition defined by a change in appearance and/or function that the self perceives to be unpleasant (Ellis et al., 2019; Fingeret et al., 2010; Rhoten et al., 2013). Up to 75% of HNC patients report having body image issues; a rise in the frequency and severity of these issues early in the survival phase is linked to social exclusion, stigma, depression, and a reduction in QOL (Fingeret et al., 2012; Graboyes et al., 2019; Rhoten et al., 2013). HNC survivors should routinely be evaluated for BID (Cohen et al., 2016). However, few patient-centered, psychometrically sound instruments are available to assess BID in HNC survivors. Better measurement techniques are a demand in both clinical and scientific settings (Ellis et al., 2019). One of the most crucial aspects of HNC survival care is still BID management (Cohen et al., 2016). Affected patients should be referred for psycho-oncologic care; however, more research is necessary to create efficient interventions that target BID in HNC survivors in particular (Chen et al., 2017; Cohen et al., 2016; Fingeret et al., 2014; Huang & Liu, 2008).

11.4.6.2 Distress, Anxiety, and Depression

Compared to survivors of other cancer types, HNC survivors are more likely to present psychological aftereffects, and symptoms of distress, anxiety, and depression are more common among them (Lydiatt et al., 2009). Therefore, utilizing validated screening instruments (e.g., Hospital Anxiety and Depression Scale, NCCN Distress Thermometer, Beck Depression or Generalized Anxiety Disorder-7, Anxiety Inventories, and Patient Health Questionnaire–9), HNC survivors should be evaluated regularly for distress, anxiety, and depression (Beck et al., 1993; Cohen et al., 2016; Denlinger et al., 2017; Kroenke et al., 2001). Treatments for survivors who exhibit clinical signs of anxiety, sadness, or discomfort include medication, psychotherapy, and referral to psycho-oncology. Sadly, mental health services are often underutilized (Chen et al., 2013; Cohen et al., 2016). Evidence suggests that preventing HNC survivors from developing depression before starting treatment may reduce this risk. Prophylactic escitalopram administered to HNC patients at treatment commencement reduced the incidence of depression by > 50% according to a landmark trial. The favorable benefits were mostly shown in patients treated with definitive radiation-based treatments (Lydiatt et al., 2013). Health psychologists have been incorporated into the multidisciplinary treatment team in other multidisciplinary HNC programs to support pre-treatment screening and the identification of psychosocial risk factors, with careful monitoring and intervention as necessary. Medical professionals, caregivers, and patients have all praised this integration (Jesse et al., 2015).

Support group involvement has been reported to reduce anxiety and depression in patients with breast, lung, and colon cancer, even though the volume of research on HNC is very small (Schou et al., 2008). Furthermore, virtual support groups have been linked to lower levels of psychological and physiological stress since the development of internet technology (Golant et al., 2004). Online meetings can lessen feelings of social isolation, mental anguish, despair, and helplessness while also boosting functional status, self-worth, and personal empowerment (Algtewi et al., 2015). Better health-related QOL was linked to a longer duration of membership in an online support group ($B = 0.07$, $p < .05$) in a study including 199 patients with HNC (Algtewi et al., 2015). Given these noteworthy advantages, medical professionals should recommend patients to look for local support groups, especially those created for their specific clinical condition (Goyal et al., 2022).

Suicide is an extremely serious issue, especially considering the heavy psychological toll that HNC takes on its survivors (Zeller, 2006). Within the first year, up to 16% of HNC survivors report having considered suicide; individuals with drug misuse histories and a history of psychiatric problems are most at risk (Henry et al., 2018). In the United States, HNC survivors have an adjusted suicide risk of 38 to 60/100,000 person-years; they have a suicide risk that is two times higher than that of patients with other cancers and three times higher than that of the US population as a whole (Henry et al., 2018; Kam et al., 2015). Even more worrisome is that HNC survivors are becoming more likely to commit suicide (Osazuwa-Peters et al., 2018). Therefore, it is imperative to create new approaches and include them in standard clinical care to prevent suicide among HNC survivors (Henry et al., 2018).

11.4.7 Fatigue

An unpleasant, persistent, and subjective feeling of emotional, physical, and/or cognitive tiredness or exhaustion that is unrelated to recent activity and that interferes with normal function is known as *cancer-related fatigue*. It can be brought on by either cancer or oncologic treatment (National Comprehensive Cancer Network [NCCN], 2019). Usually, sleep or rest do not make cancer-related weariness go away. Cancer-related fatigue affects most patients with HNC, especially if they are receiving radiation therapy or chemoradiation (Jereczek-Fossa et al., 2007; Spratt et al., 2012). An important loss of QOL is caused by fatigue symptoms, which peak early (i.e., within 8 weeks) when radiation therapy begins and continue or deteriorate for the first 2 years after treatment (Spratt et al., 2012).

Numerous underlying medical disorders that may coexist with an HNC diagnosis can cause fatigue, such as anemia, anxiety, sadness, low cardiopulmonary reserve, malnourishment, psychological distress, sleep disorders, thyroid dysfunction, a pro-inflammatory or catabolic condition, pain associated with cancer and/or its treatment, and substance addiction. This list also includes baseline frailty (Bower et al., 2014). Patients with a history of HNC may receive counseling and weariness screening at the time of their initial assessment and then on a recurrent basis throughout their survival (NCCN, 2019). When a patient is found to be experiencing fatigue, they should have their medical history thoroughly reviewed, undergo a physical examination, receive relevant biochemical and hematology testing (e.g., complete blood count, comprehensive metabolic panel, thyroid function testing, and nutritional markers), be administered screening tools for psychological depression and distress, and, when necessary, be referred to a specialist (Goyal et al., 2022).

Patients need to be encouraged to engage in a regular exercise program in addition to receiving treatment and counseling for any coexisting medical issues that may be causing their fatigue (NCCN, 2019; Rock et al., 2012). Physical therapists with expertise in oncology care help relieve weariness brought on by cancer. To lessen cancer-related exhaustion, doctors and patients may also think about using cognitive-behavioral therapy, yoga, massage treatment, and other methods (Gielissen et al., 2007; NCCN, 2019).

11.4.8 Return-to-Work Issues

For cancer patients, going back to work after treatment can be a difficult undertaking. Simple activities like eating in public, exhaustion, radiation dermatitis, and mouth ulcers can make it difficult and even unpleasant for HNC patients to work in a public setting. It may be challenging for the patient to communicate with coworkers and carry out regular work-related tasks because of the influence of HNC and its treatment on their speech and voice. Employers must encourage their staff members' effective return to work and give them opportunities for participation or make adjustments to alter the nature of their employment (Goyal et al., 2022). Cancelliere and colleagues showed that socioeconomic status and higher education, greater self-efficacy and optimistic expectations for recovery and return to work, lower severity of injury or illness, return to work coordination, and multidisciplinary interventions involving the workplace and stakeholders are common factors linked with positive return to work outcomes. Conversely, characteristics like older age, female gender, greater pain or disability, depression, sick leave, higher physical job demands, past unemployment, and activity limitations were linked to worse results when it came to returning to work (Cancelliere et al., 2016).

In the United States, physicians who treat HNC patients should be aware of medical disabilities and the legal safeguards provided by the law. Under two federal laws—the Family and Medical Leave Act (FMLA) and the Americans with Disabilities Act (ADA)—employees may be entitled to medical and/or disability-related leave when they are ill, injured, or become incapacitated while working. An individual is considered to have a disability if they meet any of the following three criteria: (1) have a mental or physical impairment that significantly limits one or more main activities of daily living, (2) have a record of such an impairment, or (3) are thought to have such an impairment. The ADA does not expressly require employers to offer disability- or medical-related leave. However, it does mandate that employers provide qualified workers with disabilities with reasonable accommodations if needed to carry out critical job duties or to take advantage of the same opportunities and privileges as workers without disabilities. Alterations to work schedules (e.g., 8-hour shifts instead of 12-hour shifts or a 5-day work week with no overtime), restricted duties (e.g., lifting restrictions), or medical leave are examples of accommodations (Goyal et al., 2022).

11.4.9 Financial Burden

An increasing number of people are becoming aware of the catastrophic financial toll that HNC survivors and their caregivers may face due to the convergence of better oncologic outcomes, rising cancer care costs, and ongoing patient cost-shifting (Deschler, 2019; Massa et al., 2019). The concept of "financial toxicity" has several dimensions and is based on three factors that contribute to material hardship: (1) reduced income and increased out-of-pocket expenses, (2) psychological distress brought on by material hardship, and (3) compensating coping mechanisms developed by families in reaction to the high cost of cancer and its treatment (Altice et al., 2017; Zafar & Abernethy, 2013).

In comparison to patients with other cancer types, HNC patients bear a larger share of financial toxicity's devastating effects. HNC patients are most likely to experience financial toxicity, or the financial burden of cancer therapy; cumulative incidence estimates for HNC patients range from 40% to 69% (de Souza et al., 2017; Krouse et al., 1989). Patients with Medicaid, lower wealth, greater perceived social isolation, and higher total out-of-pocket treatment costs are among those with the highest risk for financial devastation (de Souza et al., 2017); this marks another area of the cancer care continuum where there are notable and unsettling differences in outcomes (Deschler, 2019). Quantitative metrics (such as financial load and the ratio of out-of-pocket medical expenses to household income) or patient-reported metrics (like the Comprehensive Score for Financial Toxicity questionnaire) can be used to evaluate financial toxicity (Banthin et al., 2008; De Souza et al., 2014). Financial toxicity has a major knock-on effect on cancer patients since it is linked to poorer survival rates, higher unmet needs for HNC survivors, increased symptom load, decreased QOL, and decreased adherence to cancer therapy (Lathan et al., 2016; O'Brien et al., 2017; Neugut et al., 2011; Ramsey et al., 2016; Zafar et al., 2015). For HNC caretakers, financial toxicity is another prevalent issue that can have disastrous consequences (Balfe et al., 2016a; Giuliani et al., 2017).

While the multidisciplinary HNC team cannot control many sociodemographic factors that contribute to financial toxicity, providers can still make a difference by raising awareness of the fact that financial toxicity is frequent after HNC treatment, identifying patients who may be at risk, connecting patients and caregivers to resources for managing financial burdens, and referring patients to financial navigators and social workers who can help them engage with social welfare systems to evaluate and manage financial toxicity related to HNC (Balfe et al., 2016a; Deschler, 2019).

11.5 Supportive Care Interventions

11.5.1 Survivorship Care Plans

Five cancer survivorship care domains are described in the Quality of Cancer Survivorship Care Framework, and HNC survivorship care falls under each of them. Physical impacts, psychosocial effects, chronic disease management, monitoring for cancer recurrences and new cases, promotion of health and disease prevention, and contextual domains of the health care delivery system are some of these areas. Health outcomes, like function- and health-related QOL, emergency room visits and hospitalization, expenses, and death, can be used to measure the impact of survivorship care in various domains. In particular, how to provide for these demands in the long run following therapy and acute recovery is not well understood. The US Institute of Medicine (IOM) suggested that survivorship care plans (SCPs) be used to help primary care and cancer doctors better coordinate patient care (Margalit et al., 2022; Nekhlyudov et al., 2019; Salz et al., 2016). An SCP is a review of treatment, a plan of care outlining side effects, and advice for self-management and interventions that the patient receives from oncology professionals after their treatment. According to the Commission on Cancer Standard 3.3, all eligible survivors must receive a SCP by January 1, 2019, according to the IOM's recommendation that all survivors receive one following their cancer treatment. SCPs give details about the cancer diagnosis and stage, course of treatment, any side effects, and suggestions for ongoing monitoring and follow-up care (Hill et al., 2020; Salz et al., 2016). Nevertheless, there is scant proof that SCPs have an impact on outcomes as reported by patients (Brennan et al., 2014; Jacobsen et al., 2018).

To ascertain the influence of SCPs on the outcomes of survivors, a meta-analysis is needed. According to earlier evaluations, there was no difference in QOL, distress, or satisfaction with care between survivors who received a SCP and those who did not. On the other hand, according to one review, SCPs seemed to enhance the quality and frequency of communication between patients, medical specialists, and primary care physicians, as well as the quantity of information survivors received about their condition and testing. The American Society of Clinical Oncology and the American Cancer Society released the first thorough recommendations for the multidisciplinary treatment of HNC survivors. According to these guidelines, primary care should diagnose and treat low mood, manage comorbidities, adjust risk factors, do suggested screening for other malignancies, and provide preventative treatment. Survivors frequently require the assistance of healthcare professionals to participate in self-management, which includes reducing alcohol intake, quitting smoking, improving diet, exercising, and receiving symptom rehabilitation. The time and staff needed to prepare SCPs, as well as the challenge of routinely assessing their content, are the main obstacles to their adoption (Hill et al., 2020; Nekhlyudov et al., 2017; Salz et al., 2021).

11.5.2 Online Methods of Survivor Care Plans

A web-based, algorithm-driven electronic platform called the Head and Neck Survivorship Tool: Assessment and Recommendations (HN-STAR) (Salz et al., 2016, 2018, 2021) was created to solve the most important problems in giving HNC survivors full survivorship care. A patient's symptoms are directly collected, and treatment information, patient-reported outcomes, and the most recent research on survivorship care are combined to build a customized interactive discussion guide. Based on the clinic visit, the SCP is automatically generated. In response to expert and end-user comments, usability testing helps to modify the content and delivery of HN-STAR, resulting in a strong clinical platform for further clinical testing. This is a crucial first step in better treatment for complex cancer survivors, for whom it can be very challenging to provide ongoing care and administer SCPs.

The HN-STAR attempts to make the delivery of individualized care in cancer survivorship clinics easier. It consists of four interwoven components: an interactive conversation guide, an online self-assessment, a streamlined treatment summary, and a survivorship care plan created after each visit. HN-STAR standardizes complete care in routine survivorship visits by integrating clinical information, patient-reported outcomes, and evidence-based standards via an algorithmic approach. Additionally, it gives priority to the toxicities that HNC patients must deal with.

The ENHANCES trial was the only one to examine SCPs specifically for HNC survivors (Salz et al., 2016, 2018, 2021). This research looked at the viability, acceptability, and efficacy of web-based dyadic treatments for informal caregivers and cancer patients, the majority of whom are undergoing active treatment. Luo et al. (2020) conducted a critical literature analysis and found that web-based therapies were practical and improved the physical, psychological, and social functioning of cancer patients and their caregivers. Online interventions can offer adaptable platforms and programs to help fulfill the educational requirements of couples facing HNC care while enhancing their coping mechanisms, according to another assessment of online treatments (Vanstone & Fergus, 2020). The total results indicate a trend in the beneficial impacts of these interventions on cancer survivor–caregiver dyads and support the viability, applicability, and acceptability of eHealth intervention programs.

The most crucial information is that the majority of online platforms used to deliver interventions featured several functions, offering participants social networking, video, and audio in addition to textual resources. Furthermore, several online platforms offered visitors the ability to select the information they required and generated customized intervention content depending on their selections. Programs for survivorship care must consider the needs of cancer survivors as well as the supportive care requirements of those who care for them, considering their knowledge, abilities, and physical and mental well-being. In addition, physical, mental, and social issues may arise for caregivers while they are providing care. For cancer survivors and their caregivers, web-based dyadic therapies that help lower the barriers of conventional face-to-face therapy might also be essential (Akkol-Solakoglu et al., 2021; Beer et al., 2020; Chen et al., 2022a; Pauwels et al., 2012; Pekmezi et al., 2021).

A clinically led approach to supportive interventions for cancer survivors post-treatment must eventually give way to one that emphasizes supportive self-management and tailored support according to each patient's needs (Jefford et al., 2013). Enhancing survival adaptations for survivors and their caregivers can be achieved through several therapeutic elements such as psychotherapy, dyadic coping, problem-solving training, physical exercises, caring skills training, information assistance, and social support (Carmack et al., 2021; Pekmezi et al., 2021; Song et al., 2021; Winters-Stone et al., 2022). The dyadic intervention proved to be more advantageous for cancer survivor–caregiver dyads than the survivor-only intervention according to two randomized controlled trials (Carmack et al., 2021; Price-Blackshear et al., 2020). To fully meet the supportive care requirements of survivors and caregivers, future post-treatment survivorship web-based therapies might incorporate sessions with all five therapy elements. This could potentially lead to overall positive survival outcomes (Chen et al., 2022a).

Participants in dyadic interventions have the chance to boost one another's confidence, encourage one another, and set an example for one another. This enhances learning efficiency and encourages cancer survivor–caregiver dyads to finish interventions, which benefits both survivors and their caregivers. Since individual interventions solely concentrate on survivor or caregiver outcomes, future dyadic interventions must incorporate modules that support interactions between cancer survivors and their caregivers (Carmack et al., 2021; Price-Blackshear et al., 2020).

In certain patients who are at risk of pharyngoesophageal junction stricture, endoscopic dilatation may result in an improvement in dysphagia (Wu et al., 2019). Exercises designed specifically for rehabilitation that address shoulder problems can enhance function and health-related QOL (HRQOL). Programs for self-help exercises have shown that even among long-term survivors, dysphagia-related QOL may somewhat improve. Incorporating movement-based programs like Tai Chi into a survival program may be effective for maintaining overall health and preventing chronic diseases (Fong et al., 2014; Jansen et al., 2020; McNeely et al., 2015). Only two small studies (Manne et al., 2020; Sterba et al., 2019) have specifically focused on depression and unmet survival needs using internet-based technologies.

11.6 Challenges and Limitations of Survivorship Care

11.6.1 Issues with the Existing Survivorship Care Recommendations

It is difficult to define survivorship recommendations in HNC. Not only is the area of survival care extremely new, but recommendations for survivors are barely getting started when it comes to patients with HNCs. There are not many recommendations, and programs and clinics addressing these issues are still being developed (Ringash et al., 2018).

11.6.2 Clinical Load of Primary Care Physicians

From a clinical standpoint, it could be too much to ask for a primary care physician (PCP) to evaluate every potential late effect at every follow-up, as advised by the American College of Physicians (ACS). Since PCPs may offer comprehensive, patient-centered care and address long-term health issues and psychosocial requirements that may not be adequately addressed by oncology-led treatment alone, it may be advantageous to encourage PCPs to take on a greater role in the follow-up care of HNC survivors. Moreover, working together to create a practical follow-up schedule and a protocol for the transfer of care may be beneficial. According to the Australian Cancer Council, it is also important to create a method for PCPs to quickly understand the most likely late effects for a given patient, give the best estimations of their probabilities for outcomes, and to present suitable management or referrals. In the "survivorship care summary," patients' known common unmet needs may receive special attention. These include making sure there is sufficient information available to enable a smooth transition from "HNC follow-up" to "survivorship follow-up," helping with the purchase of life and/or travel insurance, and assisting with the acquisition of accessible parking if necessary. The needs of partners must be recognized and met. Solutions most likely rely on the healthcare infrastructure unique to each local/regional government, patient population, and available resources. Research is required to determine underserved areas and high-risk populations. It takes specific tactics to address complicated demands (Nguyen & Ringash, 2018).

11.6.3 Specific Knowledge Required for Head and Neck Cancer Follow-Up

Follow-up for HNC is complicated. Not all PCPs will have access to the specialist knowledge and tools needed for the physical examination. In a healthy person, vague symptoms may be deemed insignificant, but in the HNC survivor population, they can be side effects or a relapse. Two studies have demonstrated that, in the diagnostic setting, a lack of follow-up or referral can cause up to 25–50% (Alho et al., 2006; Tromp et al., 2005a) of patients to experience a delay in the initial diagnosis of HNC. This is particularly true for patients with glottis and tongue malignancies who present with hoarseness, pain, or dysphagia (Tromp et al., 2005a, 2005b). In a follow-up situation, it might even be more challenging to separate late-effect symptoms and/or recurrence indicators, particularly in patients who have undergone complicated flap reconstructions or who have severe edema or fibrosis. It could be interesting to find out if PCPs would benefit from continuing medical education where they received training on recurrence recognition for the head and neck region (Nguyen & Ringash, 2018).

11.6.4 The Presence (or Absence) of a Local Multidisciplinary Team

For many PCPs, it may be sufficient to have access to a multidisciplinary team that includes an SLP, a social worker, a nutritionist, a dentist, a physiotherapist, an occupational therapist, a rehabilitation physician, a psychiatrist, and a psychologist who are educated in caring for those with HNC. While it will not solve every problem, connecting patients to community exercise programs or general physical therapy programs will encourage healthy lifestyles and relieve symptoms, including exhaustion (Rogers et al., 2006), pain, weakness, sadness, distress, and overall low QOL (Eades et al., 2013). According to Passchier et al. (2016), involvement in a comprehensive HNC rehabilitation program enhances QOL, functioning, and social engagement, and, after a 7-month program, health-related QOL did not differ substantially from the general population. In these programs, a case manager collaborates with the patient, the multidisciplinary team, and the PCP to create personalized SMART rehabilitation goals—that is, time-bound, relevant, quantifiable, and detailed goals. More research into the particular requirements in various regions is required to assist policymakers in allocating sufficient resources. Alternatively, in places where PCPs lack access to the necessary resources, the onus of referral and assessment may need to stay with experts (Nguyen & Ringash, 2018).

11.7 Conclusion

Multicomponent intervention material spanning all five treatment elements (individual-level skills training, information support, psychotherapy, social support, and dyadic coping) is advised to address the supportive care needs of cancer survivors who have finished treatment and their caregivers. Oral cavity cancer survivors who chose not to return to work had worsened physical and socioemotional functioning and needed more positive social connections and real social support. As healthcare systems incorporate patient-reported outcomes into clinical practice, evidence-based recommendations are essential. Additionally, getting survivors to recognize their symptoms and discuss them directly with doctors enhances assessment precision, care quality, and health outcomes, including survival (Mali, 2023).

In patients with oral cancer, the psychological adjustment level is less than ideal. Compared to patients with tumors in the buccal mucosa, those with cancers in other oral cavity regions have severe psychosocial adjustment. Medical practitioners may utilize these factors to pinpoint high-risk populations needing immediate, intense intervention. Patients' and caregivers' psychological needs must be given special consideration. The likelihood that the survivor will return as a productive member of society increases with the patient's psychological strength. Therefore, action needs to be taken to address this frequently disregarded aspect of patient care. Numerous studies have shown that happier surroundings and happier patients promote faster healing. There is no better approach to ensuring the patient is content than through psychological counseling (Mali, 2023).

Current research is constrained by patient heterogeneity, sample size/power estimates, blinding, loss of follow-up, and medium to high risk of bias. Future studies are required to evaluate the viability of putting guidelines into practice; the optimal ways to coordinate treatment among the patient, specialist(s), caregivers, and PCPs; and the multidisciplinary resources that are available and their accessibility. Strategies are needed to adjust guidelines to local variables, like the prevalence of HNC, care methods, and the accessibility of specialized resources. For HNC patients who are particularly susceptible because of high labor turnover rates and gaps in dental coverage, financial toxicity, and cost are major concerns (Mali, 2023).

References

AKKOL-SOLAKOGLU, S., HEVEY, D., & RICHARDS, D. 2021. A randomised controlled trial comparing internet-delivered cognitive behavioural therapy (iCBT) with and without main carer access versus treatment-as-usual for depression and anxiety among breast cancer survivors: Study protocol. *Internet Interv*, 24, 100367.

ALGTEWI, E. E., OWENS, J., & BAKER, S. R. 2015. Analysing people with head and neck cancers' use of online support groups. *Cyberpsychology*, 9, 1–20.

ALHO, O.-P., TEPPO, H., MÄNTYSELKÄ, P., & KANTOLA, S. 2006. Head and neck cancer in primary care: Presenting symptoms and the effect of delayed diagnosis of cancer cases. *Cmaj*, 174, 779–84.

ALTICE, C. K., BANEGAS, M. P., TUCKER-SEELEY, R. D., & YABROFF, K. R. 2017. Financial hardships experienced by cancer survivors: A systematic review. *J Nati Cancer Instit*, 109, djw205.

AMERICAN ACADEMY OF PEDIATRICS SECTION ON HEMATOLOGY/ONCOLOGY CHILDREN'S ONCOLOGY GROUP. 2009. Long-term follow-up care for pediatric cancer survivors. *Pediatrics*, 123(3), 906–15.

AMERICAN SOCIETY OF CLINICAL ONCOLOGY. 1997. Recommended breast cancer surveillance guidelines. *J Clin Oncol*, 15, 2149–56.

ARMES, J., CROWE, M., COLBOURNE, L., MORGAN, H., MURRELLS, T., OAKLEY, C., PALMER, N., REAM, E., YOUNG, A., & RICHARDSON, A. 2009. Patients' supportive care needs beyond the end of cancer treatment: A prospective, longitudinal survey. *J Clin Oncol*, 27, 6172.

BALFE, M., BUTOW, P., O'SULLIVAN, E., GOOBERMAN-HILL, R., TIMMONS, A., & SHARP, L. 2016a. The financial impact of head and neck cancer caregiving: A qualitative study. *Psycho-oncology*, 25, 1441–7.

BALFE, M., O'BRIEN, K., TIMMONS, A., BUTOW, P., O'SULLIVAN, E., GOOBERMAN-HILL, R., & SHARP, L. 2016b. The unmet supportive care needs of long-term head and neck cancer caregivers in the extended survivorship period. *J Clin Nurs*, 25, 1576–86.

BANTHIN, J. S., CUNNINGHAM, P., & BERNARD, D. M. 2008. Financial burden of health care, 2001–2004. *Health Aff*, 27, 188–95.

BAR AD, V. 2010. Gabapentin for the treatment of cancer-related pain syndromes. *Rev Recent Clin Trials*, 5, 174–8.

BAR AD, V., WEINSTEIN, G., DUTTA, P. R., CHALIAN, A., BOTH, S., & QUON, H. 2010. Gabapentin for the treatment of pain related to radiation-induced mucositis in patients with head and neck tumors treated with intensity-modulated radiation therapy. *Head Neck*, 32, 173–7.

BECK, A. T., EPSTEIN, N., BROWN, G., & STEER, R. 1993. Beck anxiety inventory. *J Consult Clin Psychol*. https://doi.org/10.1037/t02025-000

BEER, J. M., SMITH, K. N., KENNEDY, T., MOIS, G., ACENA, D., GALLERANI, D. G., MCDONNELL, K. K., & OWENS, O. L. 2020. A focus group evaluation of breathe easier: A mindfulness-based mHealth app for survivors of lung cancer and their family members. *Am J Health Promot*, 34, 770–8.

BHANDARE, N., ANTONELLI, P. J., MORRIS, C. G., MALAYAPA, R. S., & MENDENHALL, W. M. 2007. Ototoxicity after radiotherapy for head and neck tumors. *Int J Radiat Oncol Biol Physics*, 67, 469–79.

BINCZAK, M., NAVEZ, M., PERRICHON, C., BLANCHARD, D., BOLLET, M., CALMELS, P., COUTURAUD, C., DREYER, C., ESPITALIER, F., & TESTELIN, S. 2014. Management of somatic pain induced by head-and-neck cancer treatment: Definition and assessment. Guidelines of the French Oto-Rhino-Laryngology-Head and Neck Surgery Society (SFORL). *Eur Ann Otorhinolaryngol Head Neck Dis*, 131, 243–7.

BONOMO, P., MARUELLI, A., SAIEVA, C., TAYLOR, K., SINGER, S., PATELLI, Z., ROGERS, S., MATTAVELLI, D., SIMON, C., & SCOTTÉ, F. 2020. Assessing preferences in patients with head and neck squamous cell carcinoma: Phase I and II of questionnaire development. *Cancers*, 12, 3577.

BOWER, J. E., BAK, K., BERGER, A., BREITBART, W., ESCALANTE, C. P., GANZ, P. A., SCHNIPPER, H. H., LACCHETTI, C., LIGIBEL, J. A., & LYMAN, G. H. 2014. Screening, assessment, and management of fatigue in adult survivors of cancer: An American Society of Clinical oncology clinical practice guideline adaptation. *J Clin Oncol*, 32, 1840.

BRENNAN, M., GORMALLY, J., BUTOW, P., BOYLE, F., & SPILLANE, A. 2014. Survivorship care plans in cancer: A systematic review of care plan outcomes. *Br J Cancer*, 111, 1899–908.

CANCELLIERE, C., DONOVAN, J., STOCHKENDAHL, M. J., BISCARDI, M., AMMENDOLIA, C., MYBURGH, C., & CASSIDY, J. D. 2016. Factors affecting return to work after injury or illness: Best evidence synthesis of systematic reviews. *Chiropractic Manual Ther*, 24, 1–23.

CANCER COUNCIL OF AUSTRALIA (CCA). 2016. Optimal care pathway for people with head and neck cancers. https://www.cancer.org.au/assets/pdf/head-and-neck-cancers-optimal-cancer-care-pathway

CARLSON, L. E., WALLER, A., & MITCHELL, A. J. 2012. Screening for distress and unmet needs in patients with cancer: Review and recommendations. *J Clin Oncol*, 30, 1160–77.

CARMACK, C. L., PARKER, N. H., DEMARK-WAHNEFRIED, W., SHELY, L., BAUM, G., YUAN, Y., GIORDANO, S. H., RODRIGUEZ-BIGAS, M., PETTAWAY, C., & BASEN-ENGQUIST, K. 2021. Healthy moves to improve lifestyle behaviors of cancer survivors and their spouses: Feasibility and preliminary results of intervention efficacy. *Nutrients*, 13, 4460.

CARNABY-MANN, G., CRARY, M. A., SCHMALFUSS, I., & AMDUR, R. 2012. "Pharyngocise": Randomized controlled trial of preventative exercises to maintain muscle structure and swallowing function during head-and-neck chemoradiotherapy. *Int J Radiat Oncol Biol Physics*, 83, 210–19.

CHATURVEDI, A. K., ENGELS, E. A., PFEIFFER, R. M., HERNANDEZ, B. Y., XIAO, W., KIM, E., JIANG, B., GOODMAN, M. T., SIBUG-SABER, M., & COZEN, W. 2011. Human papillomavirus and rising oropharyngeal cancer incidence in the United States. *J Clin Oncol*, 29, 4294.

CHEN, A. M., DALY, M. E., VAZQUEZ, E., COURQUIN, J., LUU, Q., DONALD, P. J., & FARWELL, D. G. 2013. Depression among long-term survivors of head and neck cancer treated with radiation therapy. *JAMA Otolaryngol Head Neck Surg*, 139, 885–9.

CHEN, M., GONG, J., & LI, Q. 2022a. The application of eHealth in cancer survivorship care: A review of web-based dyadic interventions for post-treatment cancer survivors and caregivers. *Asia-Pacific J Oncol Nurs*, 9, 100109.

CHEN, S. C., HUANG, B. S., HUNG, T. M., LIN, C. Y., & CHANG, Y. L. 2019. Impact of physical and psychosocial dysfunction on return to work in survivors of oral cavity cancer. *Psycho-Oncology*, 28, 1910–17.

CHEN, S. C., HUANG, B. S., LIN, C. Y., FAN, K. H., CHANG, J. T. C., WU, S. C., & LAI, Y. H. 2017. Psychosocial effects of a skin camouflage program in female survivors with head and neck cancer: A randomized controlled trial. *Psycho-Oncology*, 26, 1376–83.

CHEN, Y.-W., LIN, T.-R., KUO, P.-L., LEE, S.-C., WU, K.-F., DUONG, T. V., & WANG, T.-J. 2022b. Psychosocial adjustment changes and related factors in postoperative oral cancer patients: A longitudinal study. *Biomedicines*, 10, 3231.

CIANFRONE, G., PENTANGELO, D., CIANFRONE, F., MAZZEI, F., TURCHETTA, R., ORLANDO, M. P., & ALTISSIMI, G. 2011. Pharmacological drugs inducing ototoxicity, vestibular symptoms and tinnitus: A reasoned and updated guide. *Eur Rev Med Pharmacol Sci*, 15, 601–36.

CLARKE, P., RADFORD, K., COFFEY, M., & STEWART, M. 2016. Speech and swallow rehabilitation in head and neck cancer: United Kingdom National Multidisciplinary Guidelines. *J Laryngol Otol*, 130, S176–80.

COHEN, E. E., LAMONTE, S. J., ERB, N. L., BECKMAN, K. L., SADEGHI, N., HUTCHESON, K. A., STUBBLEFIELD, M. D., ABBOTT, D. M., FISHER, P. S., & STEIN, K. D. 2016. American Cancer Society head and neck cancer survivorship care guideline. *CA: Cancer J*, 66, 203–39.

CRAMER, J. D., JOHNSON, J. T., & NILSEN, M. L. 2018. Pain in head and neck cancer survivors: Prevalence, predictors, and quality-of-life impact. *Otolaryngol Head Neck Surg*, 159, 853–8.

DE SOUZA, J. A., KUNG, S., O'CONNOR, J., & YAP, B. J. 2017. Determinants of patient-centered financial stress in patients with locally advanced head and neck cancer. *J Oncol Pract*, 13, e310–18.

DE SOUZA, J. A., YAP, B. J., HLUBOCKY, F. J., WROBLEWSKI, K., RATAIN, M. J., CELLA, D., & DAUGHERTY, C. K. 2014. The development of a financial toxicity patient-reported outcome in cancer: The COST measure. *Cancer*, 120, 3245–53.

DENG, J., RIDNER, S. H., & MURPHY, B. A. 2011. Lymphedema in patients with head and neck cancer: Oncology Nursing Society forum. *Oncology Nurs*, E1, 1–10.

DENLINGER, C. S., SANFT, T., BAKER, K. S., BAXI, S., BRODERICK, G., DEMARK-WAHNEFRIED, W., FRIEDMAN, D. L., GOLDMAN, M., HUDSON, M., & KHAKPOUR, N. 2017. Survivorship, version 2.2017, NCCN clinical practice guidelines in oncology. *J Nat Comp Cancer Netw*, 15, 1140–63.

DESCHLER, D. G. 2019. Head and neck cancer compared with other cancers: Does the great equalizer equalize equally? *JAMA Otolaryngol Head Neck Surg*, 145, 249–50.

DESHPANDE, A., & GHOOI, R. 2017. Narrative: The fear of disfigurement in cancer patients. *Indian J Palliat Care*, 23, 347.

DEWA, C. S., TROJANOWSKI, L., TAMMINGA, S. J., RINGASH, J., MCQUESTION, M., & HOCH, J. S. 2018. Work-related experiences of head and neck cancer survivors: An exploratory and descriptive qualitative study. *Disabil Rehabil*, 40, 1252–8.

DIJKSTRA, P., KALK, W., & ROODENBURG, J. 2004. Trismus in head and neck oncology: A systematic review. *Oral Oncol*, 40, 879–89.

DIJKSTRA, P. U., VAN WILGEN, P. C., BUIJS, R. P., BRENDEKE, W., DE GOEDE, C. J., KERST, A., KOOLSTRA, M., MARINUS, J., SCHOPPINK, E. M., & STUIVER, M. M. 2001. Incidence of shoulder pain after neck dissection: A clinical explorative study for risk factors. *Head Neck*, 23, 947–53.

DILLE, M. F., ELLINGSON, R. M., MCMILLAN, G. P., & KONRAD-MARTIN, D. 2013. ABR obtained from time-efficient train stimuli for cisplatin ototoxicity monitoring. *J Am Acad Audiol*, 24, 769–81.

DIXIT J, GUPTA N, KATAKI A, ROY P, MEHRA N, KUMAR L, *et al.* (2024). Health-related quality of life and its determinants among cancer patients: Evidence from 12,148 patients of Indian database. *Health Qual Life Outcomes* 22, 26. https://doi.org/10.1186/s12955-024-02227-0

DOSS, J., GHANI, W., RAZAK, I., YANG, Y., ROGERS, S., & ZAIN, R. 2017. Changes in health-related quality of life of oral cancer patients treated with curative intent: Experience of a developing country. *Int J Oral Maxillofacial Surg*, 46, 687–98.

DOWELL, D., HAEGERICH, T. M., & CHOU, R. 2016. CDC guideline for prescribing opioids for chronic pain—United States, 2016. *JAMA*, 315, 1624–45.

EADES, M., MURPHY, J., CARNEY, S., AMDOUNI, S., LEMOIGNAN, J., JELOWICKI, M., NADLER, M., CHASEN, M., & GAGNON, B. 2013. Effect of an interdisciplinary rehabilitation program on quality of life in patients with head and neck cancer: Review of clinical experience. *Head Neck*, 35, 343–9.

ELLIS, M. A., STERBA, K. R., DAY, T. A., MARSH, C. H., MAURER, S., HILL, E. G., & GRABOYES, E. M. 2019. Body image disturbance in surgically treated head and neck cancer patients: A patient-centered approach. *Otolaryngol Head Neck Surg*, 161, 278–87.

EMERY, J., BUTOW, P., LAI-KWON, J., NEKHLYUDOV, L., RYNDERMAN, M., & JEFFORD, M. 2022. Management of common clinical problems experienced by survivors of cancer. *Lancet*, 399, 1537–50.

ÉSIK, O., CSERE, T., STEFANITS, K., LENGYEL, Z., SÁFRÁNY, G., VÖNÖCZKY, K., LENGYEL, E., NEMESKÉRI, C., REPA, I., & TRÓN, L. 2003. A review on radiogenic Lhermitte's sign. *Pathol Oncol Res*, 9, 115–20.

FAN, E., CIESLA, N. D., TRUONG, A. D., BHOOPATHI, V., ZEGER, S. L., & NEEDHAM, D. M. 2010. Inter-rater reliability of manual muscle strength testing in ICU survivors and simulated patients. *Intens Care Med*, 36, 1038–43.

FERRELL, B. R., TEMEL, J. S., TEMIN, S., ALESI, E. R., BALBONI, T. A., BASCH, E. M., FIRN, J. I., PAICE, J. A., PEPPERCORN, J. M., & PHILLIPS, T. 2017. Integration of palliative care into standard oncology care: American Society of Clinical Oncology clinical practice guideline update. *J Clin Oncol*, 35, 96–112.

FINGERET, M. C., HUTCHESON, K. A., JENSEN, K., YUAN, Y., URBAUER, D., & LEWIN, J. S. 2013. Associations among speech, eating, and body image concerns for surgical patients with head and neck cancer. *Head Neck*, 35, 354–60.

FINGERET, M. C., TEO, I., & EPNER, D. E. 2014. Managing body image difficulties of adult cancer patients: Lessons from available research. *Cancer*, 120, 633–41.

FINGERET, M. C., VIDRINE, D. J., REECE, G. P., GILLENWATER, A. M., & GRITZ, E. R. 2010. Multidimensional analysis of body image concerns among newly diagnosed patients with oral cavity cancer. *Head Neck*, 32, 301–9.

FINGERET, M. C., YUAN, Y., URBAUER, D., WESTON, J., NIPOMNICK, S., & WEBER, R. 2012. The nature and extent of body image concerns among surgically treated patients with head and neck cancer. *Psycho-Oncol*, 21, 836–44.

FONG, S. S., NG, S. S., LUK, W., CHUNG, J. W., LEUNG, J. C., & MASTERS, R. S. 2014. Effects of a 6-month Tai Chi Qigong program on arterial hemodynamics and functional aerobic capacity in survivors of nasopharyngeal cancer. *J Cancer Survivorship*, 8, 618–26.

FRISINA, R. D., WHEELER, H. E., FOSSA, S. D., KERNS, S. L., FUNG, C., SESSO, H. D., MONAHAN, P. O., FELDMAN, D. R., HAMILTON, R., & VAUGHN, D. J. 2016. Comprehensive audiometric analysis of hearing impairment and tinnitus after cisplatin-based chemotherapy in survivors of adult-onset cancer. *J Clin Oncol*, 34, 2712.

GANE, E., MICHALEFF, Z., COTTRELL, M., MCPHAIL, S., HATTON, A., PANIZZA, B., & O'LEARY, S. 2017. Prevalence, incidence, and risk factors for shoulder and neck dysfunction after neck dissection: A systematic review. *Eur J Surg Oncol*, 43, 1199–218.

GARTON, E. M., ALI, Z., CIRA, M. K., HASKINS, L., JACOBSEN, P. B., KAYIIRA, A., LASEBIKAN, N., ONYEKA, T., ROMERO, Y., & SHIRIMA, S. 2023. An analysis of survivorship care strategies in national cancer control plans in Africa. *J Cancer Survivorship*, 17, 634–45.

GEERSE, O. P., LAKIN, J. R., BERENDSEN, A. J., ALFANO, C. M., & NEKHLYUDOV, L. 2018. Cancer survivorship and palliative care: Shared progress, challenges, and opportunities. *Cancer*, 124, 4435–41.

GEMICI, C. 2010. Lhermitte's sign: Review with special emphasis in oncology practice. *Crit Rev Oncol/Hematol*, 74, 79–86.

GIELISSEN, M., VERHAGEN, C., & BLEIJENBERG, G. 2007. Cognitive behaviour therapy for fatigued cancer survivors: Long-term follow-up. *Br J Cancer*, 97, 612–18.

GILLESPIE, M. B., BRODSKY, M. B., DAY, T. A., LEE, F. S., & MARTIN-HARRIS, B. 2004. Swallowing-related quality of life after head and neck cancer treatment. *Laryngoscope*, 114, 1362–7.

GILLISON, M. L., CHATURVEDI, A. K., ANDERSON, W. F., & FAKHRY, C. 2015. Epidemiology of human papillomavirus–positive head and neck squamous cell carcinoma. *J Clin Oncol*, 33, 3235.

GINSBERG, J. P., HOBBIE, W. L., CARLSON, C. A., & MEADOWS, A. T. 2006. Delivering long-term follow-up care to pediatric cancer survivors: Transitional care issues. *Pediatr Blood Cancer*, 46, 169–73.

GIRGIS, A., LAMBERT, S., & LECATHELINAIS, C. 2011. The supportive care needs survey for partners and caregivers of cancer survivors: Development and psychometric evaluation. *Psycho-oncology*, 20, 387–93.

GIULIANI, M., MCQUESTION, M., JONES, J., PAPADAKOS, J., LE, L. W., ALKAZAZ, N., CHENG, T., WALDRON, J., CATTON, P., & RINGASH, J. 2016. Prevalence and nature of survivorship needs in patients with head and neck cancer. *Head Neck*, 38, 1097–103.

GIULIANI, M., MILNE, R., MCQUESTION, M., SAMPSON, L., LE, L. W., JONES, J., CHENG, T., WALDRON, J., & RINGASH, J. 2017. Partner's survivorship care needs: An analysis in head and neck cancer patients. *Oral Oncol*, 71, 113–21.

GIULIANI, M., PAPADAKOS, J., BROADHURST, M., JONES, J., MCQUESTION, M., LE, L. W., BECK, L., WALDRON, J., & RINGASH, J. 2019. The prevalence and determinants of return to work in head and neck cancer survivors. *Support Care Cancer*, 27, 539–46.

GOLANT, M., LIEBERMAN, M., GIESE-DAVIS, J., WINZELBERG, A., & ELLIS, W. 2004. Emotional expression and facilitation of online vs. face-to-face breast cancer support groups. *Psycho-Oncology*, 13(1), S18–19.

GOLDSTEIN, D. P., RINGASH, J., BISSADA, E., JAQUET, Y., IRISH, J., CHEPEHA, D., & DAVIS, A. M. 2014. Evaluation of shoulder disability questionnaires used for the assessment of shoulder disability after neck dissection for head and neck cancer. *Head Neck*, 36, 1453–8.

GOYAL, N., DAY, A., EPSTEIN, J., GOODMAN, J., GRABOYES, E., JALISI, S., KIESS, A. P., KU, J. A., MILLER, M. C., & PANWAR, A. 2022. Head and neck cancer survivorship consensus statement from the American Head and Neck Society. *Laryngoscope Invest Otolaryngol*, 7, 70–92.

GRABOYES, E. M., HILL, E. G., MARSH, C. H., MAURER, S., DAY, T. A., & STERBA, K. R. 2019. Body image disturbance in surgically treated head and neck cancer patients: A prospective cohort pilot study. *Otolaryngol Head Neck Surg*, 161, 105–10.

HENRY, M., FUEHRMANN, F., HIER, M., ZEITOUNI, A., KOST, K., RICHARDSON, K., MLYNAREK, A., BLACK, M., MACDONALD, C., & CHARTIER, G. 2019. Contextual and historical factors for increased levels of anxiety and depression in patients with head and neck cancer: A prospective longitudinal study. *Head Neck*, 41, 2538–48.

HENRY, M., HABIB, L.-A., MORRISON, M., YANG, J., LI, X., LIN, S., ZEITOUNI, A., PAYNE, R., MACDONALD, C., & MLYNAREK, A. 2014. Head and neck cancer patients went us to support them psychologically in the posttreatment period: Survey results. *Palliat Support Care*, 12, 1–13.

HENRY, M., ROSBERGER, Z., BERTRAND, L., KLASSEN, C., HIER, M., ZEITOUNI, A., KOST, K., MLYNAREK, A., RICHARDSON, K., & BLACK, M. 2018. Prevalence and risk factors of suicidal ideation among patients with head and neck cancer: Longitudinal study. *Otolaryngol Head Neck Surg*, 159, 843–52.

HILL, R. E., WAKEFIELD, C. E., COHN, R. J., FARDELL, J. E., BRIERLEY, M. E. E., KOTHE, E., JACOBSEN, P. B., HETHERINGTON, K., & MERCIECA-BEBBER, R. 2020. Survivorship care plans in cancer: A meta-analysis and systematic review of care plan outcomes. *Oncologist*, 25, e351–72.

HITCHCOCK, Y. J., TWARD, J. D., SZABO, A., BENTZ, B. G., & SHRIEVE, D. C. 2009. Relative contributions of radiation and cisplatin-based chemotherapy to sensorineural hearing loss in head-and-neck cancer patients. *Int J Radiat Oncol Biol Physics*, 73, 779–88.

HODGKINSON, K., BUTOW, P., HOBBS, K., HUNT, G., LO, S. K., & WAIN, G. 2007. Assessing unmet supportive care needs in partners of cancer survivors: The development and evaluation of the Cancer Survivors' Partners Unmet Needs measure (CaSPUN). *Psycho-Oncology*, 16, 805–13.

HOFFMAN, B. S., ELLEN & STOVALL, E. 2006. Survivorship perspectives and advocacy. *J Clin Oncol*, 24, 5154–9.

HUANG, S., & LIU, H.-E. 2008. Effectiveness of cosmetic rehabilitation on the body image of oral cancer patients in Taiwan. *Support Care Cancer*, 16, 981–6.

HUTCHESON, K. A., BHAYANI, M. K., BEADLE, B. M., GOLD, K. A., SHINN, E. H., LAI, S. Y., & LEWIN, J. 2013. Eat and exercise during radiotherapy or chemoradiotherapy for pharyngeal cancers: Use it or lose it. *JAMA Otolaryngol Head Neck Surg*, 139, 1127–34.

HUTCHESON, K. A., NURGALIEVA, Z., ZHAO, H., GUNN, G. B., GIORDANO, S. H., BHAYANI, M. K., LEWIN, J. S., & LEWIS, C. M. 2019. Two-year prevalence of dysphagia and related outcomes in head and neck cancer survivors: An updated SEER-Medicare analysis. *Head neck*, 41, 479–87.

JACOBSEN, P. B., DEROSA, A. P., HENDERSON, T. O., MAYER, D. K., MOSKOWITZ, C. S., PASKETT, E. D., & ROWLAND, J. H. 2018. Systematic review of the impact of cancer survivorship care plans on health outcomes and health care delivery. *J Clin Oncol*, 36, 2088.

JACOBSON, M. C. 2018. The experience of head and neck cancer survivorship (including laryngectomy): An integrated biopsychosocial model. *Curr Opin Support Palliat Care*, 12, 65–73.

JANSEN, F., EERENSTEIN, S. E., CNOSSEN, I. C., LISSENBERG-WITTE, B. I., DE BREE, R., DOORNAERT, P., HALMOS, G. B., HARDILLO, J. A., VAN HINTE, G., & HONINGS, J. 2020. Effectiveness of a guided self-help exercise program tailored to patients treated with total laryngectomy: Results of a multi-center randomized controlled trial. *Oral Oncol*, 103, 104586.

JEFFORD, M., ROWLAND, J., GRUNFELD, E., RICHARDS, M., MAHER, J., & GLASER, A. 2013. Implementing improved post-treatment care for cancer survivors in England, with reflections from Australia, Canada and the USA. *Br J Cancer*, 108, 14–20.

JEPSEN, J., LAURSEN, L., LARSEN, A., & HAGERT, C.-G. 2004. Manual strength testing in 14 upper limb muscles A study of inter-rater reliability. *Acta Orthopaedica Scandinavica*, 75, 442–8.

JERECZEK-FOSSA, B. A., SANTORO, L., ALTERIO, D., FRANCHI, B., FIORE, M. R., FOSSATI, P., KOWALCZYK, A., CANINO, P., ANSARIN, M., & ORECCHIA, R. 2007. Fatigue during head-and-neck radiotherapy: Prospective study on 117 consecutive patients. *Int J Radiat Oncol Biol Physics*, 68, 403–15.

JESSE, M. T., RYAN, M. E., ESHELMAN, A., GHANEM, T., WILLIAMS, A. M., MILLER-MATERO, L. R., & YAREMCHUK, K. 2015. Integrated psychological care in head and neck cancer: Views from health care providers, patients, and supports. *Laryngoscope*, 125, 1345–51.

KAM, D., SALIB, A., GORGY, G., PATEL, T. D., CARNIOL, E. T., ELOY, J. A., BAREDES, S., & PARK, R. C. W. 2015. Incidence of suicide in patients with head and neck cancer. *JAMA Otolaryngol Head Neck Surg*, 141, 1075–81.

KAMSTRA, J. I., VAN LEEUWEN, M., ROODENBURG, J. L., & DIJKSTRA, P. U. 2017. Exercise therapy for trismus secondary to head and neck cancer: A systematic review. *Head Neck*, 39, 2352–62.

KATZ, J., WEINRIB, A., FASHLER, S. R., KATZNELZON, R., SHAH, B. R., LADAK, S. S., JIANG, J., LI, Q., MCMILLAN, K., & MINA, D. S. 2015. The Toronto General Hospital Transitional Pain Service: Development and implementation of a multidisciplinary program to prevent chronic postsurgical pain. *J Pain Res*, 695–702.

KEAN, S., DONAGHY, E., BANCROFT, A., CLEGG, G., & RODGERS, S. 2021. Theorising survivorship after intensive care: A systematic review of patient and family experiences. *J Clin Nurs*, 30, 2584–2610.

KHAN, N., HARRISON, S., ROSE, P., WARD, A., & EVANS, J. 2012. Interpretation and acceptance of the term "cancer survivor": A United Kingdom-based qualitative study. *Eur J Cancer Care*, 21, 177–86.

KHATCHERESSIAN, J. L., WOLFF, A. C., SMITH, T. J., GRUNFELD, E., MUSS, H. B., VOGEL, V. G., HALBERG, F., SOMERFIELD, M. R., & DAVIDSON, N. E. 2006. American

Society of Clinical Oncology 2006 update of the breast cancer follow-up and management guidelines in the adjuvant setting. *J Clin Oncol*, 24, 5091–7.

KIRKPATRICK, J. P., VAN DER KOGEL, A. J., & SCHULTHEISS, T. E. 2010. Radiation dose–volume effects in the spinal cord. *Int J Radiat Oncol Biol Physics*, 76, S42–9.

KLERNÄS, P., JOHNSSON, A., HORSTMANN, V., & JOHANSSON, K. 2018. Health-related quality of life in patients with lymphoedema: A cross-sectional study. *Scand J Caring Sci*, 32, 634–44.

KOTZ, T., FEDERMAN, A. D., KAO, J., MILMAN, L., PACKER, S., LOPEZ-PRIETO, C., FORSYTHE, K., & GENDEN, E. M. 2012. Prophylactic swallowing exercises in patients with head and neck cancer undergoing chemoradiation: A randomized trial. *Arch Otolaryngol Head Neck Surg*, 138, 376–82.

KRAUS, D. H. 2016. Living in a patient-centric universe. *JAMA Otolaryngol Head Neck Surg*, 142, 1231–2.

KROENKE, K., SPITZER, R. L., & WILLIAMS, J. B. 2001. The PHQ-9: Validity of a brief depression severity measure. *J Gen Intern Med*, 16, 606–13.

KROUSE, J. H., KROUSE, H. J., & FABIAN, R. L. 1989. Adaptation to surgery for head and neck cancer. *Laryngoscope*, 99, 789–94.

KUMAR, C. D., JOSEPH, J., JANAKIRAM, C., & GOPINATH, M. 2017. Health-related quality of life and the perceived palliative care needs among oral cancer patients. *J Indian Assoc Public Health Dentistry*, 15, 327–33.

LANDIER, W., BHATIA, S., ESHELMAN, D. A., FORTE, K. J., SWEENEY, T., HESTER, A. L., DARLING, J., ARMSTRONG, F. D., BLATT, J., & CONSTINE, L. S. 2004. Development of risk-based guidelines for pediatric cancer survivors: The Children's Oncology Group long-term follow-up guidelines from the Children's Oncology Group Late Effects Committee and Nursing Discipline. *J Clin Oncol*, 22, 4979–90.

LANGMORE, S. E. 2001. Normal swallowing: The endoscopic perspective. *Endoscopic Eval Treat Swallowing Dis*, 37–59.

LATHAN, C. S., CRONIN, A., TUCKER-SEELEY, R., ZAFAR, S. Y., AYANIAN, J. Z., & SCHRAG, D. 2016. Association of financial strain with symptom burden and quality of life for patients with lung or colorectal cancer. *J Clin Oncol*, 34, 1732.

LIN, Y. S., JEN, Y. M., & LIN, J. C. 2002. Radiation-related cranial nerve palsy in patients with nasopharyngeal carcinoma. *Cancer*, 95, 404–9.

LIST, M. A., D'ANTONIO, L. L., CELLA, D. F., SISTON, A., MUMBY, P., HARAF, D., & VOKES, E. 1996. The performance status scale for head and neck cancer patients and the functional assessment of cancer therapy-head and neck scale: A study of utility and validity. *Cancer*, 77, 2294–301.

LUO, X., GAO, L., LI, J., LIN, Y., ZHAO, J., & LI, Q. 2020. A critical literature review of dyadic web-based interventions to support cancer patients and their caregivers, and directions for future research. *Psycho-Oncology*, 29, 38–48.

LYDIATT, W. M., BESSETTE, D., SCHMID, K. K., SAYLES, H., & BURKE, W. J. 2013. Prevention of depression with escitalopram in patients undergoing treatment for head and neck cancer: Randomized, double-blind, placebo-controlled clinical trial. *JAMA Otolaryngol Head Neck Surg*, 139, 678–86.

LYDIATT, W. M., MORAN, J., & BURKE, W. J. 2009. A review of depression in the head and neck cancer patient. *Clin Adv Hematol Oncol*, 7, 397–403.

MALI, S. B. 2023. Survivorship care in head neck cancer. *Oral Oncol Rep*, 6, 100029.

MALLOY, K. M., & POU, A. M. 2017. Survivorship: Morbidity, mortality, malignancy. *Otolaryngol Clin N Am*, 50, 853–66.

MANNE, S., HUDSON, S., FREDERICK, S., MITAROTONDO, A., BAREDES, S., KALYOUSSEF, E., OHMAN-STRICKLAND, P., & KASHY, D. A. 2020. e-Health self-management intervention for oral and oropharyngeal cancer survivors: Design and single-arm pilot study of empowered survivor. *Head Neck*, 42, 3375–88.

MARGALIT, D. N., SALZ, T., VENCHIARUTTI, R., MILLEY, K., MCNAMARA, M., CHIMA, S., WONG, J., DRUCE, P., & NEKHLYUDOV, L. 2022. Interventions for head and neck cancer survivors: Systematic review. *Head Neck*, 44, 2579–99.

MASSA, S. T., OSAZUWA-PETERS, N., BOAKYE, E. A., WALKER, R. J., & WARD, G. M. 2019. Comparison of the financial burden of survivors of head and neck cancer with other cancer survivors. *JAMA Otolaryngol Head Neck Surg*, 145, 239–49.

MAURER, J., HIPP, M., SCHÄFER, C., & KÖLB, O. 2011. Impact on quality of life after radio (chemo) therapy of head and neck cancer. *Strahlenther Onkol*, 187, 744–9.

MCDERMOTT, J. D., EGUCHI, M., STOKES, W. A., AMINI, A., HARARAH, M., DING, D., VALENTINE, A., BRADLEY, C. J., & KARAM, S. D. 2019. Short-and long-term opioid use in patients with oral and oropharynx cancer. *Otolaryngol Head Neck Surg*, 160, 409–19.

MCDOWELL, L. J., ROCK, K., XU, W., CHAN, B., WALDRON, J., LU, L., EZZAT, S., POTHIER, D., BERNSTEIN, L. J., & SO, N. 2018. Long-term late toxicity, quality of life, and emotional distress in patients with nasopharyngeal carcinoma treated with intensity modulated radiation therapy. *Int J Radiat Oncol Biol Physics*, 102, 340–52.

MCDOWELL, M. E., OCCHIPINTI, S., FERGUSON, M., DUNN, J., & CHAMBERS, S. 2010. Predictors of change in unmet supportive care needs in cancer. *Psycho-oncology*, 19, 508–16.

MCELDUFF, P., BOYES, A., ZUCCA, A., & GIRGIS, A. 2004. *Supportive Care Needs Survey: A Guide to Administration, Scoring and Analysis*. Newcastle: Centre for Health Research & Psycho-oncology.

MCGARVEY, A. C., CHIARELLI, P. E., OSMOTHERLY, P. G., & HOFFMAN, G. R. 2011. Physiotherapy for accessory nerve shoulder dysfunction following neck dissection surgery: A literature review. *Head Neck*, 33, 274–80.

MCGARVEY, A. C., HOFFMAN, G. R., OSMOTHERLY, P. G., & CHIARELLI, P. E. 2015. Maximizing shoulder function after accessory nerve injury and neck dissection surgery: A multicenter randomized controlled trial. *Head Neck*, 37, 1022–31.

MCNEELY, M. L., PARLIAMENT, M. B., SEIKALY, H., JHA, N., MAGEE, D. J., HAYKOWSKY, M. J., & COURNEYA, K. S. 2015. Sustainability of outcomes after a randomized crossover trial of resistance exercise for shoulder dysfunction in survivors of head and neck cancer. *Physiother Canada*, 67, 85–93.

MELARIRI, H., ELS, T., OYEDELE, O., SUTTLE, T. K., BERMOSKY, K. T., DE FREITAS, A., MURTAZA, A., MOOSAJEE, M., & MELARIRI, P. E. 2023. Prevalence of locoregional recurrence and survival post-treatment of head and neck cancers in Africa: A systematic review and meta-analysis. *EClinicalMedicine*, 59. https://www.thelancet.com/journals/eclinm/article/PIIS2589-5370(23)00141-4/fulltext

MEYERHARDT, J. A., MANGU, P. B., FLYNN, P. J., KORDE, L., LOPRINZI, C. L., MINSKY, B. D., PETRELLI, N. J., RYAN, K., SCHRAG, D. H., & WONG, S. L. 2013. Follow-up care, surveillance protocol, and secondary prevention measures for survivors of colorectal cancer: American Society of Clinical Oncology clinical practice guideline endorsement. *J Clin Oncol*, 31, 4465–70.

MILAS, Z. L., NEELANDS, B., TRUFAN, S. J., BENBOW, J., CARRIZOSA, D., BRICKMAN, D. S., FRENKEL, C. H., SUMRALL, A. L., SUDHAKAR, S. M., & WARD, M. C. 2022. Survivorship care plans improve the identification of post-radiation hypothyroidism after head and neck cancer treatment. *Anticancer Res*, 42, 4429–37.

MILLER, K. D., SIEGEL, R. L., LIN, C. C., MARIOTTO, A. B., KRAMER, J. L., ROWLAND, J. H., STEIN, K. D., ALTERI, R., & JEMAL, A. 2016. Cancer treatment and survivorship statistics, 2016. *CA: Cancer J*, 66, 271–89.

MURPHY, B. A., & GILBERT, J. 2009. Dysphagia in head and neck cancer patients treated with radiation: Assessment, sequelae, and rehabilitation. *Semin Radiat Oncol*, 35–42.

NADER, M.-E., & GIDLEY, P. W. 2019. Challenges of hearing rehabilitation after radiation and chemotherapy. *J Neurol Surg Part B: Skull Base*, 80, 214–24.

NATIONAL COMPREHENSIVE CANCER NETWORK. 2019. NCCN guidelines version 1.2019. Cancer-related fatigue. Available at: https://www.nccn.org/professionals/physician_gls/pdf/fatigue.pdf [Accessed May 30, 2019.]

NATIONAL RESEARCH COUNCIL. 2006. *From Cancer Patient to Cancer Survivor: Lost in Transition. An American Society of Clinical Oncology and Institute of Medicine Symposium*. Washington, DC: National Academies Press.

NEKHLYUDOV, L., LACCHETTI, C., DAVIS, N. B., GARVEY, T. Q., GOLDSTEIN, D. P., NUNNINK, J. C., NINFEA, J. I. R., SALNER, A. L., SALZ, T., & SIU, L. L. 2017. Head and neck cancer survivorship care guideline: American Society of Clinical Oncology clinical practice guideline endorsement of the American Cancer Society guideline. *J Clin Oncol*, 35, 1606–21.

NEKHLYUDOV, L., MOLLICA, M. A., JACOBSEN, P. B., MAYER, D. K., SHULMAN, L. N., & GEIGER, A. M. 2019. Developing a quality of cancer survivorship care framework: Implications for clinical care, research, and policy. *JNCI*, 111, 1120–30.

NEUGUT, A. I., SUBAR, M., WILDE, E. T., STRATTON, S., BROUSE, C. H., HILLYER, G. C., GRANN, V. R., & HERSHMAN, D. L. 2011. Association between prescription co-payment amount and compliance with adjuvant hormonal therapy in women with early-stage breast cancer. *J Clin Oncol*, 29, 2534.

NGUYEN, N.-T. A., & RINGASH, J. 2018. Head and neck cancer survivorship care: A review of the current guidelines and remaining unmet needs. *Curr Treat Opt Oncol*, 19, 1–20.

NIELSEN-SCOTT, M., FELLMETH, G., OPONDO, C., & ALDERDICE, F. 2022. Prevalence of perinatal anxiety in low-and middle-income countries: A systematic review and meta-analysis. *J Affect Dis*, 306, 71–9.

NIGHTINGALE, C. L., CURBOW, B. A., WINGARD, J. R., PEREIRA, D. B., & CARNABY, G. D. 2016. Burden, quality of life, and social support in caregivers of patients undergoing radiotherapy for head and neck cancer: A pilot study. *Chronic Illness*, 12, 236–45.

O'BRIEN, K. M., TIMMONS, A., BUTOW, P., GOOBERMAN-HILL, R., O'SULLIVAN, E., BALFE, M., & SHARP, L. 2017. Associations between neighbourhood support and financial burden with unmet needs of head and neck cancer survivors. *Oral Oncol*, 65, 57–64.

OJO, B., GENDEN, E. M., TENG, M. S., MILBURY, K., MISIUKIEWICZ, K. J., & BADR, H. 2012. A systematic review of head and neck cancer quality of life assessment instruments. *Oral Oncol*, 48, 923–37.

OKOTURO, E., OSASUYI, A., & OPALEYE, T. 2020. Genetic polymorphism of head and neck cancers in African populations: A systematic review. *OTO Open*, 4, 2473974X20942202.

OSAZUWA-PETERS, N., SIMPSON, M. C., ZHAO, L., BOAKYE, E. A., OLOMUKORO, S. I., DESHIELDS, T., LOUX, T. M., VARVARES, M. A., & SCHOOTMAN, M. 2018. Suicide risk among cancer survivors: Head and neck versus other cancers. *Cancer*, 124, 4072–9.

PAK, D., VINEBERG, K., FENG, F., TEN HAKEN, R. K., & EISBRUCH, A. 2012. Lhermitte sign after chemo-IMRT of head-and-neck cancer: Incidence, doses, and potential mechanisms. *Int J Radiat Oncol Biol Physics*, 83, 1528–33.

PALERI, V., & ROLAND, N. 2016. Introduction to the United Kingdom national multidisciplinary guidelines for head and neck cancer. *J Laryngol Otol*, 130, S3–S4.

PANG, J., TRINGALE, K. R., TAPIA, V. J., MOSS, W. J., MAY, M. E., FURNISH, T., BARNACHEA, L., BRUMUND, K. T., SACCO, A. G., & WEISMAN, R. A. 2017. Chronic opioid use following surgery for oral cavity cancer. *JAMA Otolaryngol Head Neck Surg*, 143, 1187–94.

PASSCHIER, E., STUIVER, M. M., VAN DER MOLEN, L., KERKHOF, S. I., VAN DEN BREKEL, M. W., & HILGERS, F. J. 2016. Feasibility and impact of a dedicated multidisciplinary rehabilitation program on health-related quality of life in advanced head and neck cancer patients. *Eur Arch Oto-Rhino-Laryngol*, 273, 1577–87.

PAULI, N., JOHNSON, J., FINIZIA, C., & ANDRELL, P. 2013. The incidence of trismus and long-term impact on health-related quality of life in patients with head and neck cancer. *Acta Oncologica*, 52, 1137–45.

PAULOSKI, B. R., RADEMAKER, A. W., LOGEMANN, J. A., STEIN, D., BEERY, Q., NEWMAN, L., HANCHETT, C., TUSANT, S., & MACCRACKEN, E. 2000. Pretreatment swallowing function in patients with head and neck cancer. *Head Neck*, 22, 474–82.

PAUWELS, E., VAN HOOF, E., CHARLIER, C., LECHNER, L., & DE BOURDEAUDHUIJ, I. 2012. Design and process evaluation of an informative website tailored to breast cancer survivors' and intimate partners' post-treatment care needs. *BMC Res Notes*, 5, 1–13.

PEKMEZI, D. W., CRANE, T. E., OSTER, R. A., ROGERS, L. Q., HOENEMEYER, T., FARRELL, D., COLE, W. W., WOLIN, K., BADR, H., & DEMARK-WAHNEFRIED, W. 2021. Rationale and methods for a randomized controlled trial of a dyadic, web-based, weight loss intervention among cancer survivors and partners: The DUET study. *Nutrients*, 13, 3472.

PENNER, J. L. 2009. Psychosocial care of patients with head and neck cancer. *Semin Oncol Nurs*, 25, 231–41.

POULSEN, M. G., RIDDLE, B., KELLER, J., PORCEDDU, S. V., & TRIPCONY, L. 2008. Predictors of acute grade 4 swallowing toxicity in patients with stages III and IV squamous carcinoma of the head and neck treated with radiotherapy alone. *Radiother Oncol*, 87, 253–9.

PRICE-BLACKSHEAR, M. A., PRATSCHER, S. D., OYLER, D. L., ARMER, J. M., CHENG, A.-L., CHENG, M. X., RECORDS, K., UDMUANGPIA, T., CARSON, J. W., & ANN BETTENCOURT, B. 2020. Online couples mindfulness-based intervention for young breast cancer survivors and their partners: A randomized-control trial. *J Psychosoc Oncol*, 38, 592–611.

RAMSEY, S. D., BANSAL, A., FEDORENKO, C. R., BLOUGH, D. K., OVERSTREET, K. A., SHANKARAN, V., & NEWCOMB, P. 2016. Financial insolvency as a risk factor for early mortality among patients with cancer. *J Clin Oncol*, 34, 980.

RESNICK, M. J., LACCHETTI, C., BERGMAN, J., HAUKE, R. J., HOFFMAN, K. E., KUNGEL, T. M., MORGANS, A. K., & PENSON, D. F. 2015. Prostate cancer survivorship care guideline: American Society of Clinical Oncology clinical practice guideline endorsement. *J Clin Oncol*, 33, 1078–85.

RHOTEN, B. A., MURPHY, B., & RIDNER, S. H. 2013. Body image in patients with head and neck cancer: A review of the literature. *Oral Oncol*, 49, 753–60.

RIDNER, S. H., DIETRICH, M. S., NIERMANN, K., CMELAK, A., MANNION, K., & MURPHY, B. 2016. A prospective study of the lymphedema and fibrosis continuum in patients with head and neck cancer. *Lymphatic Res Biol*, 14, 198–205.

RIEKE, K., SCHMID, K. K., LYDIATT, W., HOUFEK, J., BOILESEN, E., & WATANABE-GALLOWAY, S. 2017. Depression and survival in head and neck cancer patients. *Oral Oncol*, 65, 76–82.

RIFKIN, W. J., KANTAR, R. S., ALI-KHAN, S., PLANA, N. M., DIAZ-SISO, J. R., TSAKIRIS, M., & RODRIGUEZ, E. D. 2018. Facial disfigurement and identity: A review of the literature and implications for facial transplantation. *AMA J Ethics*, 20, 309–23.

RINGASH, J., BERNSTEIN, L. J., DEVINS, G., DUNPHY, C., GIULIANI, M., MARTINO, R., & MCEWEN, S. 2018. Head and neck cancer survivorship: Learning the needs, meeting the needs. *Semin Radiat Oncol*, 28, 64–74.

ROBINSON, M., WARD, L., MEHANNA, H., PALERI, V., & WINTER, S. 2018. Provision of physiotherapy rehabilitation following neck dissection in the UK. *J Laryngol Otol*, 132, 624–7.

ROCK, C. L., DOYLE, C., DEMARK-WAHNEFRIED, W., MEYERHARDT, J., COURNEYA, K. S., SCHWARTZ, A. L., BANDERA, E. V., HAMILTON, K. K., GRANT, B., & MCCULLOUGH, M. 2012. Nutrition and physical activity guidelines for cancer survivors. *CA: Cancer J*, 62, 242–74.

ROGERS, L. Q., COURNEYA, K. S., ROBBINS, K. T., MALONE, J., SEIZ, A., KOCH, L., RAO, K., & NAGARKAR, M. 2006. Physical activity and quality of life in head and neck cancer survivors. *Support Care Cancer*, 14, 1012–19.

ROSENBERG-YUNGER, Z. R., KLASSEN, A. F., AMIN, L., GRANEK, L., D'AGOSTINO, N. M., BOYDELL, K. M., GREENBERG, M., BARR, R. D., & NATHAN, P. C. 2013. Barriers and facilitators of transition from pediatric to adult long-term follow-up care in childhood cancer survivors. *J Adolesc Young Adult Oncol* 2, 104–11.

ROSENTHAL, D. I., MENDOZA, T. R., CHAMBERS, M. S., ASPER, J. A., GNING, I., KIES, M. S., WEBER, R. S., LEWIN, J. S., GARDEN, A. S., & ANG, K. K. 2007. Measuring head and neck cancer symptom burden: The development and validation of the MD Anderson symptom inventory, head and neck module. *Head Neck*, 29, 923–31.

RUNOWICZ, C. D., LEACH, C. R., HENRY, N. L., HENRY, K. S., MACKEY, H. T., COWENS-ALVARADO, R. L., CANNADY, R. S., PRATT-CHAPMAN, M. L., EDGE, S. B., & JACOBS, L. A. 2016. American Cancer Society/American Society of Clinical Oncology breast cancer survivorship care guideline. *CA: Cancer J*, 66, 43–73.

SALVESTRINI, V., BECHERINI, C., DESIDERI, I., CAPRARA, L., MARIOTTI, M., BANINI, M., PIEROSSI, N., SCOTTI, V., LIVI, L., & BONOMO, P. 2022. The impact of patient preference in the treatment algorithm for recurrent/metastatic head and neck squamous cell carcinoma. *La Radiologia Medica*, 127, 866–71.

SALZ, T., MCCABE, M. S., OEFFINGER, K. C., CORCORAN, S., VICKERS, A. J., SALNER, A. L., DORNELAS, E., SCHNALL, R., RAGHUNATHAN, N. J., & FORTIER, E. 2016. A head and neck cancer intervention for use in survivorship clinics: A protocol for a feasibility study. *Pilot Feasibility Studies*, 2, 1–13.

SALZ, T., OSTROFF, J. S., NIGHTINGALE, C. L., ATKINSON, T. M., DAVIDSON, E. C., JINNA, S. R., KRIPLANI, A., LESSER, G. J., LYNCH, K. A., & MAYER, D. K. 2021. The Head and Neck Survivorship Tool (HN-STAR) Trial (WF-1805CD): A protocol for a cluster-randomized, hybrid effectiveness-implementation, pragmatic trial to improve the follow-up care of head and neck cancer survivors. *Contemp Clin Trials*, 107, 106448.

SALZ, T., SCHNALL, R. B., MCCABE, M. S., OEFFINGER, K. C., CORCORAN, S., VICKERS, A. J., SALNER, A. L., DORNELAS, E., RAGHUNATHAN, N. J., & FORTIER, E. 2018. Incorporating multiple perspectives into the development of an electronic survivorship platform for head and neck cancer. *JCO Clin Cancer Informatics*, 2, 1–15.

SANDERS, J. G., & DAWES, P. J. 2016. Gabapentin for perioperative analgesia in otorhinolaryngology–head and neck surgery: Systematic review. *Otolaryngol Head Neck Surg*, 155, 893–903.

SCHERPENHUIZEN, A., VAN WAES, A. M., JANSSEN, L. M., VAN CANN, E. M., & STEGEMAN, I. 2015. The effect of exercise therapy in head and neck cancer patients in the treatment of radiotherapy-induced trismus: A systematic review. *Oral Oncol*, 51, 745–50.

SCHOU, I., EKEBERG, O., KARESEN, R., & SORENSEN, E. 2008. Psychosocial intervention as a component of routine breast cancer care: Who participates and does it help? *Psycho-Oncology*, 17, 716–20.

SILVER, N., DOURADO, J., HITCHCOCK, K., FULLERTON, A., FREDENBURG, K., DZIEGIELEWSKI, P., DANAN, D., TIGHE, P., MORRIS, C., & AMDUR, R. 2019. Chronic opioid use in patients undergoing treatment for oropharyngeal cancer. *Laryngoscope*, 129, 2087–93.

SKOLARUS, T. A., WOLF, A. M., ERB, N. L., BROOKS, D. D., RIVERS, B. M., UNDERWOOD III, W., SALNER, A. L., ZELEFSKY, M. J., ARAGON-CHING, J. B., & SLOVIN, S. F. 2014. American Cancer Society prostate cancer survivorship care guidelines. *CA: Cancer J*, 64, 225–49.

SMIT, M., BALM, A. J., HILGERS, F. J., & TAN, I. B. 2001. Pain as sign of recurrent disease in head and neck squamous cell carcinoma. *Head Neck*, 23, 372–5.

SMITH, B. G., HUTCHESON, K. A., LITTLE, L. G., SKORACKI, R. J., ROSENTHAL, D. I., LAI, S. Y., & LEWIN, J. S. 2015. Lymphedema outcomes in patients with head and neck cancer. *Otolaryngol Head Neck Surg*, 152, 284–91.

SMITH, B. G., & LEWIN, J. S. 2010. Lymphedema management in head and neck cancer. *Curr Opin Otolaryngol Head Neck Surg*, 18, 153–8.

SMITH, T. J., DAVIDSON, N. E., SCHAPIRA, D. V., GRUNFELD, E., MUSS, H. B., VOGEL III, V. G., & SOMERFIELD, M. R. 1999. American Society of Clinical Oncology 1998 update of recommended breast cancer surveillance guidelines. *J Clin Oncol*, 17, 1080.

SMITH, W. H., LUSKIN, I., SALGADO, L. R., SCARBOROUGH, B. M., LIN, J.-Y., ÖZBEK, U., MILES, B. A., GUPTA, V., & BAKST, R. L. 2019. Risk of prolonged opioid use among cancer patients undergoing curative intent radiation therapy for head and neck malignancies. *Oral Oncology*, 92, 1–5.

SO, W. K., CHOI, K., CHEN, J. M., CHAN, C. W., CHAIR, S., FUNG, O. W., WAN, R. W., MAK, S. S., LING, W., & NG, W. 2014. Quality of life in head and neck cancer survivors at 1 year after treatment: The mediating role of unmet supportive care needs. *Support Care Cancer*, 22, 2917–26.

SONG, L., GUO, P., TAN, X., CHEN, R. C., NIELSEN, M. E., BIRKEN, S. A., KOONTZ, B. F., NORTHOUSE, L. L., & MAYER, D. K. 2021. Enhancing survivorship care planning for patients with localized prostate cancer using a couple-focused web-based, mHealth program: The results of a pilot feasibility study. *J Cancer Survivorship*, 15, 99–108.

SPRATT, D. E., SAKAE, M., RIAZ, N., LOK, B. H., ESSANDOH, S., HSU, M., ZHANG, Z., SCHUPAK, K., SETTON, J., & LEE, N. Y. 2012. Time course and predictors for cancer-related fatigue in a series of oropharyngeal cancer patients treated with chemoradiation therapy. *oncologist*, 17, 569–76.

STERBA, K. R., ARMESON, K., ZAPKA, J., SCALLION, M. A., GARRIS, T. K., GRABOYES, E. M., RUGGIERO, K., & DAY, T. A. 2019. Evaluation of a survivorship needs assessment planning tool for head and neck cancer survivor-caregiver dyads. *J Cancer Survivorship*, 13, 117–29.

STROJAN, P., HUTCHESON, K. A., EISBRUCH, A., BEITLER, J. J., LANGENDIJK, J. A., LEE, A. W., CORRY, J., MENDENHALL, W. M., SMEE, R., & RINALDO, A. 2017. Treatment of late sequelae after radiotherapy for head and neck cancer. *Cancer Treat Rev*, 59, 79–92.

SUN, D. Q., WARD, B. K., SEMENOV, Y. R., CAREY, J. P., & DELLA SANTINA, C. C. 2014. Bilateral vestibular deficiency: Quality of life and economic implications. *JAMA Otolaryngol Head Neck Surg*, 140, 527–34.

TERKAWI, A. S., TSANG, S., ALSHEHRI, A. S., MULAFIKH, D. S., ALGHULIKAH, A. A., & ALDHAHRI, S. F. 2017. The burden of chronic pain after major head and neck tumor therapy. *Saudi J Anaesthesia*, 11, S71–9.

TROMP, D. M., BROUHA, X. D., HORDIJK, G.-J., WINNUBST, J. A., & DE LEEUW, J. R. J. 2005a. Patient factors associated with delay in primary care among patients with head and neck carcinoma: A case-series analysis. *Fam Pract*, 22, 554–9.

TROMP, D. M., BROUHA, X. D., HORDIJK, G.-J., WINNUBST, J. A., & DE LEEUW, R. J. 2005b. Patient and tumour factors associated with advanced carcinomas of the head and neck. *Oral Oncol*, 41, 313–19.

TSATSOU, I., KONSTANTINIDIS, T., KALEMIKERAKIS, I., ADAMAKIDOU, T., VLACHOU, E., & GOVINA, O. 2021. Unmet supportive care needs of patients with hematological malignancies: A systematic review. *Asia-Pacific J Oncol Nurs* 8, 5–17.

VAN DER GEER, S. J., VAN RIJN, P. V., KAMSTRA, J. I., LANGENDIJK, J. A., VAN DER LAAN, B. F., ROODENBURG, J. L., & DIJKSTRA, P. U. 2018. Prevalence and prediction of trismus in patients with head and neck cancer: A cross-sectional study. *Head Neck*, 41, 64–71.

VAN DER GEER, S. J., VAN RIJN, P. V., KAMSTRA, J. I., ROODENBURG, J. L., & DIJKSTRA, P. U. 2019. Criterion for trismus in head and neck cancer patients: A verification study. *Support Care Cancer*, 27, 1129–37.

VANSTONE, R., & FERGUS, K. D. 2020. Online couple interventions in cancer. *Curr Opin Support Palliat Care*, 14, 67–73.

WAKISAKA, H., YAMADA, H., MOTOYOSHI, K., UGUMORI, T., TAKAHASHI, H., & HYODO, M. 2011. Incidence of long-term ipsilateral and contralateral ototoxicity following radiotherapy for nasopharyngeal carcinoma. *Auris Nasus Larynx*, 38, 95–100.

WALL, L. R., WARD, E. C., CARTMILL, B., & HILL, A. J. 2013. Physiological changes to the swallowing mechanism following (chemo) radiotherapy for head and neck cancer: A systematic review. *Dysphagia*, 28, 481–93.

WANG, T.-J., LU, M.-H., KUO, P.-L., CHEN, Y.-W., LEE, S.-C., & LIANG, S.-Y. 2018. Influences of facial disfigurement and social support for psychosocial adjustment among patients with oral cancer in Taiwan: A cross-sectional study. *BMJ Open*, 8, e023670.

WEBER, C., DOMMERICH, S., PAU, H. W., & KRAMP, B. 2010. Limited mouth opening after primary therapy of head and neck cancer. *Oral Maxillofac Surg*, 14, 169–73.

WINDON, M. J., D'SOUZA, G., FARAJI, F., TROY, T., KOCH, W. M., GOURIN, C. G., KIESS, A. P., PITMAN, K. T., EISELE, D. W., & FAKHRY, C. 2019. Priorities, concerns, and regret among patients with head and neck cancer. *Cancer*, 125, 1281–9.

WINTERS-STONE, K. M., BOISVERT, C., LI, F., LYONS, K. S., BEER, T. M., MITRI, Z., MEYERS, G., ECKSTROM, E., & CAMPBELL, K. L. 2022. Delivering exercise medicine to cancer survivors: Has COVID-19 shifted the landscape for how and who can be reached with supervised group exercise? *Support Care Cancer*, 30, 1903–6.

WU, P., SZCZESNIAK, M., MACLEAN, J., GRAHAM, P., QUON, H., CHOO, L., & COOK, I. 2019. Endoscopic dilatation improves long-term dysphagia following head and neck cancer therapies: A randomized control trial. *Dis Esophagus*, 32, doy087.

WU, Y.-S., LIN, P.-Y., CHIEN, C.-Y., FANG, F.-M., CHIU, N.-M., HUNG, C.-F., LEE, Y., & CHONG, M.-Y. 2016. Anxiety and depression in patients with head and neck cancer: 6-month follow-up study. *Neuropsychiatric Dis Treat*, 1029–36.

YAO, T., BEADLE, B., HOLSINGER, C. F., & STARMER, H. M. 2020. Effectiveness of a home-based head and neck lymphedema management program: A pilot study. *Laryngoscope*, 130, E858–62.

ZAFAR, S. Y., & ABERNETHY, A. P. 2013. Financial toxicity, part I: A new name for a growing problem. *Oncology (Williston Park, NY)*, 27, 80.

ZAFAR, S. Y., MCNEIL, R. B., THOMAS, C. M., LATHAN, C. S., AYANIAN, J. Z., & PROVENZALE, D. 2015. Population-based assessment of cancer survivors' financial burden and quality of life: A prospective cohort study. *J Oncol Pract*, 11, 145–50.

ZAHID, N., ZAHID, W., KHALID, W., AZAM, I., IKRAM, M., HASSAN, A., IFTIKAR, H., BHAMANI, S. S., JABBAR, A. A., & AKHTAR, S. 2021. Resilience and its associated factors in head and neck cancer patients in Pakistan: An analytical cross-sectional study. *BMC Cancer*, 21, 888.

ZELLER, J. L. 2006. High suicide risk found for patients with head and neck cancer. *JAMA*, 296, 1716–17.

ZHI, W. I., & SMITH, T. J. 2015. Early integration of palliative care into oncology: Evidence, challenges and barriers. *Ann Palliat Med*, 4, 12231.

ZUUR, C. L., SIMIS, Y. J., LAMERS, E. A., HART, A. A., DRESCHLER, W. A., BALM, A. J., & RASCH, C. R. 2009. Risk factors for hearing loss in patients treated with intensity-modulated radiotherapy for head-and-neck tumors. *Int J Radiat Oncol Biol Physics*, 74, 490–6.

12

Emerging Technologies and Future Directions

Tsholofelo Kungoane, Zarah Yakoob, Diana Mavuso, Melvin Ambele, Oluwatoyin A. Asojo, and Zodwa Dlamini

12.1 Introduction

Head and neck cancers (HNCs) encompass a diverse group of malignancies originating in the oral cavity, pharynx, larynx, nasal cavity, and paranasal sinuses. The complex anatomy and heterogeneous nature of HNCs pose significant challenges in diagnosis, staging, and treatment planning (Balgobind et al., 2024; Basheeth & Patil, 2019; Chiu et al., 2020). Traditional diagnostic approaches, including clinical examination, imaging, and tissue biopsy, often provide limited information and may be invasive or insufficiently sensitive. However, recent advancements in diagnostic technologies are revolutionizing the diagnostic workup of HNCs, offering more precise, comprehensive, and less invasive methods to assess these tumors (Balgobind et al., 2024; Basheeth & Patil, 2019; Chiu et al., 2020). Emerging technologies such as advanced imaging modalities, molecular profiling techniques, liquid biopsy, and artificial intelligence (AI) are transforming the landscape of HNC diagnosis. Advanced imaging techniques, including positron emission tomography-computed tomography (PET-CT) and magnetic resonance imaging (MRI), provide high-resolution, functional, and anatomical information, improving the accuracy of tumor localization and staging (Balgobind et al., 2024).

Molecular profiling techniques, including next-generation sequencing (NGS) and transcriptomics, enable detailed characterization of tumors' genetic and molecular landscape and facilitate personalized treatment strategies based on specific molecular aberrations (Balgobind et al., 2024; Basheeth & Patil, 2019; Chiu et al., 2020). Liquid biopsy represents a significant breakthrough in non-invasive diagnostics, allowing for the detection and analysis of circulating tumor DNA (ctDNA), circulating tumor cells (CTCs), and other tumor-derived components in bodily fluids. This approach offers real-time insights into tumor dynamics, treatment response, and emerging resistance mechanisms (Balgobind et al., 2024; Basheeth & Patil, 2019; Chiu et al., 2020). Additionally, AI and machine learning algorithms are increasingly being integrated into diagnostic processes, enhancing the interpretation of complex data, predicting disease progression, and aiding in clinical decision-making (Balgobind et al., 2024; Basheeth & Patil, 2019; Chiu et al., 2020).

Integrating these emerging technologies into the diagnostic workup of HNCs holds great promise for improving early detection, accurate staging, and personalized treatment planning (Balgobind et al., 2024; Basheeth & Patil, 2019; Chiu et al., 2020). By providing a more detailed and dynamic understanding of tumor biology, these innovations can enhance patient outcomes, reduce treatment-related morbidity, and ultimately improve survival rates (Balgobind et al., 2024; Basheeth & Patil, 2019; Chiu et al., 2020). This chapter focuses on the technologies in the diagnostic work-up and treatment of HNCs. It sets the stage for a comprehensive review of the cutting-edge diagnostic technologies transforming HNC management, highlighting their applications, benefits, and potential to address existing diagnostic challenges.

12.2 Emerging Technologies in Histological and Molecular Diagnosis of Head and Neck Tumors

Histological diagnosis of head and neck tumors relies on examining and/or selecting appropriate histochemical and immunohistochemical (IHC) staining and molecular testing. Most neoplasms express biomarkers that aid in the diagnosis, treatment, and prognosis. The biomarkers in HNCs can be associated with immunological, infectious, and genetic aberrations. Biomarkers are molecules expressed in serum and tumors that are a sign of a normal or abnormal process of a condition or disease and are used to guide the management of disease and recurrence (Balgobind et al., 2024; Henry & Hayes, 2012). Tumor-specific biomarkers can be detected using IHC, in-situ hybridization (ISH), polymerase chain reaction (PCR), florescent in-situ hybridization (FISH), and genetic sequencing (Balgobind et al., 2024; Spence et al., 2016). This can be done on fresh tissue, cytology specimens, and formalin-fixed paraffin-embedded (FFPE) tissue. These modalities are used in the histological and molecular diagnosis of tumors to assess for predictive markers and prognostication (Balgobind et al., 2024; Filippini et al., 2023; Gavrielatou et al., 2020).

12.2.1 Immunohistochemistry in the Era of Personalized Medicine

IHC is a histopathology technique that utilizes binding specific antibodies to antigens in tissue and using light microscopy to visualize the localization of the staining pattern. The use of IHC in histopathology includes determining tumor histogenesis, therapeutic targets, and predictive and prognostic markers (Balgobind et al., 2024; Zhu et al., 2015). The principle of IHC involves using chromogen/enzyme-labeled probes to identify the staining patterns. The use of IHC in diagnostic histopathology depends on the IHC clone, tissue fixation and processing, antigen retrieval methods, and the interpretation of results (Oumarou Hama et al., 2022; Tsutsumi, 2021). The benefits of IHC include low cost, quick turnaround time, and visual interpretation by pathologists, and, most importantly, the staining can be performed on FFPE tissue and cell blocks. Limitations to IHC include interobserver interpretation and variability and the labeling of up to two markers per tissue section. The use of IHC has evolved. The most important use of IHC in oncology is for prognostic and predictive tumor biomarkers (Balgobind et al., 2024; Basheeth & Patil, 2019; Chiu et al., 2020). Table 12.1 summarizes the predictive and prognostic IHC head and neck biomarkers. Also, IHC is used to detect molecular alterations in tumors and infections (Balgobind et al., 2024; Bishop et al., 2017; Spence et al., 2016; Zaborowski et al., 2020). Table 12.2 summarizes the head and neck neoplasms with their IHC stains and molecular alterations.

12.2.2 Human Papillomavirus Infection in the Head and Neck

The head and neck is a hotspot for human papillomavirus (HPV) infection. The sites for HPV infection include the oropharynx, oral cavity, and sinonasal cavity.

Table 12.1 Predictive and prognostic immunohistochemical biomarkers in the head and neck

Immunohistochemistry	Diagnostic utility	Diagnosis
P16	Human papillomavirus (HPV)	Oropharyngeal carcinoma
PDL	Immunotherapy	Squamous cell carcinoma
Ki-67	Tumor differentiation/tumor grade	Neuroendocrine tumors
		Lymphomas
		Sarcomas
		Salivary gland neoplasm

Source: Balgobind et al., 2024; Basheeth and Patil, 2019; Chiu et al., 2020.

Table 12.2 Head and neck neoplasms and their associated molecular alterations

Diagnosis	Immunohistochemistry stain	Genetic aberration
	Salivary gland pathology	
Pleomorphic adenoma	Plag1	PLAG1 gene abnormalities
Carcinoma ex pleomorphic adenoma	Plag1	PLAG1 gene abnormalities
Adenoid cystic carcinoma	MYB	MYB-NFIB t(6;9)(q22-23;p23-24)
Secretory carcinoma	pan-Trk	ETV6-NTRK3 t(12;15)(p13;q25)
Acinic cell carcinoma	NR4A3	SCPP::NR4A3 fusion t(4;9)(q13;q31)
Mucoepidermoid carcinoma	MAML2	CRTC1-MAML2 t(11:19)(q14-21;p12-13)
	Sinonasal pathology	
Adenoid cystic carcinoma	MYB	MYB-NFIB t(6;9)(q22-23;p23-24)
NUT midline carcinoma	NUT	NUT-BRD4 t(15;19)(q14;p13) NUT-BRD3 and NUT-NSD3
HPV-related multiphenotypic sinonasal carcinoma	P16, LEF-1	High-risk HPV genotypes (33, 35, 52 and 56)
Teratocarcinosarcoma	Loss of SMARCA4 expression	SMARCA4-deficient sinonasal carcinomas
SMARCB1-deficient sinonasal carcinomas	Loss of SMARCB1 (INI1) expression	SWI/SNF complex located at 22q11.2
Biphenotypic sinonasal sarcoma	S100, SOX10, desmin	PAX3-MAML3 t(2;4)(q35;q31.1)
Synovial sarcoma	SS18	SS18–SSX1 (X;18)(p11;q11), SS18–SSX2 or SS18–SSX4
Solitary fibrous tumour	STAT6	NAB2-STAT6 gene fusion
	Oral cavity	
Oropharyngeal carcinoma	P16	High-risk HPV genotypes (16, 18, 33, 35, 52 and 56)
DEK-AFF2 non-keratinizing SCC	AFF2	DEK::AFF2 fusion t(6;X)(q28;p22.3)

Source: Zaborowski et al., 2020; Balgobind et al., 2024; Spence et al., 2016; Bishop et al., 2017.

HPV-associated oropharyngeal carcinomas have a better prognosis compared to conventional tobacco-related carcinomas (Mirghani & Blanchard, 2018; Perri et al., 2020). In the oral cavity proper, the overall prevalence of HPV was reported at 6% (Katirachi et al., 2023). HPV-related sinonasal carcinomas include nonkeratinizing, papillary, and HPV-related multiphenotypic sinonasal carcinomas (Bishop et al., 2017).

p16 is a tumor suppressor gene that inhibits cyclin-dependent kinase 4. HPV oncoproteins E6 and E7 inactivate the Rb protein and degrade the p53 protein, leading to p16 overexpression (Keller et al., 2014). IHC staining for p16 is a cost-effective method of assessing high-risk HPV and triaging tissue for HPV-ISH testing (Singhi & Westra, 2010; Spence et al., 2016; Wang et al., 2020). P16 IHC staining can be performed on FFPE tissue and cytology cell blocks. A positive test result requires that p16 IHC should be positive with a 70% nuclear and cytoplasmic staining cutoff of tumor cells (Lewis et al., 2017) (Figure 12.1).

Also, p16 is used to diagnose carcinoma of unknown primary (CUP) of oropharyngeal origin (Fotopoulos & Pavlidis, 2015; Keller et al., 2014) and a subset of HPV koilocytic dysplasia. In addition, the expression of p16 in the tumor is used for prognosis and in selecting patients for de-escalation therapy (Bishop et al., 2017; Bouland et al., 2021; Mirghani & Blanchard, 2018; Paver et al., 2020).

12.2.3 Pan-Trk Immunohistochemistry in Head and Neck Tumors

Pan-TrK IHC staining is used as a surrogate marker for screening and detection of the NTRK1, NTRK2, and NTRK3 fusions in various tumors (Hechtman et al., 2017; Solomon et al., 2020). Depending on the fusion partner, the staining pattern includes nuclear, cytoplasmic, membranous, or a combination (Hechtman et al., 2017). Nuclear staining for pan-Trk is highly specific for secretory carcinoma, which harbors the ETV6-NTRK3 fusion (Csanyi-Bastien et al., 2021; Xu et al., 2020). Recently, $S100^{+}/CD34^{+}/SOX10$ spindle cell neoplasms with perivascular hyalinization and staghorn vessels have been added to the NTRK-rearranged spindle cell neoplasms (Xu et al., 2023). These tumours show diverse morphological patterns and have been reported from a wide range of anatomical sites. Molecular confirmation is mandatory for IHC-positive NTRK cases for patients to be eligible for TRK inhibitors such as crizotinib, larotrectinib, and entrectinib.

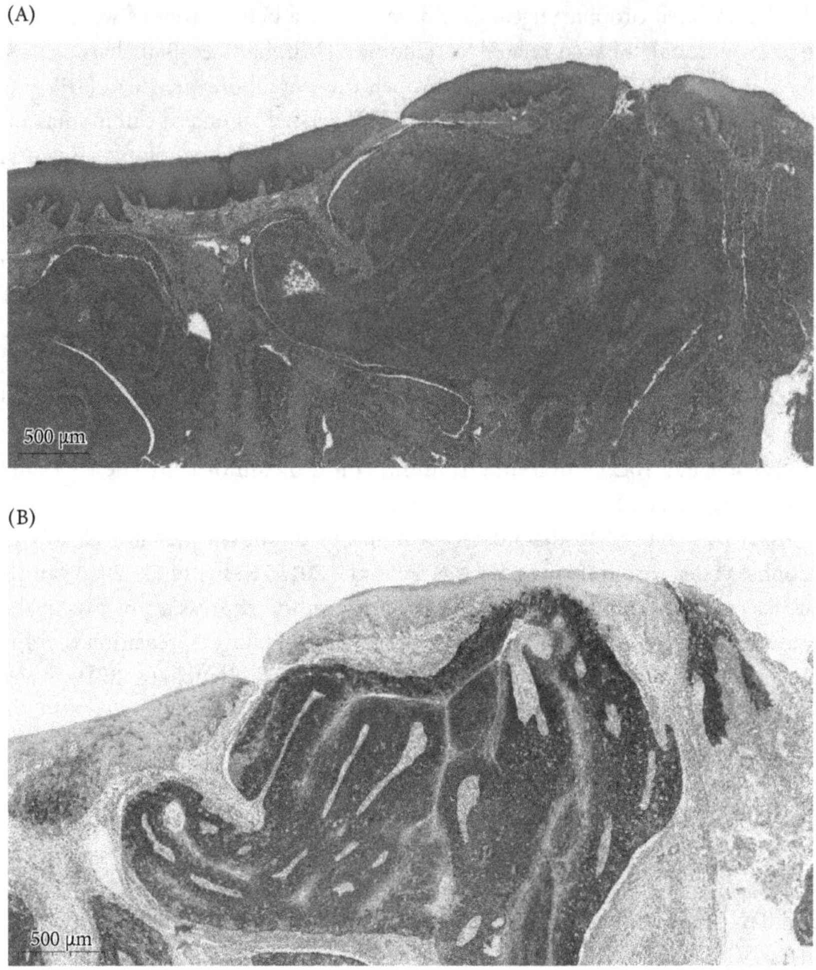

Figure 12.1 Non-keratinizing squamous cell carcinoma (SCC) (A, H&E) with a strong nuclear and cytoplasmic expression of p16 in > 70% of tumor cells (B). Immunohistochemical staining for p16 is a cost-effective method of assessing high-risk human papillomavirus (HPV) infection and triaging tissue for HPV-ISH testing.

12.3 Multiplex Immunohistochemistry/ Immunofluorescence (mIHC/IF) Technologies

A tumor interacts with its microenvironment, which comprises immune cells and stromal cells. The tumor microenvironment predicts the tumor's responsiveness to immunotherapy (De Keukeleire et al., 2021; Obradovic et al., 2022).

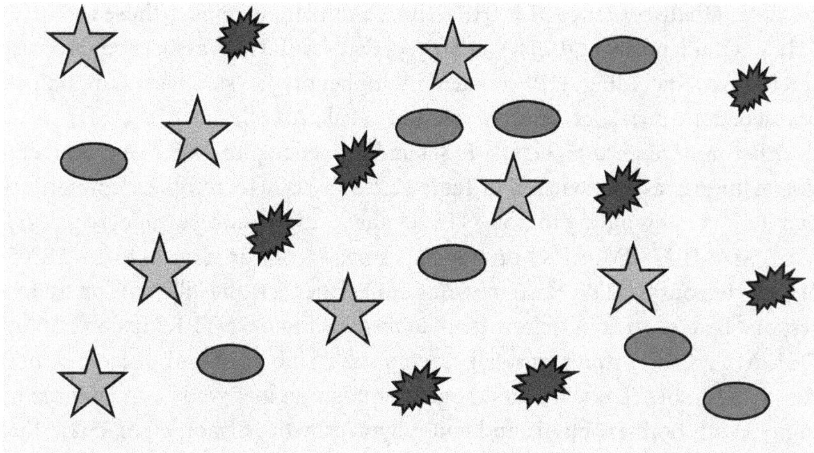

Figure 12.2 Multiplex chromogenic immunohistochemistry staining. Triplex staining with green, yellow, and blue chromogens.

Multiplex IHC/immunofluorescence (mIHC/IF) technologies allow tissue examination to detect multiple cell compositions, functional state, and cell–cell interactions (Tan et al., 2020; Taube et al., 2020). The mIHC/IF techniques involve using multiple chromogenic IHC on the same slide with different chromogens (colors) (Figure 12.2). Importantly, mIHC/IF facilitates evaluating the diagnostic and prognostic biomarkers in a single slide using light microscopy. Microscopy multiplexed IHC consecutive staining on a single slide (MICSSS) uses iterative cycles of tagging, image scanning, and destaining of chromogen substrate on a single slide to generate multiplex imaging (Taube et al., 2020).

12.4 Molecular Testing in Diagnosis

Molecular methods such as FISH, ISH, PCR, and RNA/DNA-based sequencing are used to assess tumors at RNA and DNA levels. Although IHC staining is a cost-effective way of diagnosis, molecular testing is still mandatory in some cases. ISH is the commonly cost-effective molecular testing method in head and neck tumors. The molecular method is mostly used for Epstein-Barr virus (EBER-ISH) and HPV (HPV-ISH) infections in the diagnosis of EBV-related and HPV-related tumors, respectively. ISH is mandatory in tumors with p16-positive IHC staining from smokers and p16-negative oropharyngeal carcinomas. Recent data suggest that patients with concordance p16$^+$/HPV$^+$ have a better prognosis compared to discordance patients (Mehanna et al., 2023). Nonsmoker patients with discordance p16$^+$/HPV$^-$ have a similar outcome to those with p16$^+$ / HPV$^+$ (Bouland et al., 2021). Similarly, patients with HPV-associated sinonasal carcinomas, including HPV-related multiphenotypic sinonasal carcinomas, have a better clinical outcome (Chowdhury et al., 2017).

Other molecular tests include FISH and sequencing to detect genetic alteration in tumors, as summarized in Table 12.2. Subsets of secretory carcinoma lack pan-TrK, corresponding to non-NTRK3 alternative fusion partners (e.g., RET, MET, MAML3, VIM, ALK) or atypical exons 4 to 14 or exons 5 to 14, ETV6-NTRK3 fusions (Csanyi-Bastien et al., 2021). Patients with NTRK fusion tumors respond better to Trk inhibitors than do those with non-NTRK3 fusion tumors. DEK-AFF2 fusion squamous cell carcinomas of the head and neck are a new subset of tumors. These tumors range from high- to low-grade nonkeratinizing tumors with both exophytic and endophytic growth (Bishop et al., 2021; Kuo et al., 2021). These tumors show a response to immune checkpoint inhibitor therapy.

12.5 Biomarkers in Head and Neck Squamous Cell Carcinoma

Standard practice in head and neck squamous cell carcinoma (HNSCC) diagnosis is histological examination of biopsy. This method is invasive and may have some drawbacks in diagnosing HNSCC at an early stage. In this light, newer approaches for diagnosing HNSCC that will use less invasive methods, such as liquid biopsies, are currently being explored due to the inaccessibility of pathology lab facilities and the complex nature of histological examination of biopsy in diagnosing the different types of HNSCC. Despite liquid biopsy biomarkers' promising use in diagnosis, they are not utilized in routine clinical practice because more research is required to assess their diagnostic efficacy in HNSCC (Guerra et al., 2016). Nevertheless, diagnosing a tumor is only possible through identifying quantifiable or semi-quantifiable biomarkers that can differentiate between tumor and normal tissue (Basheeth & Patil, 2019).

12.5.1 Immunological Biomarkers

The programmed cell death protein 1 (PD-1) and programmed death ligand 1 (PD-L1) are tumor microenvironment immune markers used in HNSCC. IHC assessment of PD-L1 expression in tumor samples is both a diagnostic and prognostic biomarker for using PD-1/PD-L1 inhibitors targeted to treat HNSCC (Economopoulou et al., 2019). The clinical use of PD-L1 inhibitors is based on

PD-1/PD-L1, tumor mutation burden (TMB), and tumor microsatellite instability (MSI), although for HNSCC treatment, MSI testing is not required. This is based on a 2018 recommendation by the Society for Immunotherapy of Cancer consensus statement on immunotherapy for the treatment of HNSCC (Cohen et al., 2019a) since IHC of (TPS and CPS) to determine PDL-1 expression levels has successfully been used for pre-treatment screening. The $CD3^+$, $CD4^+$, and $CD8^+$ T cells are the most clinically relevant subset of tumor-infiltrating lymphocytes (TILs) investigated in HNSCC with both diagnostic and prognostic biomarker potential.

12.5.2 Infectious Biomarkers

HPV and EBV are the most common infectious identifiable risk factors for HNSCC. EBV DNA load is a potential biomarker for nasopharyngeal carcinoma with a sensitivity for diagnosis of 95% (95% confidence interval [CI], 91–98%). When combined with anti-EBV capsid antigen IgA (IgA VCA), the overall sensitivity for positive diagnosis by either marker is 99% (Leung et al., 2004). This suggests that a combination of EBV DNA and IgA VCA may show promising diagnostic value for nasopharyngeal carcinoma, with high sensitivity and specificity of this biomarker panel (Leung et al., 2004). It is well-established in HNSCC that HPV^+ oropharyngeal SCC (OPSCC) shows better treatment response and disease-specific and disease-free survival (DFS) (De Keukeleire et al., 2021). There are currently 12 high-risk cancer-causing HPV strains (types 16, 18, 31, 33, 35, 39, 45, 51, 52, 56, 58, and 59), with HPV 16 being the main cause of OPSCC development (Elrefaey et al., 2014; Tanaka & Alawi, 2018). IHC expression of P16 is used as a surrogate marker in HNSCC to determine HPV infection. However, this is mostly true for OPSCC rather than for OSCC (Ambele et al., 2019). E6 and E7 are the common high-risk HPV oncoproteins involved in HNSCC development, and these oncoproteins promote the degradation of Retinoblastoma protein (RB) and P53, which are regulated by P16 to drive tumorigenesis (Wai et al., 2020).

The direct detection of HPV infection in HNSCC is either by ISH or PCR. RT-qPCR detection of E6/E7 mRNA is considered the gold standard in detecting clinically significant HPV infection (Bernadt & Collins, 2017), although the sensitivity of this technique decreases with the quality of the sample. The DNA ISH showed high specificity in detecting the presence of HPV in pathological samples, ensuring positive stains are from tumor samples and not surrounding tissues, but it is less sensitive (Venuti & Paolini, 2012). Notwithstanding, E6/E7-mRNA ISH of processed FFPE tissues allows for direct visualization of viral transcripts with high sensitivity similar to p16 IHC and qRT-PCR (Kang et al.,

2015). The sensitivity and specificity of P16 expression in OPSCC are about 94% and 83% for HPV positivity, respectively, while the specificity of P16 expression for HPV positivity is lower in non-oropharyngeal HNSCC (Elrefaey et al., 2014). Nevertheless, HPV status and its surrogate marker, P16, remain a valuable diagnostic tool in HNSCC, with p16 IHC routinely used in clinical practice owing to its simplicity and high sensitivity for detecting all high-risk types of HPV.

12.5.3 Genetic Biomarkers

The TMB determined by either whole-exome or whole-genome DNA sequencing of tumor tissue is a quantitative measure of the number of coding mutations present in a specific tumor genome (mut/mB) that represents a genetic biomarker with application in HNSCC, which shows one of the highest TMBs of all solid malignancies (Oliva et al., 2019). HNSCC is genetically very heterogeneous, and several studies have attempted to uncover genetic signatures as biomarkers for diagnosis, tumorigenesis, and antitumor immune response (Ambele et al., 2020; Lawrence et al., 2015; She et al., 2020). Among the immune-related genes, the interferon (IFN)-α response, the IFN-γ response, IL-6/JAK/STAT3, and IL-2/STAT5 signaling pathways correlate negatively with immune risk, while high CD8 T cell, memory-activated CD4 T cell, and Treg cell infiltration correlate strongly with low immune risk groups (She et al., 2020). In addition to the amplification of genes in chromosomal regions 3q26.2, 5q14.3, 8q24.3, 8q22.3, and 14q32.33 reported as common genetic markers in OSCC, other known genetic markers frequently observed in HNSCC include loss of heterozygosity or deletion in 17p (*TP53*), 9p (*CDKN2A*), and 3p (*FHIT* & *RSSFIA*) (Ambele et al., 2020).

The Cancer Genome Atlas Network reported gains of 3q, 5p, and 8q and losses of 3p and 8p chromosomal regions as common copy number alterations (CNAs) present in the genome of most HNSCCs (Lawrence et al., 2015). Furthermore, both positive and negative HPV HNSCC showed amplifications of the region 3q26/28 containing the transcription factors *TP63* and *SOX2* for squamous lineage and the *PIK3CA* oncogene (Lawrence et al., 2015). HPV-positive HNSCC showed amplification of *E2F1* and an intact 9p21.3 (CDKN2A) in addition to deletion or truncating mutations in tumor necrosis factor (TNF) receptor-associated factor 3 (*TRAF3*), which is implicated in innate and acquired antiviral response to EBV, HPV, and HIV, thus providing evidence linking *TRAF3* to HPV-positive HNSCC (Lawrence et al., 2015). On the other hand, HPV-negative HNSCC showed amplification of 11q13 (*CCND1*, *FADD*, and *CTTN*) and 11q22 (*BIRC2* and *YAP1*) as well as deletion of tumor suppressor genes (*FAT1*, *NOTCH1*, *SMAD4*, and *CDKN2A*) and *NSD1* (Lawrence et al., 2015).

12.5.4 Emerging Approaches to New Biomarker Discovery from Liquid Biopsy

Liquid biopsies constitute various biological fluids ranging from blood (plasma and serum) to saliva or urine and have emerged as exciting noninvasive tools for the discovery of biomarkers such as metabolites, proteins, ctDNA, CTCs, mRNA, and miRNAs in cancer diagnosis, treatment response, and progression (Kong & Birkeland, 2021). In the case of HNSCC, many studies have explored liquid biopsy for biomarker identification, including the identification of four measurable serum metabolites—glutamine, acetone, acetate, and choline—in a cohort study as potential biomarkers to distinguish 92.4% of oral leukoplakia from OSCC with a high-level sensitivity and specificity that is similar to the gold standard histological examination for oral cancer diagnosis (Gupta et al., 2015). Additionally, a cohort study showed plasma levels of gelsolin are significantly lower in people with HNSCC than in healthy controls and showed high sensitivity (82.7%) and specificity (95.6%) levels as diagnostic biomarkers. The sensitivity was increased to 90.6% when combined with soluble Fas ligand for early disease detection.

ctDNA, broadly referred to as *cell-free DNA* (cfDNA), is released from cells via pathological and physiological mechanisms such as apoptosis and necrosis into blood circulation. In cancer patients, cfDNA comprises those from tumor cells (ctDNA) and normal cells, with the proportion of ctDNA ranging from < 0.1% to > 10% based on the cancer stage, tumor burden, response to treatment, and cellular turnover (Diehl et al., 2008). ctDNA could serve as a potential blood biomarker for cancer but its detection and quantification via sequencing is very challenging, thus new digital technologies that employ targeted and untargeted ctDNA approaches are being studied and optimized to address this challenge (Siravegna et al., 2017). The targeted approach uses droplet digital PCR (ddPCR) or beads, emulsion, amplification, and magnetic (BEAMing) to optimize samples with low ctDNA counts.

In addition, sequencing techniques like AmpliSeq, cancer personalized profiling by deep sequencing (CAPP-Seq), tagged amplicon deep sequencing (TAm-Seq), and safe sequencing system (Safe-Seq) are also being used to isolate and capture ctDNA. Meanwhile, the "untarget approach" includes methods that do not require prior knowledge of genetic mutations, such as whole-exome sequencing and whole-genome sequencing (Kong & Birkeland, 2021). Whole-genome sequencing, TAm-Seq, AmpliSeq, and ddPCR have been used in HNSCC to quantify CNAs and somatic mutations in low-level ctDNA (Kong & Birkeland, 2021; Mes et al., 2020). Notwithstanding limitations in the sensitivity of ctDNA as a biomarker, further technological advances will improve its sensitivity and specificity, which will facilitate its clinical application in HNSCC.

Integrins are commonly expressed by tumor cells, including HNSCC, and therefore, using specific ligands to target integrins could prove beneficial to isolate and capture rare CTCs, especially with the use of the CellSearch system platform (de Wit et al., 2014; Kong & Birkeland, 2021), approved by the US Food and Drug Administration (FDA). Notwithstanding, the expression of integrins and other epithelial cell adhesion molecules decreases as cells undergo epithelial-mesenchymal transition, thereby introducing bias in its usage (Zeisberg & Neilson, 2009). Depletion by negative selection of blood cell markers such as CD45 and CD235a has been suggested as a viable alternative to remove bias and select for CTCs since they do not express these markers (Lu et al., 2015a). Achieving better cell purity despite the optimized capture efficiency remains a challenge (Shen et al., 2017). A new technology, *label-free inertial microfluidics*, outperformed the CellSearch system; it was developed to detect a larger CTC pool of 3–133 CTC/mL of blood (Onidani et al., 2019). Furthermore, a two-step isolation and purification method that uses a negative selection-based CTC isolation scheme followed by an 8-day spheroid cell culture to further purify CTCs to yield cells of higher purity has been developed (Liao et al., 2019) with potential for use in HNSCC.

Noncoding RNAs are another class of molecular factors measured in serum and that have diagnostic potential in HNSCC. The expression of serum exosomal miR-21 and HOTAIR was significantly higher in people with laryngeal SCC (LSCC) compared to those with vocal cord polyps (Wang et al., 2014). Expression levels of miR-21 and HOTAIR in serum were also significantly different between clinical stages III/IV and the early stage, as patients with lymph node metastasis had higher expression of these factors. The receiver-operating characteristic (ROC) curve of miR-21 and HOTAIR combined for diagnosing LSCC was 87.6%, with 94.2% and 73.5% sensitivity and specificity, respectively, to distinguish between malignant and benign disease, which was found to correlate significantly with clinical parameters of LSCC (Wang et al., 2014). Patients with oral cancers, as well as those with oral precancerous lesions, are reported to have significantly high plasma levels of circulating miR-196a and miR-196b.

The high levels of these miRNAs were able to differentiate precancer or cancer patients from healthy subjects (Lu et al., 2015b). The specificity and sensitivity of combining both miR-196a and miR-196b in diagnosing precancer or oral cancer and predicting possible malignancy was high (91% sensitivity and 85% specificity). This indicates that a panel of miR-196a and miR-196b levels with high sensitivity and specificity could serve as a potential biomarker for early detection of oral cancer (Lu et al., 2015b). lncRNA LOC284454 is dysregulated in HNSCC, with higher expression in patients compared to healthy controls, and it showed good diagnostic potential for these cancers as evaluated by ROC (Fan et al., 2020).

Patients with OSCC have high expression of galectin-1 (gal-1) and galectin-3 (gal-3) in both serum and tumor tissue compared to healthy subjects, and these levels were significantly higher with higher tumor burden than with lower tumor burden (Aggarwal et al., 2015). The ROC showed > 80% sensitivity and specificity for gal-1 and gal-3 serum levels to discriminate patients from healthy subjects, suggesting a potential biomarker for screening high-risk populations for OSCC (Aggarwal et al., 2015). Serum levels of Cyfra 21-1 showed high sensitivity (96%) and specificity (87%) in subjects with mucosal oral SCC, and these levels were significantly reduced by 47% ($P \leq 0.003$) within 3 weeks post tumor resection (Nagler et al., 1999). Cyfra 21-1 levels were significantly higher in subjects with SCC compared to those with benign tumors, in healthy subjects, or in those in disease remission, suggesting a possible clinical use of this factor as a possible biomarker in the early detection of oral SCC lesions (Nagler et al., 1999). Serum fascin is reported to be significantly higher in people with HNSCC and to correlate with pathological lymph node metastasis. It was shown to discriminate people with HNSCC and healthy subjects with an area under the curve in ROC of 0.808 (95% CI 0.723–0.901) (Lee et al., 2015).

Flow cytometric analysis of immune cell dysregulation has diagnostic and prognostic potential in HNSCC, which has an immunosuppressive environment characterized by lower $CD4^+$ and $CD8^+$ T-cell counts and elevated Tregs and myeloid-derived stem cells (MDSCs) (Takahashi et al., 2016). The $CD4^+$ T cells in tumors are of the subtype Tregs and can be subdivided into three groups based on their immunophenotypic surface markers and function as CD45RA-positive $FoxP3^{low}$ (immunosuppressive resting), CD45RA-negative $FoxP3^{low}$ (nonimmunosuppressive), and CD45RA-negative $FoxP3^{high}$ (activating) Tregs (Miyara et al., 2009). Flow cytometric analysis of peripheral blood from oropharyngeal and laryngeal cancer patients in a prospective study reported a shift from naïve $CD8^+$ T cells into effector memory T cells, which was shown to be higher in HPV-positive HNSCC compared to HPV-negative HNSCC (Takahashi et al., 2022). This suggests a diagnostic potential of this technique. Furthermore, it has also been observed that HPV-positive HNSCC with low TILs (cytotoxic $CD8^+$) showed no survival advantage compared to HPV-negative counterparts, while only HPV-positive HNSCC with high TILs showed superior survival advantage compared to HPV-negative HNSCC (Ou et al., 2017; Ward et al., 2014). This suggests cytotoxic $CD8^+$ as a potential biomarker for patient treatment selection in HPV-positive HNSCC.

Recent studies have implicated oral microbiome dysbiosis in HNSCC development (Sarkar et al., 2021; Su et al., 2021), with a high abundance of *Fusobacterium* and a low abundance of *Streptococcus* reported in primary and metastatic tumors (Shin et al., 2017). Nonetheless, more studies are required to determine the diagnostic and prognostic performance of the oral microbiome in

HNSCC, considering the multiple intrinsic and extrinsic factors influencing its composition.

12.5.5 Biomarkers in Treatment Response

12.5.5.1 Immunological Biomarkers

High levels of TILs in HNSCC patients relate to better prognostic value in terms of longer overall survival (OS), DFS, and better locoregional control (de Ruiter et al., 2017; Xu et al., 2017). $CD8^+$ TILs kill tumor cells by directly targeting PD-L1 on tumor cells, thereby maintaining immune surveillance and extending OS (Solomon et al., 2018). A tumor model established to predict response to immunotherapy revealed a better response to PD-1/PD-L1 inhibitor therapy if both TILs and PD-L1 are expressed, while negative expression of both shows resistance to PD-1/PD-L1 inhibitor therapy (Teng et al., 2015). Pembrolizumab and nivolumab are immunotherapies developed to target PD-1 (PD-1 inhibitor) in recurrent or metastatic HNSCC, which, when compared to standard chemotherapy, provides longer OS (Burtness et al., 2019). Compared to standard chemotherapy, PD-L1 inhibitors showed little prolonged progression-free survival (PFS) in multiple clinical trials (Burtness et al., 2019; Cohen et al., 2019b; Ferris et al., 2018; Seiwert et al., 2016). Tumor proportion score (TPS) and combined positive score (CPS) are the two immune indicators used to evaluate treatment options with the PD-1 inhibitor, pembrolizumab. However, only CPS values have a better prognosis in HNSCC because they have been shown to correlate positively with OS (Burtness et al., 2019).

The prognostic value of $CD3^+$ IHC staining in HNSCC remains contradictory because some studies have reported beneficial clinical outcomes with high compared to low $CD3^+$ infiltrated tumors, while another study reported no difference in OS in primary or metastatic lesions in highly $CD3^+$ infiltrated HNSCC tissues (De Keukeleire et al., 2021; Lechner et al., 2017). Also, retrospective analyses of $CD4^+$ $FoxP3^+$ infiltration into OPSCC demonstrated no effect on clinical outcome with this Treg cell density, while a significantly better prognosis was obtained in HNSCC with high $CD8^+$ lymphocyte infiltration (De Keukeleire et al., 2021). Nevertheless, a systematic meta-analysis review revealed high $CD3^+$ and $CD8^+$ infiltration correlates with better prognosis in HNSCC independent of HPV status (de Ruiter et al., 2017).

IFN-γ acts upstream of PD-L1 to drive its expression (Abiko et al., 2015) and can, therefore, be a potential predictor of PD-1 treatment response (Ayers et al., 2017). In HNSCC, CXCL9, IDO1, HLA-DRA, CXCL10, STAT1, and IFN-γ constitute a six-gene interferon-γ signature panel shown to be statistically related to best Overall Survival and PFS, making it a potential biomarker for use in excluding immunotherapy because it has a negative predictive value of about 95% (Seiwert et al., 2016). The expression of the CXC chemokine family is known to increase in HNSCC, with CXCL9 and CXCL10 being significantly expressed in the Tumor Microenvironment (TME), which, indicates a therapeutic benefit from immunotherapy (Seiwert et al., 2016; Uppaluri et al., 2020). Although not in HNSCC, CXCL-related inhibitors have been successfully used to suppress growth and metastasis (Cambien et al., 2009) and should, therefore, be considered a viable treatment option in combination with PD-1 inhibitors for HNSCC. Cancer-associated fibroblasts (CAFs) are known to always be present in TME, with recognizable head and neck CAF subtypes (HNCAF-0/3) present as a predictive biomarker for nivolumab treatment response in HNSCC, while immune suppression was associated with the presence of HNCAF-1. This suggests that HNCAF subtypes are potential biomarkers of response and resistance in HNSCC (Obradovic et al., 2022).

12.5.5.2 Infectious Biomarkers

HPV positivity and/or P16 expression in OPSCC is associated with better response to chemo- and radiotherapy, with a more favorable prognosis compared to negative HPV/P16 status. It is worth mentioning that the relationship between P16/HPV status and TILs remains unclear since better OS and DFS (in OPSCC) are observed in patients with high lymphocyte infiltration independent of HPV status (Wai et al., 2020). Overall, HPV-positive HNSCC showed an intact *p53* gene, making it more amendable to treatment compared to HPV-negative HNSCC, which has a mutated *TP53* with high TMB and may thus account for the better prognosis seen with HPV-positive HNSCC than HPV-negative HNSCC (Andersen et al., 2014). Studies looking at HPV/P16 status with PD-1 inhibitor treatment outcomes have produced contradictory reports (Bauml et al., 2017; Segal et al., 2019), which therefore requires further investigation on the effect of HPV/P16 status on the prognosis of overall response rate (ORR) in patients treated with PD-1 inhibitors.

12.5.5.3 Genetic Biomarkers

HNSCC tumors with wild-type *P53* showed favorable outcomes compared to those with *TP53* mutants and amplification of 11q13/*CCND1*, irrespective of HPV status (Lawrence et al., 2015). Also notable in HNSCC are tumors primarily driven by mutation rather than CNAs, known as *M class tumors* (Ambele et al., 2020; Ciriello et al., 2013). This class of tumors with few CNAs showed favorable clinical outcomes compared to those with high CNAs (Lawrence et al., 2015). Furthermore, high TMB HNSCC showed a better prognosis in clinical trials when treated with PD-1/PD-L1 inhibitors, particularly in cases of virus-negative (HPV^-/EBV^-) HNSCC (Hanna et al., 2018). Although there is much interest in using TMB as a biomarker for prognosis in HNSCC before treatment initiation with PD-1 inhibitors, research studies into its validity still need to be conducted in prospective trial studies.

12.5.5.4 Circulating Biomarkers in Liquid Biopsy

Several studies have explored the quantitative counts of CTCs and survival outcomes in HNSCC, with one study showing improved DFS with no CTCs present, while a count of >25 CTCs/mL indicates worse clinical outcomes; this study further reported a significant correlation between DFS and CTC counts (Jatana et al., 2010). In contrast, CTC counts did not correlate with DFS and OS in advanced HNSCC because the presence of CTCs correlated with improved DFS and OS in OPSCC and a prognostic marker for worse DFS and OS in non-OPSCC HNSCC (Tinhofer et al., 2014). Despite showing potential as a prognostic marker, contradictory reports suggest that more research still needs to be done to improve the prognostic potential of liquid biopsy. Additionally, a cohort study has shown that higher levels of gelsolin were predictive of improved prognosis in the overall 5-year survival and PFS in HNSCC, making it a strong independent biomarker predictor of favorable clinical outcomes (Chiu et al., 2020).

12.6 Emerging Technologies in Radiological Diagnosis and Treatment

Since the first discovery of x-rays by Wilhelm Roentgen in 1895, the field of radiology has evolved to include not only diagnostic workups but also the therapeutic landscape. This section highlights the most popular forms of radiological systems and the latest technological trends.

12.6.1 Computed Tomography

Since its introduction, CT has progressively evolved and now forms an integral component of head and neck oncology diagnosis and treatment planning. Sliced, high-resolution, multiplanar images in CT are used to assess the primary tumor site, evaluate nodal involvement, and determine TNM staging. Additionally, the use of CT for radiotherapy planning remains highly valuable. Due to the rapid acquisition time, CT has minimal artifact movement compared to MRI (Burkill et al., 2016).

12.6.2 Positron Emission Tomography

PET imaging is important in managing HNCs. The most commonly used tracer for PET-CT imaging is 18F-FDG, a glucose analog that travels from the blood into the cells via membrane glucose transporters. The principle of PET-CT is based on the premise that malignant cells have an increased glucose metabolism. One advantage of this modality is the ability to capture the whole body, and, in this way, it can detect distant metastasis and secondary primary tumors. A small percentage of patients may initially present with cervical lymph node metastasis and with no detectable primary tumor. In such cases, PET-CT is useful in detecting the primary tumor through a whole-body scan (Burkill et al., 2016). The assessment of chemotherapy response through PET-CT has become more popular, and increasing evidence supports PET in identifying complete responders and detecting residual or recurrent disease. Because 18F-FDG may still have uptake months after chemotherapy, it is suggested that the timing of the scans is important and should only be considered after 3 months. These findings of chemotherapy response are important because response may prevent unnecessary neck dissection after radiotherapy or chemotherapy. Therefore, the use of PET-CT as a surveillance strategy is supported (Burkill et al., 2016).

12.6.3 Adaptive Radiotherapy

Over the past few decades, the standard care in radiotherapy for HNCs has progressed from 2D radiotherapy to 3D-conformal radiotherapy and the most recent intensity-modulated radiation therapy (IMRT). These improvements in radiotherapy were introduced over time to minimize radiation-induced toxicities while improving the accuracy and efficiency of radiation treatment. Many patients undergo internal anatomic changes during radiotherapy due to weight loss, inflammation, muscle atrophy, and tumor size reduction, which can show effects as soon as 2 weeks into treatment. Although the dose given may be constant, these anatomical changes affect the patient's dose because the overall environment may differ from that used in initial planning. As a result, a patient may receive an overdose to normal tissues or an underdose to targeted tissues. To address this challenge, adaptive radiotherapy (ART) has been developed (Morgan & Sher, 2020).

ART can be categorized into three broad categories, namely, offline ART, online ART, and real-time ART. Offline ART involves scheduled imaging between fractions, and online ART involves the manual adjustment of a treatment plan while the patient is in treatment by accounting for inter-fraction changes. Real-time ART, however, accounts for intra-fractional changes and allows automatic plan adjustments during the radiation treatment. Over the years, both offline and online ART have succeeded in improving target coverage and sparing organs at risk (OAR) (Liu et al., 2023). ART is a process whereby a patient's treatment plan is adjusted during their treatment as a response to a stimulus or change, or it may also be performed at predefined intervals. This allows the radiation plan to be adjusted as the normal and tumor tissue anatomy changes to allow a reduction in dose to radiation-sensitive areas such as the salivary glands, an OAR in head and neck treatment. In this instance, the term "anatomy-adaptive radiotherapy" (A-ART) is used (Liu et al., 2023; Morgan & Sher, 2020).

An emerging trend is to utilize diagnostic imaging such as PET-CT or MRI during treatment to identify treatment response on the tumor tissue. The term "response-adapted adaptive radiotherapy" (R-ART) is used in this setting. Unlike A-ART, R-ART is a process of changing the radiation target and doses based on how the body responds to treatment. Depending on imaging findings, it may lead to dose escalation or de-escalation (Morgan & Sher, 2020). PET-guided ART is a promising area under investigation that is expected to improve radiotherapy protocols. This is built on the principle that there will be persistent radiotracer uptake during the early stages of the treatment, which may represent radioresistance. While A-ART and R-ART both have promising outcomes for patients undergoing head and neck radiotherapy, there is no established protocol for its application. As some patients undergo minimal anatomical change during treatment, the time burden of A-ART may not be beneficial for this subgroup. Therefore, more research is needed in identifying individuals who will benefit.

12.6.4 Flash Therapy

As highlighted previously, dose reduction to normal surrounding tissues is an ongoing challenge and has therefore always been an area of interest in radiotherapy research. Flash radiotherapy is a novel technology that has been conducted on animals, with promising results. This technology uses a single ultra-high dose of ≥40 Gy/s, 400-fold more than traditional radiation. This technology is based on the principle that normal tissues will be spared while preserving antitumor activity. In 2018, the first patient to receive flash radiotherapy showed long-lasting successful results with very little effect in the surrounding tissues. In addition, the treatment was received in a shorter time frame and was therefore advantageous. Currently, there is a clear understanding that flash radiotherapy causes a rapid depletion of hypoxia that results in transient hypoxia. However, the exact mechanisms of responses between normal and tumor tissues are not fully understood. Further studies are required to better understand this novel technology and its application in HNC treatment (Bourhis et al., 2019; Hughes & Parsons, 2020; Lin et al., 2021).

12.6.5 Cone Beam Computed Tomography and Adaptive Radiotherapy

Cone beam CT (CBCT), since its inception in the late 1990s, has advanced in many ways and now finds many uses in dentistry. Initially, CBCT was primarily used in a dental setting to evaluate hard tissues and for implant planning. Current CBCT technology is available in a larger field of view with multiple thin-slice thickness, making it ideal for bony assessment and to discern involvement in head and neck tumors. CBCT is often preferred over medical CT due to its fast acquisition time, lower radiation dose, high resolution, and minimal distortion. One major drawback of CBCT in HNCs is the lack of soft tissue detail. In cases where the soft tissue involvement needs to be assessed, a CT or MRI is preferred. A novel technology is currently being explored whereby kilovoltage CBCT (kV-CBCT) and machine learning are used in ART for HNC patients (Liu et al., 2023). kV-CBCT is integrated into the system as a tool to guide radiation therapy. The fast gantry movement allows for a single scan while the patient holds their breath.

Recent advances in online ART technology include the use of guided CBCT technology, MRI, and linear accelerators. Ethos is a recent kV-CBCT system introduced in 2020 that utilizes AI and machine learning to perform ART and provide automated treatment planning. This technology requires high-quality images that are acquired quickly, allowing for autosegmentation and real-time treatment adaptation. Studies conducted in abdominal, head and neck, breast, bladder, and cervical cancers that used the Ethos system found a significant dose improvement and increased sparing of OAR. In addition, there is evidence of improvement in target coverage (Liu et al., 2023). Currently, there are limited studies on the clinical benefit of the use of Ethos; however, the clinical gain and significance are actively being explored.

12.6.6 Ultrasound

Ultrasound is a simple and inexpensive technology continuously used in the initial triage of HNC diagnosis. One important role is in the support of image-guided biopsies and the identification of malignant nodes. Fine needle aspiration (FNA) and core biopsies are the two main variants available. The differentiation between benign lymphadenopathy and pathological nodal masses can be discerned using ultrasound imaging, and the morphological pattern can be visualized. Malignant nodes tend to appear more rounded and often without a hilus because the central architecture is destroyed by the malignancy. Another important feature that may be seen is the presence of necrosis. However, it is important to note that false positives may occur, as in the case of necrosis due to tuberculosis (Burkill et al., 2016). An advantage of ultrasound imaging is the ability to assess dynamic blood flow in real time. Malignant nodes often have additional feeding vessels, unlike benign ones with central feeding vessels. Ultrasound provides a simple, easy, and affordable method of visualizing the vascular makeup of nodes.

Tongue cancers are often detected in the early stages, and, depending on tumor thickness, the treatment of choice is resection. Determining the tumor margin is imperative for a successful outcome. The consensus is to obtain at least a 5 mm clear margin. In cases where clear margins cannot be achieved, adjuvant treatment is necessary (either re-resection, chemotherapy, or radiotherapy). Precise surgical management is important to avoid the drawbacks associated with adjuvant treatment. Tumor thickness and depth of invasion have traditionally been guided by visual inspection and by touch. MRI and intraoral ultrasound have been used to measure tissue thickness in recent years. Recent studies have found that preoperative intraoral ultrasound successfully measured tumor thickness in a large cohort of patients and was more accurate than MRI (Noorlag et al., 2020). Studies that compared the accuracy of intraoral ultrasound to CT and MRI found that intraoral ultrasound was the most accurate, and CT and MRI tended to have an overestimation of 2–3 mm (Takamura et al., 2022). Therefore, with the ability to measure tumors of <10 mm, intraoral ultrasound should be explored and considered for use during surgical excision to better guide the surgeon.

12.6.7 Magnetic Resonance Imaging

MRI has played an important role in staging HNC. MRI's advantage over CT is its ability to detect perineural invasion. Historically, a disadvantage of MRI is the long acquisition time. In recent years, acquisition times have been shorted as the hardware of MRI systems continuously improves and the choice of sequences expands. Although this varies, typical MRI protocol sequences for HNC diagnosis include (but are not limited to) T1 weighted pre- and post-gadolinium contrast, T1 fat-saturated post-contrast sequence, T2 weighted, short tau inversion recovery (STIR), and diffusion-weighted sequences (Burkill et al., 2016; Touska & Connor, 2019).

Diffusion-weighted imaging (DWI) is a complementary MRI approach that depicts the tumor microstructure. Highly cellular tumors will display restricted diffusion and an increased signal on the DWI sequence due to the impeded motion of water molecules. In post-treatment patients, DWI is useful in detecting high signal-viable tumors because the signal intensity can be compared from pre- to post-treatment. Still in its infancy, DWI is a promising prognostic imaging biomarker for HNCs (Boeke et al., 2021; Burkill et al., 2016). The quantitative application of the apparent diffusion coefficient (ADC) has become increasingly popular in characterizing lesions and acts as a biomarker for predicting chemotherapy response. A challenge in the post-treatment phase is distinguishing between viable tumors and post-treatment changes such as fibrosis and inflammation. ADC values may be beneficial in these instances, making it more useful than PET-CT due to the frequent number of false-positive changes found on PET (Boeke et al., 2021; Burkill et al., 2016).

12.6.8 Synthetic Magnetic Resonance Imaging

MRI has become the imaging modality of choice for assessing soft tissues in the head and neck. As this modality has advanced, there have been numerous investigations in quantitative MR techniques. To date, these have included DWI, intravoxel incoherent motion, and dynamic contrast-enhanced quantitative analysis. These quantitative techniques, through clinical trials, have proved to improve preoperative tumor characterization. However, the major drawbacks are long scanning times and complex post-processing. As discussed earlier, the ADC values are the most widely accepted and used quantitative parameter that can differentiate between benign and malignant lesions by measuring the diffusion of water molecules within tumor tissue.

Conventional quantitative techniques require a long acquisition time. To overcome this challenge, recent technological advances have explored the possibility of using synthetic MRI to assess head and neck tumors. Synthetic MRI is a novel technology that has been explored in the breast, brain, prostate, and rectum. Synthetic MRI generates quantitative maps and multiple contrast images simultaneously, resulting in reduced scan time. Recent preliminary studies have been conducted using synthetic MRI for the quantitative characterization of head and neck tumors, and the results indicate that T1 and T2 values may provide added information to improve differentiating between benign and malignant lesions (Zhang et al., 2023). The novel technology of synthetic MRI applications is currently in its infancy, and the preliminary results motivate an area for future research.

12.6.9 Magnetic Resonance-Guided Radiotherapy

In recent years image-guided therapy has expanded and resulted in improvements in cancer treatment. Magnetic resonance guidance (MRg) has been utilized to better visualize tumor tissues without providing additional radiation exposure. Due to the superior soft tissue contrast provided by MRI, it remains beneficial in precisely delineating tumor margins. Daily adaptive online MRg can be beneficial for tumors that are fast responding, such as HPV-positive oropharyngeal cancers. Presently, a hybrid platform MR-guided linear accelerator (MR-Linac) is used that combines MRI with radiation therapy to adjust the treatment in real time while providing an accurate depiction of the soft tissues. While this technology is well-established in lung and prostate cancers, implementation in HNC is not as established (Boeke et al., 2021).

Offline MRg has shown positive outcomes; however, online MRg radiotherapy is a recent area of research. One of the challenges currently experienced by MR-Linac is the *electron return effect*, which results in secondary electrons being influenced by the magnetic field. This effect is more pronounced at higher magnetic field strengths and involves dose enhancement between high density and low density tissues. As air–tissue interfaces are common in HNC targets, this may result in variation in dose deposits and the risk of hotspots where the beams move from air to tissue. While there are still challenges to overcome before the widespread application of MRg radiotherapy for HNCs, the rapid rate at which technology is evolving is likely to solve these challenges shortly (Boeke et al., 2021).

12.7 Technologies in Intraoperative Surgical Techniques

Intraoperative consultation in HNC is important for immediate patient management. Frozen sections are utilized in head and neck surgical pathology mostly to assess margin status intraoperatively before reconstruction (Meier et al., 2005). Positive margins are associated with locoregional recurrence and may contribute to deciding whether the patient will receive postoperative adjuvant therapy (Loree, 1991). The use of frozen sections has gradually increased and has been regarded as an invaluable tool by different specialties of head and neck surgery. Table 12.3 summarizes the indications for requesting and performing intraoperative frozen sections in the head and neck region.

Table 12.3 Indications for requesting and performing intraoperative frozen sections

Indications for frozen sections	Illegitimate reasons for requesting a frozen section	Limitations of the frozen section
Provide a diagnosis that equips the surgeon to make an intraoperative decision	Curiosity	Only a few samples are examined, which may lead to false negative results
To assess margin status	To provide a preliminary report	Tissue shrinkage
To assess for perineural involvement	If the frozen section results do not change the intraoperative surgical management	Time constraints (may extend anesthesia duration by 15–45 min)
To assess for sentinel lymph nodes	For the diagnosis of infections in tissue	Cannot freeze and cut bone on the cryostat

12.7.1 Current Techniques in Frozen Section and Margin Assessment

The foremost reasons for requesting frozen sections in academic hospitals include margin assessment, malignancy exclusion, and tumor classification (Hinni et al., 2013; Kain et al., 2020; Thomas Robbins et al., 2019). The standard frozen section technique consists of the following process:

- The specimen is delivered from the operating room to the pathology laboratory.
- Resection specimens submitted en bloc must be anatomically oriented and have visible landmarks. Direct face-to-face consultation between the surgeon and pathologist may enhance the accuracy of specimen orientation.
- Intraoperative and radiographic information should also be shared with the pathologist.
- Any supplemental margins taken from the surgical defect must be oriented, and this orientation must be communicated to the pathologist.

A timeline highlighting the progression of frozen section analysis in surgical pathology demonstrates the crucial dates when distinctive changes were made (Figure 12.3). The first documented frozen section technique was performed by William Welch, in 1891, for a suspected breast cancer case (Urken et al., 2023;

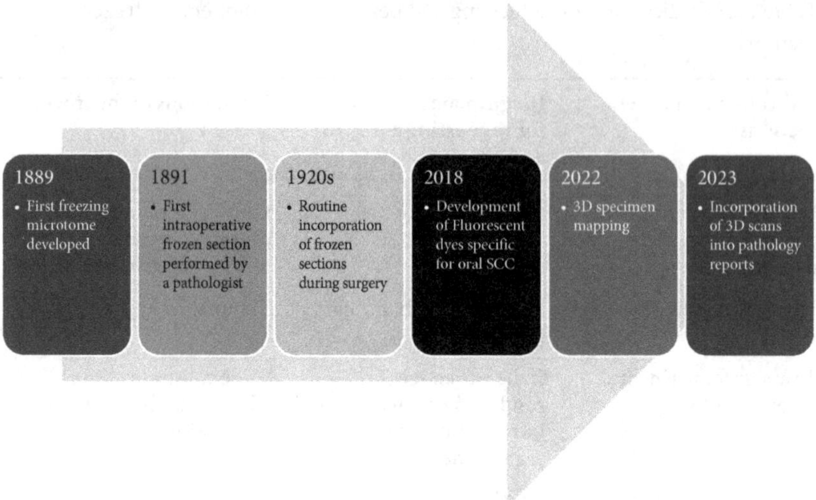

Figure 12.3 Timeline showing the history of frozen section analysis and pertinent dates in head and neck surgical pathology. The timeline highlights the progression of frozen section analysis in surgical pathology demonstrating the crucial dates when distinctive changes were made to improve outcomes of the procedure.

Lechago, 2005). Welch prepared the slide using a carbon dioxide freezing microtome. It is generally accepted that the standard cryostat method used to date was initially published in the *Journal of the American Medical Association* in 1905, by Louis Wilson of the Mayo Clinic (Gal & Cagle, 2005). Controversy regarding the importance of the frozen section was seen in the literature during the period from 1925 to 1935 (Urken et al., 2023).

Intraoperative turnaround times for head and neck frozen sections average 19.7 minutes, with a mean technical time of 13.7 minutes and a mean interpretive time of 6.0 minutes (Laakman et al., 2021). Complex en bloc specimens have a longer turnaround time, sometimes up to 45 minutes for the entire intraoperative consultation (Laakman et al., 2021). Frozen section analysis presents interpretive, sampling, technical, and communication limitations. Consideration must be given to the freezing process causing diminished cytologic quality, which may lead to interpretive error. The inability to evaluate the entire continuous margin creates a sampling dilemma. Decalcification of bony specimens usually requires approximately 24 hours, thus excluding bone margins from routine frozen section analysis (Weinstock et al., 2014).

The majority of frozen section requests are for the evaluation of surgical margins. There is no consensus on the true universal definition of positive, clear, or close head and neck surgical margins (Bulbul et al., 2021; Hinni et al.,

2013). A widely accepted definition states that a clear margin is a radial distance of at least 5 mm between the carcinoma and the resection edge on microscopic evaluation (Urken et al., 2023). According to National Comprehensive Cancer Network (NCCN) Guidelines, Version 1. 2022, a clear margin is a distance of 5 mm or more from the invasive tumor front to the resected margin. A positive margin is defined as the "cut-through" of either carcinoma in-situ or frank invasive carcinoma. A close margin is defined as 2–5 mm from the invasive tumor front to the resected margin, depending on the anatomic site involved. The NCCN guidelines make an exception for glottic cancers, in which 1–2 mm margins are acceptable (Hinni et al., 2013). When a specimen has been removed from the body, it shrinks linearly by 25–75% depending on tissue composition (Cheng et al., 2008; Mistry et al., 2005). The 5 mm histologic margin clearance measured on a microscopic slide roughly corresponds to 1 cm of gross tissue in the operative field (Wenig, 2008).

Tumors in the oropharynx, hypopharynx, and larynx produce three-dimensionally challenging resection specimens. Biological factors also add to the complexity of head and neck surgical specimens and their intraoperative pathologic analysis (Smits et al., 2016; Weinstock et al., 2014). Bone margins represent a technical challenge because calcified bone requires decalcification, so accepted methods include frozen section analysis of cancellous bone scrapings: small bony trabeculae can be cut on a cryostat. Sampling periosteal tissue and inferior alveolar nerve may also show the state of the bone margin (Bilodeau & Chiosea, 2011; Nieberler et al., 2020).

12.7.2 Novel Approaches in Intraoperative Pathology and Surgical Navigation

Several recent innovations have attempted to improve intraoperative margin analysis and surgical navigation in HNC (Rosenthal et al., 2015; Singhal, 2016). Due to the challenges encountered in the accuracy of frozen specimen navigation, a novel virtual 3D specimen mapping technique that optimizes intraoperative consultations was developed (Urken et al., 2023). 3D scanning technology is now entering the healthcare realm and anatomic pathology, with a recent case report demonstrating the 3D scanning of a fresh glossectomy specimen before formalin fixation (Farahani et al., 2017). Using a commercially available, structured light desktop 3D scanner (Einscan-SP, Shining 3D, Hangzhou, China), researchers have produced 55 virtual models of head and neck specimens, showing the ability to reliably capture the 3D surface topography of a fresh surgical specimen. This scanner readily scans specimens from the facial skin, larynx, oral cavity, oropharynx, mandible, palatomaxillary, and parotid regions.

After fresh, ex vivo surgical specimens were taken from the operating room to the pathology lab, the specimens were rinsed, dried, and placed on a turntable platform. Optical scans were then produced by capturing two 360-degree scans, each from a different orientation. The two 3D scans were then manually aligned to render a virtual model of the specimen (Saturno et al., 2023). 3D image acquisition time was consistently <12 minutes. The scan data were processed and imported into a graphics workspace (Paint 3D, Microsoft, Redmond, WA) as a 3D object file. After 3D scanning, the frozen section process was carried out as described above. The virtual 3D representation was then used to convey the results. The pathologist directly annotated the 3D specimen representation, illustrating regions of concern. The 3D representation was displayed by videoconferencing on overhead monitors in the operating room, thus becoming the reference point for discussion rather than the inked, dissected resection specimen, which would be unrecognizable to the surgeon, or the crude specimen sketch.

The surgeon need no longer break the sterile field, and the 3D scan of the specimen can serve as a permanent reference point in the patient's electronic medical record (Urken et al., 2023). After ex vivo surgical specimens are scanned using a structured light desktop 3D scanner, computer-aided design (CAD) software can be used to document sites of margin sampling and to graphically demonstrate inked surfaces on the specimen to give valuable insight to surgeons in cases where re-resection is necessary. Mixed-media pathology reports also are being discussed whereby 3D scans and CAD technology are incorporated into final pathology reports (Alexander et al., 2023). Since patients usually require adjuvant radiation therapy following positive margins in oral cavity SCC resections, 3D models with annotated surgical resection margins may be correlated with radiologic images to optimize radiation field planning (Urken et al., 2023).

12.8 Artificial Intelligence in the Diagnosis of Head and Neck Lesions

Traditionally, the diagnosis of head and neck tumors involves clinical, radiological, and histopathological examinations. There is a direct correlation between the stage of diagnosis and the prognosis; early detection of tumors improves patients' outcomes. In recent years, AI has gained popularity in all fields of medicine. There are multiple studies conducted that assessed the accuracy and efficiency of AI in HNC diagnosis in the field of histopathology and radiology (Bassani et al., 2022; Mahmood et al., 2020, 2021). Machine learning and medical image analysis detect patterns and use these to make predictions regarding tumor prognosis (Mahmood et al., 2021; Peng et al., 2021).

Digital pathology (DP) using high-resolution scanners has revolutionized histopathology diagnosis and collaboration. *Pathomics* involves the use of AI in digital pathology. Whole-slide imaging (WSI) is used in DP for routine diagnosis, tumor grading, biomarker evaluation, and tumor microenvironment description (Classe et al., 2021). In pathomics, WSI with machine learning can be used to evaluate prognostic and predictive markers such as Ki-67 and PDL because these have a high rate of interobserver reliability. In radiology, AI has been used in the form of radionics to extract mathematically defined radiological features from radiological medical images to generate analyzable data (Peng et al., 2021). The generated data can be used to construct models that predict tumor stage, recurrence, metastasis, and progression.

12.9 Challenges and Limitations

Translational research has advanced precision medicine and oncological treatments (De Maria Marchiano et al., 2021). However, economic discrepancies exist that present a barrier to acquiring and implementing these technologies, especially in low-income countries. These challenges are seen in clinical, radiological, and histological diagnosis, as well as in oncological care. Most of the challenges are a result of the lag in multi-institutional and multipopulation data validation, retrospective study designs, low sample sizes, patient selection biases, and, most importantly, patient-related factors (Alberti et al., 2022; Haider et al., 2020; Muniz et al., 2024; Tortora et al., 2023). Given the cost of precision medicine, few patients can afford these treatments, even with the right diagnosis.

12.10 Conclusion

Early diagnosis and treatment of HNCs are of paramount importance in the current era of personalized medicine and targeted therapy. Appropriate clinical, radiological, and histological diagnosis is imperative in selecting patients for appropriate targeted treatment. As new technology in head and neck oncology advances, it will improve patient outcomes.

References

ABIKO, K., MATSUMURA, N., HAMANISHI, J., HORIKAWA, N., MURAKAMI, R., YAMAGUCHI, K., YOSHIOKA, Y., BABA, T., KONISHI, I., & MANDAI, M. 2015. IFN-γ from lymphocytes induces PD-L1 expression and promotes progression of ovarian cancer. *Br J Cancer*, 112, 1501–9.

AGGARWAL, S., SHARMA, S. C., & DAS, S. N. 2015. Galectin-1 and galectin-3: plausible tumour markers for oral squamous cell carcinoma and suitable targets for screening high-risk population. *Clin Chim Acta*, 442, 13–21.

ALBERTI, A., LORINI, L., RAVANELLI, M., PERRI, F., VINCHES, M., RONDI, P., ROMANI, C., & BOSSI, P. 2022. New challenges in evaluating outcomes after immunotherapy in recurrent and/or metastatic head and neck squamous cell carcinoma. *Vaccines*, 10, 885.

ALEXANDER, N. P., KAYVON, F. S., ERICA, G., SOPHIE, L., ALEXIS, M., KAVITA, P., ROBERT, J. S., JAMES S. LEWIS, JR., & MICHAEL, C. T. 2023. Ex vivo 3D scanning and specimen mapping in anatomic pathology. *J Pathol Informatics*, 14. Available at: http://dx.doi.org/10.1016/j.jpi.2022.100186

AMBELE, M. A., PEPPER, M. S., VAN HEERDEN, M. B., & VAN HEERDEN, W. F. 2019. Heterozygosity of p16 expression in an oral squamous cell carcinoma with associated loss of heterozygosity and copy number alterations. *Head Neck*, 41, E62–5.

AMBELE, M. A., VAN ZYL, A., PEPPER, M. S., VAN HEERDEN, M. B., & VAN HEERDEN, W. F. 2020. Amplification of 3q26. 2, 5q14. 3, 8q24. 3, 8q22. 3, and 14q32. 33 are possible common genetic alterations in oral cancer patients. *Front Oncol*, 10, 683.

ANDERSEN, A. S., KOLDJAER SØLLING, A. S., OVESEN, T., & RUSAN, M. 2014. The interplay between HPV and host immunity in head and neck squamous cell carcinoma. *Int J Cancer*, 134, 2755–63.

AYERS, M., LUNCEFORD, J., NEBOZHYN, M., MURPHY, E., LOBODA, A., KAUFMAN, D. R., ALBRIGHT, A., CHENG, J. D., KANG, S. P., SHANKARAN, V., PIHA-PAUL, S. A., YEARLEY, J., SEIWERT, T. Y., RIBAS, A., & MCCLANAHAN, T. K. 2017. IFN-γ-related mRNA profile predicts clinical response to PD-1 blockade. *J Clin Invest*, 127, 2930–40.

BALGOBIND, S., CHEUNG, V. K. Y., LUK, P., LOW, T.-H. H., WYKES, J., WU, R., LEE, J., CH'NG, S., PALME, C. E., CLARK, J. R., & GUPTA, R. 2024. Prognostic and predictive biomarkers in head and neck cancer: Something old, something new, something borrowed, something blue and a sixpence in your shoe. *Pathology*, 56, 170–85.

BASHEETH, N., & PATIL, N. 2019. Biomarkers in head and neck cancer: An update. *Indian J Otolaryngol Head Neck Surg*, 71, 1002–11.

BASSANI, S., SANTONICCO, N., ECCHER, A., SCARPA, A., VIANINI, M., BRUNELLI, M., BISI, N., NOCINI, R., SACCHETTO, L., MUNARI, E., PANTANOWITZ, L., GIROLAMI, I., & MOLTENI, G. 2022. Artificial intelligence in head and neck cancer diagnosis. *J Pathol Inform*, 13, 100153.

BAUML, J., SEIWERT, T. Y., PFISTER, D. G., WORDEN, F., LIU, S. V., GILBERT, J., SABA, N. F., WEISS, J., WIRTH, L., SUKARI, A., KANG, H., GIBSON, M. K., MASSARELLI, E., POWELL, S., MEISTER, A., SHU, X., CHENG, J. D., & HADDAD, R. 2017. Pembrolizumab for platinum- and cetuximab-refractory head and neck cancer: Results from a single-arm, phase II study. *J Clin Oncol*, 35, 1542–9.

BERNADT, C. T., & COLLINS, B. T. 2017. Fine-needle aspiration biopsy of HPV-related squamous cell carcinoma of the head and neck: Current ancillary testing methods for determining HPV status. *Diagn Cytopathol*, 45, 221–9.

BILODEAU, E. A., & CHIOSEA, S. 2011. Oral squamous cell carcinoma with mandibular bone invasion: Intraoperative evaluation of bone margins by routine frozen section. *Head Neck Pathol*, 5, 216–20.

BISHOP, J. A., ANDREASEN, S., HANG, J.-F., BULLOCK, M. J., CHEN, T. Y., FRANCHI, A., GARCIA, J. J., GNEPP, D. R., GOMEZ-FERNANDEZ, C. R., & IHRLER, S. 2017. HPV-related multiphenotypic sinonasal carcinoma: An expanded series of 49 cases of the tumor formerly known as HPV-related carcinoma with adenoid cystic carcinoma-like features. *Am J Surg Pathol*, 41, 1690–701.

BISHOP, J. A., GAGAN, J., PATERSON, C., MCLELLAN, D., & SANDISON, A. 2021. Nonkeratinizing squamous cell carcinoma of the sinonasal tract with DEK-AFF2: Further solidifying an emerging entity. *Am J Surg Pathol*, 45, 718–20.

BOEKE, S., MONNICH, D., VAN TIMMEREN, J. E., & BALERMPAS, P. 2021. MR-guided radiotherapy for head and neck cancer: Current developments, perspectives, and challenges. *Front Oncol*, 11, 616156.

BOULAND, C., DEQUANTER, D., LECHIEN, J. R., HANSSENS, C., DE SAINT AUBAIN, N., DIGONNET, A., JAVADIAN, R., YANNI, A., RODRIGUEZ, A., & LOEB, I. 2021. Prognostic significance of a scoring system combining p16, smoking, and drinking status in a series of 131 patients with oropharyngeal cancers. *Int J Otolaryngol*, 2021, 8020826.

BOURHIS, J., SOZZI, W. J., JORGE, P. G., GAIDE, O., BAILAT, C., DUCLOS, F., PATIN, D., OZSAHIN, M., BOCHUD, F., GERMOND, J. F., MOECKLI, R., & VOZENIN, M. C. 2019. Treatment of a first patient with FLASH-radiotherapy. *Radiother Oncol*, 139, 18–22.

BULBUL, M. G., ZENGA, J., TARABICHI, O., PARIKH, A. S., SETHI, R. K., ROBBINS, K. T., PURAM, S. V., & VARVARES, M. A. 2021. Margin practices in oral cavity cancer resections: Survey of American Head and Neck Society members. *Laryngoscope*, 131, 782–7.

BURKILL, G. J., EVANS, R. M., RAMAN, V. V., & CONNOR, S. E. 2016. Modern radiology in the management of head and neck cancer. *Clin Oncol (R Coll Radiol)*, 28, 440–50.

BURTNESS, B., HARRINGTON, K. J., GREIL, R., SOULIÈRES, D., TAHARA, M., DE CASTRO, G., JR., PSYRRI, A., BASTÉ, N., NEUPANE, P., BRATLAND, Å., FUEREDER, T., HUGHES, B. G. M., MESÍA, R., NGAMPHAIBOON, N., RORDORF, T., WAN ISHAK, W. Z., HONG, R. L., GONZÁLEZ MENDOZA, R., ROY, A., ZHANG, Y., GUMUSCU, B., CHENG, J. D., JIN, F., & RISCHIN, D. 2019. Pembrolizumab alone or with chemotherapy versus cetuximab with chemotherapy for recurrent or metastatic squamous cell carcinoma of the head and neck (KEYNOTE-048): A randomised, open-label, phase 3 study. *Lancet*, 394, 1915–28.

CAMBIEN, B., KARIMDJEE, B. F., RICHARD-FIARDO, P., BZIOUECH, H., BARTHEL, R., MILLET, M. A., MARTINI, V., BIRNBAUM, D., SCOAZEC, J. Y., ABELLO, J., AL SAATI, T., JOHNSON, M. G., SULLIVAN, T. J., MEDINA, J. C., COLLINS, T. L., SCHMID-ALLIANA, A., & SCHMID-ANTOMARCHI, H. 2009. Organ-specific inhibition of metastatic colon carcinoma by CXCR3 antagonism. *Br J Cancer*, 100, 1755–64.

CHENG, A., COX, D., & SCHMIDT, B. L. 2008. Oral squamous cell carcinoma margin discrepancy after resection and pathologic processing. *J Oral Maxillofac Surg*, 66, 523–9.

CHIU, C. T., WANG, P. W., ASARE-WEREHENE, M., TSANG, B. K., & SHIEH, D. B. 2020. Circulating plasma gelsolin: A predictor of favorable clinical outcomes in head and neck cancer and sensitive biomarker for early disease diagnosis combined with soluble fas ligand. *Cancers (Basel)*, 12(6), 1569.

CHOWDHURY, N., ALVI, S., KIMURA, K., TAWFIK, O., MANNA, P., BEAHM, D., ROBINSON, A., KERLEY, S., & HOOVER, L. 2017. Outcomes of HPV-related nasal squamous cell carcinoma. *Laryngoscope*, 127, 1600–3.

CIRIELLO, G., MILLER, M. L., AKSOY, B. A., SENBABAOGLU, Y., SCHULTZ, N., & SANDER, C. 2013. Emerging landscape of oncogenic signatures across human cancers. *Nat Genet*, 45, 1127–33.

CLASSE, M., LEROUSSEAU, M., SCOAZEC, J. Y., & DEUTSCH, E. 2021. Perspectives in pathomics in head and neck cancer. *Curr Opin Oncol*, 33, 175–83.

COHEN, E. E. W., BELL, R. B., BIFULCO, C. B., BURTNESS, B., GILLISON, M. L., HARRINGTON, K. J., LE, Q. T., LEE, N. Y., LEIDNER, R., LEWIS, R. L., LICITRA, L., MEHANNA, H., MELL, L. K., RABEN, A., SIKORA, A. G., UPPALURI, R., WHITWORTH, F., ZANDBERG, D. P., & FERRIS, R. L. 2019a. The Society for Immunotherapy of Cancer consensus statement on immunotherapy for the treatment of squamous cell carcinoma of the head and neck (HNSCC). *J Immunother Cancer*, 7, 184.

COHEN, E. E. W., SOULIÈRES, D., LE TOURNEAU, C., DINIS, J., LICITRA, L., AHN, M. J., SORIA, A., MACHIELS, J. P., MACH, N., MEHRA, R., BURTNESS, B., ZHANG, P., CHENG, J., SWABY, R. F., & HARRINGTON, K. J. 2019b. Pembrolizumab versus methotrexate, docetaxel, or cetuximab for recurrent or metastatic head-and-neck squamous cell carcinoma (KEYNOTE-040): A randomised, open-label, phase 3 study. *Lancet*, 393, 156–67.

CSANYI-BASTIEN, M., LANIC, M.-D., BEAUSSIRE, L., FERRIC, S., FRANÇOIS, A., MESEURE, D., JARDIN, F., WASSEF, M., RUMINY, P., & LAÉ, M. 2021. Pan-TRK immunohistochemistry is highly correlated with NTRK3 gene rearrangements in salivary gland tumors. *Am J Surg Pathol*, 45, 1487–1498.

DE KEUKELEIRE, S. J., VERMASSEN, T., HILGERT, E., CREYTENS, D., FERDINANDE, L., & ROTTEY, S. 2021. Immuno-oncological biomarkers for squamous cell cancer of the head and neck: Current state of the art and future perspectives. *Cancers (Basel)*, 13(7), 1714.

DE MARIA MARCHIANO, R., DI SANTE, G., PIRO, G., CARBONE, C., TORTORA, G., BOLDRINI, L., PIETRAGALLA, A., DANIELE, G., TREDICINE, M., & CESARIO, A. 2021. Translational research in the era of precision medicine: Where we are and where we will go. *J Personalized Med*, 11, 216.

DE RUITER, E. J., OOFT, M. L., DEVRIESE, L. A., & WILLEMS, S. M. 2017. The prognostic role of tumor infiltrating T-lymphocytes in squamous cell carcinoma of the head and neck: A systematic review and meta-analysis. *Oncoimmunology*, 6, e1356148.

DE WIT, S., VAN DALUM, G., & TERSTAPPEN, L. W. 2014. Detection of circulating tumor cells. *Scientifica (Cairo)*, 2014, 819362.

DIEHL, F., SCHMIDT, K., CHOTI, M. A., ROMANS, K., GOODMAN, S., LI, M., THORNTON, K., AGRAWAL, N., SOKOLL, L., SZABO, S. A., KINZLER, K. W., VOGELSTEIN, B., & DIAZ, L. A., JR. 2008. Circulating mutant DNA to assess tumor dynamics. *Nat Med*, 14, 985–90.

ECONOMOPOULOU, P., DE BREE, R., KOTSANTIS, I., & PSYRRI, A. 2019. Diagnostic tumor markers in head and neck squamous cell carcinoma (HNSCC) in the clinical setting. *Front Oncol*, 9, 827.

ELREFAEY, S., MASSARO, M. A., CHIOCCA, S., CHIESA, F., & ANSARIN, M. 2014. HPV in oropharyngeal cancer: The basics to know in clinical practice. *Acta Otorhinolaryngol Ital*, 34, 299–309.

FAN, C., WANG, J., TANG, Y., ZHANG, S., XIONG, F., GUO, C., ZHOU, Y., LI, Z., LI, X., LI, Y., LI, G., ZENG, Z., & XIONG, W. 2020. Upregulation of long non-coding RNA LOC284454 may serve as a new serum diagnostic biomarker for head and neck cancers. *BMC Cancer*, 20, 917.

FARAHANI, N., BRAUN, A., JUTT, D., HUFFMAN, T., REDER, N., LIU, Z., YAGI, Y., & PANTANOWITZ, L. 2017. Three-dimensional imaging and scanning: Current and future applications for pathology. *J Pathol Informatics*, 8, 36.

FERRIS, R. L., BLUMENSCHEIN, G., JR., FAYETTE, J., GUIGAY, J., COLEVAS, A. D., LICITRA, L., HARRINGTON, K. J., KASPER, S., VOKES, E. E., EVEN, C., WORDEN, F., SABA, N. F., DOCAMPO, L. C. I., HADDAD, R., RORDORF, T., KIYOTA, N., TAHARA, M., LYNCH, M., JAYAPRAKASH, V., LI, L., & GILLISON, M. L. 2018. Nivolumab vs investigator's choice in recurrent or metastatic squamous cell carcinoma of the head and neck: 2-year long-term survival update of CheckMate 141 with analyses by tumor PD-L1 expression. *Oral Oncol*, 81, 45–51.

FILIPPINI, D. M., BROSEGHINI, E., CAROSI, F., MOLIN, D. D., RIEFOLO, M., FABBRI, L., ABESHI, A., FERNANDEZ, I. J., & FERRACIN, M. 2023. A systematic review of diagnostic and prognostic biomarkers for head and neck cancer of unknown primary: An unmet clinical need. *Diagnostics*, 13, 1492.

FOTOPOULOS, G., & PAVLIDIS, N. 2015. The role of human papilloma virus and p16 in occult primary of the head and neck: A comprehensive review of the literature. *Oral Oncol* 51, 119–23.

GAL, A. A., & CAGLE, P. T. 2005. The 100-year anniversary of the description of the frozen section procedure. *JAMA*, 294, 3135–7.

GAVRIELATOU, N., DOUMAS, S., ECONOMOPOULOU, P., FOUKAS, P. G., & PSYRRI, A. 2020. Biomarkers for immunotherapy response in head and neck cancer. *Cancer Treat Rev*, 84, 101977.

GUERRA, E. N., RÊGO, D. F., ELIAS, S. T., COLETTA, R. D., MEZZOMO, L. A., GOZAL, D., & DE LUCA CANTO, G. 2016. Diagnostic accuracy of serum biomarkers for head and neck cancer: A systematic review and meta-analysis. *Crit Rev Oncol Hematol*, 101, 93–118.

GUPTA, A., GUPTA, S., & MAHDI, A. A. 2015. ^{1}H NMR-derived serum metabolomics of leukoplakia and squamous cell carcinoma. *Clin Chim Acta*, 441, 47–55.

HAIDER, S. P., BURTNESS, B., YARBROUGH, W. G., & PAYABVASH, S. 2020. Applications of radiomics in precision diagnosis, prognostication and treatment planning of head and neck squamous cell carcinomas. *Cancers Head Neck*, 5, 1–19.

HANNA, G. J., LIZOTTE, P., CAVANAUGH, M., KUO, F. C., SHIVDASANI, P., FRIEDEN, A., CHAU, N. G., SCHOENFELD, J. D., LORCH, J. H., UPPALURI, R., MACCONAILL, L. E., & HADDAD, R. I. 2018. Frameshift events predict anti-PD-1/L1 response in head and neck cancer. *JCI Insight*, 3(4), e98811.

HECHTMAN, J. F., BENAYED, R., HYMAN, D. M., DRILON, A., ZEHIR, A., FROSINA, D., ARCILA, M. E., DOGAN, S., KLIMSTRA, D. S., LADANYI, M., & JUNGBLUTH, A. A. 2017. Pan-Trk immunohistochemistry is an efficient and reliable screen for the detection of NTRK fusions. *Am J Surg Pathol*, 41, 1547–51.

HENRY, N. L., & HAYES, D. F. 2012. Cancer biomarkers. *Mol Oncol*, 6, 140–6.

HINNI, M. L., FERLITO, A., BRANDWEIN-GENSLER, M. S., TAKES, R. P., SILVER, C. E., WESTRA, W. H., SEETHALA, R. R., RODRIGO, J. P., CORRY, J., BRADFORD, C. R., HUNT, J. L., STROJAN, P., DEVANEY, K. O., GNEPP, D. R., HARTL, D. M., KOWALSKI, L. P., RINALDO, A., & BARNES, L. 2013. Surgical margins in head and neck cancer: A contemporary review. *Head Neck*, 35, 1362–70.

HUGHES, J. R., & PARSONS, J. L. 2020. FLASH radiotherapy: Current knowledge and future insights using proton-beam therapy. *Int J Mol Sci*, 21.

JATANA, K. R., BALASUBRAMANIAN, P., LANG, J. C., YANG, L., JATANA, C. A., WHITE, E., AGRAWAL, A., OZER, E., SCHULLER, D. E., TEKNOS, T. N., & CHALMERS, J. J. 2010. Significance of circulating tumor cells in patients with squamous cell carcinoma of the head and neck: Initial results. *Arch Otolaryngol Head Neck Surg*, 136, 1274–9.

KAIN, J. J., BIRKELAND, A. C., UDAYAKUMAR, N., MORLANDT, A. B., STEVENS, T. M., CARROLL, W. R., ROSENTHAL, E. L., & WARRAM, J. M. 2020. Surgical margins in oral cavity squamous cell carcinoma: Current practices and future directions. *Laryngoscope*, 130, 128–38.

KANG, H., KIESS, A., & CHUNG, C. H. 2015. Emerging biomarkers in head and neck cancer in the era of genomics. *Nat Rev Clin Oncol*, 12, 11–26.

KATIRACHI, S. K., GRØNLUND, M. P., JAKOBSEN, K. K., GRØNHØJ, C., & VON BUCHWALD, C. 2023. The prevalence of HPV in oral cavity squamous cell carcinoma. *Viruses*, 15, 451.

KELLER, L. M., GALLOWAY, T. J., HOLDBROOK, T., RUTH, K., YANG, D., DUBYK, C., FLIEDER, D., LANGO, M. N., MEHRA, R., & BURTNESS, B. 2014. p16 status, pathologic and clinical characteristics, biomolecular signature, and long-term outcomes in head and neck squamous cell carcinomas of unknown primary. *Head Neck*, 36, 1677–84.

KONG, L., & BIRKELAND, A. C. 2021. Liquid biopsies in head and neck cancer: current state and future challenges. *Cancers (Basel)*, 13(8), 1874.

KUO, Y.-J., LEWIS JR, J. S., ZHAI, C., CHEN, Y.-A., CHERNOCK, R. D., HSIEH, M.-S., LAN, M.-Y., LEE, C.-K., WEINREB, I., & HANG, J.-F. 2021. DEK-AFF2 fusion-associated papillary squamous cell carcinoma of the sinonasal tract: Clinicopathologic characterization of seven cases with deceptively bland morphology. *Modern Pathol*, 34, 1820–30.

LAAKMAN, J. M., CHEN, S. J., LAKE, K. S., BLAU, J. L., RAJAN, D. A., SAMUELSON, M. I., & ROBINSON, R. A. 2021. Frozen section quality assurance: Using separate frozen section slide preparation times and interpretative time measurements to improve process. *Am J Clin Pathol*, 156, 461–70.

LAWRENCE, M. S., SOUGNEZ, C., LICHTENSTEIN, L., CIBULSKIS, K., LANDER, E., GABRIEL, S. B., GETZ, G., ALLY, A., BALASUNDARAM, M., BIROL, I., BOWLBY, R., BROOKS, D., BUTTERFIELD, Y. S. N., CARLSEN, R., CHENG, D., CHU, A., DHALLA, N., GUIN, R., HOLT, R. A., JONES, S. J. M., LEE, D., LI, H. I., MARRA, M. A., MAYO, M., MOORE, R. A., MUNGALL, A. J., GORDON ROBERTSON, A., SCHEIN, J. E., SIPAHIMALANI, P., TAM, A., THIESSEN, N., WONG, T., PROTOPOPOV, A., SANTOSO, N., LEE, S., PARFENOV, M., ZHANG, J., MAHADESHWAR, H. S., TANG, J., REN, X., SETH, S., HASELEY, P., ZENG, D., YANG, L., XU, A. W., SONG, X., PANTAZI, A., BRISTOW, C. A., HADJIPANAYIS, A., SEIDMAN, J., CHIN, L., PARK, P. J., KUCHERLAPATI, R., AKBANI, R., CASASENT, T., LIU, W., LU, Y., MILLS, G., MOTTER, T., WEINSTEIN, J., DIAO, L., WANG, J., HONG FAN, Y., LIU, J., WANG, K., TODD AUMAN, J., BALU, S., BODENHEIMER, T., BUDA, E., NEIL HAYES, D., HOADLEY, K. A., HOYLE, A. P., JEFFERYS, S. R., JONES, C. D., KIMES, P. K., LIU, Y., MARRON, J. S., MENG, S., MIECZKOWSKI, P. A., MOSE, L. E., PARKER, J. S., PEROU, C. M., PRINS, J. F., ROACH, J., SHI, Y., SIMONS, J. V., SINGH, D., SOLOWAY, M. G., TAN, D., VELUVOLU, U., WALTER, V., WARING, S., WILKERSON, M. D., WU, J., ZHAO, N., CHERNIACK, A. D., HAMMERMAN, P. S., TWARD, A. D., SEKHAR PEDAMALLU, C., SAKSENA, G., et al. 2015. Comprehensive genomic characterization of head and neck squamous cell carcinomas. *Nature*, 517, 576–82.

LECHAGO, J. 2005. The frozen section: Pathology in the trenches. *Arch Pathol Lab Med*, 129, 1529–31.

LECHNER, A., SCHLÖßER, H., ROTHSCHILD, S. I., THELEN, M., REUTER, S., ZENTIS, P., SHIMABUKURO-VORNHAGEN, A., THEURICH, S., WENNHOLD, K., GARCIA-MARQUEZ, M., THARUN, L., QUAAS, A., SCHAUSS, A., ISENSEE, J., HUCHO, T., HUEBBERS, C., VON BERGWELT-BAILDON, M., & BEUTNER, D. 2017. Characterization of tumor-associated T-lymphocyte subsets and immune checkpoint molecules in head and neck squamous cell carcinoma. *Oncotarget*, 8, 44418–33.

LEE, L. Y., CHEN, Y. J., LU, Y. C., LIAO, C. T., CHEN, I. H., CHANG, J. T., HUANG, Y. C., CHEN, W. H., HUANG, C. C., TSAI, C. Y., & CHENG, A. J. 2015. Fascin is a circulating tumor marker for head and neck cancer as determined by a proteomic analysis of interstitial fluid from the tumor microenvironment. *Clin Chem Lab Med*, 53, 1631–41.

LEUNG, S. F., TAM, J. S., CHAN, A. T., ZEE, B., CHAN, L. Y., HUANG, D. P., VAN HASSELT, A., JOHNSON, P. J., & LO, Y. M. 2004. Improved accuracy of detection of nasopharyngeal carcinoma by combined application of circulating Epstein-Barr virus DNA and anti-Epstein-Barr viral capsid antigen IgA antibody. *Clin Chem*, 50, 339–45.

LEWIS, J. S., JR, BEADLE, B., BISHOP, J. A., CHERNOCK, R. D., COLASACCO, C., LACCHETTI, C., MONCUR, J. T., ROCCO, J. W., SCHWARTZ, M. R., SEETHALA, R. R., THOMAS, N. E., WESTRA, W. H., & FAQUIN, W. C. 2017. Human papillomavirus testing in head and neck carcinomas: Guideline from the College of American Pathologists. *Arch Pathol Lab Med*, 142, 559–97.

LIAO, C. J., HSIEH, C. H., HUNG, F. C., WANG, H. M., CHOU, W. P., & WU, M. H. 2019. The integration of a three-dimensional spheroid cell culture operation in a circulating tumor cell (CTC) isolation and purification process: A preliminary study of the clinical significance and prognostic role of the CTCs isolated from the blood samples of head and neck cancer patients. *Cancers (Basel)*, 11(6), 783.

LIN, B., GAO, F., YANG, Y., WU, D., ZHANG, Y., FENG, G., DAI, T., & DU, X. 2021. FLASH Radiotherapy: History and Future. *Front Oncol*, 11, 644400.

LIU, H., SCHAAL, D., CURRY, H., CLARK, R., MAGLIARI, A., KUPELIAN, P., KHUNTIA, D., & BERIWAL, S. 2023. Review of cone beam computed tomography based online adaptive radiotherapy: Current trend and future direction. *Radiat Oncol*, 18, 144.

LOREE, T. R., & STRONG, E. W. 1991. Significance of positive margins in oral cavity squamous carcinoma. *Am J Otolaryngol*, 12, 179.

LU, Y., LIANG, H., YU, T., XIE, J., CHEN, S., DONG, H., SINKO, P. J., LIAN, S., XU, J., WANG, J., YU, S., SHAO, J., YUAN, B., WANG, L., & JIA, L. 2015a. Isolation and characterization of living circulating tumor cells in patients by immunomagnetic negative enrichment coupled with flow cytometry. *Cancer*, 121, 3036–45.

LU, Y. C., CHANG, J. T., HUANG, Y. C., HUANG, C. C., CHEN, W. H., LEE, L. Y., HUANG, B. S., CHEN, Y. J., LI, H. F., & CHENG, A. J. 2015b. Combined determination of circulating miR-196a and miR-196b levels produces high sensitivity and specificity for early detection of oral cancer. *Clin Biochem*, 48, 115–21.

MAHMOOD, H., SHABAN, M., INDAVE, B. I., SANTOS-SILVA, A. R., RAJPOOT, N., & KHURRAM, S. A. 2020. Use of artificial intelligence in diagnosis of head and neck precancerous and cancerous lesions: A systematic review. *Oral Oncol*, 110, 104885.

MAHMOOD, H., SHABAN, M., RAJPOOT, N., & KHURRAM, S. A. 2021. Artificial Intelligence-based methods in head and neck cancer diagnosis: An overview. *Br J Cancer*, 124, 1934–40.

MEHANNA, H., TABERNA, M., VON BUCHWALD, C., TOUS, S., BROOKS, J., MENA, M., MOREY, F., GRØNHØJ, C., RASMUSSEN, J. H., & GARSET-ZAMANI, M. 2023. Prognostic implications of p16 and HPV discordance in oropharyngeal cancer (HNCIG-EPIC-OPC): A multicentre, multinational, individual patient data analysis. *Lancet Oncol*, 24, 239–51.

MEIER, J. D., OLIVER, D. A., & VARVARES, M. A. 2005. Surgical margin determination in head and neck oncology: Current clinical practice. The results of an International American Head and Neck Society Member Survey. *Head Neck*, 27, 952–8.

MES, S. W., BRINK, A., SISTERMANS, E. A., STRAVER, R., OUDEJANS, C. B. M., POELL, J. B., LEEMANS, C. R., & BRAKENHOFF, R. H. 2020. Comprehensive multiparameter genetic analysis improves circulating tumor DNA detection in head and neck cancer patients. *Oral Oncol*, 109, 104852.

MIRGHANI, H., & BLANCHARD, P. 2018. Treatment de-escalation for HPV-driven oropharyngeal cancer: Where do we stand? *Clin Translat Radiat Oncol*, 8, 4–11.

MISTRY, R. C., QURESHI, S. S., & KUMARAN, C. 2005. Post-resection mucosal margin shrinkage in oral cancer: Quantification and significance. *J Surg Oncol*, 91, 131–3.

MIYARA, M., YOSHIOKA, Y., KITOH, A., SHIMA, T., WING, K., NIWA, A., PARIZOT, C., TAFLIN, C., HEIKE, T., VALEYRE, D., MATHIAN, A., NAKAHATA, T., YAMAGUCHI, T., NOMURA, T., ONO, M., AMOURA, Z., GOROCHOV, G., & SAKAGUCHI, S. 2009. Functional delineation and differentiation dynamics of human CD4+ T cells expressing the FoxP3 transcription factor. *Immunity*, 30, 899–911.

MORGAN, H. E., & SHER, D. J. 2020. Adaptive radiotherapy for head and neck cancer. *Cancers Head Neck*, 5, 1.

MUNIZ, I. D. A. F., ARAUJO, M., BOUASSALY, J., FARSHADI, F., ATIQUE, M., ESFAHANI, K., BONAN, P. R. F., HIER, M., MASCARELLA, M., & MLYNAREK, A. 2024. Therapeutic advances and challenges for the management of HPV-associated oropharyngeal cancer. *Int J Mol Sci*, 25, 4009.

NAGLER, R. M., BARAK, M., PELED, M., BEN-ARYEH, H., FILATOV, M., & LAUFER, D. 1999. Early diagnosis and treatment monitoring roles of tumor markers Cyfra 21-1 and TPS in oral squamous cell carcinoma. *Cancer*, 85, 1018–25.

NIEBERLER, M., STIMMER, H., RASTHOFER, D., NENTWIG, K., WEIRICH, G., & WOLFF, K. D. 2020. Defining secure surgical bone margins in head and neck squamous cell carcinomas: The diagnostic impact of intraoperative cytological assessment of bone resection margins compared with preoperative imaging. *Oral Oncol*, 102, 104579.

NOORLAG, R., KLEIN NULENT, T. J. W., DELWEL, V. E. J., PAMEIJER, F. A., WILLEMS, S. M., DE BREE, R., & VAN ES, R. J. J. 2020. Assessment of tumour depth in early tongue cancer: Accuracy of MRI and intraoral ultrasound. *Oral Oncol*, 110, 104895.

OBRADOVIC, A., GRAVES, D., KORRER, M., WANG, Y., ROY, S., NAVEED, A., XU, Y., LUGINBUHL, A., CURRY, J., GIBSON, M., IDREES, K., HURLEY, P., JIANG, P., LIU, X. S., UPPALURI, R., DRAKE, C. G., CALIFANO, A., & KIM, Y. J. 2022. Immunostimulatory cancer-associated fibroblast subpopulations can predict immunotherapy response in head and neck cancer. *Clin Cancer Res*, 28, 2094–109.

OLIVA, M., SPREAFICO, A., TABERNA, M., ALEMANY, L., COBURN, B., MESIA, R., & SIU, L. L. 2019. Immune biomarkers of response to immune-checkpoint inhibitors in head and neck squamous cell carcinoma. *Ann Oncol*, 30, 57–67.

ONIDANI, K., SHOJI, H., KAKIZAKI, T., YOSHIMOTO, S., OKAYA, S., MIURA, N., SEKIKAWA, S., FURUTA, K., LIM, C. T., SHIBAHARA, T., BOKU, N., KATO, K., & HONDA, K. 2019. Monitoring of cancer patients via next-generation sequencing of patient-derived circulating tumor cells and tumor DNA. *Cancer Sci*, 110, 2590–9.

OU, D., ADAM, J., GARBERIS, I., BLANCHARD, P., NGUYEN, F., LEVY, A., CASIRAGHI, O., GORPHE, P., BREUSKIN, I., JANOT, F., TEMAM, S., SCOAZEC, J. Y., DEUTSCH, E., & TAO, Y. 2017. Clinical relevance of tumor infiltrating lymphocytes, PD-L1 expression and correlation with HPV/p16 in head and neck cancer treated with bio- or chemo-radiotherapy. *Oncoimmunology*, 6, e1341030.

OUMAROU HAMA, H., ABOUDHARAM, G., BARBIERI, R., LEPIDI, H., & DRANCOURT, M. 2022. Immunohistochemical diagnosis of human infectious diseases: A review. *Diagn Pathol*, 17, 17.

PAVER, E. C., CURRIE, A. M., GUPTA, R., & DAHLSTROM, J. E. 2020. Human papilloma virus related squamous cell carcinomas of the head and neck: Diagnosis, clinical implications and detection of HPV. *Pathology*, 52, 179–91.

PENG, Z., WANG, Y., WANG, Y., JIANG, S., FAN, R., ZHANG, H., & JIANG, W. 2021. Application of radiomics and machine learning in head and neck cancers. *Int J Biol Sci*, 17, 475–86.

PERRI, F., LONGO, F., CAPONIGRO, F., SANDOMENICO, F., GUIDA, A., DELLA VITTORIA SCARPATI, G., OTTAIANO, A., MUTO, P., & IONNA, F. 2020. Management of HPV-related squamous cell carcinoma of the head and neck: Pitfalls and caveat. *Cancers*, 12, 975.

ROSENTHAL, E. L., WARRAM, J. M., BLAND, K. I., & ZINN, K. R. 2015. The status of contemporary image-guided modalities in oncologic surgery. *Ann Surg*, 261, 46–55.

SARKAR, P., MALIK, S., LAHA, S., DAS, S., BUNK, S., RAY, J. G., CHATTERJEE, R., & SAHA, A. 2021. Dysbiosis of oral microbiota during oral squamous cell carcinoma development. *Front Oncol*, 11, 614448.

SATURNO, M. P., BRANDWEIN-WEBER, M., GREENBERG, L., SILBERZWEIG, A., BUCHBINDER, D., DOWLING, E. M., KHAN, M. N., CHAI, R., & URKEN, M. L. 2023. Utilizing 3D head and neck specimen scanning for intraoperative margin discussions: Proof of concept of our novel approach. *Head Neck*, 45, 10–21.

SEGAL, N. H., OU, S. I., BALMANOUKIAN, A., FURY, M. G., MASSARELLI, E., BRAHMER, J. R., WEISS, J., SCHÖFFSKI, P., ANTONIA, S. J., MASSARD, C., ZANDBERG, D. P., KHLEIF, S. N., XIAO, F., REBELATTO, M. C., STEELE, K. E., ROBBINS, P. B., ANGRA, N., SONG, X., ABDULLAH, S., & BUTLER, M. 2019. Safety and efficacy of durvalumab in patients with head and neck squamous cell carcinoma: Results from a phase I/II expansion cohort. *Eur J Cancer*, 109, 154–61.

SEIWERT, T. Y., BURTNESS, B., MEHRA, R., WEISS, J., BERGER, R., EDER, J. P., HEATH, K., MCCLANAHAN, T., LUNCEFORD, J., GAUSE, C., CHENG, J. D., & CHOW, L. Q. 2016. Safety and clinical activity of pembrolizumab for treatment of recurrent or metastatic squamous cell carcinoma of the head and neck (KEYNOTE-012): An open-label, multicentre, phase 1b trial. *Lancet Oncol*, 17, 956–65.

SHE, Y., KONG, X., GE, Y., YIN, P., LIU, Z., CHEN, J., GAO, F., & FANG, S. 2020. Immune-related gene signature for predicting the prognosis of head and neck squamous cell carcinoma. *Cancer Cell Int*, 20, 22.

SHEN, Z., WU, A., & CHEN, X. 2017. Current detection technologies for circulating tumor cells. *Chem Soc Rev*, 46, 2038–56.

SHIN, J. M., LUO, T., KAMARAJAN, P., FENNO, J. C., RICKARD, A. H., & KAPILA, Y. L. 2017. Microbial communities associated with primary and metastatic head and neck squamous cell carcinoma: A high fusobacterial and low streptococcal signature. *Sci Rep*, 7, 9934.

SINGHAL, S. 2016. The future of surgical oncology: Image-guided cancer surgery. *JAMA Surg*, 151, 184–5.

SINGHI, A. D., & WESTRA, W. H. 2010. Comparison of human papillomavirus in situ hybridization and p16 immunohistochemistry in the detection of human papillomavirus-associated head and neck cancer based on a prospective clinical experience. *Cancer*, 116, 2166–73.

SIRAVEGNA, G., MARSONI, S., SIENA, S., & BARDELLI, A. 2017. Integrating liquid biopsies into the management of cancer. *Nat Rev Clin Oncol*, 14, 531–48.

SMITS, R. W. H., KOLJENOVIĆ, S., HARDILLO, J. A., TEN HOVE, I., MEEUWIS, C. A., SEWNAIK, A., DRONKERS, E. A. C., BAKKER SCHUT, T. C., LANGEVELD, T. P. M., MOLENAAR, J., HEGT, V. N., PUPPELS, G. J., & BAATENBURG DE JONG, R. J. 2016. Resection margins in oral cancer surgery: Room for improvement. *Head Neck*, 38, E2197–203.

SOLOMON, B., YOUNG, R. J., BRESSEL, M., URBAN, D., HENDRY, S., THAI, A., ANGEL, C., HADDAD, A., KOWANETZ, M., FUA, T., CORRY, J., FOX, S., & RISCHIN, D. 2018. Prognostic significance of PD-L1(+) and CD8(+) immune cells in HPV(+) oropharyngeal squamous cell carcinoma. *Cancer Immunol Res*, 6, 295–304.

SOLOMON, J. P., LINKOV, I., ROSADO, A., MULLANEY, K., ROSEN, E. Y., FROSINA, D., JUNGBLUTH, A. A., ZEHIR, A., BENAYED, R., DRILON, A., HYMAN, D. M., LADANYI, M., SIRECI, A. N., & HECHTMAN, J. F. 2020. NTRK fusion detection across multiple assays and 33,997 cases: Diagnostic implications and pitfalls. *Modern Pathol*, 33, 38–46.

SPENCE, T., BRUCE, J., YIP, K. W., & LIU, F.-F. 2016. HPV associated head and neck cancer. *Cancers*, 8, 75.

SU, S. C., CHANG, L. C., HUANG, H. D., PENG, C. Y., CHUANG, C. Y., CHEN, Y. T., LU, M. Y., CHIU, Y. W., CHEN, P. Y., & YANG, S. F. 2021. Oral microbial dysbiosis and its performance in predicting oral cancer. *Carcinogenesis*, 42, 127–35.

TAKAHASHI, H., SAKAKURA, K., IDA, S., KAWABATA-IWAKAWA, R., MATSUYAMA, T., TADA, H., MITO, I., & CHIKAMATSU, K. 2022. Circulating naïve and effector memory T cells correlate with prognosis in head and neck squamous cell carcinoma. *Cancer Sci*, 113, 53–64.

TAKAHASHI, H., SAKAKURA, K., MITO, I., IDA, S., & CHIKAMATSU, K. 2016. Dynamic changes in immune cell profile in head and neck squamous cell carcinoma: Immunomodulatory effects of chemotherapy. *Cancer Sci*, 107, 1065–71.

TAKAMURA, M., KOBAYASHI, T., NIKKUNI, Y., KATSURA, K., YAMAZAKI, M., MARUYAMA, S., TANUMA, J. I., & HAYASHI, T. 2022. A comparative study between CT, MRI, and intraoral US for the evaluation of the depth of invasion in early stage (T1/T2) tongue squamous cell carcinoma. *Oral Radiol*, 38, 114–25.

TAN, W. C. C., NERURKAR, S. N., CAI, H. Y., NG, H. H. M., WU, D., WEE, Y. T. F., LIM, J. C. T., YEONG, J., & LIM, T. K. H. 2020. Overview of multiplex immunohistochemistry/immunofluorescence techniques in the era of cancer immunotherapy. *Cancer Commun (Lond)*, 40, 135–53.

TANAKA, T. I., & ALAWI, F. 2018. Human papillomavirus and oropharyngeal cancer. *Dent Clin North Am*, 62, 111–20.

TAUBE, J. M., AKTURK, G., ANGELO, M., ENGLE, E. L., GNJATIC, S., GREENBAUM, S., GREENWALD, N. F., HEDVAT, C. V., HOLLMANN, T. J., JUCO, J., PARRA, E. R., REBELATTO, M. C., RIMM, D. L., RODRIGUEZ-CANALES, J., SCHALPER, K. A., STACK, E. C., FERREIRA, C. S., KORSKI, K., LAKO, A., RODIG, S. J., SCHENCK, E., STEELE, K. E., SURACE, M. J., TETZLAFF, M. T., VON LOGA, K., WISTUBA, II & BIFULCO, C. B. 2020. The Society for Immunotherapy of Cancer statement on best practices for multiplex immunohistochemistry (IHC) and immunofluorescence (IF) staining and validation. *J Immunother Cancer*, 8(1), e000155.

TENG, M. W., NGIOW, S. F., RIBAS, A., & SMYTH, M. J. 2015. Classifying cancers based on T-cell infiltration and PD-L1. *Cancer Res*, 75, 2139–45.

THOMAS ROBBINS, K., TRIANTAFYLLOU, A., SUAREZ, C., LOPEZ, F., HUNT, J. L., STROJAN, P., WILLIAMS, M. D., BRAAKHUIS, B. J. M., DE BREE, R., HINNI, M. L., KOWALSKI, L. P., RINALDO, A., RODRIGO, J. P., VANDER POORTEN, V., NIXON, I. J., TAKES, R. P., SILVER, C. E., & FERLITO, A. 2019. Surgical margins in head and neck cancer: Intra- and postoperative considerations. *Auris Nasus Larynx*, 46, 10–17.

TINHOFER, I., KONSCHAK, R., STROMBERGER, C., RAGUSE, J. D., DREYER, J. H., JÖHRENS, K., KEILHOLZ, U., & BUDACH, V. 2014. Detection of circulating tumor cells for prediction of recurrence after adjuvant chemoradiation in locally advanced squamous cell carcinoma of the head and neck. *Ann Oncol*, 25, 2042–7.

TORTORA, M., GEMINI, L., SCARAVILLI, A., UGGA, L., PONSIGLIONE, A., STANZIONE, A., D'ARCO, F., D'ANNA, G., & CUOCOLO, R. 2023. Radiomics applications in head and neck tumor imaging: A narrative review. *Cancers*, 15, 1174.

TOUSKA, P., & CONNOR, S. E. J. 2019. Recent advances in MRI of the head and neck, skull base and cranial nerves: new and evolving sequences, analyses and clinical applications. *Br J Radiol*, 92, 20190513.

TSUTSUMI, Y. 2021. Pitfalls and caveats in applying chromogenic immunostaining to histopathological diagnosis. *Cells*, 10, 1501.

UPPALURI, R., CAMPBELL, K. M., EGLOFF, A. M., ZOLKIND, P., SKIDMORE, Z. L., NUSSENBAUM, B., PANIELLO, R. C., RICH, J. T., JACKSON, R., PIPKORN, P., MICHEL, L. S., LEY, J., OPPELT, P., DUNN, G. P., BARNELL, E. K., SPIES, N. C., LIN, T., LI, T., MULDER, D. T., HANNA, Y., CIRLAN, I., PUGH, T. J., MUDIANTO, T., RILEY, R., ZHOU, L., JO, V. Y., STACHLER, M. D., HANNA, G. J., KASS, J., HADDAD, R., SCHOENFELD, J. D., GJINI, E., LAKO, A., THORSTAD, W., GAY, H. A., DALY, M., RODIG, S. J., HAGEMANN, I. S., KALLOGJERI, D., PICCIRILLO, J. F., CHERNOCK, R. D., GRIFFITH, M., GRIFFITH, O. L., & ADKINS, D. R. 2020. Neoadjuvant and adjuvant pembrolizumab in resectable locally advanced, human papillomavirus-unrelated head and neck cancer: A multicenter, phase II trial. *Clin Cancer Res*, 26, 5140–52.

URKEN, M. L., YUN, J., SATURNO, M. P., GREENBERG, L. A., CHAI, R. L., SHARIF, K., & BRANDWEIN-WEBER, M. 2023. Frozen section analysis in head and neck surgical pathology: A narrative review of the past, present, and future of intraoperative pathologic consultation. *Oral Oncol*, 143, 106445.

VENUTI, A., & PAOLINI, F. 2012. HPV detection methods in head and neck cancer. *Head Neck Pathol*, 6 Suppl 1, S63–74.

WAI, K. C., STROHL, M. P., VAN ZANTE, A., & HA, P. K. 2020. Molecular diagnostics in human papillomavirus-related head and neck squamous cell carcinoma. *Cells*, 9.

WANG, H., ZHANG, Y., BAI, W., WANG, B., WEI, J., JI, R., XIN, Y., DONG, L., & JIANG, X. 2020. Feasibility of immunohistochemical p16 staining in the diagnosis of human papillomavirus infection in patients with squamous cell carcinoma of the head and neck: A systematic review and meta-analysis. *Front Oncol*, 10, 524928.

WANG, J., ZHOU, Y., LU, J., SUN, Y., XIAO, H., LIU, M., & TIAN, L. 2014. Combined detection of serum exosomal miR-21 and HOTAIR as diagnostic and prognostic biomarkers for laryngeal squamous cell carcinoma. *Med Oncol*, 31, 148.

WARD, M. J., THIRDBOROUGH, S. M., MELLOWS, T., RILEY, C., HARRIS, S., SUCHAK, K., WEBB, A., HAMPTON, C., PATEL, N. N., RANDALL, C. J., COX, H. J., JOGAI, S., PRIMROSE, J., PIPER, K., OTTENSMEIER, C. H., KING, E. V., & THOMAS, G. J. 2014. Tumour-infiltrating lymphocytes predict for outcome in HPV-positive oropharyngeal cancer. *Br J Cancer*, 110, 489–500.

WEINSTOCK, Y. E., ALAVA, I., 3RD & DIERKS, E. J. 2014. Pitfalls in determining head and neck surgical margins. *Oral Maxillofac Surg Clin North Am*, 26, 151–62.

WENIG, B. M. 2008. Intraoperative consultation (IOC) in mucosal lesions of the upper aerodigestive tract. *Head Neck Pathol*, 2, 131–44.

XU, B., HAROON AL RASHEED, M. R., ANTONESCU, C. R., ALEX, D., FROSINA, D., GHOSSEIN, R., JUNGBLUTH, A. A., & KATABI, N. 2020. Pan-Trk immunohistochemistry is a sensitive and specific ancillary tool for diagnosing secretory carcinoma of the salivary gland and detecting ETV6–NTRK3 fusion. *Histopathology*, 76, 375–82.

XU, B., SUURMEIJER, A. J., AGARAM, N. P., & ANTONESCU, C. R. 2023. Head and neck mesenchymal tumors with kinase fusions: A report of 15 cases with emphasis on wide anatomic distribution and diverse histologic appearance. *Am J Surg Pathol*, 47, 248–58.

XU, Q., WANG, C., YUAN, X., FENG, Z., & HAN, Z. 2017. Prognostic value of tumor-infiltrating lymphocytes for patients with head and neck squamous cell carcinoma. *Transl Oncol*, 10, 10–16.

ZABOROWSKI, M., VARGAS, A. C., PULVERS, J., CLARKSON, A., DE GUZMAN, D., SIOSON, L., MACLEAN, F., CHOU, A., & GILL, A. J. 2020. When used together SS18–SSX fusion-specific and SSX C-terminus immunohistochemistry are highly specific and sensitive for the diagnosis of synovial sarcoma and can replace FISH or molecular testing in most cases. *Histopathology*, 77, 588–600.

ZEISBERG, M., & NEILSON, E. G. 2009. Biomarkers for epithelial-mesenchymal transitions. *J Clin Invest*, 119, 1429–37.

ZHANG, Z., LI, S., WANG, W., ZHANG, Y., WANG, K., CHENG, J., & WEN, B. 2023. Synthetic MRI for the quantitative and morphologic assessment of head and neck tumors: A preliminary study. *Dentomaxillofac Radiol*, 52, 20230103.

ZHU, S., SCHUERCH, C., & HUNT, J. 2015. Review and updates of immunohistochemistry in selected salivary gland and head and neck tumors. *Arch Pathol Lab Med*, 139, 55–66.

13

Biomarkers and Predictive Modeling

Rahaba Marima, Pontsho Molela, Ntlotlang Mokgautsi, Olalekan Fadebi, Sheefa Mirza, Amahle Nyalambisa, Clement Penny, Jyotsna Batra, and Zodwa Dlamini

13.1 Introduction

Head and neck cancer (HNC) ranks as the seventh most common cancer worldwide and is responsible for > 680,000 new diagnoses each year (Gormley et al., 2022). HNC includes various tumors that develop in the head and neck area, such as those that arise from the epithelial lining of the oral cavity, mouth, throat, larynx, pharynx, and adjacent structures (Dive et al., 2014; Leemans et al., 2011). Precise diagnosis of HNC in its early stages, when patients are more responsive to treatments with potential for cure, is crucial in reducing mortality rates and improving clinical outcomes associated with the disease. The treatment modalities for HNC may include surgical resection, radiotherapy (RT), chemotherapy (CT), targeted therapy, or a combination of these options. The choice of treatment approach or combination depends on the stage at which the cancer is detected (Huang & O'Sullivan, 2013; Rivera, 2015). However, the majority of HNC cases are diagnosed at an advanced stage (III and IV) (Du et al., 2019), thus limiting the effectiveness of therapeutic intervention. Patients with HNC generally have a poor prognosis in terms of survival, and, depending on the stage and location of the tumor, the 5-year survival rate varies between 30% and 70% (Warnakulasuriya, 2009). HNC racial disparities further exacerbate this poor patient outcome. In addition, there is a lack of HNC biomarkers and reliable predictive modeling in HNC management and improving patient outcomes. The poor prognosis of HNC patients is driven by a multifactorial landscape involving genetic factors as well as inequitable access to healthcare and other social constructs. This chapter discusses current advances in HNC biomarkers, predictive modeling in HNC, and the impact of these tools in redefining the landscape of HNC clinical management.

13.2 Biomarkers in Head and Neck Cancer and Predictive Modeling

13.2.1 Head and Neck Cancer Diagnostic, Prognostic, and Predictive Biomarkers

Diagnostic biomarkers can either confirm the presence of a disease or distinguish among different subtypes of a disease in patients (Califf, 2018). Several diagnostic biomarkers have been identified for HNC that aid in early detection, prognosis, and treatment planning. For example, human papillomavirus (HPV) infection is the most common sexually transmitted infection (STI) globally and is associated with cancers affecting both the anogenital region and the oropharynx (Scott-Wittenborn & Fakhry, 2021). Since 1983, when Syrjänen initially linked HPV infection with HNC, extensive research has ensued (Deneka et al., 2018). HPV infection, particularly with high-risk HPV16, accounts for the overwhelming majority (> 90%) of HPV-related HNC cases, especially as a key prognosis for oropharyngeal cancer (OPC) (Syrjänen, 2018; Syrjänen et al., 2021). OPC occurs mainly on the tonsils and base of the tongue (Kaneko et al., 2021; Lim & D'Silva, 2024). The sexually transmitted virus causes HPV-positive HNC (HPV-HNC), a distinct subset of HNCs that occur primarily in the oropharynx and arise from the lymphoid tissues of the palatine and lingual tonsils (Begum et al., 2005). HNC/OPC has been classified as either HPV-negative and HPV-positive among men and women (Agrawal et al., 2011; Ang et al., 2010).

Interestingly, recent studies have shown that patients with HPV-positive OPC respond better to treatment, resulting in > 50% improvements in both overall survival and disease-specific survival (Masterson et al., 2014; Straetmans et al., 2009). This prognosis may differ depending on the HPV genotype, suggesting a preference for type-specific HPV detection methods in the future (Agrawal et al., 2011; Ang et al., 2010). HPV-positive tumors often have a better prognosis and may respond differently to treatment compared to HPV-negative tumors (Nogues et al., 2021; Tumban, 2019). Studies reveal that HPV-negative tumors exhibit significant dysregulation in the copy numbers of the epidermal growth factor receptor (EGFR) family, a subclass of receptor tyrosine kinase (RTK) (Seiwert et al., 2015). EGFR is a 170 kDa transmembrane glycoprotein cell surface receptor that constitutes the ErbB/HER family, together with ErbB2 (HER2/neu), ErbB3 (HER3), and ErbB4 (HER4) (Furuuchi et al., 2007; Kalyankrishna & Grandis, 2006). A reliable biomarker is indicative of disease onset, prognosis, and treatment outcome (Figure 13.1).

Overexpression of EGFR is prevalent in HNC and is associated with tumor progression and a poor prognosis. Moreover, targeting EGFR can lead to various biological and cellular effects, including the potential to restore apoptotic

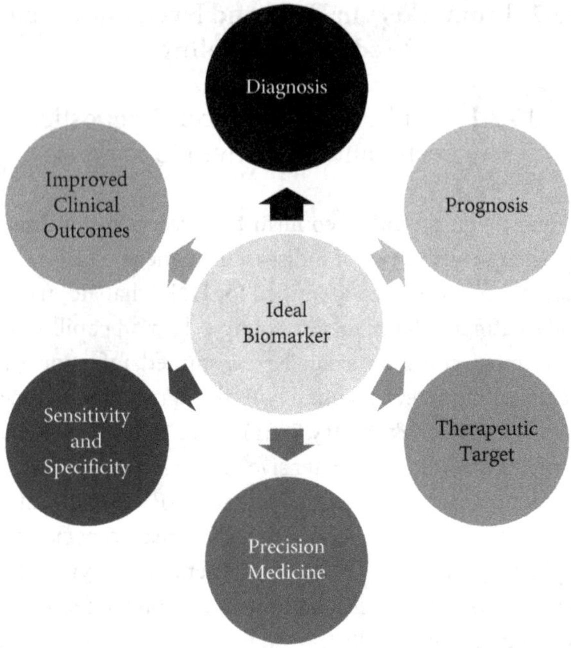

Figure 13.1 An ideal biomarker. Reliable biomarkers are critical in head and neck cancer (HNC) for diagnosis, prognosis, and treatment selection. They provide valuable insights into tumor biology, predict therapeutic responses, and help tailor personalized treatment strategies.

capabilities, reduce DNA-repair activity, inhibit angiogenesis, and hinder tumor cell migration (Bourhis et al., 2007). The EGFR inhibitor cetuximab, a monoclonal antibody approved by the US Food and Drug Administration (FDA), as HNC therapy, has demonstrated enhanced efficacy in tumors characterized by increased levels of EGFR expression. However, the emergence of resistance to anti-EGFR agents remains a significant obstacle, limiting survival rates in advanced HNC. EGFR overexpression in cancers is associated with poor clinical outcomes, therapeutic resistance, and distant metastasis in HNC.

The cell cycle is an intricate process in which a cell duplicates its components and divides into two identical daughter cells. It is vital for cell growth and reproduction and involves various regulatory proteins (Wenzel & Singh, 2018). One of the critical regulators within the cell cycle is cyclin D1, which has been extensively reported for its role in the nucleus and cytoplasmic membrane (Montalto & De Amicis, 2020b). Cyclin D also plays a critical role in the pathogenesis of cancer proliferation; particularly, the overexpression of cyclin D1 has been associated with tumor aggressiveness and poor prognosis in head and neck, esophagus, breast, ovary, lung and colon cancers. Furthermore, the elevated expression of this regulator is associated with the development of regional lymph node metastases in HNC. Additionally, cyclin D1 also regulates the expression of specific micro-RNAs (miRNAs) (also implicated in the development and progression of HNC) (El-Mahdy et al., 2023; Nagadia et al., 2013; Thomaidou et al., 2022) and plays a crucial role in tumor–stroma interactions, potentiating most cancer hallmarks (Montalto & De Amicis, 2020a). Another crucial biomarker commonly elevated in HNC is Bcl-2, an anti-apoptotic protein commonly linked to resistance against chemotherapy and radiation treatment when expressed at elevated levels in HNC (Yang et al., 2019; Zhang et al., 2023). Additionally, p16, a protein involved in the regulation of the cell cycle, has been reported to be highly expressed in HNC, and its expression is indicative of HPV positivity in the disease. Since HPV-positive tumors generally respond better to treatment, p16 status can help predict which patients are more likely to respond favorably to standard therapies (Adilbay et al., 2018). Table 13.1 describes HNC biomarkers.

13.2.2 Advances and Integrated Approaches in Head and Neck Cancer Biomarker Discovery and Applications

Advanced molecular technologies like gene expression and proteome profiling are used to identify novel biomarkers. Finding variations in gene expression before an oncological transformation is a vital initial phase in searching for biomarkers that aid in early cancer detection. These biomarkers aid in targeted therapy by predicting the behavior of different tumors (Lutzky et al., 2008). Automating laboratory processes into tiny cards or chips facilitates the advancement and simplification of HNC diagnostic techniques. These methods have been used for microarray analysis, product sizing, polymerase chain reaction (PCR), and cell lysis. Based on several indicators, analysis of a saliva sample put on the chip can identify specific malignant cells (Basheeth & Patil, 2019). The intricacy of metastasis makes it highly improbable that a single sign can determine it with absolute certainty, but several markers combined may aid in a more accurate prognosis than a single, solitary sign.

Almost all expressed genes can be profiled at the RNA and DNA levels using next-generation sequencing (NGS), which makes it possible to concurrently examine the therapeutic or prognostic implications of many biomarkers in head and neck squamous cell cancer (HNSCC) (Basheeth & Patil, 2019). Advances in multiomics profiling have led to the identification of proteins linked to HNC carcinogenesis and the measurement of their expression from tissue, blood, or saliva samples. Proteins are desirable biomarkers since they can be found in bodily fluids using enzyme-linked immunosorbent assay (ELISA) or in tissue

Table 13.1 Head and neck cancer biomarkers

Biomarker	Description	References
HPV	A diverse group of viruses transmitted through direct skin-to-skin contact, is associated with various cancers, including head and neck cancer, particularly oropharyngeal cancer, with HPV type 16 being a significant risk factor	Brianti et al., 2017
Cyclin D1	Regulates the G1 checkpoint in cell division and is associated with the development of tumors in several areas, including the esophagus, ovaries, breast, colon, lungs, and HNC	Eberly et al., 2024
Bcl-2	A critical protein within mitochondria regulates apoptosis by inhibiting pro-apoptotic proteins when overexpressed, thus blocking cell death	Deveraux et al., 2001
P16	An indirect indicator of HPV infection in oropharyngeal squamous cell carcinomas, serving as a surrogate marker for HPV-positive disease	Nava-Villalba et al., 2014
EGFR	Commonly elevated in solid tumors, including HNC, and exerting a significant influence on tumor development	Eberly et al., 2024
miRNAs	MicroRNAs are molecules of noncoding DNA that regulate gene expression and dysregulation	Kaikkonen et al., 2011
PD-L1 expression	PD-L1 is an immune checkpoint regulator and immunomodulatory protein expressed in various immune cells	Dermani et al., 2019

using immunohistochemistry (IHC). ELISA and IHC are widely used, simple, and economical methods in clinical pathology (Schaaij-Visser et al., 2010).

Selected reaction monitoring (SRM), a mass spectrometry (MS)-based technique, has proved helpful in identifying, measuring, and validating possible biomarkers (Schaaij-Visser et al., 2010). Based on mass spectrometry, protein profiling was recently discovered when HNSCC cell lines (FaDu, UTSCC8, and UTSCC42a) were cultured in a conditioned medium (secretome). Proteomic and genomic profiling revealed overexpressed MMP14, PLAU, THBS1, and IGFBP7 levels in tumors. The results showed a relationship between a higher risk of recurrence and a lower rate of disease-free survival (Sepiashvili et al., 2012).

Positron emission tomography and computed tomography (PET/CT) scans as imaging biomarker tools are being developed owing to the development of innovative 18F-based radiotracers. Complementary mechanism-specific disease characterization is used for this purpose. The proliferation tracer 30-deoxy-30-18F fluorothymidine and the hypoxia tracer 18F-fluoromisonodazole (F-MISO) are two of the radiotracers of HNSCC that are being studied. Diffusion-weighted magnetic resonance imaging (MRI) and dynamic contrast-enhanced MRI (DCE-MRI) can quantify vascular integrity and tumor perfusion changes and analyze the tumor's response through localization and recurrence detection (Basheeth & Patil, 2019).

Furthermore, it is proposed that anti-PD-1/PD-L1 efficaciousness can be predicted as biomarkers using PD-L1 expression and $CD8^+$ T cell density. The density of $CD8^+$ lymphocytes and PD-L1 positivity on tumor-infiltrating immune cells are correlated with docetaxel, platinum, and fluorouracil (TPF) induction CT in advanced HNSCC. These characteristics imply that combination treatments using concurrent cytotoxic treatment and anti-PD-1/PD-L1 therapy may be pertinent for HNSCC (Adam et al., 2018).

13.2.3 Predictive Modeling in Head and Neck Cancer

A few isolated studies have demonstrated HNC predictive modeling. However, there is a lack of these tools in HNC care. To aid in the early detection of HNC, risk prediction models are key. HPV is reported as an oncovirus in HNC (Gillison et al., 2000; International Agency for Research on Cancer, 1988; Kreimer et al., 2018). For instance, the E6 protein of HPV 16 is a very sensitive and specific marker for HPV-positive oropharyngeal cancers, while E6 HPV antibodies can be found in HPV16-positive people a number of years before cancer diagnosis (Hibbert et al., 2021; Kreimer et al., 2013, 2017, 2019). While HPV infection, tobacco use, and alcohol consumption are key risk predictors, a predictive model should not only be based on genetic and epidemiological factors, but also on a variety of factors that include socioeconomic and education status, social determinants of health, social constructs, genetic markers, oncogenic virus (e.g., HPV), and serological markers (Budhathoki et al., 2023).

13.2.4 Artificial Intelligence in Cancer Risk Prediction Modeling

Risk prediction models, which use known or probable risk variables for a variety of malignancies including HNC, have been created as a tool to aid in risk stratification. Risk prediction models provide a chance to improve HNC patient care. To help with early detection (McCarthy et al., 2020), the results of personalized risk calculators can be used during patient consultations to help explain risk levels to specific patients and support risk behavior counseling (prevention). Additionally, they can be used to increase patient awareness of the disease's signs and symptoms (Sherratt et al., 2018) with the aim of promoting early detection (McCarthy et al., 2020). Additionally, a risk calculator could be used to help design clinical trials by facilitating the recruitment of patient subgroups with the highest risk of illness. Risk models have been successfully developed and implemented in this context in other cancer types, such as breast (Pfeiffer et al., 2013), colorectal (Tammemagi et al., 2011), and lung cancer (Marcus et al., 2015). There are limited previous work reported for risk prediction of HNC (Iwasaki et al., 2020; Koyanagi et al., 2017; Lee et al., 2020; McCarthy et al., 2020), and none of the existing risk prediction models considered all potential major risk factors, including HPV seropositivity and genetic susceptibility (Iwasaki et al., 2020; Koyanagi et al., 2017). As a result, several promising studies emphasizing the diagnostic and prognostic potentials of artificial intelligence (AI) models as an assistant decision-making tool have been reported during the past decade (Bejnordi et al., 2017; Kourou et al., 2015; Mahmood et al., 2020). Machine learning (ML) analyzes large amounts of empirical data using computational algorithms to automatically extract distinguishing characteristics and recognize intricate patterns (Giraud et al., 2019; Parmar et al., 2015). Developments in ML and deep learning (DL) have generated great interest in the idea of a "rapid learning health system." By examining large patient datasets, this method allows for customized decision-making (Lambin et al., 2013). AI offers a unique opportunity for the development of predictive models that can help stratify individual patient risk and guide therapeutic decisions for optimal patient outcomes and quality of life in HNC (Figure 13.2) (Bang et al., 2023). It is hypothesized that ML-based models can more accurately predict outcomes than existing models by combining clinical, biological, genomic, and radiologic data (Chinnery et al., 2021).

13.3 Tumor Microenvironment and Predictive Factors

It has become clear that finding biomarkers as a stratification tool for HNC patients is crucial to predicting the advance of the illness, the prognosis of the patient, or the patient's response to therapy (Corredor et al., 2019). Digital pathology has significantly improved our understanding of the pathogenies of many tumors by helping to quantify various biomarkers such as morphological, immunological, and behavioral indicators. To help in early cancer detection and

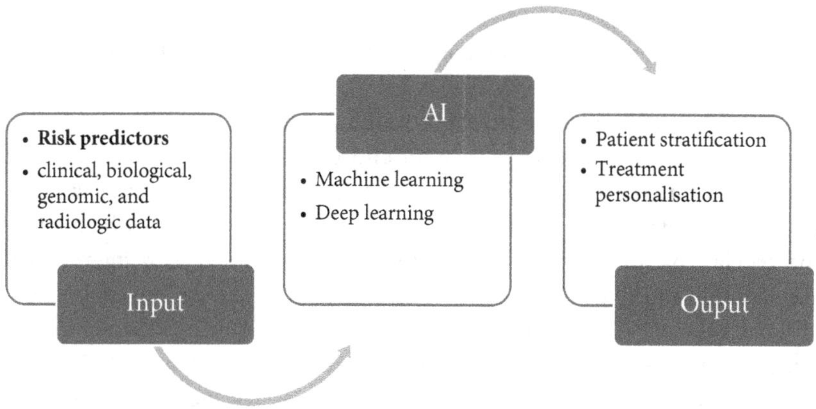

Figure 13.2 Head and neck cancer (HNC) risk prediction using artificial intelligence (AI). AI can be used as a powerful tool for improved patient risk stratification.

eventually improve patient prognosis, it is crucial to identify markers that can predict the course of the illness (Hijazi et al., 2024). To diagnose head and neck lesions that may be cancerous, changes in tissue and cellular shape are crucial indicators (Peltanova et al., 2019). It is vital to comprehend these modifications to find indicators of malignant transformation. To enhance the classification techniques employed for these lesions, many tissue and cell architectural characteristics in normal, premalignant, and malignant oral tissues can be quantified by image analysis. Changes in the basement membrane's complexity and several cellular morphological characteristics can be assessed by fractal geometry (Eid & Landini, 2003). The size can be measured objectively to identify changes in cell morphology, and a progressive rise in irregularity in the basement membrane is linked to the development of the illness (Eid & Landini, 2003).

A major challenge in treating HNC is its high rate of recurrence and metastasis, reflecting the intricate molecular landscape of the disease (Johnson et al., 2020; Morris et al., 2017). This complexity is attributed to dynamic interactions within the tumor microenvironment (TME), where the surrounding tissue matrix and immune cells play pivotal roles. The TME dictates treatment response and tumor progression, representing a complex ecosystem wherein various cellular and noncellular components interact (Chen et al., 2020; Qin et al., 2021). Traditionally, cancer was viewed solely as a mass of undifferentiated tumor cells, a stance that overlooked the critical influence of stromal cells in the microenvironment. However, the TME is recognized as a highly intricate network comprising cellular and noncellular components. This multifaceted environment consists of cellular constituents like natural killer (NK) cells, T cells, myeloid-derived suppressor cells (MDSCs), B cells, macrophages, dendritic cells (DCs), and one of the major components—cancer-associated fibroblasts (CAFs) (Bhat et al., 2021; Cristina et al., 2019; Jumaniyazova et al., 2023; Wu & Dai, 2017).

Noncellular components include extracellular matrix (ECM) proteins like fibronectin, laminin, collagen, tenascin and elastin, as well as chemical and physical factors such as pH, interstitial pressure, oxygen levels, and fluid dynamics (Bhat et al., 2021; Du et al., 2024). Recent investigations have highlighted the crucial role of stromal cells in supplying tumor cells with intermediate metabolites, nutrients, hormones, cytokines/chemokines, and growth factors, all of which support tumor proliferation, invasion, metastasis, and survival, thus underscoring the need for a comprehensive understanding of the TME in HNC. Moreover, stromal cells facilitate the recruitment of CAFs and immune cells that promote tumor growth while aiding in immune evasion, thus fostering an immunosuppressive microenvironment for tumor progression, metastasis, and resistance to therapy (Bilotta et al., 2022; Castells et al., 2012; Elmusrati et al., 2021; Hanahan, 2022; Wang et al., 2021). Hence, understanding the TME in HNC is crucial due to its significant influence on tissue function and its role in driving the progression of advanced malignancies. Thus, targeting the TME is an emerging and a promising therapeutic strategy for HNC patients.

Identifying predictive factors in HNC therapy response by targeting TME is crucial for optimizing patient selection and treatment strategies. These factors may include the expression levels of specific immune checkpoint molecules, the abundance and activation state of tumor-infiltrating lymphocytes, the presence of tumor-associated macrophages and other immune cells, the degree of angiogenesis within the TME, and the levels of cytokines and chemokines known to modulate immune responses (Kotoula et al., 2016; Martinez & Gordon, 2014; Wondergem et al., 2020). Likewise, biomarkers including PD-1/PD-L1 expression, tumor mutational burden (TMB), and immune cell infiltration, hold potential for predicting response to immune checkpoint inhibitors (ICIs). Unfortunately, the inability to accurately predict the success of ICI therapy for individual patients remains a challenge.

In recent years, growing evidence indicates that extracellular vesicles (EVs) play critical roles in tumor development and progression by regulating components in the TME (Kumar et al., 2024; Patel et al., 2022; Van Niel et al., 2018). In addition, EVs also contribute to drug resistance and hinder effective immunotherapy response by releasing various molecules thus lead to poorer clinical outcomes. It has been reported that EVs carry molecules and factors that are able to suppress the functions of immune cells in their TME (Chang et al., 2021; Reale et al., 2022). EVs have been known to modify the transcriptional landscape of recipient cells by delivering immune suppressive signals. Data from both laboratory experiments and animal studies suggest that tumor growth factor (TGF) carried by EVs originating from HNC plays a significant role in stimulating tumor growth by fostering angiogenesis within TME and aiding in immune evasion (Ludwig et al., 2022).

EV-encapsulated TGFβ1 has the capability to transform normal fibroblasts (NFs) into CAFs both in vitro and in vivo through the activation of the TGFβ-Smad signaling pathway, thereby facilitating cancer progression (Ringuette Goulet et al., 2018). Moreover, EVs carry immunosuppressive molecules such as PD-L1, TGFβ1, FasL, TRAIL, and NKG2D ligands, which make them important mediators of immune evasion and possible targets for immunotherapy (Mathew et al., 2020). According to one study, TGF-1 carried by EVs initiated the transformation of NFs by regulating fibronectin expression rather than modulating the classical TGF-Smad signaling pathway. These EVs derived from HNSCC exhibited distinct features compared to TGF-activated CAFs because they induced the upregulation of pro-inflammatory gene IL-6 and hypoxia-related genes such as *HIF1*, *PFKL*, *NF-B*, and *HK2* (Arebro et al., 2023).

Nevertheless, a comprehensive understanding of the microenvironmental interactions between EVs and their surrounding immune cells is still lacking, although recently substantial attention is being directed toward EVs and their immunomodulatory effects to identify predictive factors for therapeutic responses. Collectively, understanding the therapeutic implications and predictive factors in targeting TME in HNSCC is essential for developing personalized treatment strategies that maximize efficacy and improve patient outcomes. Further research is needed to validate predictive biomarkers, identify novel therapeutic targets, and overcome resistance mechanisms to enhance the effectiveness of TME-based therapies in HNSCC. The TME in HNCs is complex, and understanding it is key because it may be exacerbated by racial disparities in immunological responses.

13.4 Disparities and Other Factors

The pattern of HNC racial disparities is similar in developed countries and in low- and middle-income countries (LMICs). This HNC racial disparity can be attributed to inequitable socioeconomic status and inaccessibility to healthcare. These disparities are also associated with the social determinants of health, such as higher population density, lifestyle factors, pollution, nutrition, and the built environment within communities with lower income and education levels (Figure 13.3) (Whitehead et al., 2024). The biological, genetic, and immunological differences between races also lead to HNC disparities. These factors, unfortunately, may lead to differential patterns in treatment response. Genetic polymorphisms are also reported to contribute to HNC racial disparities. For example, Whitehead et al. (2024) revealed that in HNC the African DNA

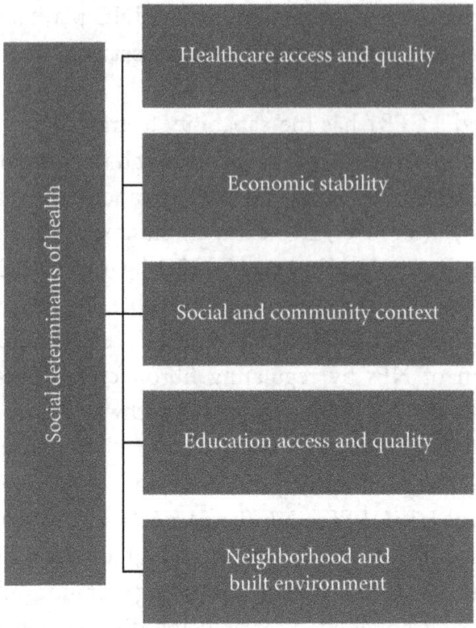

Figure 13.3 Social determinants of health contributing to head and neck cancer (HNC) racial disparities. Various social determinants of health lead to disparities in HNC patient care and outcomes.

polymerase β (POLB) gene is overexpressed, and the gene alleles promote resistance to cisplatin compared to the white ancestry alleles. POLB is involved in DNA repair. A correlation between POLB expression and poorer HNC overall survival was also reported (Ramakodi et al., 2017).

In addition to germline differences, somatic changes were also reported to contribute to HNC racial disparities. These included mutations in tumor suppressor genes, transcription factors, and cancer signaling pathways. Furthermore, genes involved in immune response, such as antigen-presenting regulation and T-cell activation, were found to be enriched in patients of African origin (Liu et al., 2023). The biological, genetic, social deterministic, and other extrinsic factors all contribute to HNC racial disparities. Biomarker discovery and predictive modeling for HNCs will be impactful when addressing and integrating solutions to addressing these disparities.

13.5 Challenges and Limitations

Cancer biomarkers and predictive modeling are at the forefront of precision medicine, but there is a current lack of such markers and modeling in HNC.

HNC is highly heterogenous and therefore requires specific biomarkers and predictive factors. Thus, employing a panel of biomarkers instead of using one may aid to overcome this challenge. HNC racial disparities due to genetic and nongenetic factors also contribute to the challenge of HNC biomarker clinical utility and predictive factors application. Developing and validating biomarkers and predictive modeling across different races may be beneficial to all HNC patients. Additionally, the inability to accurately predict the success of ICI therapy for individual patients remains a challenge, particularly considering the racial disparities in immune response observed in the HNCs. The lack of large and inclusive HNC datasets also impedes the identification of reliable HNC biomarkers and predictive values. Even when biomarkers are available, their lack of HNC sensitivity and specificity poses as a challenge. The independence of clinicopathological features and sample type, breaking beyond racial disparities will permit reproducibility and this is key in biomarker HNC application and predictive modeling. Often these limiting factors necessitate resources that are beyond the reach of initial preclinical studies. However, augmenting these resources with AI tools has the potential to yield impactful outcomes.

13.6 Conclusion

HNC patients have a poor prognosis despite therapeutic advances. This is partly due to the lack of reliable diagnostic and prognostic biomarkers. The lack of predictive modeling is also a problem, and racial disparities in HNC aggravate this public health problem. These disparities are driven by genetic and nongenetic factors, and addressing the social determinants of health potentially holds the key to unlocking these disparities. Biological and immunological factors have also been identified to play a role and could potentially be targeted for biomarker and therapeutic purposes. For instance, immune-related biomarkers in the HNC TME hold prognostic and predictive values. However, challenges associated with the clinical utility of these biomarkers exists and need to be overcome.

The precision oncology approach in HNC is fundamental to providing optimum solutions for non-white HNC patients who seem to bear the brunt of this disease due to both genetic predispositions and nongenetic external factors. Disparities in HNC biomarkers, predictive factors, and predictive modeling pose a real challenge. Overcoming these barriers will improve the impact of these tools in refining their clinical applications and improving HNC patient outcome, irrespective of race and socioeconomic status. Proper application of AI tools may aid in overcoming these challenges (Figure 13.4).

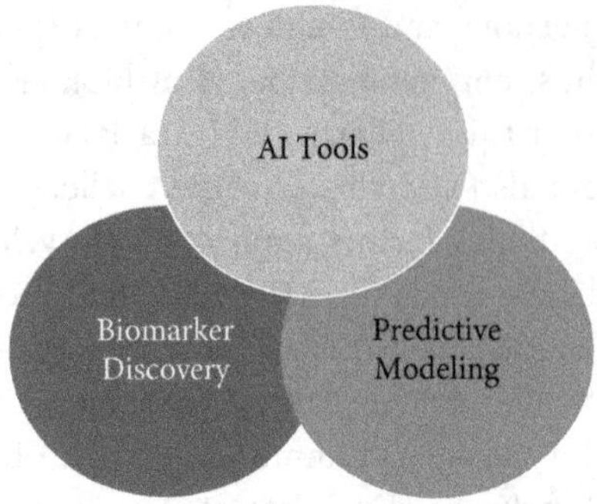

Figure 13.4 Artificial intelligence (AI). AI integrated approaches toward head and neck cancer (HNC) clinical utility of biomarkers and predictive modeling.

References

ADAM, J., LOUVET, E., SOURISSEAU, T., DORVAULT, N., BERNARD, M., MAINGOT, E., FAIVRE, L., CASSIN-KUO, M.-S., BOISSIER, E. & DESSOLIERS, M.-C. 2018. TPF induction chemotherapy increases PD-L1 expression in tumour cells and immune cells in head and neck squamous cell carcinoma. *ESMO Open*, 3, e000257.

ADILBAY, D., ADILBAYEV, G., KIDIRBAYEVA, G., SHIPILOVA, V., SADYK, Z., KOYANBEKOVA, G., SOKOLENKO, E., & KLOZAR, J. 2018. HPV infection and P16 expression in oral and oropharyngeal cancer in Kazakhstan. *Infect Agent Cancer*, 13, 2.

AGRAWAL, N., FREDERICK, M. J., PICKERING, C. R., BETTEGOWDA, C., CHANG, K., LI, R. J., FAKHRY, C., XIE, T. X., ZHANG, J., WANG, J., ZHANG, N., EL-NAGGAR, A. K., JASSER, S. A., WEINSTEIN, J. N., TREVIÑO, L., DRUMMOND, J. A., MUZNY, D. M., WU, Y., WOOD, L. D., HRUBAN, R. H., WESTRA, W. H., KOCH, W. M., CALIFANO, J. A., GIBBS, R. A., SIDRANSKY, D., VOGELSTEIN, B., VELCULESCU, V. E., PAPADOPOULOS, N., WHEELER, D. A., KINZLER, K. W., & MYERS, J. N. 2011. Exome sequencing of head and neck squamous cell carcinoma reveals inactivating mutations in NOTCH1. *Science*, 333, 1154–7.

ANG, K. K., HARRIS, J., WHEELER, R., WEBER, R., ROSENTHAL, D. I., NGUYEN-TÂN, P. F., WESTRA, W. H., CHUNG, C. H., JORDAN, R. C., LU, C., KIM, H., AXELROD, R., SILVERMAN, C. C., REDMOND, K. P., & GILLISON, M. L. 2010. Human papillomavirus and survival of patients with oropharyngeal cancer. *N Engl J Med*, 363, 24–35.

AREBRO, J., TOWLE, R., LEE, C.-M., BENNEWITH, K. L., & GARNIS, C. 2023. Extracellular vesicles promote activation of pro-inflammatory cancer-associated fibroblasts in oral cancer. *Front Cell Developm Biol*, 11, 1240159.

BANG, C., BERNARD, G., LE, W. T., LALONDE, A., KADOURY, S., & BAHIG, H. 2023. Artificial intelligence to predict outcomes of head and neck radiotherapy. *Clin Transl Radiat Oncol*, 39, 100590.

BASHEETH, N., & PATIL, N. 2019. Biomarkers in head and neck cancer: An update. *Indian J Otolaryngol Head Neck Surg*, 71, 1002–11.

BEGUM, S., CAO, D., GILLISON, M., ZAHURAK, M., & WESTRA, W. H. 2005. Tissue distribution of human papillomavirus 16 DNA integration in patients with tonsillar carcinoma. *Clin Cancer Res*, 11, 5694–9.

BEJNORDI, B. E., VETA, M., VAN DIEST, P. J., VAN GINNEKEN, B., KARSSEMEIJER, N., LITJENS, G., VAN DER LAAK, J. A., HERMSEN, M., MANSON, Q. F., & BALKENHOL,

M. 2017. Diagnostic assessment of deep learning algorithms for detection of lymph node metastases in women with breast cancer. *JAMA*, 318, 2199–210.

BHAT, A. A., YOUSUF, P., WANI, N. A., RIZWAN, A., CHAUHAN, S. S., SIDDIQI, M. A., BEDOGNETTI, D., EL-RIFAI, W., FRENNEAUX, M. P., & BATRA, S. K. 2021. Tumor microenvironment: An evil nexus promoting aggressive head and neck squamous cell carcinoma and avenue for targeted therapy. *Signal Transduct Targeted Therap*, 6, 12.

BILOTTA, M. T., ANTIGNANI, A., & FITZGERALD, D. J. 2022. Managing the TME to improve the efficacy of cancer therapy. *Front Immunol*, 13, 954992.

BOURHIS, J., TAO, Y. G., ZHANG, P., & DEUTSCH, E. 2007. [Epidermal growth factor receptor (EGF) in head-and-neck cancers]. *Bull Cancer*, 94, F189–91.

BRIANTI, P., DE FLAMMINEIS, E., & MERCURI, S. R. 2017. Review of HPV-related diseases and cancers. *New Microbiol*, 40, 80–5.

BUDHATHOKI, S., DIERGAARDE, B., LIU, G., OLSHAN, A., NESS, A., WATERBOER, T., VIRANI, S., BASTA, P., BENDER, N., & BRENNER, N. 2023. A risk prediction model for head and neck cancers incorporating lifestyle factors, HPV serology and genetic markers. *Int J Cancer*, 152, 2069–80.

CALIFF, R. M. 2018. Biomarker definitions and their applications. *Exp Biol Med (Maywood)*, 243, 213–21.

CASTELLS, M., THIBAULT, B., DELORD, J.-P., & COUDERC, B. 2012. Implication of tumor microenvironment in chemoresistance: Tumor-associated stromal cells protect tumor cells from cell death. *Int J Mol Sci*, 13, 9545–71.

CHANG, W.-H., CERIONE, R. A., & ANTONYAK, M. A. 2021. Extracellular vesicles and their roles in cancer progression. *Cancer Cell Signal Methods Protocols*, 2174, 143–70.

CHEN, S. M., KRINSKY, A. L., WOOLAVER, R. A., WANG, X., CHEN, Z., & WANG, J. H. 2020. Tumor immune microenvironment in head and neck cancers. *Mol Carcinogenesis*, 59, 766–74.

CHINNERY, T., ARIFIN, A., TAY, K. Y., LEUNG, A., NICHOLS, A. C., PALMA, D. A., MATTONEN, S. A., & LANG, P. 2021. Utilizing artificial intelligence for head and neck cancer outcomes prediction from imaging. *Can Assoc Radiol J*, 72, 73–85.

CORREDOR, G., WANG, X., ZHOU, Y., LU, C., FU, P., SYRIGOS, K., RIMM, D. L., YANG, M., ROMERO, E., & SCHALPER, K. A. 2019. Spatial architecture and arrangement of tumor-infiltrating lymphocytes for predicting likelihood of recurrence in early-stage non-small cell lung cancer. *Clin Cancer Res*, 25, 1526–34.

CRISTINA, V., HERRERA-GÓMEZ, R. G., SZTURZ, P., ESPELI, V., & SIANO, M. 2019. Immunotherapies and future combination strategies for head and neck squamous cell carcinoma. *Int J Mol Sci*, 20, 5399.

DENEKA, A. Y., LIU, J. C., & RAGIN, C. C. 2018. Biology and epidemiology of human papillomavirus-related head and neck cancer. *Mol Determinants Head Neck Cancer*, 545–83.

DERMANI, F. K., SAMADI, P., RAHMANI, G., KOHLAN, A. K., & NAJAFI, R. 2019. PD-1/PD-L1 immune checkpoint: Potential target for cancer therapy. *J Cell Physiol*, 234, 1313–25.

DEVERAUX, Q. L., SCHENDEL, S. L., & REED, J. C. 2001. Antiapoptotic proteins: The bcl-2 and inhibitor of apoptosis protein families. *Cardiol Clin*, 19, 57–74.

DIVE, A. M., BODHADE, A. S., MISHRA, M. S., & UPADHYAYA, N. 2014. Histological patterns of head and neck tumors: An insight to tumor histology. *J Oral Maxillofac Pathol*, 18, 58–68.

DU, E., MAZUL, A. L., FARQUHAR, D., BRENNAN, P., ANANTHARAMAN, D., ABEDI-ARDEKANI, B., WEISSLER, M. C., HAYES, D. N., OLSHAN, A. F., & ZEVALLOS, J. P. 2019. Long-term survival in head and neck cancer: Impact of site, stage, smoking, and human papillomavirus status. *Laryngoscope*, 129, 2506–13.

DU, W., XIA, X., HU, F., & YU, J. 2024. Extracellular matrix remodeling in the tumor immunity. *Front Immunol*, 14, 1340634.

EBERLY, H. W., SCISCENT, B. Y., LORENZ, F. J., RETTIG, E. M., & GOYAL, N. 2024. Current and emerging diagnostic, prognostic, and predictive biomarkers in head and neck cancer. *Biomedicines*, 12, 415.

EID, R. A., & LANDINI, G. 2003. Quantification of the global and local complexity of the epithelial-connective tissue interface of normal, dysplastic, and neoplastic oral mucosae using digital imaging. *Pathol Res Pract*, 199, 475.

EL-MAHDY, H. A., MOHAMADIN, A. M., ABULSOUD, A. I., KHIDR, E. G., EL-HUSSEINY, A. A., ISMAIL, A., ELSAKKA, E. G. E., MOKHLIS, H. A., EL-HUSSEINY, H. M., & DOGHISH, A. S. 2023. miRNAs as potential game-changers in head and neck cancer: Future clinical and medicinal uses. *Pathol Res Pract*, 245, 154457.

ELMUSRATI, A., WANG, J., & WANG, C.-Y. 2021. Tumor microenvironment and immune evasion in head and neck squamous cell carcinoma. *Int J Oral Sci*, 13, 24.

FURUUCHI, K., BEREZOV, A., KUMAGAI, T., & GREENE, M. I. 2007. Targeted antireceptor therapy with monoclonal antibodies leads to the formation of inactivated tetrameric forms of ErbB receptors. *J Immunol*, 178, 1021–9.

GILLISON, M. L., KOCH, W. M., CAPONE, R. B., SPAFFORD, M., WESTRA, W. H., WU, L., ZAHURAK, M. L., DANIEL, R. W., VIGLIONE, M., & SYMER, D. E. 2000. Evidence for a causal association between human papillomavirus and a subset of head and neck cancers. *J Nat Cancer Instit*, 92, 709–20.

GIRAUD, P., GIRAUD, P., GASNIER, A., EL AYACHY, R., KREPS, S., FOY, J.-P., DURDUX, C., HUGUET, F., BURGUN, A., & BIBAULT, J.-E. 2019. Radiomics and machine learning for radiotherapy in head and neck cancers. *Front Oncol*, 9, 174.

GORMLEY, M., CREANEY, G., SCHACHE, A., INGARFIELD, K., & CONWAY, D. I. 2022. Reviewing the epidemiology of head and neck cancer: Definitions, trends and risk factors. *Br Dent J*, 233, 780–6.

HANAHAN, D. 2022. Hallmarks of cancer: New dimensions. *Cancer Disc*, 12, 31–46.

HIBBERT, J., HALEC, G., BAAKEN, D., WATERBOER, T., & BRENNER, N. 2021. Sensitivity and specificity of human papillomavirus (HPV) 16 early antigen serology for HPV-driven oropharyngeal cancer: A systematic literature review and meta-analysis. *Cancers*, 13, 3010.

HIJAZI, A., BIFULCO, C., BALDIN, P., & GALON, J. 2024. Digital pathology for better clinical practice. *Cancers*, 16, 1686.

HUANG, S. H., & O'SULLIVAN, B. 2013. Oral cancer: Current role of radiotherapy and chemotherapy. *Med Oral Patol Oral Cir Bucal*, 18, e233–40.

INTERNATIONAL AGENCY FOR RESEARCH ON CANCER. 1988. *IARC Monographs on the Evaluation of Carcinogenic Risks to Humans*. Geneva: International Agency for Research on Cancer, World Health Organization.

IWASAKI, M., BUDHATHOKI, S., YAMAJI, T., TANAKA-MIZUNO, S., KUCHIBA, A., SAWADA, N., GOTO, A., SHIMAZU, T., INOUE, M., & TSUGANE, S. 2020. Inclusion of a gene-environment interaction between alcohol consumption and the aldehyde dehydrogenase 2 genotype in a risk prediction model for upper aerodigestive tract cancer in Japanese men. *Cancer Sci*, 111, 3835–44.

JOHNSON, D. E., BURTNESS, B., LEEMANS, C. R., LUI, V. W. Y., BAUMAN, J. E., & GRANDIS, J. R. 2020. Head and neck squamous cell carcinoma. *Nat Rev Dis Primers*, 6, 92.

JUMANIYAZOVA, E., LOKHONINA, A., DZHALILOVA, D., KOSYREVA, A., & FATKHUDINOV, T. 2023. Role of microenvironmental components in head and neck squamous cell carcinoma. *J Personalized Medi*, 13, 1616.

KAIKKONEN, M. U., LAM, M. T., & GLASS, C. K. 2011. Non-coding RNAs as regulators of gene expression and epigenetics. *Cardiovasc Res*, 90, 430–40.

KALYANKRISHNA, S., & GRANDIS, J. R. 2006. Epidermal growth factor receptor biology in head and neck cancer. *J Clin Oncol*, 24, 2666–72.

KANEKO, T., SUEFUJI, H., KOTO, M., DEMIZU, Y., SAITOH, J. I., TSUJI, H., OKIMOTO, T., OHNO, T., SHIOYAMA, Y., NEMOTO, K., NAKANO, T., & KAMADA, T. 2021.

Multicenter study of carbon-ion radiotherapy for oropharyngeal non-squamous cell carcinoma. *In Vivo*, 35, 2239–45.

KOTOULA, V., CHATZOPOULOS, K., LAKIS, S., ALEXOPOULOU, Z., TIMOTHEADOU, E., ZAGOURI, F., PENTHEROUDAKIS, G., GOGAS, H., GALANI, E., & EFSTRATIOU, I. 2016. Tumors with high-density tumor infiltrating lymphocytes constitute a favorable entity in breast cancer: A pooled analysis of four prospective adjuvant trials. *Oncotarget*, 7, 5074.

KOUROU, K., EXARCHOS, T. P., EXARCHOS, K. P., KARAMOUZIS, M. V., & FOTIADIS, D. I. 2015. Machine learning applications in cancer prognosis and prediction. *Comput Struct Biotechnol J*, 13, 8–17.

KOYANAGI, Y. N., ITO, H., OZE, I., HOSONO, S., TANAKA, H., ABE, T., SHIMIZU, Y., HASEGAWA, Y., & MATSUO, K. 2017. Development of a prediction model and estimation of cumulative risk for upper aerodigestive tract cancer on the basis of the aldehyde dehydrogenase 2 genotype and alcohol consumption in a Japanese population. *Eur J Cancer Prevent*, 26, 38–47.

KREIMER, A. R., FERREIRO-IGLESIAS, A., NYGARD, M., BENDER, N., SCHROEDER, L., HILDESHEIM, A., ROBBINS, H. A., PAWLITA, M., LANGSETH, H., & SCHLECHT, N. F. 2019. Timing of HPV16-E6 antibody seroconversion before OPSCC: Findings from the HPVC3 consortium. *Ann Oncol*, 30, 1335–43.

KREIMER, A. R., JOHANSSON, M., WATERBOER, T., KAAKS, R., CHANG-CLAUDE, J., DROGEN, D., TJØNNELAND, A., OVERVAD, K., QUIRÓS, J. R., & GONZÁLEZ, C. A. 2013. Evaluation of human papillomavirus antibodies and risk of subsequent head and neck cancer. *J Clin Oncol*, 31, 2708.

KREIMER, A. R., JOHANSSON, M., YANIK, E. L., KATKI, H. A., CHECK, D. P., LANG KUHS, K. A., WILLHAUCK-FLECKENSTEIN, M., HOLZINGER, D., HILDESHEIM, A., & PFEIFFER, R. 2017. Kinetics of the human papillomavirus type 16 E6 antibody response prior to oropharyngeal cancer. *JNCI*, 109, djx005.

KREIMER, A. R., SHIELS, M. S., FAKHRY, C., JOHANSSON, M., PAWLITA, M., BRENNAN, P., HILDESHEIM, A., & WATERBOER, T. 2018. Screening for human papillomavirus-driven oropharyngeal cancer: Considerations for feasibility and strategies for research. *Cancer*, 124, 1859–66.

KUMAR, M. A., BABA, S. K., SADIDA, H. Q., MARZOOQI, S. A., JEROBIN, J., ALTEMANI, F. H., ALGEHAINY, N., ALANAZI, M. A., ABOU-SAMRA, A.-B., & KUMAR, R. 2024. Extracellular vesicles as tools and targets in therapy for diseases. *Signal Transduct Targeted Ther*, 9, 27.

LAMBIN, P., ROELOFS, E., REYMEN, B., VELAZQUEZ, E. R., BUIJSEN, J., ZEGERS, C. M., CARVALHO, S., LEIJENAAR, R. T., NALBANTOV, G., & OBERIJE, C. 2013. Rapid Learning health care in oncology: An approach towards decision support systems enabling customised radiotherapy. *Radiother Oncol*, 109, 159–64.

LEE, Y.-C. A., AL-TEMIMI, M., YING, J., MUSCAT, J., OLSHAN, A. F., ZEVALLOS, J. P., WINN, D. M., LI, G., STURGIS, E. M., & MORGENSTERN, H. 2020. Risk prediction models for head and neck cancer in the US population from the INHANCE consortium. *Am J Epidemiol*, 189, 330–42.

LEEMANS, C. R., BRAAKHUIS, B. J., & BRAKENHOFF, R. H. 2011. The molecular biology of head and neck cancer. *Nat Rev Cancer*, 11, 9–22.

LIM, Y. X., & D'SILVA, N. J. 2024. HPV-associated oropharyngeal cancer: In search of surrogate biomarkers for early lesions. *Oncogene*, 43, 543–54.

LIU, Y., KRAMER, J. R., SANDULACHE, V. C., YU, R., LI, G., CHEN, L., YUSUF, Z. I., SHI, Y., PYARAJAN, S., & TSAVACHIDIS, S. 2023. Immunogenetic determinants of susceptibility to head and neck cancer in the Million Veteran Program cohort. *Cancer Res*, 83, 386–97.

LUDWIG, N., YERNENI, S. S., AZAMBUJA, J. H., PIETROWSKA, M., WIDŁAK, P., HINCK, C. S., GŁUSZKO, A., SZCZEPAŃSKI, M. J., KÄRMER, T., & KALLINGER, I. 2022. TGFβ+

small extracellular vesicles from head and neck squamous cell carcinoma cells reprogram macrophages towards a pro-angiogenic phenotype. *J Extracell Vesicles*, 11, 12294.

LUTZKY, V. P., MOSS, D. J., CHIN, D., COMAN, W. B., PARSONS, P. G., & BOYLE, G. M. 2008. Biomarkers for cancers of the head and neck. *Clin Med Ear Nose Throat*, 1, CMENT. S1051.

MAHMOOD, H., SHABAN, M., INDAVE, B., SANTOS-SILVA, A., RAJPOOT, N., & KHURRAM, S. 2020. Use of artificial intelligence in diagnosis of head and neck precancerous and cancerous lesions: A systematic review. *Oral Oncol*, 110, 104885.

MARCUS, M. W., CHEN, Y., RAJI, O. Y., DUFFY, S. W., & FIELD, J. K. 2015. LLPi: Liverpool lung project risk prediction model for lung cancer incidence. *Cancer Prevent Res*, 8, 570–5.

MARTINEZ, F. O., & GORDON, S. 2014. The M1 and M2 paradigm of macrophage activation: Time for reassessment. *F1000prime Rep*, 6, 13.

MASTERSON, L., MOUALED, D., LIU, Z. W., HOWARD, J. E., DWIVEDI, R. C., TYSOME, J. R., BENSON, R., STERLING, J. C., SUDHOFF, H., JANI, P., & GOON, P. K. 2014. De-escalation treatment protocols for human papillomavirus-associated oropharyngeal squamous cell carcinoma: A systematic review and meta-analysis of current clinical trials. *Eur J Cancer*, 50, 2636–48.

MATHEW, M., ZADE, M., MEZGHANI, N., PATEL, R., WANG, Y., & MOMEN-HERAVI, F. 2020. Extracellular vesicles as biomarkers in cancer immunotherapy. *Cancers*, 12, 2825.

MCCARTHY, C. E., BONNET, L. J., MARCUS, M. W., & FIELD, J. K. 2020. Development and validation of a multivariable risk prediction model for head and neck cancer using the UK Biobank. *Int J Oncol*, 57, 1192–202.

MONTALTO, F. I., & DE AMICIS, F. 2020a. Cyclin D1 in cancer: A molecular connection for cell cycle control, adhesion and invasion in tumor and stroma. *Cells*, 9, 2648.

MONTALTO, F. I., & DE AMICIS, F. 2020b. Cyclin D1 in cancer: A molecular connection for cell cycle control, adhesion and invasion in tumor and stroma. *Cells*, 9(12), 2648.

MORRIS, L. G., CHANDRAMOHAN, R., WEST, L., ZEHIR, A., CHAKRAVARTY, D., PFISTER, D. G., WONG, R. J., LEE, N. Y., SHERMAN, E. J., & BAXI, S. S. 2017. The molecular landscape of recurrent and metastatic head and neck cancers: Insights from a precision oncology sequencing platform. *JAMA Oncol*, 3, 244–55.

NAGADIA, R., PANDIT, P., COMAN, W. B., COOPER-WHITE, J., & PUNYADEERA, C. 2013. miRNAs in head and neck cancer revisited. *Cell Oncol (Dordr)*, 36, 1–7.

NAVA-VILLALBA, M., ARANDA-ROMO, S., & MEZA-GARCÍA, G. 2014. p16INK4 as a biomarker in oropharyngeal squamous cell carcinoma. *Recent Patents on Biomarkers*, 4, 75–84.

NOGUES, J. C., FASSAS, S., MULCAHY, C., & ZAPANTA, P. E. 2021. Human papillomavirus-associated head and neck cancer. *J Am Board Fam Med*, 34, 832–37.

PARMAR, C., GROSSMANN, P., BUSSINK, J., LAMBIN, P., & AERTS, H. J. 2015. Machine learning methods for quantitative radiomic biomarkers. *Sci Rep*, 5, 1–11.

PATEL, A., PATEL, S., PATEL, P., & TANAVDE, V. 2022. Saliva based liquid biopsies in head and neck cancer: how far are we from the clinic? *Front Oncol*, 12, 828434.

PELTANOVA, B., RAUDENSKA, M., & MASARIK, M. 2019. Effect of tumor microenvironment on pathogenesis of the head and neck squamous cell carcinoma: A systematic review. *Mol Cancer*, 18, 63.

PFEIFFER, R. M., PARK, Y., KREIMER, A. R., LACEY JR, J. V., PEE, D., GREENLEE, R. T., BUYS, S. S., HOLLENBECK, A., ROSNER, B., & GAIL, M. H. 2013. Risk prediction for breast, endometrial, and ovarian cancer in white women aged 50 y or older: derivation and validation from population-based cohort studies. *PLoS Med*, 10, e1001492.

QIN, Y., ZHENG, X., GAO, W., WANG, B., & WU, Y. 2021. Tumor microenvironment and immune-related therapies of head and neck squamous cell carcinoma. *Mol Ther Oncolytics*, 20, 342–51.

RAMAKODI, M. P., DEVARAJAN, K., BLACKMAN, E., GIBBS, D., LUCE, D., DELOUMEAUX, J., DUFLO, S., LIU, J. C., MEHRA, R., & KULATHINAL, R. J. 2017. Integrative genomic analysis identifies ancestry-related expression quantitative trait loci on

DNA polymerase β and supports the association of genetic ancestry with survival disparities in head and neck squamous cell carcinoma. *Cancer*, 123, 849–60.

REALE, A., KHONG, T., & SPENCER, A. 2022. Extracellular vesicles and their roles in the tumor immune microenvironment. *J Clin Med*, 11, 6892.

RINGUETTE GOULET, C., BERNARD, G., TREMBLAY, S., CHABAUD, S., BOLDUC, S., & POULIOT, F. 2018. Exosomes induce fibroblast differentiation into cancer-associated fibroblasts through TGFβ signaling. *Mol Cancer Res*, 16, 1196–204.

RIVERA, C. 2015. Essentials of oral cancer. *Int J Clin Exp Pathol*, 8, 11884–94.

SCHAAIJ-VISSER, T. B., BRAKENHOFF, R. H., LEEMANS, C. R., HECK, A. J., & SLIJPER, M. 2010. Protein biomarker discovery for head and neck cancer. *J Proteomics*, 73, 1790–803.

SCOTT-WITTENBORN, N., & FAKHRY, C. 2021. Epidemiology of HPV related malignancies. *Semin Radiat Oncol*, 31, 286–96.

SEIWERT, T. Y., ZUO, Z., KECK, M. K., KHATTRI, A., PEDAMALLU, C. S., STRICKER, T., BROWN, C., PUGH, T. J., STOJANOV, P., CHO, J., LAWRENCE, M. S., GETZ, G., BRÄGELMANN, J., DEBOER, R., WEICHSELBAUM, R. R., LANGERMAN, A., PORTUGAL, L., BLAIR, E., STENSON, K., LINGEN, M. W., COHEN, E. E., VOKES, E. E., WHITE, K. P., & HAMMERMAN, P. S. 2015. Integrative and comparative genomic analysis of HPV-positive and HPV-negative head and neck squamous cell carcinomas. *Clin Cancer Res*, 21, 632–41.

SEPIASHVILI, L., HUI, A., IGNATCHENKO, V., SHI, W., SU, S., XU, W., HUANG, S. H., O'SULLIVAN, B., WALDRON, J., & IRISH, J. C. 2012. Potentially novel candidate biomarkers for head and neck squamous cell carcinoma identified using an integrated cell line-based discovery strategy. *Mol Cell Proteomics*, 11, 1404–15.

SHERRATT, F. C., MARCUS, M. W., ROBINSON, J., & FIELD, J. K. 2018. Utilizing lung Cancer risk prediction models to promote smoking cessation: Two randomized controlled trials. *Am J Health Promot*, 32, 1196–205.

STRAETMANS, J. M., OLTHOF, N., MOOREN, J. J., DE JONG, J., SPEEL, E. J., & KREMER, B. 2009. Human papillomavirus reduces the prognostic value of nodal involvement in tonsillar squamous cell carcinomas. *Laryngoscope*, 119, 1951–7.

SYRJANEN, J., MICHALSKI, K., KAWATE, T., & FURUKAWA, H. 2021. On the molecular nature of large-pore channels. *J Mol Biol*, 433, 166994.

SYRJÄNEN, S. 2018. Oral manifestations of human papillomavirus infections. *Eur J Oral Sci*, 126 Suppl 1, 49–66.

TAMMEMAGI, C. M., PINSKY, P. F., CAPORASO, N. E., KVALE, P. A., HOCKING, W. G., CHURCH, T. R., RILEY, T. L., COMMINS, J., OKEN, M. M., & BERG, C. D. 2011. Lung cancer risk prediction: prostate, lung, colorectal and ovarian cancer screening trial models and validation. *J Nat Cancer Instit*, 103, 1058–68.

THOMAIDOU, A. C., BATSAKI, P., ADAMAKI, M., GOULIELMAKI, M., BAXEVANIS, C. N., ZOUMPOURLIS, V., & FORTIS, S. P. 2022. Promising biomarkers in head and neck cancer: The most clinically important miRNAs. *Int J Mol Sci*, 23(15), 8257.

TUMBAN, E. 2019. A current update on human papillomavirus-associated head and neck cancers. *Viruses*, 11(10), 922.

VAN NIEL, G., D'ANGELO, G., & RAPOSO, G. 2018. Shedding light on the cell biology of extracellular vesicles. *Nat Rev Mol Cell Biol*, 19, 213–28.

WANG, G., ZHANG, M., CHENG, M., WANG, X., LI, K., CHEN, J., CHEN, Z., CHEN, S., CHEN, J., & XIONG, G. 2021. Tumor microenvironment in head and neck squamous cell carcinoma: Functions and regulatory mechanisms. *Cancer Lett*, 507, 55–69.

WARNAKULASURIYA, S. 2009. Global epidemiology of oral and oropharyngeal cancer. *Oral Oncol*, 45, 309–16.

WENZEL, E. S., & SINGH, A. T. K. 2018. Cell-cycle checkpoints and aneuploidy on the path to cancer. *In Vivo*, 32, 1–5.

WHITEHEAD, R. A., PATEL, E. A., LIU, J. C., & BHAYANI, M. K. 2024. Racial disparities in head and neck cancer: It's not just about access. *Otolaryngol Head Neck Surg*, 170(4), 1032–44.

WONDERGEM, N. E., NAUTA, I. H., MUIJLWIJK, T., LEEMANS, C. R., & VAN DE VEN, R. 2020. The immune microenvironment in head and neck squamous cell carcinoma: On subsets and subsites. *Curr Oncol Rep*, 22, 1–14.

WU, T., & DAI, Y. 2017. Tumor microenvironment and therapeutic response. *Cancer Lett*, 387, 61–8.

YANG, G. D., WANG, Z. C., CHEN, Q. Y., ZHANG, H. L., LIN, X. G., HUANG, T. J., QIAN, C. N., & HUANG, B. J. 2019. p53, latent membrane protein 1, bcl-2, and prognosis in nasopharyngeal carcinoma: A meta-analysis. *Histol Histopathol*, 34, 103–10.

ZHANG, Q., LUO, S., LUO, Y., HUANG, Y., WANG, Z., & XIE, X. 2023. Upregulation of KHDC1L promotes the proliferation and inhibits apoptosis in head and neck squamous cell carcinoma. *Epigenetics*, 18, 2175168.

14
Artificial Intelligence in Head and Neck Cancer

Rodney Hull, Shamlan K. Naidoo, Rupert C. Ecker, and Zodwa Dlamini

14.1 Introduction

Artificial intelligence (AI) describes the use of computers to emulate human intelligence through the use of algorithms. The aim is to allow computers to perform tasks that are normally performed by human beings. AI relies on machine learning (ML), the ability of computers to learn and alter these algorithms as a means to adapt to the conditions described by new data in new conditions. Finally, deep learning (DL) is a type of ML that mimics the neural networks in the human brain by using artificial neural networks (Chen et al., 2022). Despite the idea and initial work on AI occurring in 1956, and nearly two decades of subsequent research on the topic, interest waned as development stalled, leading to interest and funding in AI dropping off in the 1970s. However, with the development of increased computing power and new techniques, research was reinvigorated. This was also largely due to the use of new forms of statistical reduction. This ability to reduce data to forms that computers could analyze in a way resembling human intelligence led to AI being applied to predictive medicine (Müller & Bostrom, 2016; Nilsson, 1998). These techniques rely on using the frequencies of variables within medical data to create predictive models. Further developments led to the emergence of ML algorithms, including but not limited to random forests (RF), support vector machines (SVM), and gradient boosting (GB).

As the technologies of AI continue to develop there is increasing interest in the use of AI to analyze clinical, epidemiologic, radiomic, histologic, and genomic data. In oncology, this analysis can be applied to research, diagnosis, prognosis, and the prediction of treatment response as well as the prediction of malignant transformation of precancerous lesions. This has been applied to head and neck cancer (HNC) to improve research, screening, and prognosis (Mahmood et al., 2020; Mäkitie et al., 2023; Resteghini et al., 2018).

14.2 Machine Learning Algorithms

ML requires the use of training data for the algorithm to learn from as well as development and fine-tuning the modeling algorithm. The more training data available to the AI, the more accurate and efficient the ML algorithm (LeCun et al., 2015). Initial construction of the ML model requires that the entire data cohort be split into training data (~60%) and testing data (~40%). The performance of the ML model can be assessed using validation datasets employing the area under the receiving operator characteristic curve measure. The area under the curve (AUC) is the area on a graph representing the data analysis; it is bounded by the x axis (i.e., the function of the analysis), and vertical lines delineate the function's boundaries. Essentially it allows for the identification of the probability at which most of the data are correctly classified by a model into one of two classes (binary classification) (Narkhede, 2018).

ML algorithms use various learning models to create prediction models to both diagnose HNC and predict HNC outcomes (Figure 14.1). These can be either supervised or unsupervised learning models (Parmar et al., 2015). *Supervised learning* uses labeled data to teach the computer the relationship between the input and output data (Figure 14.2). In this way, the computer learns from data that already has been linked through specific parameters (e.g., "Samples containing these specific markers always have certain survival rates"). The algorithms then learn these relationships and how to come to conclusions

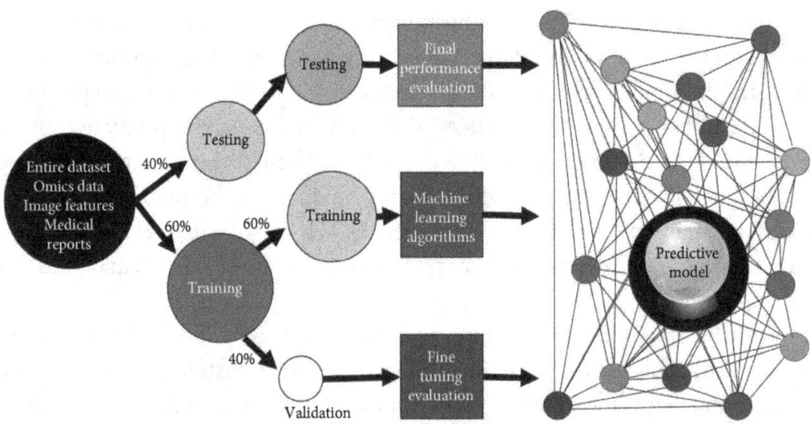

Figure 14.1 Teaching an algorithm in machine learning means creating models. Input data is split into testing and training data with about 60% of the data being used to train the model. The training data can be further divided into training and validation data. The training data are used to construct the model and the validation data are run afterward to fine-tune the model. Once the model has been taught and fine-tuned, the testing data are run on the model to confirm if the output is accurate.

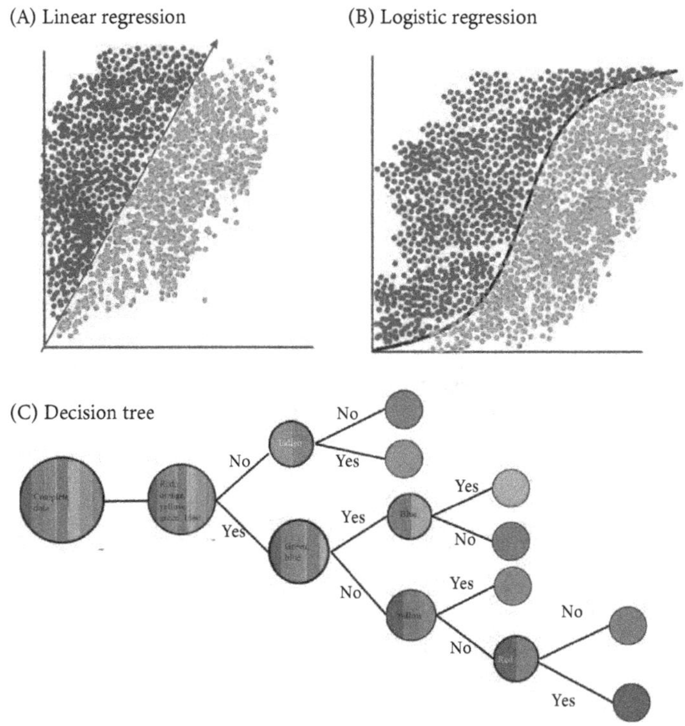

Figure 14.2 Supervised machine learning models. Supervised learning models use labeled data; these are paired data where *n* inputs are matched to an output. The algorithm then learns these associations and applies them to new data. Regression uses inputs to predict continuous numerical values by establishing a functional relationship between independent and dependent variables. Alternatively they can remain where they are since they depict regression either linear or logistic (A and B). (C) Decision trees model decisions and their possible outcomes, with each internal node representing the result of a decision as well as a subsequent question that is joined by branches representing the decision. (D) Support vector machines identify a hyperplane or boundary that maximizes the distance between different groups of data and uses this line to rank data into each separate class. (E) Bayesian networks are graphical representations showing causes and their probable effects. (F) K nearest neighbor uses a single data point and then determines the distance of that datapoint to other datapoints in various classes. The class determined to have the most members within a cutoff distance to the point then adds that point to the same class. (G) Neural networks are an artificial mathematical approximation of biological neural networks that aim to mimic the human brain. (H) Random forests use multiple decision trees that sample different subsets of the data and use different terms as questions to come to different decisions. The results of all the trees are then combined and the most common outcome is selected as the output.

(D) Support vector machines

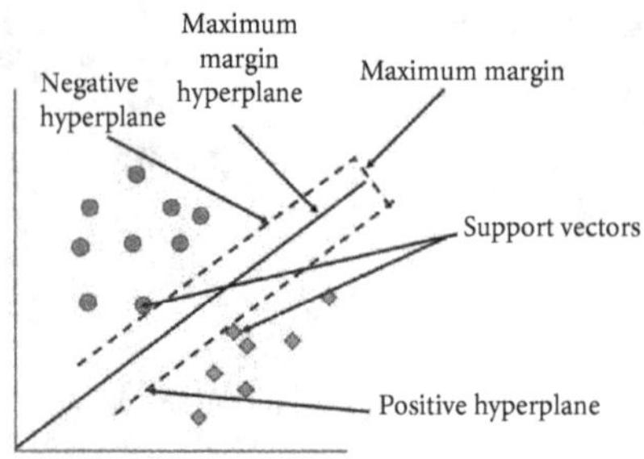

(E) K-Nearest neighbor

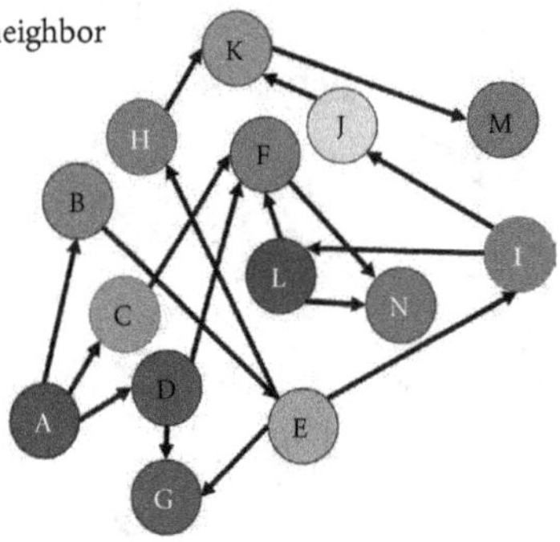

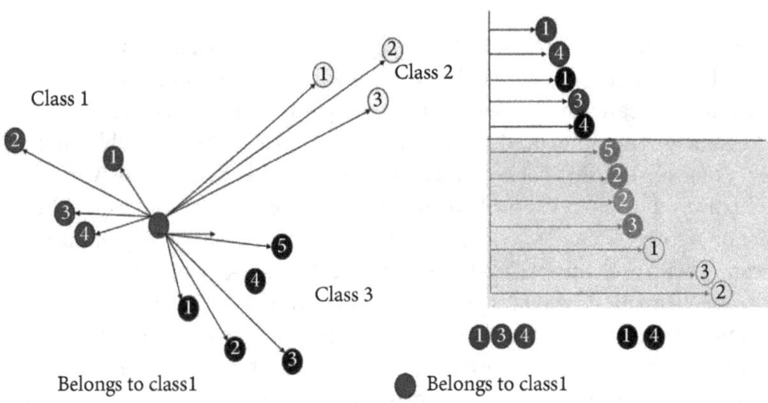

Figure 14.2 Continued

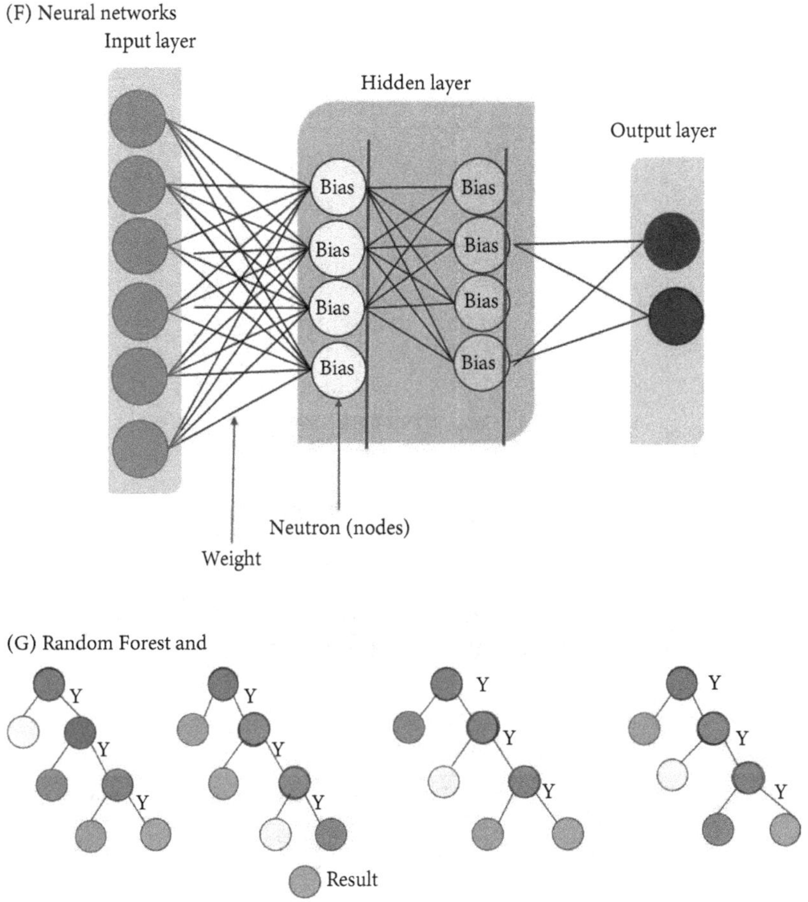

Figure 14.2 Continued

using new input data. In *unsupervised learning*, unlabeled data are given to the AI, which then identifies patterns in the data and creates its own rules to distinguish separate patterns (Figure 14.3). As it is given more data to analyze, these rules become stronger and more precise (Parmar et al., 2015).

Supervised models include linear regression, logistic regression, decision trees, support vector machines, Bayesian networks, neural networks, K nearest neighbor, and random forests (Murali et al., 2020). Linear egression estimates a linear relationship between a dependent and independent variable (Binson et al., 2024). Logistic regression establishes the relationship between an independent variable and a dependent variable that can only have two values and is used to classify data into classes (Valle et al., 2015). Decision trees can accomplish both classification and regression by splitting the data into branches based on a classification parameter. This gives rise to a tree structure (Binson et al., 2024). Support vector

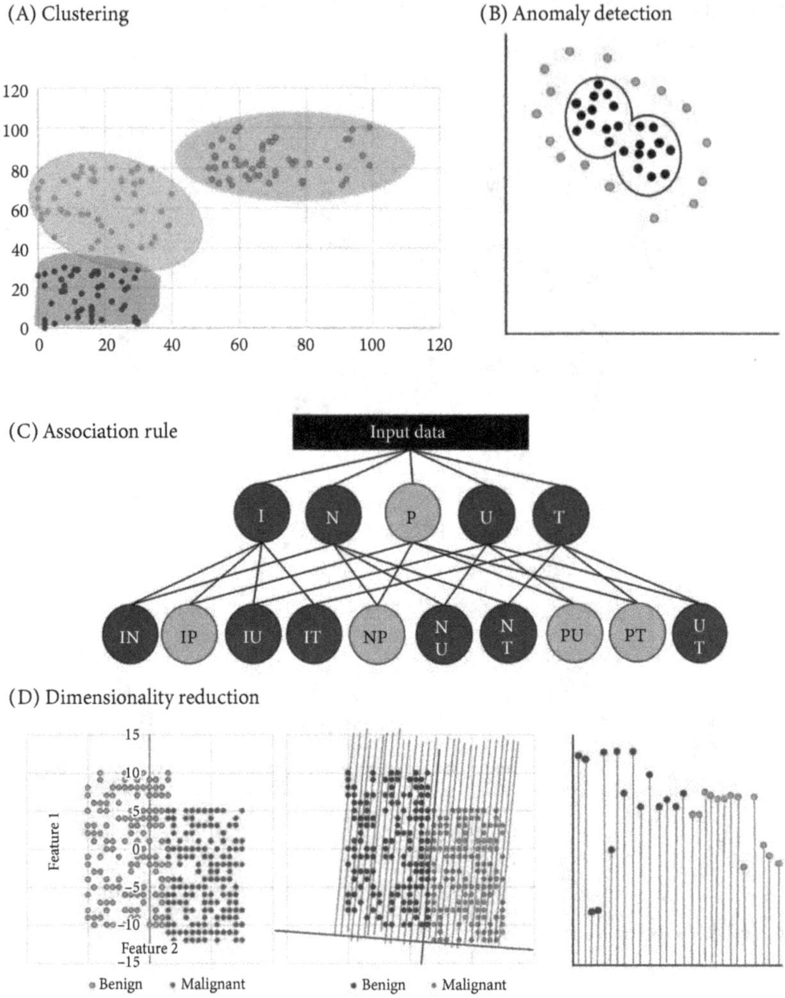

Figure 14.3 Unsupervised machine learning models. Unsupervised learning models use unlabeled data to detect patterns without the need for human intervention. They do this by learning to classify data themselves as opposed to needing labeled data that has been classified before being entered into the model. (A) Clustering groups use data based on shared characteristics or separate them based on differences. (B) Anomaly detection identifies data points that are significantly different from the rest of the dataset. (C) Association rule uses predefined rules to find associations between different data. (D) Dimensionality reduction simplifies complex data to allow machine algorithms to operate more effectively while preserving data integrity. (E) Self-organizing maps are a method of dimensionality reduction that groups observations or data of a similar value and represents them as a single data point.

(E) Self-organizing Map

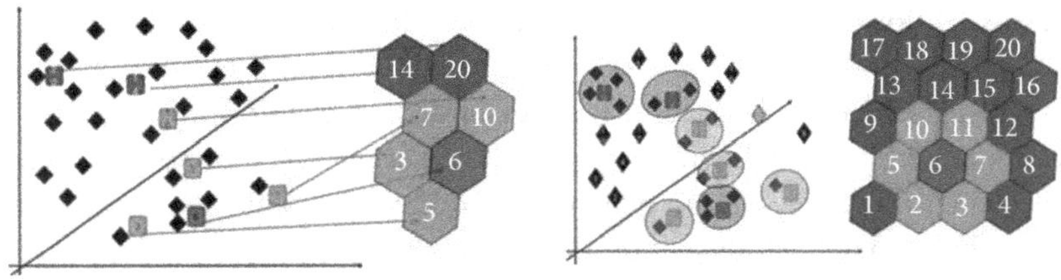

Figure 14.3 Continued

machines can classify data by establishing the best boundary between distinct classes of data. This boundary is known as the *hyperplane* (Murali et al., 2020). Bayesian networks use probability models that use graphical representations. This graphical representation of Bayesian probabilities consists of a directed acyclic graph with nodes and edges, in which the nodes represent relationships detailing cause and effect. The relationships between some of these nodes can be established based on prior knowledge, while the values of others can be inferred. This allows AI to simulate scenarios (Xue et al., 2022). Neural networks are a computer simulation of biological neural networks. The neurons in this network (nodes) are arranged into layers, and information moves from layer to layer. The data that move to the subsequent node are the output of the analysis performed by a previous node. This output is calculated by a threshold value known as the *activation function* of that node. The channels connecting the nodes of each layer are assigned a value known as the *weight*. The input data are multiplied by the weight, and this value is added to a numerical value associated with the neuron or node, known as the *bias*. If this value exceeds the activation function, then the neuron is activated and the result is passed on to the next layer (Murali et al., 2020). K-nearest network neighbors classify data based on similarities in the data using a distance function. One data point is assigned as the starting point, and the algorithm identifies points near to it using a specified distance cutoff value (Murali et al., 2020). A random forest is a collection of decision trees with each tree using a random subset of the whole data and running a different decision tree with multiple different random subsets of the data and different node criteria. Random forests reduce overfitting and bias (Gonzalez et al., 2024).

Unsupervised methods include clustering, association rule, manifold learning/dimensionality reduction, and anomaly detection. In clustering, algorithms divide the data into specific groups based on shared characteristics. Data may be placed in more than one group, and then groups may be related to each other. Association rule algorithms attempt to identify connected data points. This may involve relationships between single datasets, groups of datasets (used in conjunction with clustering), or even relationships between different datasets. Dimensionality reduction functions to simplify data without the loss of information. This is useful when analyzing large and complex datasets. This method aims to simplify data by decreasing the number of data points but preserving the accuracy and consistency of the data. The self-organizing map is a type of dimension-simplifying technique. This clusters data based on data similarity. Finally, anomaly detection involves identification of data that are different from other data within a dataset (outliers) (Binson et al., 2024).

Despite the advantages offered by ML models over manual data interpretation in using various forms of data for the diagnosis, prognosis, and treatment monitoring of HNC, it has been superseded by DL, which has been shown to outperform ML in the construction of predictive models. DL algorithms use artificial neural networks (ANNs) and convoluted neural networks (CNNs) (Goldemberg et al., 2019).

14.3 Large Dataset Interpretation

HNCs are one of the many cancers that have been used in various studies to assess the use of "big data" in oncology to increase the accuracy, reliability. and speed of diagnosis, prognosis, treatment effectiveness, treatment outcome, and the use of targeted therapies. The use of AI to analyze large datasets can contribute to the use of big data in HNC management by examining patterns in omics data to identify the molecular mechanisms driving HNC pathogenesis. AI can also identify molecules that can serve as biomarkers for diagnosis, prognosis, and prediction. Finally, computer-assisted large data studies can identify new therapeutic targets for the development of new treatments for various HNCs. The sources of big data that can be used by AI vary from radiomic data, genomic data, patterns in histopathological images, and clinical-epidemiological data (Resteghini et al., 2018).

Initially HNC was treated as a single disease, and only the development of methods allowing for the recognition of patterns based on clinical-pathological features and molecular changes has shown how complex HNC is. Cancers at different subsites, such as those in the oral cavity, oropharynx, larynx, or hypopharynx, can be treated as separate diseases despite all of them arising from common epithelial tissue (Leemans et al., 2018). New high-throughput technologies such as next-generation sequencing and databases such as the Cancer Genome Atlas have allowed researchers to access large amounts of molecular data specific to these heterogenous forms of cancer. "Omics" is the name given to the analysis and use of these data (Tonella et al., 2017). Omics data can include genomics (DNA sequence analysis), transcriptomics (mRNA sequence and level as well as ncRNA sequences and levels), epigenomics (alterations in markers on DNA changing transcription), proteomics (presence and levels of proteins

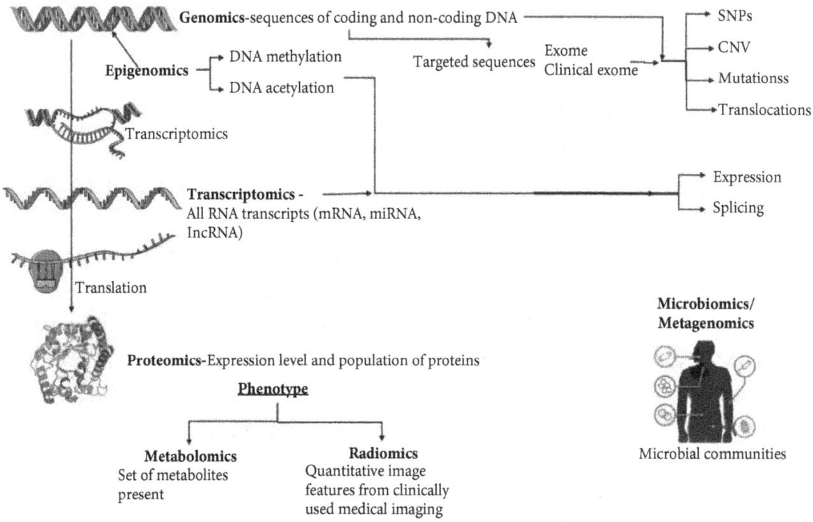

Figure 14.4 Large datasets. High throughput technologies such as next-generation sequencing and mass spectroscopy have given rise to large collections of omics datasets. These range from DNA sequence data (genomics, epigenomics) over RNA sequence data (transcriptomics and protein expression data) to proteomics and data linked to the phenotype of the individual, such as metabolomics and radiomic image data. In addition to these there are also databases concerning the population of microbes within the individual, referred to as microbiomics. All these omics data can be mined for disease-specific patterns as well as patterns that give information concerning disease and treatment outcomes.

present), metabolomics (presence of different metabolites), and microbiomics (microbiome makeup) (Figure 14.4). Artificial intelligence is the only way to make full use of these large datasets as their size and complexity make manual analysis too slow, the results may be influenced by user bias, and many important patterns or features in the data may be missed by human observers or analysis.

ML requires large datasets to learn from, and this creates a paradox: large data requires AI and AI requiring large datasets (Dlamini et al., 2020). An analysis of 61 HNC omics studies, including 57 transcriptomic and 4 epigenomic studies, showed that more than 10 of these studies identified HNC-specific molecular patterns enabling the different subtypes of HNC to be distinguished. These studies also indicated that specific gene expression signatures could be used for prognosis/prediction in a clinical setting (Lee et al., 2024). Various omics studies on HNC have sought to discover the molecular basis behind the link between human papillomavirus (HPV) infection and the development of HNC (Cancer Genome Atlas Network, 2015). These studies have indicated a link between HPV, prognosis (Locati et al., 2019) and carcinogenesis in HPV-related HNC

(Orlandi & Licitra, 2018). However, these approaches have not yet identified the precise underlying basis for this relationship, despite omics data providing the best hope of achieving this. It is expected that the use of more advanced AI to analyze these large and diverse omics datasets might lead to the full integration of large multiomics datasets, which would provide the most comprehensive understanding of the effective molecular relationships and regulatory networks in place (Resteghini et al., 2018).

Microarray and RNAseq data from hundreds of patients and containing the transcription of thousands of genes have recently been analyzed using ML self-organizing maps (SOM) (Kristensen et al., 2014). This mapping relies on the clustering of data, which are assigned to neurons (or nodes) based on their position, with datasets near to each other being assigned to the same neuron or to adjacent neurons; this leads the system to be self-organizing. This results in clusters of data with reduced dimensionality, making data interpretation easier and more accurate, and it allows for pattern recognition in the data. SOMs have been used to examine the pattern of gene expression in HPV-positive HNC cases, and this was used to group these cases into three subtypes of HPV-linked HNCs that can be used for prognostic purposes. These three groups were Cl1, immune-related: Cl2, epithelial–mesenchymal transition-related; and Cl3, proliferation-related. The Cl1 group had the best prognosis, while the Cl2 group had the worst (Locati et al., 2019).

14.4 Digital Twins

AI-based prediction models that are constructed using radiomics or molecular patterns can be used to both choose the appropriate treatment as well as predict treatment outcome. These models can also be used to make the decision to either escalate or de-escalate treatment. Both molecular signatures and radiomics can be used to create models that can be used to design prophylactic measures and advise on the best supportive care. A *digital twin* is a digital model representing a specific physical object. In medical terms, it normally refers to a digital representation of a patient. This model can be built with various data ranging from omics, medical images, medical history, or demographic data to name a few. This digital copy of the patient can contain as much data as possible to create a comprehensive digital duplicate of the patient, or it can use only data pertinent to the factor being modeled. The digital twin can then be duplicated, and each twin is used to run a model for a particular treatment option. The digital twin produces a patient-specific prediction that can be used to provide informed treatment options (Kaul et al., 2023).

Digital twins have been utilized to predict shape and position changes that will take place in soft tissue as a result of surgical interventions to treat HNC.

In one application, a 3D scan of the patient's head was used to create the digital twin. A Bayesian algorithm was trained to model the effects of surgery on these soft tissues (Männle et al., 2023).

14.5 Artificial Intelligence-Empowered Tissue Cytometry

While AI can be used in many areas of biomedical research, from predicting 3D protein structure and function to simulating vaccine efficacy, the analysis of real cells in tissue context is of particular importance to understand carcinogenesis and tumor progression. Tissue is the place where diseases occur, so understanding that particular place will help to answer questions that remain beyond the scope of cell cultures and in vitro experiments. Quantifying multiple markers on individual cells in the tissue context allows us to understand the complex interplay between cancer cells, the tumor microenvironment, and the body's immune response. The technology that permits this type of tissue analysis is referred to as *tissue cytometry* (Mungenast et al., 2021). This in situ analysis allows the identification and quantification of molecular markers on the protein level, referred to as *cellular phenotypes*, but may also include data on DNA and mRNA expression profiles.

A central aspect of tissue cytometry lies in computer-assisted image analysis, which includes ML and DL algorithms for analyzing microscopic images, segmenting cells and tumor regions in situ, and classifying tissue regions on glass slides (Meshcheryakova et al., 2021). Tissue cytometry can be used to understand both the physiological function of tissue as well as the interplay of tumor cells with the normal adjacent tissue in which they are embedded after loss of control and malignant transformation (Gonçalves-Alves et al., 2022).

Tissue cytometry allows researchers to extract observer-independent and standardized in situ data in a reproducible manner and in an automated fashion, which is a prerequisite for precision diagnostics. It allows us to determine molecular processes that trigger HNC, how the immune system responds (or fails to respond) to the cancer cells, which molecular mechanism are active in a particular patient, and, thereby, what is the best therapeutic approach.

Cells not only form tissue structures with respect to morphology. Any tissue also constitutes an interwoven cellular network where cells form functional elements that communicate to each other and respond to various internal as well as external stimuli. Cells are organized in regulatory networks, which themselves are governed through signal transduction cascades. Such regulatory networks are formed through the molecular interactions of dozens to hundreds of partners (molecules) at least. Cells go through multiple checkpoints to ensure their genetic and molecular integrity. Extensive repair mechanisms are in place to correct errors that constantly occur in our highly active cells. If cancer forms in any given patient, this must be considered an unfortunate (and actually unlikely) event. Prior to that "regrettable mistake" made possibly by a single cell, billions of other cells succeeded in regulating their physiological functions for billions of times, maybe over decades. The formation of cancer is similar to the crash of an airplane. Neither does an airplane crash "just because" nor does cancer form without reason. Understanding the complex interplay of regulatory networks and where in the network the error has occurred that caused a particular cancer in an individual patient requires the analysis of many molecular, sometime even multimodal data. This is a task that can hardly be performed manually by humans, not even by trained experts, and can definitely not be financed by contemporary healthcare systems.

If a systemic failure occurs at a particular point in the regulatory network that frequently causes a certain form of cancer to occur, we refer to this point, molecule, or irregular protein expression downstream of the actual molecular cause of regulatory derailing as a *biomarker*.

Tissue cytometry is an approach that permits researchers to determine protein expression signatures, in particular biomarkers, in situ and, through this, to elucidate the molecular mechanism of cancer formation in any particular patient. Further combination with data from other modalities in advanced AI solutions supports researchers in establishing novel and targeted treatment regimens based on precision diagnostics.

The application of AI methods for establishing novel biomarkers and the development of new therapeutic approaches in HNC are not only questions of higher diagnostic precision and more optimized therapies for patients, but also a critical strategy to employ in facing the increasing problem in most healthcare systems of limited diagnostic capacity. Tissue cytometry is an important step toward automated quantification of cell populations in the spatial context of tissue by means of computer-assisted analysis to overcome procedural as well as resource limitations in HNC research and diagnosis.

Combining such innovative AI tools has the potential to make possible what was once considered an analysis too complex for the human mind.

14.6 Artificial Intelligence in Head and Neck Cancer Diagnosis and Screening

The early diagnosis of HNC is predicted to have the greatest positive effects on its management. This can be approached from multiple angles. The first is through the use of molecular biomarkers to identify patterns of molecules linked to the development of the disease or, in the case of prevention, to identify high-risk patients. Delays in effective HNC diagnosis and detection contribute greatly to its high mortality rate and difficulties in treating the disease because delays can result in the disease only being diagnosed at an advanced stage (Alabi et al., 2019). Histopathological assessment is the gold standard for developing a prognosis and treatment plans in HNC. AI and ML and DL models can be developed for the analysis of biomarkers, images, and histopathology slides for diagnosis, risk stratification, and management guidance (Alabi et al., 2021; Kourou et al., 2015). AI has been used to develop a home diagnostic tool for use with mobile phones. This allows individuals to take an image of the inside of their mouth and analyze this image using an AI tool on their phone. This can aid in the early detection of oral, tongue, lip, and gum cancers (Dailah, 2022).

14.6.1 Radiomics

Radiomics describes the use of quantitative imaging markers for diagnosis, treatment, outcome prediction, and prognosis. However, radiomics requires the use of multiple image markers in combination since the predictive power of a single feature is insufficient to guide care. AI can help integrate these diverse features and use them to create prediction models (Ansari et al., 2024). These prediction models can be used to predict patient overall survival, progression-free survival, local-regional relapse, distant metastases, the choice of the best treatment, and pathological findings (Jiang et al., 2023).

The analysis of medical images from positron emission tomography-computed tomography (PET-CT), CT, and magnetic resonance imaging (MRI) scans is a useful tool for cancer diagnosis and prognosis. HNC is usually diagnosed using radiological examination and confirmed using histopathology to analyze tissue sections that are obtained from patient biopsies or tissue obtained from surgical resections. PET-CT and PET-MRI data are now the standard for the diagnosis and imaging of HNCs (Schlumpf & Haerle, 2014; Tshering Vogel & Thoeny, 2016). These images were traditionally analyzed manually. Visual and semi-quantitative analysis of the image involves the assessment of the standardized uptake value (SUV) of the radiotracer by regions or lesions. Elevated SUVs are associated with malignant tissue or inflamed areas. The assignment of cutoff points to define high SUVs is unclear, and no definite values exist (Riegel et al., 2006). The interpretation of results from these methods is prone to errors, biases, and inter-person variations (Schlumpf & Haerle, 2014; Tshering Vogel & Thoeny, 2016). Next-generation digital pathology, also referred to as *computational pathology*, involves the use of computers to analyze these images and provide more reliable, accurate, and reproducible analysis to improve diagnosis and prognosis. Digital and computational pathology (Mungenast et al., 2021) can form part of a cellular pathology workflow by combining it with electronic patient records and barcoding to ensure sample tracking (Hanna et al., 2022).

AI algorithms have been developed to assist in the use of digital and computational pathology, including head and neck pathology. This includes the use of AI for the analysis of medical imaging, histopathology, and in situ hybridization (Bassani et al., 2022; De Meulenaere et al., 2018). The use of AI in digital pathology requires validation and previous studies testing the accuracy of prognostic and diagnostic predictions made by AI and requires slides to be scanned at a higher magnification and sometimes even at different focusing planes to achieve confident digital reporting. The use of AI is further enhanced in the diagnosis and prognosis of HNC by using ML and, more recently, DL technologies. In these cases, the ability of an AI to learn can improve the power of prediction, the creation of prognostic models, and the development of automated diagnosis (reviewed in Mahmood et al., 2021). ML algorithms were originally applied to HNC diagnosis with the hopes of providing diagnostic accuracy that is equal or superior to that performed by health professionals (Kim et al., 2020).

These methods have also gained significant popularity in recent years due to their achieving relatively high accuracy of prediction. AI algorithms have been shown to be able to perform well as a tool to predict treatment outcomes and recurrence, evaluate clinical endpoints, and predict metastasis in HNC (Abdel Razek et al., 2022; Chinnery et al., 2021; Zhang et al., 2023). These and other studies also indicated that these algorithms make more accurate predictions than imaging methods that rely on classical TNM staging. HNC tumors can also be classified by site and stratified based on ML and DL algorithms by analyzing medical images (Abdel Razek et al., 2022; Kourou et al., 2015). This stratification and classification can help healthcare professionals to target patients for more aggressive treatment (Michelutti et al., 2023). The final aim of computational pathology is to extract information from the image to segment or classify these data, which can be associated with outcomes, stage, or even subtype of HNC (Shen et al., 2017).

14.6.2 Segmentation

Image segmentation involves the delineation of different structures or areas within an image; in oncology, image segmentation involves separating the tumor from the normal tissue in the image (Bousselham et al., 2019). Segmentation relies on the selection of pixels the belong to a defined region of interest (ROI) and/or a specific object. This selection relies on defining similar properties shared by these pixels. The process of image selection involves the preprocessing of the image after its acquisition, followed by segmentation (Pan, 2007). In terms of accuracy, manual segmentation is still considered the most accurate and referred to as "ground truth." However, this is only true for limited image datasets. When looking across a variety of images of the same subject, manual segmentation is prone to bias and inaccuracy—and it is extremely tedious and time-consuming. This fact is particularly important in medical imaging since accurate cancer imaging involves multiple images—sometimes entire digital samples, referred to as *virtual slides*—with varying contrasts. As such the segmentation of images is affected by both inter- and intra-rater variability (Philip et al., 2023), these limitations have led to the adoption of AI ML and DL to perform rapid, reproducible, and unbiased image segmentation (Mahbod et al., 2021; Moe et al., 2021). DL algorithms for object segmentation perform either *semantic segmentation* (i.e., assigns each pixel to a class or background) or *instance segmentation*, which in addition assigns a unique label (index) to each object of the same class and is thus able to distinguish between multiple occurrences of the same object type (Mahbod et al., 2021).

Specific methods of image segmentation include region, edge, fuzzy theory, partial differential equation (PDE) and threshold-based. Region-based segmentation involves the use of a reference pixel within the ROI to compare its features to neighboring pixels. It continues to identify similar pixels and thereby expands the ROI. The ROI stops growing when no neighboring pixels are similar to the seed pixel (Preetha et al., 2012). Edge-based segmentation not only segments an image but also reduces its size and storage requirements by only retaining important features in the image and removing the background (Iannizzotto & Vita, 2000). fuzzy theory–based image segmentation combines region and edge-based segmentation (Basir et al., 2003). In partial differential equation (PDE) image segmentation, the equation is a parametric function that describes the energy (localized changes) of the image function. It allows objects within an image to be tracked, extracted, and reconstituted (Sliz & Mikulka, 2016). Threshold-based methods are simple and widely used; they convert an image to grayscale. The resulting binary images have reduced complexity, making it easier to select image areas. A threshold value is established and all pixels below this achieved value are removed. The greatest difficulty in this method is establishing the threshold value (Bhargavi et al., 2014).

Specific CNNs have been developed to carry out image segmentation in medical images. Competitions are held by companies such as IBM to select the best models. In 2015, a specific CNN won this prize and was specifically designed for image segmentation in medical images. This model is known as a *U net model* and is designed to use a large number of annotated training samples. This model architecture consists of a contracting path that captures the context of the samples and a symmetrical expanding path that precisely locates the sample (Kamnitsas et al., 2017). These 2D U-nets were shown to efficiently and accurately segment HNC PET-MRI images (Liedes et al., 2023). In the U-network architecture, the contracting path is mirrored by the expansive path. The contracting path consists of two 3 × 3 convolution networks. Each network is followed by an activation value consisting of a rectified linear unit. Rectified linear units allow for only positive values to act as outputs; a negative value will be given as zero. Following this the output is entered into a 2 × 2 max pooling operation. This operation analyses the image by taking 2 × 2 neighboring pixels from the pixels of interest using a filter that is moved by 2 pixels (stride 2). This stride 2 function allows for downsampling of the image while the pooling leads to an increase in the channel size (doubling the image features) (Figure 14.5). The mirrored expansive pathway is an upsampling pathway where each upsampling function is followed by a 2 × 2 convolution network. Each channel is halved at each upsampling step. This involves the concatenation of data followed by a rectified linear unit function (Figure 14.5) (Ronneberger et al., 2015).

14.7 Artificial Intelligence in Head and Neck Cancer Treatment

Personalized medicine can be enhanced through the selection of the best treatment based on patient-specific characteristics and features ranging from genetics, phenotype, and demographics, to medical history. Based on these signatures, an AI model can be used to predict the best treatment for a patient using the predicted and modeled outcomes of these treatments. The quality of results heavily depends on proper models that can provide accurate predictions of oncologic outcomes (Jayawickrama et al., 2024). In the treatment of HNC, two of the most important variables to be modeled are disease control and acceptable treatment toxicity, along with the relationship between these two factors (Jayawickrama et al., 2024).

Predictions can be used to either escalate or de-escalate treatment. For example, in at least 10–15% of cases, patients do not respond well to treatment, and, in these cases, treatment should be escalated (Huang et al., 2015). These patients' treatment can be modified before treatment begins based on the predictions provided by AI models. These models can predict the presence of radioresistant HNCs and indicate the use of increased radiation doses. In other cases, these models may indicate that the treatment would be improved through the use of immunotherapy or chemotherapy in conjunction with radiation therapy (Manukian et al., 2019). The models can also predict potential tissue damage or toxicity risks that arise due to increasing radiation dosage or combination with chemoradiation therapy.

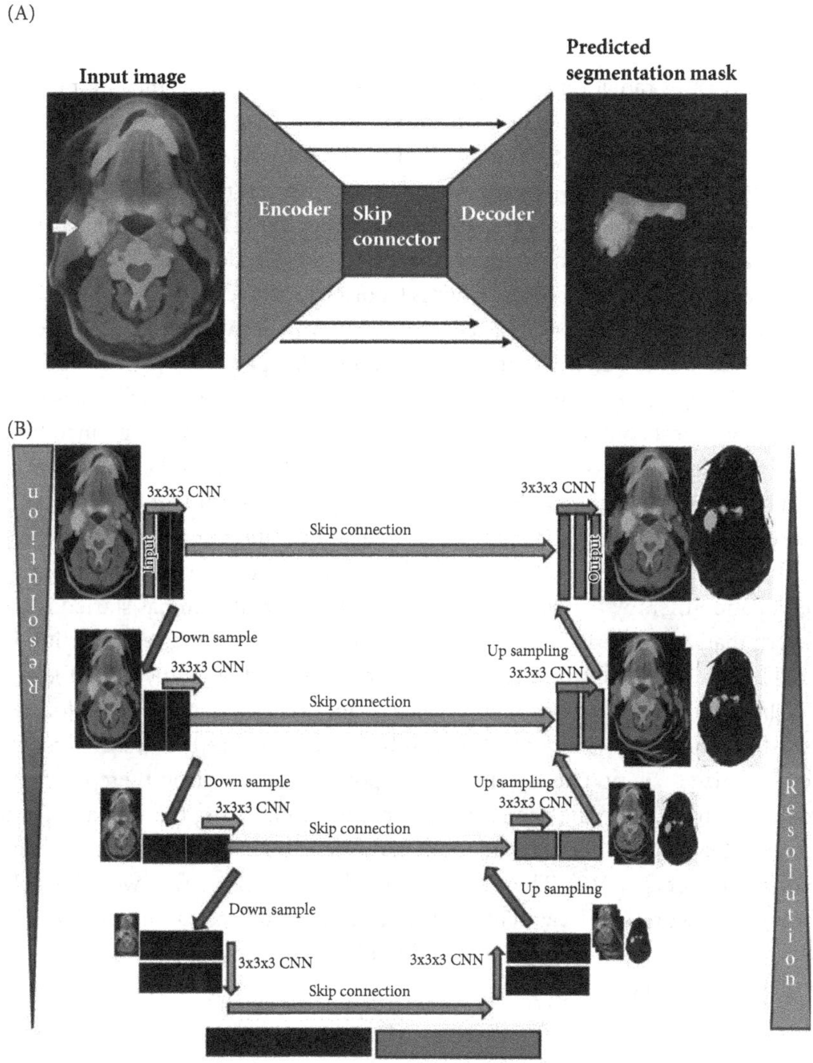

Figure 14.5 Image segmentation by the U-net architecture. (A) Using the overall architecture of the U-net, an image is fed into the network, which extracts useful features from the image through the use of multiple convolutional layers. (B) The U-network is a convolutional neural network with an encoder–decoder type architecture. Each black or brown box represents a multichannel feature map, with each stage containing a repeated 3 × 3 convolutional layer. Skip connections skip some of the layers in the neural network and feed image features directly into the decoder.

14.7.1 Radiotherapy

For many cases radiation therapy is the first-line treatment for the treatment of HNC (Figen et al., 2020). One of the most important aspects in the use of radiation therapy is the accurate targeting of the tumor while sparing surrounding normal tissue, especially organs close to the tumor that may be affected by the radiation therapy. These are known as organs at risk (OAR). To achieve this the tumor and the surrounding tissues and organs need to be delineated. Historically, this was done manually, however, this is laborious and the outcome can vary between different radiologists (Castelli et al., 2018; van der Veen et al., 2019; Vogin et al., 2021). This has led to the automation of this procedure using mechanical modeling. An example of this is *atlas-based contouring*, which relies on a library of expert contoured images as a reference for comparison with incoming patient images (Lim & Leech, 2016). AI techniques to accomplish this use ML and DL models, which have been predicted to provide advantages, in particular increases in automation, accuracy, reproducibility, and consistency (Almberg et al., 2022; D'Aviero et al., 2022; Rigaud et al., 2021). Another important aspect of radiation therapy that requires prediction before treatment has started is the determination of dosage level, and AI can be used for such dose prediction in HNC. This is especially true for intensity modulated radiotherapy (IMRT).

The ability to predict treatment toxicity is another task that can be performed by AI algorithms. This information can be used to choose the best treatments to minimize toxicity. This is especially important for radioiron therapy, where toxicity can decrease the chances of the patient completing the treatment and tissue damage can occur that will result in the need for extensive supportive care (Muzumder et al., 2019). These models can identify patients who would benefit from more aggressive treatment, which patients would require more care, and what lifestyle changes the patient could implement to help cope with treatment toxicity (Sheikh et al., 2019).

14.7.2 Dose Determination

To plan IMRT, defining a proper treatment program requires the expertise of multiple clinical personnel. It also requires prior knowledge of the patient, their medical history, size, weight, comorbidities, and nutritional level (Valdes et al., 2017). Prediction models to decide on radiation therapy dosage in HNC include atlas-based methods, fully connected neural networks, and convolutional neural networks. As previously stated, atlas-based methods use historical data collected from previous patient responses to different dosages. By comparing the current HNC patient's details to historic patient details, the volume of the dose can be determined (D'Aviero et al., 2022). This technique is also known as *data-driven knowledge-based planning* (KBP) and requires the assumption that the dose required or the dose that can be tolerated is related to the patient's anatomical geometry (tissue structure location and dynamic movement) and the required/tolerated radiation dose. This assumption accounts for the proximity of OARs to the tumor site where radiation will be delivered. To use AI-based analysis the volumetric information in an image needs to be reduced to structured input data (Osman et al., 2023). This can be achieved by reducing medical images to dose-volume data (Ziemer et al., 2017). These 3D predicted dose distributions for previous cases are used for *inverse optimization*; that is, using these patient decisions as input, with the output being the objectives, constraints, and conditions (Babier et al., 2020).

The use of dosage prediction DL algorithms has been widely studied using HNCs (Momin et al., 2021). This is due to the complexity of radiation therapy for these cancers since major OARs are in close proximity to tumor sites. Many algorithms have proved effective in dose prediction, including various types of modified U-net models as well as residual net (res-net) models and generative adversarial network (GAN) models. Despite the successes achieved with these models, their performance greatly depends on the databases used to train them (Osman et al., 2023).

Regression forest models augmented with density estimation have been tested for their ability to predict dosage in the treatment of HNC with radiation therapy. This model was applied to an atlas of previous treatments to select the plan best suited to a novel patient geometry. This model resulted in a spatial dose objective giving a prediction of the correct dose for the patient. Tests of this model gave promising results to a small sample of HNC patients. The voxel-based dose mimicking system can then be used to convert the dose distribution to a complete treatment plan. Specifically, the predicted per-voxel dose distribution can be used to predict the per voxel dose and use this to create beam geometries to best treat a patient with specific target tissues and OARs (McIntosh et al., 2017). These regression forests are an attempt to mimic an expert radiologist examining these images and comparing them to and matching them with similar historic cases and adopting the dosage used in these historic cases to the new one. Regression trees achieve this by modeling the relationship between the features on a patient's imaging scan and the per-voxel dose distribution. This is then fed into a second model, which is used to select the best regression tree (Lafferty et al., 2001).

ANNs can also be used to learn from an atlas of previous cases by classifying the features in these cases into a hierarchy of features. A simple example of this was an ANN that used an algorithm based on the distance between tumors and OARs in HNC cases and a subsequent layer of neurons specifying beam intersection information (Shiraishi et al., 2006). CNNs have now largely replaced standard ANNs to predict volumetric information (Milletari et al., 2016). Two different types of CNN have been considered for this purpose. The first is the tiramisu-based network, which is a type of U-network specific for dosage prediction. The simplification steps involve the removal of volume data and a focus on feature classification into hierarchies. The ascending complexity stage restores the volumetric data to these features and can predict the dosage required for each feature (Kajikawa et al., 2019). Dilated CNNs encode certain information while skipping over other information. This pixel skipping allows the model to cover larger areas of the image. They are particularly useful in predicting changes in dosage to target specific tissues in the complex anatomies characteristic of HNCs (Zhao et al., 2023).

14.7.3 Surgery

Surgery is the first treatment option normally adopted for the treatment of various HNCs. However, it is not without risks because surgery can leave a patient disfigured or with impaired body functions that lead to a decrease in the quality of life. This can also result in the need for temporary or permanent use of feeding tubes and lifestyle changes to account for changes or difficulties in breathing, swallowing, and eating as well as speech (Crowson et al., 2020). AI can be used to improve surgical outcomes by assessing the surgical margins (the noncancerous tissues surrounding a tumor). This margin is dictated by both the type and nature of the tumor as well as the surgical approach being used. Enough of the tissue surrounding the HNC needs to be removed to reduce the chances of recurrence, but not so much to increase disfigurement or hamper function of the remaining tissue (Baddour et al., 2016). Traditionally the surgeon would consult with a pathologist to come to an agreement regarding the surgical margin based on tissue samples taken from the tumor. However, these tissue samples may not be indicative of the tumor as a whole. ML can be used to create risk models that take into account the histopathological imaging of these tissues along with the gene and protein expression profiles of the tumor and its radiomic features (Kubik et al., 2020).

AI can also be used to run risk assessment models to predict possible surgical complications. These models can also be used to account for increased risk factors that could contribute to poor surgical outcomes, such as the presence of comorbidities. Additionally, these models can be used to predict the complexity of the surgery and the required duration of anesthesia (Ferrier et al., 2005). Often it is necessary to perform reconstructive surgery following the removal of HNC tumors. Reconstructive surgery can involve microvascular free flap transfer.

This process can be negatively affected by comorbidities, other treatments for the tumor, lifestyle factors such as smoking, and the age of the patient (Crawley et al., 2019). Risk models constructed using ML or DL can take all these risk factors into account to provide the best predictions of both the outcome and the extent of each reconstructive procedure.

14.8 Artificial Intelligence in Head and Neck Cancer Prognosis and Outcomes

AI can be used to mimic treatment planning, the course of treatment, and outcomes using digital twins of the patient. These can be used to select the best treatment based on the patient's modeled response to these various therapies. AI models can also be used to predict the likelihood of locally advanced HNC developing metastatic disease.

14.8.1 Predicting Metastatic Potential

Lymphovascular or perineural invasion has prognostic value and can influence treatment options. These models can also predict the consequences of treating metastatic tumors, which may involve aggressive surgery and lifestyle changes such as the use of a feeding tube and changes to speech, swallowing, or even breathing. Finally these models may predict the chance of survival and in cases recommend palliative care (Ilhan et al., 2021). An example of one of these models is a CNN developed to predict the occurrence of distant metastasis as well as overall survival and recurrence in HNC. This algorithm does not select image features but rather uses whole-pixel data to predict the likelihood of metastasis (Santos et al., 2019).

Another study sought to predict the metastatic risk and prognosis for laryngeal cancer. Variations in both the metastatic potential and prognosis for laryngeal cancer depend on the source of the tumor, which allows laryngeal cancer to be classified into different subtypes. Two of these subtypes are glottic and nonglottic carcinoma. A large study of patients with both types of laryngeal cancer was conducted using a random survival forest to analyze different clinicopathological characteristics. Each subtype was shown to produce separate models that were more accurate in predicting the survival and treatment outcomes of each. By combining these models, the researchers were able to effectively predict the survival, prognosis, and relative contribution of various risk factors to the development of each subtype (Wang et al., 2024).

14.8.2 Predicting Overall Survival

The use of overall survival predictions to help select the best treatment choice is now well established. AI algorithms can be used to develop accurate scoring systems that can be more accurate than previous methods to predict survival. An example of this is the subtype of salivary gland cancer, parotid mucoepidermoid carcinoma (P-MEC). P-MEC has a heterogenous and complex histopathology, and, as such, current clinical models are not able to recommend effective options for the personalized treatment of these patients. A retrospective study was conducted using data from 882 postoperative P-MEC patients obtained from the SEER database. The study aimed to assess if various ML models could accurately predict the overall survival of these patients. These models included random forest, LASSO, XGBoost, and best subset regression. The models were used to select for specific variables in the data. The model was shown to perform well and surpassed previous methods in its ability to identify key factors that contributed to overall survival. The regression forest performed the worst of the four (Huang et al., 2024).

An example of a model that was created to predict both overall and progression-free survival in oropharyngeal cancer was developed by Tosado et al. in 2020. This model uses CT scan data and a baseline mode consisting of patient demographic data. The model then employed clustering algorithms to analyze staging and radiomic features. This resulted in patients being grouped based on their radiomic and clinical features. By carrying out a retrospective study with past patient data, it was shown that this model was better able to predict survival (Tosado et al., 2020).

14.9 Limitations

Many people, including clinicians, have an innate mistrust of AI, especially due to the "black box" problem in many AIs at present—the user is unsure about how the AI is coming to its final conclusion. Data are entered into the model and a result is produced, all with the inner workings being a mystery to many/most users. This is especially true in the case of ML and DL, where the algorithm changes and adapts as it is fed with new data. This has slowed the uptake of AI in many clinical settings. This situation is made worse when AI makes an error, which can occur especially if it is not applied correctly. Even though it is far less prone to errors than humans analyzing the same data, people are less willing to excuse such an error in AI. This problem can be solved through increasing the transparency and interpretability of ML and DL algorithms (Poon & Sung, 2021).

As with many other types of cancer, genetic risk factors mean that ancestry may play a role in the incidence and mortality rate of HNCs. A study in the United States reported that, depending on the database being analyzed, patients with African ancestry had either the same or significantly worse survival times for various HNCs (Lin et al., 2024). This highlights the importance of the contribution of the dataset used to train a model and how the use of any model trained using specific data from one population can give erroneous results when applied to another population. This can be solved through the use of population-specific datasets. However, in many cases, assigning population membership to a patient may rely on the patient's own interpretation of their ancestry. The best solution is to construct more diverse databases that include patients with a wide range of ethnic backgrounds. The use of omics data for HNC diagnosis and prognosis is limited by the relatively low number of associations between omics signatures, such as DNA methylation and ncRNA transcript levels, and HNC outcomes and screening patterns. It is also difficult to find many databases with a high number of HNC cases with multiple omics datasets (Lee et al., 2024).

In many of the models that use prior knowledge as a tool and attempt to fit historic data to current patients using AI, accuracy can be affected by any error that occurs in any of the steps that first simplify the data by removing features and then follow subsequent steps to reinsert these features. This is especially true for densely connected ANNs, which are susceptible to overfitting. The use of these models is widespread in medicine since they are versatile, converge well, are easy to train, and have a broad perceptive field (Lee et al., 2024).

CNN-based methods are programmatically complex, difficult to train, and require special hardware. While CNN-based dose prediction methods are still in the developmental stage, they tend to prevail in industry, and thus it is likely that these methods will also soon become common in volumetric dose prediction for IMRT in treating HNC (Chen et al., 2018).

Studies that use data from a single source or institution to train their models may not represent the population in general, and while this can be overcome by using data from a variety of institutes or even countries (Bogowicz et al., 2020), this leads to additional problems. Different countries or even regions, states, or provinces may have vastly different clinical guidelines that call for different variables and features to be noted as well as different treatment and screening protocols. All of these can result in databases containing different data details or types of data (Cabitza et al., 2021). This has led to efforts to create guidelines for the standard collection of data and model development and evaluation. These guidelines would require models to be validated using the same types and quality of data (Collins et al., 2021).

Questions also surround the ethical and legal basis for the collection, use, and storage of personalized data such as genomic sequences and medical records.

Legal questions also exist around the use of AI models in a clinical setting. These questions have to do with the potential misuse of the model, for example self-diagnosis or diagnosis by an inexperienced operator. From an ethical as well as regulatory vantage point one question is essential: Who is to blame if the model is in error—the developer of the AI model or its user (Alabi et al., 2020)?

14.10 Conclusion

The use of AI is a promising development in the management of cancer, including HNC. The advantages offered by AI in the diagnosis, prognosis, and treatment management of HNC are vast and increasing as the number of omics databases with information concerning HNC increases. These omics databases contain details of the genetic makeup of patients or gene expression, transcription, or even epigenomic data. Contained within these data are molecular patterns for HNC across a wide range of omics categories. The identification of these patterns is difficult for a human user because errors, bias, and the tendency of human beings to miss small changes in large datasets are inevitable. AI can be taught to recognize these changes, and associate them with various characteristics of HNC such as various cancer sites, cancer subtypes, level of aggressiveness, propensity to develop resistance to treatment, treatment response, and survival. AI is also able to efficiently analyze medical images and select features that can be associated with outcomes, advise treatment decisions, and predict patient survival and risk. All of this implies that AI is a promising tool to help in the management of HNC. The application of AI can help realize the dream of personalized medicine, increase early detection rates, and improve survival rates. The final result may be a decrease in both incidence and mortality rates. However, despite this promise many barriers need to be overcome. These barriers are not insurmountable, and many can be overcome through increased testing, training, and validation of models. Others can be overcome through training clinicians in understanding and using these models. Perhaps the greatest and most sensitive issues revolve around the ethical use of these algorithms and, more importantly, the data used to train them and the ability of others to access patient data. Regulation of AI is necessary but also causes a "regulatory paradox"; that is, increasing regulatory constraints make the development and application of AI solutions, in particular access to the patient data needed to train and evaluate the model, increasingly difficult. A lack of data, however, puts any ML or DL model at risk of failure and/or at risk of generating unpredicted results. Hence, (over-) regulation might well cause the opposite effect and make AI more prone to errors rather than more robust and safer to use.

These problems will perhaps only be solved through the creation of forward-looking (rather than reactive) legal frameworks and appropriate guidelines surrounding their use.

References

ABDEL RAZEK, A. A. K., KHALED, R., HELMY, E., NAGLAH, A., ABDELKHALEK, A., & EL-BAZ, A. 2022. Artificial intelligence and deep learning of head and neck cancer. *Magn Reson Imaging Clin N Am*, 30, 81–94.

ALABI, R. O., ELMUSRATI, M., SAWAZAKI-CALONE, I., KOWALSKI, L. P., HAGLUND, C., COLETTA, R. D., MÄKITIE, A. A., SALO, T., LEIVO, I., & ALMANGUSH, A. 2019. Machine learning application for prediction of locoregional recurrences in early oral tongue cancer: A Web-based prognostic tool. *Virchows Arch*, 475, 489–497.

ALABI, R. O., VARTIAINEN, T., & ELMUSRATI, M. 2020. Machine learning for prognosis of oral cancer: What are the ethical challenges? CEUR Workshop Proceedings. https://osuva.uwasa.fi/handle/10024/11563

ALABI, R. O., YOUSSEF, O., PIRINEN, M., ELMUSRATI, M., MÄKITIE, A. A., LEIVO, I., & ALMANGUSH, A. 2021. Machine learning in oral squamous cell carcinoma: Current status, clinical concerns and prospects for future-A systematic review. *Artif Intell Med*, 115, 102060.

ALMBERG, S. S., LERVÅG, C., FRENGEN, J., EIDEM, M., ABRAMOVA, T. M., NORDSTRAND, C. S., ALSAKER, M. D., TØNDEL, H., RAJ, S. X., & WANDERÅS, A. D. 2022. Training, validation, and clinical implementation of a deep-learning segmentation model for radiotherapy of loco-regional breast cancer. *Radiother Oncol*, 173, 62–8.

ANSARI, G., MIRZA-AGHAZADEH-ATTARI, M., MOSIER, K. M., FAKHRY, C., & YOUSEM, D. M. 2024. Radiomics features in predicting human papillomavirus status in oropharyngeal squamous cell carcinoma: A systematic review, quality appraisal, and meta-analysis. *Diagnostics (Basel)*, 14.

BABIER, A., MAHMOOD, R., MCNIVEN, A. L., DIAMANT, A., & CHAN, T. C. Y. 2020. Knowledge-based automated planning with three-dimensional generative adversarial networks. *Med Phys*, 47, 297–306.

BADDOUR, H. M., JR., MAGLIOCCA, K. R., & CHEN, A. Y. 2016. The importance of margins in head and neck cancer. *J Surg Oncol*, 113, 248–55.

BASIR, O., ZHU, H., & KARRAY, F. 2003. Fuzzy based image segmentation. *In:* NACHTEGAEL, M., VAN DER WEKEN, D., KERRE, E. E., & VAN DE VILLE, D., eds. *Fuzzy Filters for Image Processing*. Berlin, Heidelberg: Springer.

BASSANI, S., SANTONICCO, N., ECCHER, A., SCARPA, A., VIANINI, M., BRUNELLI, M., BISI, N., NOCINI, R., SACCHETTO, L., MUNARI, E., PANTANOWITZ, L., GIROLAMI, I., & MOLTENI, G. 2022. Artificial intelligence in head and neck cancer diagnosis. *J Pathol Inform*, 13, 100153.

BHARGAVI, K., JYOTHI, S. J. I. J. O. I. R., & DEVELOPMENT 2014. A Survey on Threshold Based Segmentation Technique in Image Processing. 3, 234–9.

BINSON, V. A., THOMAS, S., SUBRAMONIAM, M., ARUN, J., NAVEEN, S., & MADHU, S. 2024. A review of machine learning algorithms for biomedical applications. *Ann Biomed Eng*, 52, 1159–83.

BOGOWICZ, M., JOCHEMS, A., DEIST, T. M., TANADINI-LANG, S., HUANG, S. H., CHAN, B., WALDRON, J. N., BRATMAN, S., O'SULLIVAN, B., RIESTERER, O., STUDER, G., UNKELBACH, J., BARAKAT, S., BRAKENHOFF, R. H., NAUTA, I., GAZZANI, S. E., CALARESO, G., SCHECKENBACH, K., HOEBERS, F., WESSELING, F. W. R., KEEK, S., SANDULEANU, S., LEIJENAAR, R. T. H., VERGEER, M. R., LEEMANS, C.

R., TERHAARD, C. H. J., VAN DEN BREKEL, M. W. M., HAMMING-VRIEZE, O., VAN DER HEIJDEN, M. A., ELHALAWANI, H. M., FULLER, C. D., GUCKENBERGER, M., & LAMBIN, P. 2020. Privacy-preserving distributed learning of radiomics to predict overall survival and HPV status in head and neck cancer. *Sci Rep*, 10, 4542.

BOUSSELHAM, A., BOUATTANE, O., YOUSSFI, M., & RAIHANI, A. 2019. Towards reinforced brain tumor segmentation on MRI images based on temperature changes on pathologic area. *Int J Biomed Imaging*, 2019, 1758948.

CABITZA, F., CAMPAGNER, A., SOARES, F., GARCÍA DE GUADIANA-ROMUALDO, L., CHALLA, F., SULEJMANI, A., SEGHEZZI, M., & CAROBENE, A. 2021. The importance of being external: Methodological insights for the external validation of machine learning models in medicine. *Comput Methods Programs Biomed*, 208, 106288.

CANCER GENOME ATLAS NETWORK. 2015. Comprehensive genomic characterization of head and neck squamous cell carcinomas. *Nature*, 517, 576–82.

CASTELLI, J., SIMON, A., LAFOND, C., PERICHON, N., RIGAUD, B., CHAJON, E., DE BARI, B., OZSAHIN, M., BOURHIS, J., & DE CREVOISIER, R. 2018. Adaptive radiotherapy for head and neck cancer. *Acta Oncol*, 57, 1284–92.

CHEN, M. C., BALL, R. L., YANG, L., MORADZADEH, N., CHAPMAN, B. E., LARSON, D. B., LANGLOTZ, C. P., AMRHEIN, T. J., & LUNGREN, M. P. 2018. Deep learning to classify radiology free-text reports. *Radiology*, 286, 845–52.

CHEN, M. M., TERZIC, A., BECKER, A. S., JOHNSON, J. M., WU, C. C., WINTERMARK, M., WALD, C., & WU, J. 2022. Artificial intelligence in oncologic imaging. *Eur J Radiol Open*, 9, 100441.

CHINNERY, T., ARIFIN, A., TAY, K. Y., LEUNG, A., NICHOLS, A. C., PALMA, D. A., MATTONEN, S. A., & LANG, P. 2021. Utilizing artificial intelligence for head and neck cancer outcomes prediction from imaging. *Can Assoc Radiol J*, 72, 73–85.

COLLINS, G. S., DHIMAN, P., ANDAUR NAVARRO, C. L., MA, J., HOOFT, L., REITSMA, J. B., LOGULLO, P., BEAM, A. L., PENG, L., VAN CALSTER, B., VAN SMEDEN, M., RILEY, R. D., & MOONS, K. G. 2021. Protocol for development of a reporting guideline (TRIPOD-AI) and risk of bias tool (PROBAST-AI) for diagnostic and prognostic prediction model studies based on artificial intelligence. *BMJ Open*, 11, e048008.

CRAWLEY, M. B., SWEENY, L., RAVIPATI, P., HEFFELFINGER, R., KREIN, H., LUGINBUHL, A., GOLDMAN, R., & CURRY, J. 2019. Factors associated with free flap failures in head and neck reconstruction. *Otolaryngol Head Neck Surg*, 161, 598–604.

CROWSON, M. G., RANISAU, J., ESKANDER, A., BABIER, A., XU, B., KAHMKE, R. R., CHEN, J. M., & CHAN, T. C. Y. 2020. A contemporary review of machine learning in otolaryngology-head and neck surgery. *Laryngoscope*, 130, 45–51.

D'AVIERO, A., RE, A., CATUCCI, F., PICCARI, D., VOTTA, C., PIRO, D., PIRAS, A., DI DIO, C., IEZZI, M., PREZIOSI, F., MENNA, S., QUARANTA, F., BOSCHETTI, A., MARRAS, M., MICCICHÈ, F., GALLUS, R., INDOVINA, L., BUSSU, F., VALENTINI, V., CUSUMANO, D., & MATTIUCCI, G. C. 2022. Clinical validation of a deep-learning segmentation software in head and neck: An early analysis in a developing radiation oncology center. *Int J Environ Res Public Health*, 19.

DAILAH, H. G. 2022. Mobile health (mHealth) technology in early detection and diagnosis of oral cancer: A scoping review of the current scenario and feasibility. *J Healthc Eng*, 2022, 4383303.

DE MEULENAERE, A., VERMASSEN, T., CREYTENS, D., ASPESLAGH, S., DERON, P., DUPREZ, F., ROTTEY, S., VAN DORPE, J. A., & FERDINANDE, L. 2018. Importance of choice of materials and methods in PD-L1 and TIL assessment in oropharyngeal squamous cell carcinoma. *Histopathology*, 73, 500–9.

DLAMINI, Z., FRANCIES, F. Z., HULL, R., & MARIMA, R. 2020. Artificial intelligence (AI) and big data in cancer and precision oncology. *Comput Struct Biotechnol J*, 18, 2300–11.

FERRIER, M. B., SPUESENS, E. B., LE CESSIE, S., & BAATENBURG DE JONG, R. J. 2005. Comorbidity as a major risk factor for mortality and complications in head and neck surgery. *Arch Otolaryngol Head Neck Surg*, 131, 27–32.

FIGEN, M., ÇOLPAN ÖKSÜZ, D., DUMAN, E., PRESTWICH, R., DYKER, K., CARDALE, K., RAMASAMY, S., MURRAY, P., & ŞEN, M. 2020. Radiotherapy for head and neck cancer: Evaluation of triggered adaptive replanning in routine practice. *Front Oncol*, 10, 579917.

GOLDEMBERG, D. C., THULER, L. C. S., & DE MELO, A. C. 2019. An update on mucosal melanoma: Future directions. *Acta Dermatovenerol Croat*, 27, 11–15.

GONÇALVES-ALVES, E., GARCIA, M., RODRÍGUEZ-HERNÁNDEZ, C. J., GÓMEZ-GONZÁLEZ, S., ECKER, R. C., SUÑOL, M., MUÑOZ-AZNAR, O., CARCABOSO, A. M., MORA, J., LAVARINO, C., & MATEO-LOZANO, S. 2022. AC-265347 inhibits neuroblastoma tumor growth by induction of differentiation without causing hypocalcemia. *Int J Mol Sci*, 23.

GONZALEZ, R., SAHA, A., CAMPBELL, C. J. V., NEJAT, P., LOKKER, C., & NORGAN, A. P. 2024. Seeing the random forest through the decision trees. Supporting learning health systems from histopathology with machine learning models: Challenges and opportunities. *J Pathol Inform*, 15, 100347.

HANNA, M. G., ARDON, O., REUTER, V. E., SIRINTRAPUN, S. J., ENGLAND, C., KLIMSTRA, D. S., & HAMEED, M. R. 2022. Integrating digital pathology into clinical practice. *Mod Pathol*, 35, 152–164.

HUANG, S. H., XU, W., WALDRON, J., SIU, L., SHEN, X., TONG, L., RINGASH, J., BAYLEY, A., KIM, J., HOPE, A., CHO, J., GIULIANI, M., HANSEN, A., IRISH, J., GILBERT, R., GULLANE, P., PEREZ-ORDONEZ, B., WEINREB, I., LIU, F. F., & O'SULLIVAN, B. 2015. Refining American Joint Committee on Cancer/Union for International Cancer Control TNM stage and prognostic groups for human papillomavirus-related oropharyngeal carcinomas. *J Clin Oncol*, 33, 836–45.

HUANG, Z., CHEN, Z., LI, Y., LIN, T., CAI, S., WU, W., WU, L., XU, S., LU, J., & QIU, S. 2024. Machine learning-based survival prediction nomogram for postoperative parotid mucoepidermoid carcinoma. *Sci Rep*, 14, 7686.

IANNIZZOTTO, G., & VITA, L. J. I. T. O. I. P. 2000. Fast and accurate edge-based segmentation with no contour smoothing in 2-D real images. 9, 1232–7.

ILHAN, B., GUNERI, P., & WILDER-SMITH, P. 2021. The contribution of artificial intelligence to reducing the diagnostic delay in oral cancer. *Oral Oncol*, 116, 105254.

JAYAWICKRAMA, S. M., RANAWEERA, P. M., PRADEEP, R., JAYASINGHE, Y. A., SENEVIRATHNA, K., HILMI, A. J., RAJAPAKSE, R. M. G., KANMODI, K. K., & JAYASINGHE, R. D. 2024. Developments and future prospects of personalized medicine in head and neck squamous cell carcinoma diagnoses and treatments. *Cancer Rep (Hoboken)*, 7, e2045.

JIANG, S., LOCATELLO, L. G., MAGGIORE, G., & GALLO, O. 2023. Radiomics-based analysis in the prediction of occult lymph node metastases in patients with oral cancer: A systematic review. *J Clin Med*, 12.

KAJIKAWA, T., KADOYA, N., ITO, K., TAKAYAMA, Y., CHIBA, T., TOMORI, S., NEMOTO, H., DOBASHI, S., TAKEDA, K., & JINGU, K. 2019. A convolutional neural network approach for IMRT dose distribution prediction in prostate cancer patients. *J Radiat Res*, 60, 685–93.

KAMNITSAS, K., LEDIG, C., NEWCOMBE, V. F., SIMPSON, J. P., KANE, A. D., MENON, D. K., RUECKERT, D., & GLOCKER, B. 2017. Efficient multi-scale 3D CNN with fully connected CRF for accurate brain lesion segmentation. *Med Image Anal*, 36, 61–78.

KAUL, R., OSSAI, C., FORKAN, A. R. M., JAYARAMAN, P. P., ZELCER, J., VAUGHAN, S., & WICKRAMASINGHE, N. 2023. The role of AI for developing digital twins in healthcare: The case of cancer care. *IREs Data Mining Knowledge Discovery*, 13, e1480.

KIM, M., YUN, J., CHO, Y., SHIN, K., JANG, R., BAE, H. J., & KIM, N. 2020. Deep learning in medical imaging. *Neurospine*, 17, 471–2.

KOUROU, K., EXARCHOS, T. P., EXARCHOS, K. P., KARAMOUZIS, M. V., & FOTIADIS, D. I. 2015. Machine learning applications in cancer prognosis and prediction. *Comput Struct Biotechnol J*, 13, 8–17.

KRISTENSEN, V. N., LINGJÆRDE, O. C., RUSSNES, H. G., VOLLAN, H. K., FRIGESSI, A., & BØRRESEN-DALE, A. L. 2014. Principles and methods of integrative genomic analyses in cancer. *Nat Rev Cancer*, 14, 299–313.

KUBIK, M. W., SRIDHARAN, S., VARVARES, M. A., ZANDBERG, D. P., SKINNER, H. D., SEETHALA, R. R., & CHIOSEA, S. I. 2020. Intraoperative margin assessment in head and neck cancer: A case of misuse and abuse? *Head Neck Pathol*, 14, 291–302.

LAFFERTY, J. E., NORTH, C. S., SPITZNAGEL, E., & ISENBERG, K. 2001. Laboratory screening prior to ECT. *J ect*, 17, 158–65.

LECUN, Y., BENGIO, Y., & HINTON, G. 2015. Deep learning. *Nature*, 521, 436–44.

LEE, T. F., HSIEH, Y. W., YANG, P. Y., TSENG, C. H., LEE, S. H., YANG, J., CHANG, L., WU, J. M., TSENG, C. D., & CHAO, P. J. 2024. Using meta-analysis and CNN-NLP to review and classify the medical literature for normal tissue complication probability in head and neck cancer. *Radiat Oncol*, 19, 5.

LEEMANS, C. R., SNIJDERS, P. J. F., & BRAKENHOFF, R. H. 2018. The molecular landscape of head and neck cancer. *Nat Rev Cancer*, 18, 269–82.

LIEDES, J., HELLSTRÖM, H., RAINIO, O., MURTOJÄRVI, S., MALASPINA, S., HIRVONEN, J., KLÉN, R., & KEMPPAINEN, J. 2023. Automatic segmentation of head and neck cancer from PET-MRI data using deep learning. *J Med Biol Engineer*, 43, 532–40.

LIM, J. Y., & LEECH, M. 2016. Use of auto-segmentation in the delineation of target volumes and organs at risk in head and neck. *Acta Oncol*, 55, 799–806.

LIN, J., ORESTES, M. I., SHRIVER, C. D., & ZHU, K. 2024. Differences in survival between black and white patients with head and neck squamous cell carcinoma: Comparison of data from the DOD Central Cancer Registry and SEER. *Cancer Epidemiol Biomarkers Prev*, 33, 426–34.

LOCATI, L. D., SERAFINI, M. S., IANNÒ, M. F., CARENZO, A., ORLANDI, E., RESTEGHIN, C., CAVALIERI, S., BOSSI, P., CANEVARI, S., LICITRA, L., & DE CECCO, L. 2019. Mining of self-organizing map gene-expression portraits reveals prognostic stratification of HPV-positive head and neck squamous cell carcinoma. *Cancers (Basel)*, 11.

MAHBOD, A., SCHAEFER, G., LÖW, C., DORFFNER, G., ECKER, R., & ELLINGER, I. 2021. Investigating the impact of the bit depth of fluorescence-stained images on the performance of deep learning-based nuclei instance segmentation. *Diagnostics (Basel)*, 11.

MAHMOOD, H., SHABAN, M., INDAVE, B. I., SANTOS-SILVA, A. R., RAJPOOT, N., & KHURRAM, S. A. 2020. Use of artificial intelligence in diagnosis of head and neck precancerous and cancerous lesions: A systematic review. *Oral Oncol*, 110, 104885.

MAHMOOD, H., SHABAN, M., RAJPOOT, N., & KHURRAM, S. A. 2021. Artificial Intelligence-based methods in head and neck cancer diagnosis: An overview. *Br J Cancer*, 124, 1934–40.

MÄKITIE, A. A., ALABI, R. O., NG, S. P., TAKES, R. P., ROBBINS, K. T., RONEN, O., SHAHA, A. R., BRADLEY, P. J., SABA, N. F., NUYTS, S., TRIANTAFYLLOU, A., PIAZZA, C., RINALDO, A., & FERLITO, A. 2023. Artificial intelligence in head and neck cancer: A systematic review of systematic reviews. *Adv Ther*, 40, 3360–80.

MÄNNLE, D., POHLMANN, J., MONJI-AZAD, S., HESSER, J., ROTTER, N., AFFOLTER, A., LAMMERT, A., KRAMER, B., LUDWIG, S., HUBER, L., & SCHERL, C. 2023. Artificial intelligence directed development of a digital twin to measure soft tissue shift during head and neck surgery. *Plos One*, 18, e0287081.

MANUKIAN, G., BAR-AD, V., LU, B., ARGIRIS, A., & JOHNSON, J. M. 2019. Combining radiation and immune checkpoint blockade in the treatment of head and neck squamous cell carcinoma. *Front Oncol*, 9, 122.

MCINTOSH, C., WELCH, M., MCNIVEN, A., JAFFRAY, D. A., & PURDIE, T. G. 2017. Fully automated treatment planning for head and neck radiotherapy using a voxel-based dose prediction and dose mimicking method. *Phys Med Biol*, 62, 5926–44.

MESHCHERYAKOVA, A., MUNGENAST, F., ECKER, R., & MECHTCHERIAKOVA, D. 2021. *Tissue Image Cytometry. Imaging Modalities for Biological and Preclinical Research: A Compendium, Volume 1: Part I: Ex vivo biological imaging*. Bristol, UK: IOP Publishing.

MICHELUTTI, L., TEL, A., ZEPPIERI, M., IUS, T., SEMBRONIO, S., & ROBIONY, M. 2023. The use of artificial intelligence algorithms in the prognosis and detection of lymph node involvement in head and neck cancer and possible impact in the development of personalized therapeutic strategy: A systematic review. *J Pers Med*, 13.

MILLETARI, F., NAVAB, N., & AHMADI, S.-A. 2016. *V-Net: Fully Convolutional Neural Networks for Volumetric Medical Image Segmentation. 2016 Fourth International Conference On 3D Vision (3DV)*. Washington, DC: IEEE, 565–71.

MOE, Y. M., GROENDAHL, A. R., TOMIC, O., DALE, E., MALINEN, E., & FUTSAETHER, C. M. 2021. Deep learning-based auto-delineation of gross tumour volumes and involved nodes in PET/CT images of head and neck cancer patients. *Eur J Nucl Med Mol Imaging*, 48, 2782–92.

MOMIN, S., FU, Y., LEI, Y., ROPER, J., BRADLEY, J. D., CURRAN, W. J., LIU, T., & YANG, X. 2021. Knowledge-based radiation treatment planning: A data-driven method survey. *J Appl Clin Med Phys*, 22, 16–44.

MÜLLER, V. C., & BOSTROM, N. 2016. Future progress in artificial intelligence: A survey of expert opinion. *Fundamental Issues Artificial Intelligence*, 555–72.

MUNGENAST, F., FERNANDO, A., NICA, R., BOGHIU, B., LUNGU, B., BATRA, J., & ECKER, R. C. 2021. Next-generation digital histopathology of the tumor microenvironment. *Genes (Basel)*, 12.

MURALI, N., KUCUKKAYA, A., PETUKHOVA, A., ONOFREY, J., & CHAPIRO, J. 2020. Supervised machine learning in oncology: A clinician's guide. *Dig Dis Interv*, 4, 73–81.

MUZUMDER, S., SRIKANTIA, N., UDAYASHANKAR, A. H., KAINTHAJE, P. B., & JOHN SEBASTIAN, M. G. 2019. Burden of acute toxicities in head-and-neck radiation therapy: A single-institutional experience. *South Asian J Cancer*, 8, 120–3.

NARKHEDE, S. 2018. Understanding AUC-ROC Curve: Towards Data Science. Available online: https://towardsdatascience.com/understanding-auc-roc-curve-68b2303cc9c5 (accessed on 27 April).

NILSSON, N. J. 1998. *Artificial Intelligence: A New Synthesis*. Burlington, MA: Morgan Kaufmann.

ORLANDI, E., & LICITRA, L. 2018. Personalized medicine and the contradictions and limits of first-generation deescalation trials in patients with human papillomavirus-positive oropharyngeal cancer. *JAMA Otolaryngol Head Neck Surg*, 144, 99–100.

OSMAN, A. F. I., TAMAM, N. M., & YOUSIF, Y. A. M. 2023. A comparative study of deep learning-based knowledge-based planning methods for 3D dose distribution prediction of head and neck. *J Appl Clin Med Phys*, 24, e14015.

PAN, Y. 2007. Image segmentation using PDE, variational, morphological and probabilistic methods. PhD diss., University of Tennessee. https://trace.tennessee.edu/utk_graddiss/261

PARMAR, C., GROSSMANN, P., BUSSINK, J., LAMBIN, P., & AERTS, H. 2015. Machine learning methods for quantitative radiomic biomarkers. *Sci Rep*, 5, 13087.

PHILIP, M. M., WELCH, A., MCKIDDIE, F., & NATH, M. 2023. A systematic review and meta-analysis of predictive and prognostic models for outcome prediction using positron emission tomography radiomics in head and neck squamous cell carcinoma patients. *Cancer Med*, 12, 16181–94.

POON, A. I. F., & SUNG, J. J. Y. 2021. Opening the black box of AI-Medicine. *J Gastroenterol Hepatol*, 36, 581–4.

PREETHA, M. M. S. J., SURESH, L. P., & BOSCO, M. J. 2012. *Image segmentation using seeded region growing. 2012 International Conference on Computing, Electronics and Electrical Technologies (ICCEET).* Washington, DC: IEEE, 576–83.

RESTEGHINI, C., TRAMA, A., BORGONOVI, E., HOSNI, H., CORRAO, G., ORLANDI, E., CALARESO, G., DE CECCO, L., PIAZZA, C., MAINARDI, L., & LICITRA, L. 2018. Big data in head and neck cancer. *Curr Treat Options Oncol*, 19, 62.

RIEGEL, A. C., BERSON, A. M., DESTIAN, S., NG, T., TENA, L. B., MITNICK, R. J., & WONG, P. S. 2006. Variability of gross tumor volume delineation in head-and-neck cancer using CT and PET/CT fusion. *Int J Radiat Oncol Biol Phys*, 65, 726–32.

RIGAUD, B., ANDERSON, B. M., YU, Z. H., GOBELI, M., CAZOULAT, G., SÖDERBERG, J., SAMUELSSON, E., LIDBERG, D., WARD, C., TAKU, N., CARDENAS, C., RHEE, D. J., VENKATESAN, A. M., PETERSON, C. B., COURT, L., SVENSSON, S., LÖFMAN, F., KLOPP, A. H., & BROCK, K. K. 2021. Automatic segmentation using deep learning to enable online dose optimization during adaptive radiation therapy of cervical cancer. *Int J Radiat Oncol Biol Phys*, 109, 1096–110.

RONNEBERGER, O., FISCHER, P., & BROX, T. 2015. U-net: Convolutional networks for biomedical image segmentation. Medical image computing and computer–assisted intervention–MICCAI 2015: 18th international conference, Munich, Germany, October 5–9, 2015, proceedings, part III 18. Berlin: Springer, 234–41.

SANTOS, A. G., DA ROCHA, G. O., & DE ANDRADE, J. B. 2019. Occurrence of the potent mutagens 2- nitrobenzanthrone and 3-nitrobenzanthrone in fine airborne particles. *Sci Rep*, 9, 1.

SCHLUMPF, M. F., & HAERLE, S. 2014. The current role of imaging in head and neck cancer: A clinician's perspective. *Swiss Med Wkly*, 144, w14015.

SHEIKH, K., LEE, S. H., CHENG, Z., LAKSHMINARAYANAN, P., PENG, L., HAN, P., MCNUTT, T. R., QUON, H., & LEE, J. 2019. Predicting acute radiation induced xerostomia in head and neck Cancer using MR and CT radiomics of parotid and submandibular glands. *Radiat Oncol*, 14, 131.

SHEN, D., WU, G., & SUK, H. I. 2017. Deep learning in medical image analysis. *Annu Rev Biomed Eng*, 19, 221–48.

SHIRAISHI, K., NAKAGAWA, K., YAMASHITA, H., NAKAMURA, N., TAGO, M., & OHTOMO, K. 2006. Treatment planning and dosimetry of a multi-axis dynamic arc technique for prostate cancer: A comparison with IMRT. *Radiat Med*, 24, 17–22.

SLIZ, J., & MIKULKA, J. 2016. Advanced image segmentation methods using partial differential equations: A concise comparison. *2016 Progress in Electromagnetic Research Symposium (PIERS)*, Shanghai, China, 1809–12.

TONELLA, L., GIANNOCCARO, M., ALFIERI, S., CANEVARI, S., & DE CECCO, L. 2017. Gene expression signatures for head and neck cancer patient stratification: Are results ready for clinical application? *Curr Treat Options Oncol*, 18, 32.

TOSADO, J., ZDILAR, L., ELHALAWANI, H., ELGOHARI, B., VOCK, D. M., MARAI, G. E., FULLER, C., MOHAMED, A. S. R., & CANAHUATE, G. 2020. Clustering of largely right-censored oropharyngeal head and neck cancer patients for discriminative groupings to improve outcome prediction. *Sci Rep*, 10, 3811.

TSHERING VOGEL, D. W., & THOENY, H. C. 2016. Cross-sectional imaging in cancers of the head and neck: How we review and report. *Cancer Imaging*, 16, 20.

VALDES, G., CHAN, M. F., LIM, S. B., SCHEUERMANN, R., DEASY, J. O., & SOLBERG, T. D. 2017. IMRT QA using machine learning: A multi-institutional validation. *J Appl Clin Med Phys*, 18, 279–84.

VALLE, D., LIMA, J. M., MILLAR, J., AMRATIA, P., & HAQUE, U. 2015. Bias in logistic regression due to imperfect diagnostic test results and practical correction approaches. *Malar J*, 14, 434.

VAN DER VEEN, J., GULYBAN, A., & NUYTS, S. 2019. Interobserver variability in delineation of target volumes in head and neck cancer. *Radiother Oncol*, 137, 9–15.

VOGIN, G., HETTAL, L., BARTAU, C., THARIAT, J., CLAEYS, M. V., PEYRAGA, G., RETIF, P., SCHICK, U., ANTONI, D., BODGAL, Z., DHERMAIN, F., & FEUVRET, L. 2021. Cranial organs at risk delineation: Heterogenous practices in radiotherapy planning. *Radiat Oncol*, 16, 26.

WANG, W., WANG, W., ZHANG, D., ZENG, P., WANG, Y., LEI, M., HONG, Y., & CAI, C. 2024. Creation of a machine learning-based prognostic prediction model for various subtypes of laryngeal cancer. *Sci Rep*, 14, 6484.

XUE, J., LI, B., WANG, Y., HUANG, Z., LIU, X., GUO, C., ZHENG, Z., LIANG, N., LE, X., & LI, S. 2022. Efficacy and safety of epidermal growth factor receptor (EGFR)-tyrosine kinase inhibitor combination therapy as first-line treatment for patients with advanced EGFR-mutated, non-small cell lung cancer: A systematic review and bayesian network meta-analysis. *Cancers (Basel)*, 14.

ZHANG, Y. P., ZHANG, X. Y., CHENG, Y. T., LI, B., TENG, X. Z., ZHANG, J., LAM, S., ZHOU, T., MA, Z. R., SHENG, J. B., TAM, V. C. W., LEE, S. W. Y., GE, H., & CAI, J. 2023. Artificial intelligence-driven radiomics study in cancer: The role of feature engineering and modeling. *Mil Med Res*, 10, 22.

ZHAO, L. M., ZHANG, H., KIM, D. D., GHIMIRE, K., HU, R., KARGILIS, D. C., TANG, L., MENG, S., CHEN, Q., LIAO, W. H., BAI, H., JIAO, Z., & FENG, X. 2023. Head and neck tumor segmentation convolutional neural network robust to missing PET/CT modalities using channel dropout. *Phys Med Biol*, 68.

ZIEMER, B. P., SHIRAISHI, S., HATTANGADI-GLUTH, J. A., SANGHVI, P., & MOORE, K. L. 2017. Fully automated, comprehensive knowledge-based planning for stereotactic radiosurgery: Preclinical validation through blinded physician review. *Pract Radiat Oncol*, 7, e569–78.

SECTION V
GLOBAL PERSPECTIVES

15
Pediatric Head and Neck Cancers
Challenges with Detection and Treatment

Zukile Mbita, Lloyd Mabonga, Nelisiwe Prenate Masuku, Thabang Marema, Ellen Mabunda, Ngoakoana Mahlachana, Ian C. Chikanza, and Zodwa Dlamini

15.1 Introduction

Pediatric head and neck cancers (HNCs) refer to a variety of tumors that occur in the head and neck regions of children ages 0–21 years. They are a diverse group of rare malignancies that pose significant challenges in both detection and treatment (Arboleda et al., 2020). Unlike their adult counterparts, these cancers require specialized approaches due to the distinct biological, developmental, and clinical characteristics of pediatric patients. Addressing these issues requires a nuanced approach to ensure accurate diagnosis, effective treatment, and minimal long-term impact on young patients (Lopez & Tufaro, 2024). Over the years the number of pediatric HNC cases has been on the rise, with related survival rates that are often poor in Africa. According to Force and coworkers, 100,000 new diagnoses of pediatric HNCs are reported per year in Africa (Force et al., 2019). Unlike in most developed countries where pediatric HNCs are manageable, in Africa, > 80% of these children have no access to curative treatment (Hadley et al., 2012). Worldwide, pediatric HNCs have become one of the main contributing causes of death among children. Pediatric HNCs comprise 2–15% of all cancer cases in the pediatric population (Arboleda et al., 2020, 2022).

Although HNCs are mostly prevalent among adults and thought to be extremely uncommon in children, the increased number of cases of HNC in children is due to challenges such as lack of information and experienced personnel in the diagnosis, treatment, and management of the condition (Hashim et al., 2019). Moreover, the initial symptoms of HNCs in children can be ambiguous, making it challenging to identify these illnesses and resulting in delayed diagnosis. Conversely, children with noncancerous (benign) conditions may undergo unnecessary tests or surgeries to exclude the possibility of malignancy (Lilja-Fischer et al., 2019). The primary risk factors for the rising incidence in this population are believed to be environmental and treatment-related exposures, which include exposure to ionizing radiation, excessive sun/ultraviolet (UV) radiation exposure, certain chemotherapeutic agents, environmental pollutions, parental contact with various toxins, infectious agents (though the evidence is not definitive), genetic disorders, and viral infections such as human papillomavirus (especially HPV16) and Epstein-Barr virus (EBV). However, the diversity seen in pediatric HNCs makes it challenging to identify specific causes (Cesmebasi et al.,2014; Lopez & Tufaro, 2024).

The diagnostic process for pediatric HNC is made more complicated by various factors such as age-related differences and challenges in diagnostic imaging, tissue sampling, and biopsy. The differences in anatomy and physiology between children and adults can allow tumors to appear in an atypical manner, making the diagnosis process difficult. In some children, tumors may not be noticeable or may have unusual symptoms due to their smaller size (Figaji, 2023; Pfister et al., 2021). Additionally, most childhood tumors develop from the mesoderm or neuroectoderm, while most adult tumors originate from epithelial tissue (Ward et al., 2014). The diagnosis of pediatric HNCs through imaging is unique due to age-related anatomical differences, efforts to minimize radiation exposure, and the utilization of imaging protocols suitable for children. Important imaging techniques such as magnetic resonance imaging (MRI), computed tomography (CT) scans, and ultrasound are crucial for diagnosing these types of pediatric HNCs, but the techniques must be tailored to fit the individual needs of the children in order to accurately diagnose and plan treatment (Figaji, 2023).

Tumor biopsies form the core of pediatric HNC diagnosis and treatment; as such, they are an important component of personalized and directed cancer medicine (Pfister et al., 2021). Tissue samples are typically needed for biopsy to confirm the diagnosis of pediatric HNC through histological examination. However, the operator performing the biopsies is required to have enough experience to obtain adequate tissue while at the same time minimizing potential risks and complications associated with the procedures (Lopez & Tufaro, 2024; Ward et al., 2014).

There are a vast number of different pediatric HNCs, and all require unique handling, whether for diagnosis or treatment. This chapter explores the unique challenges and advancements in the diagnosis and treatment of different types of pediatric HNCs (Lopez & Tufaro, 2024).

15.2 Various Pediatric Head and Neck Cancers and Their Handling

The most prevalent pediatric HNCs include lymphoma (Hodgkin [HL] and non-Hodgkin [NHL]), rhabdomyosarcoma (RMS), thyroid malignances, nasopharyngeal carcinoma (NPC), neuroblastoma, non-rhabdomyosarcoma soft-tissue sarcoma (NRSTS), salivary gland malignances, and malignant teratoma (Figure 15.1) (Orr et al., 2024). Lymphomas, including HL and NHL, are common pediatric HNCs originating from lymphoid tissues. The most common soft-tissue sarcoma in children, frequently affecting the head and neck region, is rhabdomyosarcoma. It arises from skeletal muscle progenitors (Lopez & Tufaro, 2024). Pediatric thyroid carcinoma, primarily differentiated thyroid cancer (papillary and follicular types), is relatively rare but has a generally favorable prognosis. NPC is rare in children but is more common in certain geographic regions (e.g., Southeast Asia) (Lopez & Tufaro, 2024). Salivary gland tumors are rare in children, with pleomorphic adenoma being the most common benign type and mucoepidermoid carcinoma the most common malignant type. Other malignancies, such as neuroendocrine tumors, various soft-tissue sarcomas, cutaneous tumors, and metastases, occasionally express in the head and neck region (Lopez & Tufaro, 2024).

Neuroblastoma is the most common extracranial solid tumor in children, arising from neural crest cells. While it typically occurs in the adrenal glands, about 5–15% of cases involve the head and neck region, particularly the paraspinal sympathetic ganglia (Gerges & Canning, 2024). NRSTS encompasses a diverse group of soft-tissue malignancies that occur less frequently than rhabdomyosarcoma in children. These tumors include fibrosarcoma, malignant peripheral nerve sheath tumors, and synovial sarcoma. Malignant teratomas are germ cell tumors that can contain tissues from all three germ layers (Ferrari et al., 2024). In the head and neck region, they are rare and often present in the cervical area. An exhaustive and comprehensive overview of these cancers is beyond the scope of this chapter, but Table 15.1 provides an overview of the most common types of pediatric HNCs and discusses the handling of each, from diagnosis to treatment and follow-up care. The rarity of these cancers limits the availability of pediatric-specific clinical trials, resulting in the frequent adaptation of adult treatment protocols that may not always be optimal for children (Orr et al., 2024). Additionally, the absence of established screening protocols and the need for advanced diagnostic imaging further complicate early detection. Treatment approaches must consider the developmental stage of pediatric patients to minimize long-term impacts on growth and organ function (Lopez & Tufaro, 2024).

Pediatric HNCs, though rare, require specialized diagnostic and treatment approaches tailored to the unique needs of children. The management of pediatric HNCs such as neuroblastoma, NRSTS, and malignant teratoma involves a multidisciplinary approach fitted to the specific characteristics of each tumor type (Ferrari et al., 2024). Early and accurate diagnosis is crucial, often involving advanced imaging and biopsy techniques. Treatment strategies that minimize long-term side effects must balance effective cancer control while facilitating

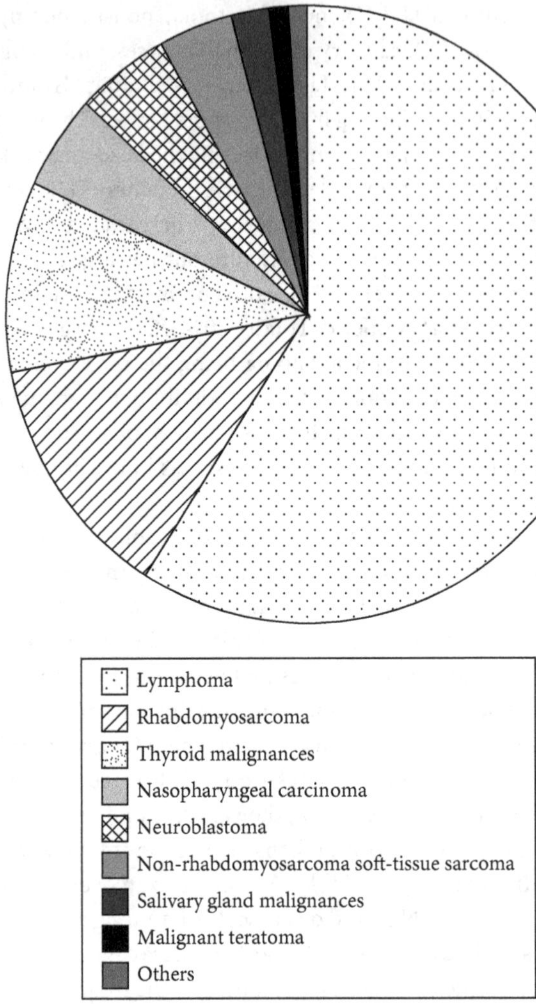

Figure 15.1 Pediatric head and neck malignancies. Pediatric head and neck cancers (HNCs) represent a rare and diverse group of malignancies that pose significant challenges in both detection and treatment. Due to their low incidence, symptoms often mimic benign conditions, leading to misdiagnosis and delays in identification. The most common pediatric HNCs include lymphoma (59%), rhabdomyosarcoma (13%), thyroid malignancies (10%), nasopharyngeal carcinoma (5%), neuroblastoma (5%), non-rhabdomyosarcoma soft-tissue sarcoma (4.5%), salivary gland malignancies (2.5%), malignant teratoma (1%) and others (1%).

Table 15.1 Common pediatric head and neck cancers and their handling

Pediatric HNC	Symptoms	Diagnosis	Treatment	References
Lymphomas	Painless lymphadenopathy, systemic symptoms (fever, weight loss, night sweats), and, in some cases, airway obstruction.	Diagnosis is confirmed through lymph node biopsy, immunophenotyping, and staging with positron emission tomography fluorodeoxyglucose computed tomography (PET FDG-CT) scans.	Chemotherapy: Multiagent chemotherapy regimens are the mainstay of treatment. For HL, protocols like ABVD (adriamycin, bleomycin, vinblastine, dacarbazine) are common. Radiation therapy: Radiation may be used for localized disease or residual masses post-chemotherapy. Follow-up: Long-term follow-up includes monitoring for relapse and managing treatment-related complications, such as cardiac and pulmonary toxicity.	Lopez & Tufaro, 2024
Rhabdomyosarcoma	Symptoms vary depending on the tumor's location but often include a palpable mass, swelling, and pain. Tumors in the orbit can cause proptosis and vision changes, while those in the nasopharynx may lead to nasal obstruction and epistaxis	Diagnosis is typically confirmed through imaging studies (MRI, CT scans) and biopsy. Immunohistochemistry and molecular testing (e.g., PAX3-FOXO1 fusion gene) are crucial for subclassification.	Surgery: Complete surgical resection is the goal but may be limited by the tumor's location and proximity to critical structures. Chemotherapy: Multi-agent chemotherapy is standard, often including vincristine, actinomycin D, and cyclophosphamide. Radiation therapy: Radiation is used for residual disease post-surgery or when surgical resection is not feasible. Follow-up: Long-term follow-up is necessary to monitor for recurrence and manage late effects of treatment, such as growth abnormalities and secondary malignancies.	Orr et al., 2024

(*continued*)

Table 15.1 Continued

Pediatric HNC	Symptoms	Diagnosis	Treatment	References
Thyroid carcinoma	Symptoms include a palpable thyroid nodule, neck swelling, and, less commonly, hoarseness or dysphagia.	Fine-needle aspiration biopsy (FNAB) is used for initial evaluation. Ultrasound and thyroid function tests aid in diagnosis and staging with PET FDG-CT scans.	Surgery: Total thyroidectomy is the standard treatment for most cases, followed by radioactive iodine ablation if indicated. Thyroid hormone suppression therapy: Lifelong thyroid hormone replacement therapy is required post-thyroidectomy to suppress TSH and reduce recurrence risk. Follow-up: Regular follow-up includes monitoring thyroid function and imaging to detect recurrence or metastasis.	Lopez & Tufaro, 2024
Nasopharyngeal carcinoma	Symptoms include nasal obstruction, epistaxis, hearing loss, and cervical lymphadenopathy.	Diagnosis is established through nasopharyngeal biopsy and imaging studies (MRI, CT). Epstein-Barr virus (EBV) serology can be supportive.	Radiation therapy: Primary treatment is radiation therapy, often combined with chemotherapy for advanced stages. Chemotherapy: Multiagent regimens, typically including cisplatin, are used concurrently with radiation or as adjuvant therapy. Follow-up: Follow-up includes regular imaging and Epstein-Barr Virus (EBV) serology to monitor for recurrence.	Shah & Nagalli, 2024
Salivary gland tumors	Symptoms include a painless mass in the parotid or submandibular gland, facial nerve palsy, and, in malignant cases, rapid growth and fixation.	Diagnosis is made through FNAB or core biopsy and imaging studies (ultrasound, MRI).	Surgery: Complete surgical resection is the primary treatment for both benign and malignant tumors. Radiation therapy: Postoperative radiation may be indicated for high-grade malignancies or incomplete resection. Follow-up: Regular follow-up is necessary to monitor for recurrence and manage any functional deficits, such as facial nerve dysfunction.	Young et al., 2024

Neuroblastoma	Symptoms vary based on the tumor's location and may include a palpable mass, Horner's syndrome (ptosis, miosis, anhidrosis), and, in some cases, respiratory distress or dysphagia due to compression of adjacent structures.	Imaging: MRI is preferred for assessing soft-tissue tumors, with CT scans used for additional detail. Biopsy: Core needle biopsy or surgical biopsy provides definitive histological diagnosis. Histopathological and molecular analysis: Detailed analysis, including immunohistochemistry and molecular studies, aids in subclassification and treatment planning.	Surgery: Complete surgical excision with clear margins is the primary treatment for localized NRSTS. Chemotherapy: Chemotherapy is used selectively, often for high-grade or metastatic disease. Regimens are tailored to the specific subtype of NRSTS. Radiation therapy: Radiation therapy is employed for local control, especially when surgical margins are inadequate or for inoperable tumors. Follow-up: Long-term follow-up includes regular imaging to monitor for recurrence and management of treatment-related side effects, such as fibrosis and secondary malignancies.	Gerges & Canning, 2024
Non-rhabdomyosarcoma soft-tissue sarcoma (NRSTS)	Symptoms depend on the tumor's location and may include a painless mass, localized pain, and functional impairment due to compression of nearby structures.	Imaging: MRI is preferred for assessing soft-tissue tumors, with CT scans used for additional detail. Biopsy: Core needle biopsy or surgical biopsy provides definitive histological diagnosis. Histopathological and molecular analysis: Detailed analysis, including immunohistochemistry and molecular studies, aids in subclassification and treatment planning.	Surgery: Complete surgical excision with clear margins is the primary treatment for localized NRSTS. Chemotherapy: Chemotherapy is used selectively, often for high-grade or metastatic disease. Regimens are tailored to the specific subtype of NRSTS. Radiation therapy: Radiation therapy is employed for local control, especially when surgical margins are inadequate or for inoperable tumors. Follow-up: Long-term follow-up includes regular imaging to monitor for recurrence and management of treatment-related side effects, such as fibrosis and secondary malignancies.	Ferrari et al., 2024

(*continued*)

Table 15.1 Continued

Pediatric HNC	Symptoms	Diagnosis	Treatment	References
Malignant teratoma	Symptoms include a neck mass, respiratory distress, dysphagia, and, occasionally, signs of Horner syndrome.	Imaging: MRI and CT scans are used to assess the extent of the tumor and its relationship to adjacent structures. Biopsy: Tissue biopsy confirms the diagnosis and allows for histological examination. Tumor markers: Serum levels of α-fetoprotein (AFP) and β-human chorionic gonadotropin (β-HCG) may be elevated and are useful for diagnosis and monitoring.	Surgery: Complete surgical resection is the primary treatment, aiming to remove all visible tumor tissue. Chemotherapy: Chemotherapy is used for malignant teratomas, particularly those with metastatic disease or incomplete resection. Common agents include cisplatin, etoposide, and bleomycin. Radiation therapy: Radiation therapy is generally reserved for cases where surgical resection is incomplete or for recurrent disease. Follow-up: Regular follow-up is essential to monitor recurrence through imaging and serum tumor marker levels. Long-term monitoring is also required to manage potential late effects of treatment.	Ferrari et al., 2024

the preservation of growth and development, utilizing a multidisciplinary approach that includes surgery, chemotherapy, radiation therapy, and comprehensive psychosocial support (Lopez & Tufaro, 2024). Comprehensive follow-up care is vital for monitoring recurrence and managing the late effects of treatment, ensuring the best possible outcomes and quality of life for young patients (Ferrari et al., 2024). And ongoing research and clinical trials are essential to refine these approaches and improve the prognosis and quality of life for children with these rare cancers.

15.3 Lymphomas

The detection and treatment of lymphomas are fraught with challenges, from the initial presentation and diagnostic work-up to the management of complex multimodal therapies and long-term survivorship issues (El-Mallawany et al., 2023; Mogensen et al., 2024). There are numerous subtypes of lymphoma, each with distinct histopathological and molecular features. Accurate diagnosis requires comprehensive pathological assessment, often involving immunohistochemistry and molecular studies (Britto et al., 2023). Obtaining an adequate biopsy sample can be difficult, particularly for deep-seated or small lymph nodes. Fine-needle aspiration (FNA) may not provide sufficient tissue for definitive diagnosis, necessitating excisional biopsy. Lymphomas can present in virtually any organ, resulting in a wide range of symptoms. For example, gastrointestinal involvement may cause abdominal pain, while central nervous system involvement may present neurological symptoms (El-Mallawany et al., 2023). Indolent lymphomas often grow slowly and may be asymptomatic for years, while aggressive lymphomas grow rapidly and require immediate attention, complicating the detection timeline (Britto et al., 2023; Mogensen et al., 2024). Staging involves imaging studies such as CT, positron emission tomography (PET), and MRI scans, which may not always clearly delineate disease extent, especially in areas like bone marrow or the central nervous system. Detecting bone marrow involvement requires biopsy, which is invasive and may miss focal disease due to sampling error (Britto et al., 2023; El-Mallawany et al., 2023).

Chemotherapy is a cornerstone of lymphoma treatment but comes with significant toxicity, including myelosuppression, infection risk, organ damage (e.g., cardiotoxicity, nephrotoxicity), and secondary malignancies (Britto et al., 2023). Children with comorbidities may have difficulty tolerating aggressive chemotherapy regimens, requiring dose adjustments that can compromise efficacy (Mogensen et al., 2024). Radiation therapy, especially when used in pediatric patients or young adults, can lead to long-term complications such as secondary cancers, cardiovascular disease, and endocrine dysfunction. Specific organs, such as the heart and lungs, are particularly sensitive to radiation, necessitating careful planning to minimize exposure (Tian et al., 2024). Lymphomas may develop resistance to targeted therapies (e.g., rituximab, a monoclonal antibody targeting CD20), thus requiring combination or sequential therapies. Targeted therapies can be expensive and may not be readily accessible to all patients, especially in low-resource settings (Britto et al., 2023). Immunotherapies, such as checkpoint inhibitors, can cause significant immune-related adverse events (e.g., colitis, pneumonitis) that require careful management. Not all lymphoma patients respond to immunotherapy, and predictive biomarkers for response are not fully established (El-Mallawany et al., 2023). Allogeneic stem cell transplantation, while potentially curative for some lymphomas, carries risks of graft-versus-host disease (GVHD) and transplant-related mortality. Autologous stem cell transplant relies on the patient's own stem cells and may be less effective for aggressive or refractory disease (Klimentova et al., 2024). Some lymphomas relapse after initial therapy or are refractory to treatment, requiring novel therapeutic strategies and clinical trial participation. Options for relapsed or refractory lymphoma can be limited and may involve more intensive regimens with higher toxicity (Tian et al., 2024).

The diagnosis and treatment of lymphoma significantly impact patients' quality of life, necessitating comprehensive supportive care, including psychological support and management of treatment-related side effects. Long-term survivors face ongoing health challenges, including monitoring for late effects of treatment and managing chronic health conditions (Mogensen et al., 2024).

HL, despite being one of the more treatable cancers, with its high cure rates, presents several challenges in both its detection and treatment. These range from the nonspecific nature of early symptoms and the complexities of accurate diagnosis and staging to the management of acute and long-term treatment-related toxicities and the need for ongoing surveillance (Mogensen et al., 2024). The heterogeneity of NHL presents numerous challenges in its detection and treatment stemming from its diverse clinical presentations, histological complexity, and the side effects of multimodal therapies (Tian et al., 2024). Table 15.2 and Table 15.3 summarize in detail the challenges in the detection and treatment of HL and NHL. Addressing these issues requires a comprehensive, multidisciplinary approach that incorporates advancements in diagnostic techniques, novel therapeutic strategies, and robust supportive care systems to optimize outcomes and improve the quality of life for patients with HL and NHL (Klimentova et al., 2024). Despite recent significant advances in medical technology and therapeutic approaches, these detection and treatment challenges remain. Continued research into the molecular underpinnings of lymphomas and the development of personalized treatment approaches hold promise for overcoming these obstacles and enhancing patient care (Britto et al., 2023).

Table 15.2 Challenges with detection and treatment of Hodgkin lymphoma

Detection challenges		
Nonspecific initial symptoms	General symptoms	Early symptoms of HL, such as persistent fatigue, fever, night sweats, and weight loss, are non-specific and can be easily mistaken for benign conditions like viral infections or autoimmune diseases.
	B symptoms	These systemic symptoms (fever, night sweats, and weight loss) often indicate advanced disease and may be absent in early stages, delaying diagnosis.
Lymphadenopathy	Painless lymph node enlargement	Swelling of lymph nodes is a common sign but can be painless and unnoticed by patients. Enlarged nodes are often initially attributed to infections or other benign causes, delaying further investigation.
	Deep-seated nodes	Lymph nodes deep within the chest or abdomen can enlarge without causing noticeable symptoms, leading to diagnostic delays until they cause significant complications, such as breathing difficulties or abdominal pain.
Imaging and biopsy challenges	Initial assessment	Initial imaging studies like chest X-rays, CT scans, and PET scans are crucial but can sometimes fail to distinguish HL from other malignancies or benign conditions, necessitating further diagnostic procedures.
	Biopsy complexity	Accurate diagnosis requires an excisional biopsy of an affected lymph node to confirm the presence of Reed-Sternberg cells, the hallmark of HL. Fine-needle aspiration (FNA) may not provide sufficient tissue for a definitive diagnosis.
Histopathological variability	Subtypes of hl	HL has different subtypes (e.g., classical HL, nodular lymphocyte-predominant HL), each with distinct histopathological features. Misclassification can occur, impacting treatment decisions and prognosis.
Staging difficulties	Comprehensive staging	Accurate staging is critical for treatment planning. It involves multiple imaging modalities and sometimes bone marrow biopsies, which are invasive and can be uncomfortable for patients.
	Detection of small disease sites	Small or early-stage disease sites may be missed by imaging, leading to under-staging and potential under-treatment.

(*continued*)

Table 15.2 Continued

Treatment challenges		
Chemotherapy toxicity	Acute side effects	Common chemotherapy regimens for HL, such as ABVD (doxorubicin, bleomycin, vinblastine, and dacarbazine), can cause acute toxicities including myelosuppression, nausea, vomiting, and risk of infections.
	Long-term effects	Long-term toxicities include cardiotoxicity, pulmonary toxicity (especially from bleomycin), and secondary malignancies, which can emerge years after treatment completion.
Radiation therapy complications	Secondary cancers	Radiation therapy, while effective, increases the risk of secondary cancers, particularly breast and lung cancer, in long-term survivors.
	Organ damage	Radiation can cause damage to nearby organs, such as the heart, lungs, and thyroid gland, leading to long-term health issues.
Treatment resistance and relapse	Primary refractory disease	Some patients do not respond to initial therapy (primary refractory disease), requiring more aggressive and experimental treatments.
	Relapse	HL can relapse after initial remission, necessitating salvage therapies that are often more toxic and less effective.
Stem cell transplantation	Autologous transplant	High-dose chemotherapy followed by autologous stem cell transplantation (ASCT) is a common approach for relapsed or refractory HL, but it comes with significant risks, including infection, bleeding, and organ toxicity.
	Allogeneic transplant	Allogeneic stem cell transplantation (allo-SCT) may be considered for patients who relapse after ASCT, but it carries a high risk of graft-versus-host disease (GVHD) and transplant-related mortality.
Pediatric and young adult considerations	Developmental impact	Pediatric and young adult patients face unique challenges, including the impact of treatment on growth, fertility, and psychological well-being.
	Long-term monitoring	Lifelong monitoring for late effects of treatment is necessary, which can be burdensome and anxiety-inducing for survivors.
Access to care and disparities	Geographic disparities	Access to advanced diagnostic and treatment facilities can be limited by geographic location, with rural or underserved areas facing significant barriers.
	Socioeconomic factors	Socioeconomic status can impact the ability to afford treatment, access supportive care, and adhere to long-term follow-up protocols.

Source: Keller et al., 2023.

Table 15.3 Challenges with detection and treatment of non-Hodgkin lymphoma (NHL)

Detection challenges		
Diverse clinical presentation	Varied symptoms	NHL can present with a wide range of symptoms depending on the subtype and the sites involved. Common symptoms include lymphadenopathy, fever, night sweats, weight loss, and fatigue, which are non-specific and can lead to misdiagnosis or delayed diagnosis.
	Extranodal involvement	NHL can affect extranodal sites (e.g., gastrointestinal tract, skin, central nervous system), leading to symptoms that may mimic other diseases and complicate the diagnostic process.
Histological and molecular heterogeneity	Subtypes of nhl	There are many subtypes of NHL, each with distinct histological, immunophenotypic, and genetic features. Accurate classification is essential for appropriate treatment planning but requires advanced diagnostic techniques and expertise.
	Complex diagnosis	Diagnosis often involves a combination of histopathology, immunohistochemistry, flow cytometry, and molecular genetic testing, which can be resource-intensive and may not be readily available in all healthcare settings.
Diagnostic procedures:	Biopsy requirements	Adequate tissue biopsy is crucial for diagnosis, but obtaining a sufficient sample can be challenging, especially for deep-seated or small lesions. Fine-needle aspiration (FNA) may be inadequate, necessitating core needle or excisional biopsy.
	Sampling error	In cases of multifocal disease, a single biopsy may not be representative of the entire disease, leading to potential underdiagnosis or misclassification.
Staging difficulties	Accurate staging	Staging NHL involves comprehensive imaging (e.g., CT, PET/CT) and sometimes bone marrow biopsy to assess the extent of disease. Small or occult lesions can be missed, impacting treatment decisions.
	Bone marrow involvement	Detecting bone marrow involvement can be challenging and may require multiple biopsy sites to confirm.

(continued)

Table 15.3 Continued

Slow-growing vs. Aggressive forms	Indolent lymphomas	Indolent (slow-growing) lymphomas may be asymptomatic for years and are often diagnosed incidentally or at an advanced stage.
	Aggressive lymphomas	Aggressive forms of NHL can progress rapidly and present with acute symptoms, requiring urgent diagnostic and therapeutic intervention.
	Treatment challenges	
Chemotherapy toxicity	Acute side effects	Chemotherapy regimens for NHL, such as CHOP (cyclophosphamide, doxorubicin, vincristine, and prednisone), are associated with significant side effects, including myelosuppression, nausea, vomiting, and increased infection risk.
	Long-term effects	Long-term toxicities include cardiotoxicity, neurotoxicity, and secondary malignancies, which necessitate ongoing monitoring and management.
Radiation therapy complications	Secondary cancers	Radiation therapy increases the risk of secondary cancers and long-term organ damage, particularly in younger patients or those receiving high-dose radiation.
	Organ sensitivity	Specific organs, such as the lungs, heart, and thyroid, are particularly sensitive to radiation damage, necessitating careful planning to minimize exposure.
Targeted therapy and resistance	Development of resistance	Targeted therapies, such as rituximab (an anti-CD20 monoclonal antibody), can initially be effective but may eventually lead to resistance, requiring alternative or combination therapies.
	Side effects	Targeted therapies have their own side effect profiles, including infusion reactions, cytopenias, and increased risk of infections.
Immunotherapy challenges	Immune-related adverse events	Immunotherapies, such as checkpoint inhibitors, can cause significant immune-related adverse events (e.g., colitis, pneumonitis), requiring careful management and sometimes discontinuation of therapy.
	Variable response	Not all patients respond to immunotherapy, and the identification of predictive biomarkers for response is an ongoing area of research.

Table 15.3 Continued

Stem cell transplantation	Transplant-related mortality	Autologous and allogeneic stem cell transplantation are options for relapsed or refractory NHL but carry significant risks, including graft-versus-host disease (GVHD) and transplant-related mortality.
	Eligibility	Not all patients are eligible for transplantation due to age, comorbidities, or disease characteristics, limiting its use.
Management of relapsed/refractory disease	Limited options	Treatment options for relapsed or refractory NHL are often limited and may involve more intensive regimens with higher toxicity.
	Salvage therapies	Salvage therapies, such as second-line chemotherapy, targeted agents, or CAR-T cell therapy, can be effective but are not universally accessible and may have significant side effects.
Psychosocial and quality of life issues	Impact on quality of life	The diagnosis and treatment of NHL significantly impact patients' quality of life, necessitating comprehensive supportive care, including psychological support and management of treatment-related side effects.
	Survivorship issues	Long-term survivors face ongoing health challenges, including monitoring for late effects of treatment and managing chronic health conditions

Source: Sapkota & Shaikh, 2023.

15.4 Rhabdomyosarcoma

The detection and treatment of RMS in children presents numerous challenges, from the initial identification of the disease to the management of complex multimodal treatment regimens (Harrison et al., 2024; Zarrabi et al., 2023). RMS can present with a wide range of symptoms that are often nonspecific and can be mistaken for benign conditions such as infections or inflammatory processes. This variability can lead to misdiagnosis or delays in diagnosis (Harrison et al., 2024). Symptoms like swelling, pain, and a localized mass can easily be confused with more common pediatric conditions, delaying further investigative steps. The head and neck region is anatomically complex, and tumors in this area can be difficult to detect and accurately diagnose due to their deep location and the presence of numerous critical structures (Carmo et al., 2023). Tumors can affect crucial functions such as vision, breathing, and swallowing, thus complicating early detection. Unlike some adult cancers, there are no established early routine screening programs for RMS, especially in asymptomatic children, making early detection reliant on clinical suspicion and prompt investigation of symptoms (Harrison et al., 2024; Zarrabi et al., 2023).

Conventional anatomic imaging techniques such as CT and MRI are useful methods for detecting RMS in pediatric patients. They are useful in capturing images of tissues, organs, and bones and are extensively used diagnostic tools for detecting or identifying injuries, tumors, diseases, or disorders inside the body (Arora et al., 2022). CT images are generated from a series of x-ray acquisitions taken from a gantry that moves completely around the patient. The image's header contains parameters that direct the capture and then reconstruction of data collected by the CT scanner into the final image. These include the distance between the slices (1 mm to 1 cm), resolution (0.5 mm^2), and filter (Carmo et al., 2023).

MRI employs a magnetic field to produce its images of tissues. MRIs are important in the medical field because they are considered safe and noninvasive, and they provide a quick way to examine the inner structures of the body (Carmo et al., 2023). MRI offers several advantages over CT scanning. MRI can be performed without ionizing radiation and contrast agents to generate images. It can provide anatomical details in multiple planes including transaxial, sagittal, and coronal. In addition, MRI is superior to CT in showing differences between tumors and normal tissues (Chang et al., 1987). Additionally, MRI is used to diagnose tumors, describe their connection with nearby tissues or organs, and detect spread to distant parts of the body (Carmo et al., 2023).

The disadvantages of MRIs include cost-effectiveness as well as longer scan times (depending on the tumor site) due to the number of images captured to generate a 3D picture for the radiologist to examine (Chang et al., 1987). While MRI and CT scans are effective in imaging RMS, access to advanced imaging techniques may be limited in some settings. MRI is most utilized in private health facilities, whereas CT scans are more commonly used in public hospitals in underresourced areas. However, the relative availability of CT in public hospitals has led to a great number of pediatric patients undergoing CT scans, with many resulting false-negative scans or inaccurate diagnoses (Fouche et al., 2021). Additionally, distinguishing between benign and malignant lesions on imaging alone can be challenging, but obtaining a biopsy from head and neck tumors can be complex due to the risk of damaging critical structures. In some cases, multiple biopsies may be necessary to obtain a definitive diagnosis (Sheng et al., 2023).

RMS treatment typically involves a combination of surgery, chemotherapy, and radiation therapy. Table 15.4 summarizes the treatment used for head and neck RMS in pediatric patients, tumor sites, median follow-up in clinical trials, age at therapy, complications, and country where the studies took place.

Table 15.4 Pediatric head and neck rhabdomyosarcoma treatments and associated late effects

Number of patients (gender)	Median age (range)	Country (period)	Tumor sites	Median follow-up (range)	Therapy used	Complications	References
8 (females) and 5 (males)	5 years (19 months–13 years)	New York (-)	Orbit ($n = 1$) Parameningeal ($n = 12$): Infratemporal fossa ($n = 5$), nasopharynx ($n = 5$), parapharyngeal ($n = 1$), and middle ear ($n = 1$)	9 years (1 – 13)	Chemotherapy (vincristine, doxorubicin, cyclophosphamide, ifosfamide, and etoposide) - Intensity-modulated radiotherapy (IMRT) Radiation dose (median 50.4 Gy, range 45–50.4 Gy)	Dentofacial abnormalities ($n = 9$): Tooth agenesis, root agenesis/stunting in the jaws, anterior and posterior teeth, and malformed enamel (hypoplastic or hypocalcified). Xerostomia or trismus ($n = 4$) Facial asymmetry and jaw hypoplasia ($n = 7$).	Owosho et al., 2016.
8 (males) and 2 (females)	4.3years(range 10 months to 19.5 years)	New York (1984–1996)	Orbit ($n = 2$) Parameningeal ($n = 6$): Nasopharynx ($n = 2$), infratemporal fossa ($n = 2$), ethmoid sinus ($n = 1$), middle ear ($n = 1$), buccal mucosa ($n = 1$), and upper lip ($n = 1$).	12.2 years (range 5.2 - 16.6)	Chemotherapy (combination of vincristine, dactinomycin, cyclophosphamide, doxorubicin, etoposide, cisplatin, ifosfamide, and methotrexate) ($n = 10$). surgery ($n = 2$) Radiation dose (median 5,400 cGy, range 5,040–6,120) ($n = 9$) External beam radiation therapy ($n = 1$).	Enamel defects ($n = 4$), agenesis ($n = 3$), trismus ($n = 2$), mandibular hypoplasia ($n = 4$), maxillary hypoplasia ($n = 5$), radiation caries ($n = 2$), xerostomia ($n = 1$), chronic facial pain ($n = 1$), delayed eruption ($n = 1$), and hypernasality ($n = 1$).	Estilo et al., 2003.

(continued)

Table 15.4 Continued

Number of patients (gender)	Median age (range)	Country (period)	Tumor sites	Median follow-up (range)	Therapy used	Complications	References
1 (female)	3.5 years	United Kingdom (2008 June–2019 October)	Embryonal RMS of the nasopharynx	8 years	Chemotherapy: 4 cycles of IVADo (I, ifosfamide; V, vincristine; A, actinomycin-D; D, doxorubicin) and 5 cycles of IVA for 25 weeks Proton beam therapy (total dose of 50.4 Gy) or 13 weeks	Dental abnormalities: Arrested root development, microdontia, failure of development UR7, UL7, and LL5; severe hypoplasia of roots (upper anterior teeth); and mild hypoplasia of lower right 6 (LR6) first molar roots	Foster-Thomas et al., 2022.
737 (female and 869 (male)	0–19 years	USA (1975–2016)	Orbital, parameningeal (*n*asal cavity, nasopharynx, paranasal sinuses, middle ear, and skull base), and non-parameningeal/non-orbital (lip, oral cavity, and pharynx)	5 years	Surgery, radiation, chemotherapy, surgery + radiation, surgery + chemotherapy, chemoradiotherapy, and surgery + chemoradiotherapy.	Increase risk of mortality in parameningeal tumors when compared to orbital and non-parameningeal/nonorbital tumors. Higher mortality risk in orbital tumors treated with chemoradiotherapy + radiation compared to surgery + radiation.	Darwish et al., 2020.
12 (male) and 8 (female)	8 years (range, 2–19)	Georgia (2000 January–2007 February)	Parameningeal ($n = 12$): Nasopharynx/nasal cavity ($n = 6$) Paranasal sinus ($n = 1$), Middle ear/mastoid ($n = 2$), Pterygopalatine/infratemporal fossa ($n = 2$), Parapharyngeal ($n = 1$), Intracranial extension ($n = 8/12$) Non-parameningeal ($n = 6$): Parotid/neck ($n = 4$), Oral cavity ($n = 1$), Larynx ($n = 1$) Orbit ($n = 2$)	29 months (range, 9 – 89)	Intensity-modulated radiotherapy with a cone-down boost	Pituitary dysfunction ($n = 1$). Bone hypoplasia ($n = 2$) Dilated cardiomyopathy was presumed due to chemotherapy and subsequently died ($n = 2$). Central nervous system (CNS) failure and death ($n = 3$). Acute toxicities include mucositis, desquamation, xerostomia, and altered taste.	McDonald et al., 2008.

7 (male) and 10 (female)	6.3years(range 8 months to 19 years)	United States (1996–2014)	Parameningeal ($n = 13$): Nasal cavity ($n = 1$), nasopharynx ($n = 6$), paranasal cavity ($n = 1$), infratemporal fossa ($n = 2$), maxillary ($n = 2$) and middle ear ($n = 1$) Non-parameningeal ($n = 4$): Nasal/cheek area ($n = 3$) and submandibular region ($n = 1$).	-	Combined chemotherapy and radiotherapy	Chemotherapy adverse effects ($n = 8$): Bacteremia, bilateral sensorineural hearing loss, cardiotoxicity, chronic weight loss, herpes zoster and severe thrombocytopenia, intracranial hemorrhage, neutropenia, peripheral neuropathy secondary to vincristine, lower extremity weakness, renal insufficiency, mucositis, and short-term memory loss. Radiotherapy adverse effects ($n = 7$) noted: Cataracts, cavernous hemangioma, chronic sinusitis, xerostomia, facial hypoplasia, fever, hypothalamic-pituitary dysfunction, growth disturbance, unilateral sensorineural hearing loss, hypothyroidism, and osteomyelitis. Secondary malignancy, acute myeloid leukemia ($n = 1$).	Reilly et al., 2015.
32	< 18 years of age)	United States of America (1955-1988)	Orbit ($n = 14$), different regions of the head and neck ($n = 8$), and parameningeal region ($n = 10$)	89 months (range, 1 – 254 months)	Chemotherapy (combined vincristine + dactinomycin + cyclophosphamide), radiation therapy (180-225 cGy/day, 5 days/week), and surgery.	Late complications identified: Cataracts ($n = 4$), Bony hypoplasia ($n = 3$) Facial asymmetry ($n = 3$) Corneal ulceration ($n = 2$) Retinopathy ($n = 2$) Blindness ($n = 1$). Visual disturbance due to cataracts ($n = 1$) Enucleation of the eye due to recurrent tumor ($n = 1$) and recurrent corneal ulceration and blindness ($n = 1$).	Sercarz et al., 1995.

(continued)

Table 15.4 Continued

Number of patients (gender)	Median age (range)	Country (period)	Tumor sites	Median follow-up (range)	Therapy used	Complications	References
12 (females) and 24 (males)	7 years (21 months–22 years)	Warsaw, Poland (January 2000 - December 2013)	Parameningeal ($n = 24$), orbit (n 3), and different regions of the head and neck ($n = 9$).	-	Surgical therapy (craniotomy, pharyngotomy, rhinotomy with partial maxillectomy, petrosectomy, adenectomy, and parotidectomy)	Early complications: Hematoma after postoperative therapy ($n = 1$) and cutaneous flap necrosis ($n = 1$). Late complications: Trismus after orbitozygomatic craniotomy ($n = 3$). Hypernasal speech due to losses of soft palate tissue ($n = 2$). Salivary fistula ending in the external acoustic meatus ($n = 1$). Orbital exenteration because of tumor infiltration of the orbit and eyeball ($n = 2$). Entire content of the orbit including bone structures removed ($n = 2$). Ocular prosthesis ($n = 1$).	Radzikowska et al., 2016.

Coordinating these treatments and managing their cumulative side effects can be challenging, especially in young children (Chen et al., 2019; von Mehren et al., 2020). Surgery is recommended when the entire tumor can be removed or resected without affecting nearby structures (Terwisscha van Scheltinga et al., 2023). Chemotherapy is used to minimize tumor size if the tumor cannot be resected completely by surgery and the surgeon is unwilling to remove the entire organ (Ning et al., 2020). Common drugs used as chemotherapy are ifosfamide, vincristine, actinomycin-D, doxorubicin, cyclophosphamide, etoposide, cisplatin, and methotrexate. They are used as a combined therapy of two or more drugs, for example, IVA (ifosfamide + vincristine + actinomycin-D) and IVADo (ifosfamide + vincristine + actinomycin-D + doxorubicin) (Casey & Wolden, 2018; Frankart et al., 2021).

Achieving complete surgical resection while preserving function and appearance is particularly challenging in the head and neck region due to the proximity of vital structures like nerves, blood vessels, and organs. Postsurgical reconstruction to restore function and appearance can be complex and may require multiple surgeries (Wen et al., 2020). For these reasons, chemotherapy is often used instead of surgery. Chemotherapy regimens, while effective, can cause significant short- and long-term side effects, including myelosuppression, cardiotoxicity, and secondary malignancies. Managing these toxicities, especially in young patients, is a significant challenge. Some RMS tumors may develop resistance to chemotherapy, thus complicating treatment and necessitating alternative therapeutic approaches (Huh & Skapek, 2010).

Radiation therapy, also known as radiotherapy, employs high doses of radiation to shrink and eradicate cancerous cells. Proton beam therapy (PBT) and intensity-modulated radiotherapy (IMRT) are emerging methods. They are applied to deliver effective radiation doses to tumor sites while reducing exposure to nearby, important normal tissues (Foster-Thomas et al., 2022). Kozak et al. (2009) compared PBT with IMRT in 10 pediatric patients with parameningeal RMS and found that PBT achieved better sparing of normal tissues compared with IMRT. PBT reduced radiation doses contralateral to the cochlea, parotid gland, entire brain, temporal lobes, hypothalamus, and pituitary compared with IMRT (Kozak et al., 2009). According to McDonald et al. (2008), treatment with IMRT in pediatric patients (2–19 years) with head and neck RMS (parameningeal, nonparameningeal, and orbital) resulted in a 3-year survival rate of 74% and an overall survival rate of 76% (McDonald et al., 2008).

The head and neck region contains many radiosensitive structures, and radiation therapy can lead to complications such as growth disturbances, endocrine dysfunction, and secondary cancers. The long-term effects of radiation on growing tissues must be carefully managed to minimize developmental and functional impairments (Miwa et al., 2020). The diagnosis and treatment of RMS can have a profound emotional and social impact on both the patient and their family. Providing adequate psychosocial support is essential but can be challenging to integrate into standard care protocols (Clemente et al., 2020). Treatment schedules and hospital stays can disrupt a child's education and social development, necessitating additional support services to help them keep up with their peers (Casey et al., 2018). Access to specialized care and advanced treatment options can be limited by geographical, socioeconomic, and healthcare system factors, and ensuring equitable access to high-quality care remains an ongoing challenge (Chen et al., 2019; Frankart et al., 2021; von Mehren et al., 2020).

15.5 Thyroid Malignances

Thyroid malignancies, which include various types of thyroid cancers such as papillary, follicular, medullary, and anaplastic, present significant challenges in both detection and treatment (Boucai et al., 2024). These challenges stem from the complex nature of thyroid cancer pathology, the limitations of current diagnostic tools, and the varied responses to treatment. Many patients remain asymptomatic for a long time, which delays diagnosis until the cancer has progressed to a more advanced stage (Raymond et al., 2024). In its early stages, thyroid cancer often presents subtle and nonspecific symptoms, such as a small, painless nodule in the thyroid gland, which can easily be overlooked or misattributed to benign conditions (Boucai et al., 2024; Raymond et al., 2024). The initial workup for every newly detected thyroid nodule should include a serum thyroid-stimulating hormone (TSH) level. The anterior pituitary releases TSH, which instructs the thyroid gland to produce thyroid hormone as needed (Cooper et al., 2009). When thyroid hormone levels are low, TSH rises in response, and vice versa; hence, monitoring TSH levels enables the distinction of functional from nonfunctional nodules. This is a significant feature because hyperfunctioning nodules are rarely cancerous (Cooper et al., 2009; Raymond et al., 2024). However, if the level of TSH is below normal, indicating an overactive gland, a nuclear medicine imaging study called a *thyroid uptake and scan* should be conducted (Nguyen et al., 2015).

This study is done to determine whether the nodule in question is functioning excessively (hot), functioning normally (warm), or not functioning at all (cold) in comparison to the surrounding thyroid tissue. If the nodule is hot or warm, no cytologic evaluation is necessary; however, if the patient is symptomatic, additional evaluation is required to rule out other causes, such as Graves disease, and to provide adequate treatment (Nguyen et al., 2015). Nonfunctional nodules necessitate the utilization of FNA for cytologic assessment. However, if the TSH level is normal or elevated, even within the upper limits of normal, then an FNA is recommended because the rate of malignancy is higher with nonfunctioning nodules and glands affected by Hashimoto's thyroiditis, a common autoimmune hypothyroid disease (Raymond et al., 2024). In addition to measuring blood TSH levels, diagnostic neck ultrasound is recommended for all individuals with suspected nodules. This ultrasound is performed to verify the presence of a nodule and to assess for any potentially concerning characteristics (Cooper et al., 2009). However, no single ultrasound feature and no combination of ultrasound features is sensitive enough or specific enough to identify malignancy. Some ultrasound features have greater correlation with certain types of cancer, such as microcalcifications with papillary thyroid cancer and its absence in follicular thyroid cancer (Nguyen et al., 2015; Raymond et al., 2024). Furthermore, certain sonographic features are highly predictive of benign nodules, such as purely cystic nodules and nodules with >50% spongiform appearance (aggregation of multiple microcystic components) (Cooper et al., 2009). Though ultrasound is the primary imaging modality used to evaluate thyroid nodules, it cannot definitively distinguish between benign and malignant lesions, leading to potential overdiagnosis and overtreatment of benign conditions (AlSaedi et al., 2024).

If the preliminary examination indicates a nonfunctional nodule with concerning sonographic characteristics, an FNA biopsy (FNAB) is recommended. This procedure is still considered the most precise, cost-efficient, and optimal diagnostic approach for assessing nodules (Cooper et al., 2009; Nguyen et al., 2015; Nikiforov et al., 2013). FNA can be conducted using either palpation or ultrasound guidance. Ultrasound-guided FNA is the recommended method, particularly when the nodules include cystic components, are positioned toward the back, or are challenging to feel by touch. Ultrasound-guided FNA also decreases the necessity for additional FNABs due to insufficient samples (Cooper et al., 2009). The goal of the FNAB is to obtain at least six follicular cell groups, each containing 10–15 cells from at least two different aspirates of a nodule for cytologic evaluation (Nguyen et al., 2015).

Typically, it is not advisable to perform routine FNA on nodules that are < 1 centimeter unless their sonographic characteristics are concerning, as previously mentioned. In that case, further assessment of the lateral and central neck lymph nodes by ultrasound is required (Cooper et al., 2009; Nguyen et al., 2015). If abnormal lymph nodes are detected, an FNAB should be performed on the lymph node in addition to the thyroid nodule. A second exception to not performing a biopsy on a subcentimeter nodule is a patient with a history of high risk for malignancy, which includes irradiation exposure, a family history of thyroid cancer, a previous hemithyroidectomy for thyroid cancer, or having positive nodules as determined by a PET scan (Cooper et al., 2009; Nguyen et al., 2015).

When conducting an FNAB, it is important to take into account certain anatomical characteristics in order to acquire the most optimal sample. Mixed cystic-solid nodules should be biopsied within the solid component, and cyst drainage may be performed if patients are symptomatic (Cooper et al., 2009). When dealing with a multinodular gland that has two or more nodules measuring > 1 cm, it is recommended to prioritize the biopsy of the nodule that exhibits suspicious sonographic characteristics (Cooper et al., 2009). Only the largest lesion should be aspirated, and the remaining nodules should be monitored with recurrent ultrasound examinations if none is questionable. A FNA should be done on the hypofunctioning nodules if nuclear imaging was performed as a result of a low serum TSH level, with a preference for those with questionable sonographic characteristics (Cooper et al., 2009; Nguyen et al., 2015).

The results of an FNAB can be classified as benign, follicular lesion of undetermined significance (5–10%), indeterminate or suspicious for neoplasm (20–30%), malignant, or suggestive for malignancy (50–75% risk) (Cooper et al., 2009). Samples that do not match the criteria for cytologic adequacy—that is, at least six follicular cell groups, each comprising 10–15 cells from at least two distinct nodule aspirates—will result in nondiagnostic cytology (Cooper et al., 2009). A second ultrasound-guided FNA ought to be performed in this situation. Nevertheless, 7% of nodules may continue to provide nondiagnostic cytology results yet could be cancerous; thus these nodules need to be surgically removed or subjected to frequent ultrasound monitoring (Cooper et al., 2009; Nguyen et al., 2015). While FNAB is a common and minimally invasive diagnostic tool, it has limitations in sensitivity and specificity. It may yield indeterminate or inconclusive results necessitating additional testing or surgical intervention for a definitive diagnosis (Boucai et al., 2024; Raymond et al., 2024).

About 25% of FNAB samples of thyroid nodules are classified as "indeterminate." With this in view, molecular tests have evolved with the goal of enhancing preoperative diagnosis in these circumstances. These tests are verified from a diagnostic perspective and have strong performance and diagnostic accuracy as well as the ability to avoid diagnostic surgeries (Ferraz, 2024). Deciphering mutations and gene rearrangement in thyroid oncogenesis is critical, and molecular markers have shifted from being solely diagnostic tools to becoming increasingly important in determining the tumor's prognostic significance in guiding target therapy (Patel et al., 2023). Although molecular testing for genetic mutations (such as BRAF, RAS, RET/PTC rearrangements) can aid in diagnosis, it is not always definitive. Not all thyroid cancers exhibit these mutations, and their presence does not always confirm malignancy. Advanced molecular testing can be expensive and may not be readily available in all healthcare settings, particularly in resource-limited regions (Ferraz, 2024; Patel et al., 2023).

Surgery should be given more serious thought when there are substantial nodules. The elevated risk of malignancy associated with indeterminate cytology (suspicious for follicular or Hürthle-cell neoplasm, or follicular lesion of unclear significance) has prompted the use of molecular markers as a therapeutic strategy (AlSaedi et al., 2024; Cooper et al., 2009). Patients with an ambiguous single nodule are advised to have a thyroid lobectomy while those with massive tumors > 4 cm or a high-risk history of malignancy are advised to have a complete thyroidectomy (Cooper et al., 2009). Therefore, unless there are contraindications or diffuse metastases, any cytology that suggests malignancy needs to be surgically treated with a lobectomy or a whole thyroidectomy (thyroid lobectomy is the surgical removal of one of the two thyroid lobes, leaving the other intact; thyroidectomy is the surgical removal of the entire gland) (Alzahrani, 2024). Thyroidectomy is the primary treatment for most thyroid cancers. However, it carries risks such as damage to the recurrent laryngeal nerve, which can affect vocal cord function, and hypoparathyroidism, which can lead to calcium metabolism disorders (AlSaedi et al., 2024; Alzahrani, 2024). Complete surgical resection may be challenging in cases where the cancer has invaded surrounding tissues or metastasized, potentially leaving residual disease that necessitates further treatment (AlSaedi et al., 2024).

Radioactive iodine (RAI) therapy is effective for treating differentiated thyroid cancers (papillary and follicular) but it is not useful for medullary and anaplastic thyroid cancers, which do not take up iodine (Zhang et al., 2024). Some thyroid cancers may be resistant to RAI, and there is a risk of recurrence even after treatment. Monitoring for recurrence requires lifelong follow-up and can be emotionally and financially burdensome for patients. For advanced or metastatic thyroid cancers, especially anaplastic thyroid cancer, treatment options are limited (Nguyen et al., 2024). Targeted therapies (e.g., tyrosine kinase inhibitors) have shown promise but are not curative and may have significant side effects. Traditional chemotherapy is generally ineffective for most thyroid cancers and is reserved for aggressive cases where other treatments have failed. Its use is limited by its toxicity and the potential for severe side effects (Guo et al., 2024). External beam radiation therapy is typically reserved for inoperable tumors or those that do not respond to RAI. Its use can be limited by the proximity of the thyroid gland to other critical structures in the neck, which increases the risk of collateral damage (Cavalcante et al., 2024).

Measurement of thyroglobulin levels is used to monitor for recurrence in differentiated thyroid cancer. However, its interpretation can be complicated by the presence of anti-thyroglobulin antibodies, which can interfere with test results (Giovanella et al., 2024). Regular imaging (e.g., ultrasound, CT scans) is required to monitor for recurrence or metastasis, but frequent imaging can be costly and expose patients to additional radiation. There are significant disparities in access to quality care, with patients in rural or low-income areas facing challenges in obtaining timely and appropriate diagnosis and treatment (Boudina et al., 2024). Limited availability of specialized healthcare providers and diagnostic tools in certain regions can delay diagnosis and treatment initiation (Ferraz, 2024). Ensuring patient compliance with follow-up appointments, medication regimens, and lifestyle modifications is crucial for effective management but can be challenging due to various socioeconomic factors. Educating patients about the importance of monitoring and potential signs of recurrence is essential but can be hampered by health literacy levels and communication barriers (Ferraz, 2024; Patel et al., 2023).

15.6 Nasopharyngeal Carcinoma

NPC is a distinct type of HNC originating in the nasopharynx, the area behind the nose and above the back of the throat. NPC is particularly prevalent in certain regions, such as Southeast Asia, North Africa, and the Arctic (Hsu et al., 2024). Despite advances in medical science, NPC presents several challenges in both detection and treatment due to its unique location, biological characteristics, and varying responses to therapy. The nasopharynx is a difficult area to examine due to its deep-seated and hidden anatomical location, which can complicate early detection (Wei et al., 2024). Traditional physical examinations may not easily reveal abnormalities in this region. NPC often goes undetected until it reaches an advanced stage because early symptoms are nonspecific or resemble common illnesses, such as nasal congestion, epistaxis (nosebleeds), or otitis media (ear infections) (Hsu et al., 2024; Wei et al., 2024).

Initial symptoms such as nasal obstruction, hearing loss, or tinnitus are nonspecific and can be mistaken for benign conditions. This leads to delays in seeking specialized medical evaluation. Symptoms like cranial nerve palsies or cervical lymphadenopathy typically appear at more advanced stages, which complicates treatment and prognosis (Shah & Nagalli, 2024). An endoscopic procedure is a minimally invasive diagnostic or surgical technique used to visualize the internal structures of the body using an endoscope. An endoscope is a flexible or rigid tube with a light source and a camera at the tip, which transmits images to a monitor, allowing the physician to examine areas inside the body without making large incisions (Wei et al., 2024). MRI and CT scans are crucial for detecting NPC and assessing its extent. However, these imaging modalities are expensive and may not be accessible in resource-limited areas. A definitive diagnosis of NPC requires a biopsy, which involves obtaining tissue from the nasopharynx. The procedure can be technically challenging due to the location and potential complications (Gong et al., 2024).

EBV infection is strongly associated with NPC. Serological tests can determine the presence of EBV antibodies and DNA, which are used as markers for screening and monitoring, but they are not definitive for all cases. False positives and false negatives can occur. Implementing effective population-wide screening programs is difficult due to variability in the prevalence of NPC and logistical challenges in high-risk areas (Chai et al., 2024).

Radiotherapy is the cornerstone of NPC treatment due to the tumor's radiosensitivity. However, delivering adequate doses while sparing surrounding critical structures (e.g., brainstem, optic nerves) is challenging. Acute and long-term side effects of radiotherapy, such as xerostomia (dry mouth), dysphagia (difficulty swallowing), and hearing loss, significantly impact patients' quality of life (Dai et al., 2024). Concurrent chemoradiotherapy is standard for advanced NPC, improving survival rates but increasing toxicity. Chemotherapy agents like cisplatin can cause severe side effects, including nephrotoxicity and ototoxicity (Xia et al., 2024).

Some NPC cases exhibit resistance to standard chemotherapeutic agents, leading to recurrence. Salvage chemotherapy options are often limited and less effective. Research into targeted therapies for NPC, such as those aimed at EBV-related pathways or specific genetic mutations, is ongoing (Xia et al., 2024). However, these treatments are still in the experimental phase and not widely available. Advanced targeted therapies can be prohibitively expensive and may not be accessible to all patients, particularly in low- and middle-income countries where NPC is more prevalent (Dai et al., 2024; Xia et al., 2024). Immunotherapy, including immune checkpoint inhibitors, shows promise for treating recurrent or metastatic NPC. However, the response rates vary, and not all patients benefit from these therapies. Immunotherapy can cause immune-related adverse events that require careful management and monitoring, thus adding complexity to treatment regimens (Gong et al., 2024).

Effective treatment of NPC requires a multidisciplinary team approach involving oncologists, radiologists, surgeons, and supportive care specialists. Coordinating care across multiple disciplines can be challenging. Long-term follow-up is essential for detecting recurrences and managing late effects of treatment (Gong et al., 2024). Ensuring patient adherence to follow-up protocols can be difficult, particularly in resource-limited settings. There are significant disparities in access to healthcare services, particularly in regions with high NPC incidence but limited medical infrastructure. Access to specialized care, including oncology and radiotherapy services, is often limited in rural or low-resource areas, delaying diagnosis and treatment (Dai et al., 2024; Xia et al., 2024). The high cost of diagnostic tests, imaging, and advanced treatments poses a significant economic burden on patients and healthcare systems, and lack of adequate insurance coverage and reimbursement policies can hinder access to necessary treatments and follow-up care (Hsu et al., 2024; Wei et al., 2024). Increasing public awareness about NPC and its symptoms is crucial for early detection. However, implementing effective awareness campaigns requires resources and sustained efforts. Educating patients about the importance of early detection, treatment adherence, and follow-up care is essential but challenging in areas with low health literacy (Shah & Nagalli, 2024).

15.7 Neuroblastoma

Neuroblastoma is a pediatric cancer arising from neural crest cells, typically affecting children under the age of 5. It is one of the most common solid tumors in children and presents unique challenges in terms of detection and treatment (Gerges & Canning, 2024). These challenges are influenced by the tumor's biological heterogeneity, the young age of affected patients, and the varying responses to therapeutic interventions. Early symptoms of neuroblastoma, such as abdominal pain, fatigue, loss of appetite, and fever, are nonspecific and can be easily mistaken for common childhood illnesses (Lopez et al., 2024). Due to the nonspecific nature of symptoms, there can be significant delays in diagnosis. By the time more specific symptoms like a palpable mass or bone pain appear, the disease may have already progressed (Johnsen & Kogner, 2024). Neuroblastoma can arise in different parts of the body, including the abdomen, chest, neck, and pelvis. This variability in location can complicate the clinical presentation and delay diagnosis. Neuroblastoma can be associated with paraneoplastic syndromes, such as opsoclonus-myoclonus syndrome, which can further obscure the diagnosis (Gerges & Canning, 2024).

Standard imaging techniques like ultrasound, CT scans, and MRIs are essential for detecting neuroblastoma but may not always provide a clear distinction between benign and malignant masses (Schäfer et al., 2023). Neuroblastoma often metastasizes to bone and bone marrow, requiring additional imaging techniques such as metaiodobenzylguanidine (MIBG) scans, which are specialized and not universally available (Vieira et al., 2023). Diagnosis of neuroblastoma typically requires a biopsy and pathological confirmation, which can be invasive and risky, especially in very young children. The tumor's histological complexity and the presence of different cellular components can make pathological interpretation challenging (Schoeman et al., 2024). Detection of v-myc myelocytomatosis viral-related oncogene and neuroblastoma-derived (avian) (MYCN) amplification, a marker of high-risk neuroblastoma, requires sophisticated molecular techniques that may not be available in all healthcare settings. The genetic heterogeneity of neuroblastoma necessitates comprehensive molecular profiling, which can be costly and time-consuming (Volegova et al., 2024).

Neuroblastoma is a heterogeneous disease with varying prognoses. Accurately stratifying patients into risk groups (low, intermediate, and high risk) is crucial but can be challenging due to overlapping clinical and molecular features (Johnsen & Kogner, 2024). The need for individualized treatment plans based on risk stratification complicates standardization of care and requires extensive resources (Gerges & Canning, 2024). Surgical removal of neuroblastoma tumors can be complex, particularly when tumors are located near vital structures or have invaded surrounding tissues. Achieving complete surgical resection without causing significant harm is often difficult, especially in high-risk or metastatic cases (Johnsen & Kogner, 2024). Chemotherapy is a cornerstone of neuroblastoma treatment, especially for high-risk cases. However, the toxicity of chemotherapy agents poses significant risks, including long-term side effects like hearing loss, kidney damage, and secondary malignancies (Gerges & Canning, 2024; Raiser et al., 2024).

Some neuroblastomas develop resistance to standard chemotherapy, necessitating the use of more intensive regimens or novel agents, which may not always be effective (Gerges & Canning, 2024). While radiation therapy can be effective in controlling localized disease, it carries risks of long-term side effects, particularly in young children, such as growth retardation, neurocognitive deficits, and increased risk of secondary cancers (Raiser et al., 2024). Precisely targeting radiation to minimize damage to surrounding healthy tissues is challenging, particularly in very young children with rapidly developing organs (Gerges & Canning, 2024).

Immunotherapy, including monoclonal antibodies and checkpoint inhibitors, is emerging as a promising treatment for neuroblastoma. However, these therapies can have severe immune-related side effects and are not yet universally effective. Immunotherapy can be extremely expensive and not universally accessible, thus limiting its use in resource-strained settings (Gerges & Canning, 2024; Raiser et al., 2024).

Autologous stem cell transplantation is often used for high-risk neuroblastoma following high-dose chemotherapy. The procedure carries significant risks, including infection and graft-versus-host disease. The long-term effects of such intensive treatment protocols are not fully understood, and survivors may face chronic health issues (Żebrowska et al., 2024). Neuroblastoma has a high rate of relapse, particularly in high-risk patients. Relapsed disease is often more resistant to treatment and has a poorer prognosis (Raiser et al., 2024). Regular monitoring and follow-up are essential for detecting recurrence, which can be logistically challenging and stressful for families. Because of significant disparities in access to specialized pediatric oncology care, particularly in low- and middle-income countries (Żebrowska et al., 2024), advanced diagnostic tools, specialized treatments, and clinical trials may not be readily available in all regions, limiting the options for optimal care (Gerges & Canning, 2024). The high cost of treating neuroblastoma, including surgery, chemotherapy, radiation, and supportive care, places a substantial economic burden on families and healthcare systems, and inadequate insurance coverage can hinder access to necessary treatments and follow-up care (Gerges & Canning, 2024; Raiser et al., 2024). The diagnosis and treatment of neuroblastoma can have a profound psychosocial impact on patients and their families, leading to significant stress, anxiety, and financial hardship. Access to comprehensive psychosocial support services, including counseling and financial assistance, is essential but may be limited (Johnsen & Kogner, 2024).

15.8 Non-Rhabdomyosarcoma Soft Tissue Sarcoma

Non-rhabdomyosarcoma soft tissue sarcomas (NRSTS) are a diverse group of rare malignancies that arise from connective tissues such as muscle, fat, nerves, and blood vessels (Ferrari et al., 2024). They present unique challenges in terms of detection and treatment due to their rarity, heterogeneity, and often complex clinical behavior (Li et al., 2023). These tumors can occur at any age, but they are particularly challenging in pediatric populations due to the need for tailored treatment approaches that balance efficacy and long-term quality of life (Vennarini et al., 2024). NRSTS encompasses a wide range of histological subtypes, including fibrosarcoma, synovial sarcoma, and malignant peripheral nerve sheath tumors, among others (Li et al., 2023). This diversity complicates the diagnostic process because each subtype can have distinct clinical and biological behaviors (Ferrari et al., 2024). Symptoms of NRSTS can vary significantly based on the tumor's location, size, and growth rate. Common symptoms like a painless mass or swelling may not immediately raise suspicion for malignancy, leading to delays in diagnosis (Vennarini et al., 2024).

Early symptoms of NRSTS are often subtle and nonspecific, such as localized pain or swelling, which can be mistaken for benign conditions or injuries. This can result in delayed medical evaluation and diagnosis (Vennarini et al., 2024). While imaging modalities such as MRI and CT scans are essential for identifying and characterizing soft tissue masses, distinguishing between benign and malignant lesions can be difficult. Imaging alone may not always provide definitive diagnostic information (Li et al., 2023). PET scans can help in assessing metabolic activity and potential malignancy, but their role in NRSTS diagnosis is not as well established as in other cancers. Obtaining a definitive diagnosis usually requires a biopsy, which is an invasive procedure (Milgrom et al., 2021). FNA or core needle biopsy is commonly used, but these procedures can sometimes yield inconclusive results (Singh et al., 2004; Vennarini et al., 2024). The histopathological examination of NRSTS can be complex due to the diverse morphological patterns. Accurate diagnosis often requires the expertise of specialized pathologists and may involve immunohistochemical staining and molecular testing (Tinkle et al., 2017; Vennarini et al., 2024).

NRSTS can be associated with various genetic alterations and molecular markers. Identifying these alterations can be crucial for diagnosis and treatment planning, but comprehensive molecular testing may not always be available or feasible in all settings (Vennarini et al., 2024). Complete surgical resection with negative margins is the primary treatment for localized NRSTS. However, achieving clear margins can be challenging due to the tumor's proximity to critical structures and the potential for extensive local invasion (Li et al., 2023). Surgery may require complex reconstructive procedures to preserve function and appearance, particularly when tumors are located in cosmetically or functionally sensitive areas (Ferrari et al., 2024). Radiation therapy is often used as an adjunct to surgery to improve local control. However, delivering effective doses while minimizing damage to surrounding normal tissues can be challenging, particularly in pediatric patients where long-term side effects such as growth disturbances and secondary malignancies are a concern (Li et al., 2023). Advanced radiation techniques like IMRT and proton therapy can help reduce toxicity, but access to these technologies may be limited (Vennarini et al., 2024).

The sensitivity of NRSTS to chemotherapy varies significantly among different subtypes. Some subtypes are relatively chemoresistant, necessitating the use of high-dose or combination regimens, which can increase the risk of severe side effects (Ferrari et al., 2024). In pediatric patients, the use of chemotherapy requires careful consideration of long-term toxicity, including potential impacts on growth, development, and fertility. Unlike other cancers where targeted therapies and immunotherapy have shown significant promise, the role of these treatments in NRSTS is still under investigation (Tinkle et al., 2017). The rarity and heterogeneity of NRSTS make it difficult to identify common molecular targets. Ongoing research is exploring the potential of targeted therapies based on specific genetic mutations or molecular pathways involved in NRSTS (Vennarini et al., 2024), and clinical trials are essential for determining the efficacy and safety of these novel treatments. Effective treatment of NRSTS often requires a multidisciplinary approach involving surgeons, medical oncologists, radiation oncologists, pathologists, and supportive care specialists. Coordinating care across these disciplines can be complex, particularly in resource-limited settings (Li et al., 2023; Vennarini et al., 2024).

Developing individualized treatment plans that consider the tumor subtype, stage, patient age, and overall health is essential but challenging. This approach requires access to comprehensive diagnostic and therapeutic resources (Vennarini et al., 2024). Long-term follow-up is crucial for monitoring potential recurrence because NRSTS can recur locally or metastasize even years after initial treatment. This requires regular imaging and clinical evaluations (Li et al., 2023). Survivors of NRSTS, particularly pediatric patients, may face long-term health issues related to their treatment, including secondary cancers, cardiovascular problems, and psychosocial challenges. Providing comprehensive survivorship care is essential but resource-intensive (Vennarini et al., 2024). Because of significant disparities in access to specialized care for NRSTS, particularly in low- and middle-income countries, limited access to advanced diagnostic tools, specialized treatments, and multidisciplinary care can adversely affect outcomes (Tinkle et al., 2017). The rarity of NRSTS means that expertise in managing these tumors may be concentrated in specialized centers, necessitating travel and potentially prolonged stays for patients and families (Vennarini et al., 2024).

The high cost of comprehensive treatment, including surgery, chemotherapy, radiation, and supportive care, places a substantial economic burden on families and healthcare systems (Li et al., 2023; Tinkle et al., 2017; Vennarini et al., 2024). Inadequate insurance coverage can hinder access to necessary treatments and follow-up care, particularly for novel therapies that may not be widely covered (Li et al., 2023; Tinkle et al., 2017). The diagnosis and treatment of NRSTS can have a profound psychosocial impact on patients and their families, leading to significant stress, anxiety, and financial hardship (Li et al., 2023; Tinkle et al., 2017). Access to comprehensive psychosocial support services, including counseling and financial assistance, is essential but may be limited (Vennarini et al., 2024).

15.9 Salivary Gland Malignances

Salivary gland malignancies (SGMs) are a diverse group of rare tumors that arise in the salivary glands, including the parotid, submandibular, sublingual, and minor salivary glands (Wai et al., 2024). These tumors present unique challenges in terms of detection and treatment due to their rarity, heterogeneity, and anatomical complexity. Early diagnosis and effective treatment are critical to improving outcomes, but these can be difficult to achieve due to various factors (Tanzawa et al., 2024). SGMs are relatively rare, accounting for only a small percentage of HNCs. This low incidence can lead to a lack of familiarity among general practitioners and even some specialists, potentially delaying diagnosis (Kucharska et al., 2024). SGMs encompass a wide variety of histological subtypes, such as mucoepidermoid carcinoma, adenoid cystic carcinoma, and acinic cell carcinoma. Each subtype has distinct biological behaviors that complicate the diagnostic process (Wai et al., 2024).

Early symptoms of SGMs, such as a painless lump or swelling in the salivary gland area, are often nonspecific and can be mistaken for benign conditions like sialadenitis or benign tumors. This can delay the consideration of malignancy (Kucharska et al., 2024). While imaging techniques like ultrasound, CT, and MRI are essential for evaluating salivary gland tumors, they sometimes cannot definitively distinguish between benign and malignant lesions (Wai et al., 2024). Advanced imaging modalities like PET scans may help but are not always conclusive. FNA biopsy is commonly used for initial assessment, but it may not always provide sufficient information for a definitive diagnosis. Core needle biopsy or open surgical biopsy might be required, and these are more invasive (Tanzawa et al., 2024). Accurate histopathological diagnosis is difficult due to the complex and varied histological features of SGMs. This requires specialized pathological expertise and sometimes additional molecular testing (Wai et al., 2024).

While molecular and genetic testing can provide valuable diagnostic and prognostic information, the specific genetic alterations in many SGMs are not well-defined, limiting the utility of these tests in clinical practice (Utsumi et al., 2024). The close proximity of salivary glands to critical structures such as facial nerves, blood vessels, and other vital organs makes surgical resection challenging. Preserving function while achieving clear margins is often difficult (Young & Okuyemi, 2023). Extensive surgeries may require complex reconstructive procedures to restore form and function, particularly when large tumors or recurrent tumors are involved (Wai et al., 2024). Radiation therapy is often used postoperatively or for inoperable tumors. Delivering effective doses while minimizing damage to adjacent critical structures like the facial nerve and the oral cavity is challenging (Young & Okuyemi, 2023). Techniques like IMRT can help reduce toxicity but require specialized equipment and expertise, which may not be available in all treatment centers (Utsumi et al., 2024).

SGMs are generally less responsive to chemotherapy compared to other HNCs. Chemotherapy is typically reserved for advanced or metastatic disease, but its effectiveness is limited and the side effects can be significant (Kucharska et al., 2024). Research into combination therapies, including chemotherapy with targeted agents, is ongoing, but the optimal regimens are not yet well established (Utsumi et al., 2024). Targeted therapies and immunotherapy are promising areas of research, but their roles in treating SGMs are still being defined. Identifying suitable targets and understanding the tumor microenvironment are ongoing challenges (Wai et al., 2024). Participation in clinical trials may provide access to novel treatments, but the rarity of SGMs means that few patients are eligible, and trial availability can be limited. Effective treatment of SGMs often requires a multidisciplinary approach involving surgeons, medical oncologists, radiation oncologists, and supportive care specialists (Young & Okuyemi, 2023). Coordinating care across these disciplines can be complex, particularly in resource-limited settings. Developing individualized treatment plans that consider tumor subtype, stage, patient age, and overall health is essential but challenging and usually requires access to comprehensive diagnostic and therapeutic resources (Utsumi et al., 2024).

SGMs can recur locally or metastasize even after initial successful treatment. Long-term follow-up with regular imaging and clinical evaluations is crucial for early detection of recurrence (Kucharska et al., 2024). Survivors may face long-term health issues related to their treatment, including xerostomia (dry mouth), dysphagia (difficulty swallowing), and facial nerve dysfunction. Providing comprehensive survivorship care is essential but resource-intensive (Utsumi et al., 2024). Significant disparities exist in access to specialized care for SGMs, particularly in low- and middle-income countries, and limited access to advanced diagnostic tools, specialized treatments, and multidisciplinary care can adversely affect outcomes. Expertise in managing SGMs may be concentrated in specialized centers, necessitating travel and potentially prolonged stays for patients and families (Wai et al., 2024). The high cost of comprehensive treatment, including surgery, radiation therapy, chemotherapy, and supportive care, places a substantial economic burden on families and healthcare systems (Tanzawa et al., 2024). Inadequate insurance coverage can hinder access to necessary treatments and follow-up care, particularly for novel therapies that may not be widely covered (Wai et al., 2024). The diagnosis and treatment of SGMs can have a profound psychosocial impact on patients and their families, leading to significant stress, anxiety, and financial hardship. Access to comprehensive psychosocial support services, including counseling and financial assistance, is essential but may be limited (Utsumi et al., 2024).

The detection and treatment of SGMs present numerous challenges due to their biological complexity, clinical heterogeneity, and the limitations of current diagnostic and therapeutic modalities. Addressing these challenges requires a multifaceted approach, including advancements in early detection techniques, the development of less toxic and more effective treatments, and improved access to specialized care. Additionally, ongoing research into the molecular underpinnings of SGMs and the integration of novel therapies hold promise for improving outcomes for patients with these challenging tumors.

15.10 Malignant Teratoma

Malignant teratomas are rare germ cell tumors that can occur in various parts of the body, including the head and neck region, where they are considered extremely rare (Salous & Adra 2024). They are characterized by the presence of tissues from all three germ layers (ectoderm, mesoderm, and endoderm) and can exhibit a wide range of differentiation (Nimodia et al., 2024). Due to their rarity and complex nature, malignant teratomas pose significant challenges in both detection and treatment. Their rarity often leads to a lack of awareness and experience among clinicians, potentially resulting in delayed diagnosis. The clinical presentation of malignant teratomas can be highly variable depending on their location and the types of tissues involved (Nimodia et al., 2024). Symptoms may be nonspecific and overlap with those of other more common conditions, making early detection difficult. Malignant teratomas can appear heterogeneously in imaging studies due to the presence of multiple tissue types. This variability can complicate the interpretation of imaging results (Saani et al., 2023). While standard imaging modalities like ultrasound, CT, and MRI are used for initial assessment, they may not always provide definitive information about the tumor's nature and extent. Advanced imaging techniques, such as PET scans, may be required but are not always readily available (Salous & Adra, 2024).

Malignant teratomas exhibit complex histological features, including the presence of immature and malignant components. Accurate diagnosis requires specialized pathological expertise and sometimes additional molecular testing (Saani et al., 2023). Obtaining a biopsy for histopathological examination can be challenging due to the tumor's location and the potential involvement of critical structures (Saani et al., 2023). The molecular and genetic characteristics of malignant teratomas are not as well understood as those of other germ cell tumors, and this limited knowledge hampers the development of specific diagnostic and prognostic biomarkers (Salous & Adra 2024). Surgical resection of malignant teratomas, especially in the head and neck region, is complicated by the proximity to vital structures such as nerves, blood vessels, and airway passages (Nimodia et al., 2024). Achieving complete resection while preserving function is a major challenge. Extensive surgery may require complex reconstructive procedures to restore form and function, which can be resource-intensive and technically demanding (Salous & Adra, 2024).

Radiation therapy can be used for malignant teratomas, particularly for residual or unresectable disease. However, delivering effective doses while minimizing damage to adjacent critical structures is challenging (Peluso et al., 2024). Radiation therapy can lead to significant long-term side effects, especially in pediatric patients, including growth retardation and secondary malignancies. Malignant teratomas may respond variably to chemotherapy, depending on the presence of immature or malignant components (Dantkale & Agrawal, 2024). Standard chemotherapy regimens used for other germ cell tumors may not be as effective. Chemotherapy can cause significant acute and long-term toxicities, necessitating careful management and supportive care (Peluso et al., 2024). Effective treatment of malignant teratomas often requires a multidisciplinary team, including surgeons, medical oncologists, radiation oncologists, and supportive care specialists (Moraru et al., 2023). Coordinating care across these disciplines can be complex and requires specialized expertise. Developing individualized treatment plans that consider the tumor's location, histological features, patient age, and overall health is essential but challenging (Dantkale & Agrawal, 2024).

Long-term follow-up is crucial for detecting recurrence, which can occur even after initial successful treatment. Regular imaging and clinical evaluations are needed but can be burdensome for patients (Peluso et al., 2024). Survivors may face long-term health issues related to their treatment, including endocrine dysfunction, fertility issues, and psychological impacts. Providing comprehensive survivorship care is essential but resource-intensive (Moraru et al., 2023). Because significant disparities exist in access to specialized care for malignant teratomas, particularly in low- and middle-income countries, limited access to advanced diagnostic tools, specialized treatments, and multidisciplinary care can adversely affect outcomes (Peluso et al., 2024). Expertise in managing malignant teratomas may be concentrated in specialized centers, necessitating travel and potentially prolonged stays for patients and families (Moraru et al., 2023). The high cost of comprehensive treatment, including surgery, radiation therapy, chemotherapy, and supportive care, places a substantial economic burden on families and healthcare systems. Inadequate insurance coverage can hinder access to necessary treatments and follow-up care, particularly for novel therapies that may not be widely covered (Peluso et al., 2024). The diagnosis and treatment of malignant teratomas can have a profound psychosocial impact on patients and their families, leading to significant stress, anxiety, and financial hardship, and access to comprehensive psychosocial support services, including counseling and financial assistance, is essential but may be limited (Dantkale & Agrawal, 2024).

15.11 Outlook and Future Perspective

The outlook and future prospectives for pediatric HNC detection and treatment is increasingly optimistic, driven by advances in precision medicine, molecular diagnostics, targeted therapies, immunotherapy, and personalized medicine (Lopez et al., 2024). Advances in next-generation sequencing and other genomic technologies allow for detailed molecular and genetic profiling of tumors. These techniques can identify specific mutations, gene fusions, and other molecular aberrations that drive cancer growth (AlSaedi et al., 2024). Early detection through these methods can lead to more accurate diagnoses and personalized treatment plans. Noninvasive techniques such as liquid biopsies are emerging as powerful tools for early cancer detection and monitoring (Utsumi et al., 2024).

By analyzing circulating tumor DNA (ctDNA) and other biomarkers in blood samples, clinicians can detect cancer at earlier stages and monitor treatment response and disease progression without the need for invasive procedures (Wai et al., 2024). Improvements in imaging technologies, such as functional MRI, PET-CT, and advanced ultrasound, provide higher-resolution images and better delineation of tumors. These advancements enable more precise localization and characterization of tumors, facilitating early diagnosis and better surgical planning (AlSaedi et al., 2024).

The development of targeted therapies that act on specific molecular pathways involved in cancer progression is a promising area in pediatric oncology (Salous & Adra, 2024). Drugs targeting specific genetic mutations, such as ALK inhibitors for anaplastic large cell lymphoma, have shown efficacy in treating certain pediatric HNCs with fewer side effects compared to traditional chemotherapy (Wai et al., 2024). Immunotherapy, including immune checkpoint inhibitors and chimeric antigen receptor (CAR)-T cell therapy, is revolutionizing cancer treatment. These therapies harness the patient's immune system to recognize and destroy cancer cells (Vennarini et al., 2024). Clinical trials are ongoing to evaluate the efficacy and safety of immunotherapy in pediatric HNCs, with early results showing promise (Wai et al., 2024). Advances in radiation therapy, such as proton therapy, offer more precise targeting of tumors with minimal damage to surrounding healthy tissues. This is particularly important in pediatric patients to reduce the risk of long-term side effects and secondary cancers (Ferraz, 2024). The integration of personalized medicine into pediatric oncology ensures that treatment plans are tailored to the individual characteristics of each patient's cancer. This approach maximizes treatment efficacy while minimizing adverse effects, thereby improving overall outcomes (Salous & Adra, 2024).

The future of pediatric HNC treatment also lies in a multidisciplinary and collaborative approach that ensures comprehensive care that addresses all aspects of the patient's health and well-being (Lopez et al., 2024). Ensuring equitable access to advanced diagnostic and treatment modalities remains a challenge, and efforts must be made to improve healthcare infrastructure and reduce disparities in access to cutting-edge care. Addressing the long-term health issues faced by survivors of pediatric HNCs is crucial (Salous & Adra, 2024). Research into minimizing treatment-related side effects and improving quality of life for survivors is needed (Lopez et al., 2024). Continued research and participation in clinical trials are essential to advance the understanding and treatment of pediatric HNCs, and a continued commitment to research, multidisciplinary care, and patient-centered approaches will be key in transforming the landscape of pediatric oncology (AlSaedi et al., 2024; Ferraz, 2024).

15.12 Conclusion

Pediatric HNCs present a unique set of challenges in both detection and treatment due to their rarity, diverse histology, and complex anatomical locations. Despite these challenges, significant advancements have been made in recent years, offering hope for improved outcomes. Early and accurate detection remains critical, with innovations in molecular and genetic profiling, liquid biopsies, and advanced imaging techniques enhancing diagnostic precision. These technologies enable earlier diagnosis and more personalized treatment plans, crucial for achieving better prognoses in young patients. On the treatment front, targeted therapies and immunotherapies are emerging as promising options, providing effective alternatives to traditional chemotherapy and radiation with fewer long-term side effects. Proton therapy represents a significant advancement in radiation treatment, offering precise targeting of tumors while sparing healthy tissues, thus reducing the risk of secondary cancers and other long-term complications. The integration of personalized medicine ensures that each patient receives tailored treatment based on their specific tumor characteristics, thus maximizing efficacy and minimizing adverse effects.

However, challenges remain in ensuring equitable access to these advanced diagnostic and treatment modalities. Addressing disparities in healthcare infrastructure and availability of cutting-edge treatments is essential to ensure all children benefit from these advancements. Additionally, long-term survivorship care is crucial to address the lasting impact of cancer treatments on pediatric patients, necessitating ongoing research and support for survivors. Pediatric HNCs pose significant detection and treatment challenges. However, the future is promising due to rapid advancements in medical science. Continued research, multidisciplinary collaboration, and a focus on personalized, patient-centered care will be key in overcoming these challenges and improving outcomes for young patients battling these complex cancers.

References

ALSAEDI, A. H., ALMALKI, D. S., & ELKADY, R. M. 2024. Approach to thyroid nodules: Diagnosis and treatment. *Cureus*, 16(1), e52232.

ALZAHRANI, H. A. 2024. Malignancy in a solitary thyroid nodule: A retrospective histopathological evaluation. *Int J Gen Med*, 17, 135–40.

ARBOLEDA, L. P. A., DE MENDONÇA, R. M. H., LOPEZ, E. E. M., ARAÚJO, A. L. D., PALMIER, N. R., DE PAULI PAGLIONI, M., FONSECA, J. M., HOFFMANN, I. L., CARDINALLI, I. A., CHAVES, A. L. F., ARANDA, S., BRANDÃO, T. B., LOPES, M. A., RIBEIRO, A. C. P., TROCONIS, C. C. M., & SANTOS-SILVA, A. R. 2020. Global frequency and distribution of HNC in pediatrics, a systematic review. *Crit Rev Oncol Hematol*, 148, 102892.

ARBOLEDA, L. P. A., HOFFMANN, I. L., CARDINALLI, I. A., GALLAGHER, K. P. D., SANTOS-SILVA, A. R., & MENDONÇA, R. M. H. 2020. Oral and maxillofacial cancer in pediatric patients: 30 years experience from a Brazilian reference center. *Int J Pediatr Otorhinolaryngol*, 131, 109879.

ARORA, V., SIDHU, B. S., & SINGH, K. 2022. Comparison of computed tomography and magnetic resonance imaging in evaluation of skull lesions. *Egyptian J Radiol Nuclear Med*, 53(1), 67.

BOUCAI, L., ZAFEREO, M., & CABANILLAS, M. E. 2024. Thyroid cancer: A review. *JAMA*, 331(5), 425–435.

BOUDINA, M., KATSAMAKAS, M., CHORTI, A., PANOUSIS, P., TZITZILI, E., TZIKOS, G., CHRISOULIDOU, A., VALERI, R., IOANNIDIS, A., & PAPAVRAMIDIS, T. 2024 Diagnostic accuracy of ultrasound and fine-needle aspiration cytology in thyroid malignancy. *Medicina (Kaunas)*, 60(5), 722.

BRITTO, T. I., FATTAH, S. A., RAHMAN, M. A. U., & CHOWDHURY, M. A. U. 2023. A systematic review on childhood non-Hodgkin lymphoma: An overlooked phenomenon in the health and research sector of Bangladesh. *Cureus*, 15(9), e45937.

CARMO, D., PINHEIRO, G., RODRIGUES, L., ABREU, T., LOTUFO, R., & RITTNER, L. 2023. Automated computed tomography and magnetic resonance imaging segmentation using deep learning: A beginner's guide. *arXiv preprint arXiv*:2304.05901.

CASEY, D. L., & WOLDEN, S. L., 2018. Rhabdomyosarcoma of the head and neck: A multimodal approach. *J Neurol Surg B: Skull Base*, 79(01), 058–064.

CAVALCANTE, L. B. C. P., TREISTMAN, N., GONZALEZ, F. M. T. T., FERNANDES, P. I. W., ALVES JUNIOR, P. A. G., ANDRADE, F. A., FERREIRA, E. N., BRITO, T. F., PANE, A., CORBO, R., ERLICH, F., BULZICO, D. A., & VAISMAN, F. 2024. External beam radiation therapy for recurrent or residual thyroid cancer: What is the best treatment time and the best candidate for long-term local disease control? *Head Neck*, 46(6), 1340–50.

CESMEBASI, A., GABRIEL, A., NIKU, D., BUKALA, K., DONNELLY, J., FIELDS, P. J., TUBBS, R. S., & LOUKAS, M. 2014. Pediatric head and neck tumors: An intra-demographic analysis using the SEER* database. *Med Sci Monit*, 20, 2536–42.

CHAI, A. W. Y., YEE, S. M., LEE, H. M., ABDUL AZIZ, N., YEE, P. S., MARZUKI, M., WONG, K. W., CHIANG, A. K. S., CHOW, L. K., DAI, W., LIU, T. F., TAN, L. P., KHOO, A. S. B., LO, K. W., LIM, P. V. H., RAJADURAI, P., LIGHTFOOT, H., BARTHORPE, S., GARNETT, M. J., & CHEONG, S. C. 2024. Establishment and characterization of an Epstein-Barr virus-positive cell line from a non-keratinizing differentiated primary nasopharyngeal carcinoma. *Cancer Res Commun*, 4(3), 645–59.

CHANG, A. E., MATORY, Y. L., DWYER, A. J., HILL, S. C., GIRTON, M. E., STEINBERG, S. M., KNOP, R. H., FRANK, J. A., HYAMS, D., & DOPPMAN, J. L. 1987. Magnetic resonance imaging versus computed tomography in the evaluation of soft tissue tumors of the extremities. *Ann Surg*, 205(4), 340.

CHEN, C., DORADO GARCIA, H., SCHEER, M., & HENSSEN, A. G. 2019. Current and future treatment strategies for rhabdomyosarcoma. *Front Oncol*, 9, 1458.

CLEMENTE, E. J., NAVALLAS, M., BARBER MARTÍNEZ DE LA TORRE, I., SUÑOL, M., MUNUERA DEL CERRO, J., TORNER, F., GARRAUS, M., & NAVARRO, O. M. 2020. MRI of rhabdomyosarcoma and other soft-tissue sarcomas in children. *Radiographics*, 40(3), 791–814.

COOPER, D. S., DOHERTY, G. M., HAUGEN, B. R., ET AL., 2009. Revised American Thyroid Association management guidelines for patients with thyroid nodules and differentiated thyroid cancer: The American Thyroid Association (ATA) Guidelines Taskforce on Thyroid Nodules and Differentiated Thyroid Cancer. *Thyroid*, 19, 1167–214.

DAI, J., ZHANG, B., SU, Y., PAN, Y., YE, Z., CAI, R., QIN, G., KONG, X., MO, Y., ZHANG, R., LIU, Z., XIE, Y., RUAN, X., & JIANG, W. 2024. Induction chemotherapy followed by radiotherapy vs chemoradiotherapy in nasopharyngeal carcinoma: A randomized clinical trial. *JAMA Oncol*, 10(4), 456–63.

DANTKALE, K. S., & AGRAWAL, M. 2024. A comprehensive review of current trends in the diagnosis and treatment of ovarian germ cell tumors. *Cureus*, 16(1), e52650.

DARWISH, C., SHIM, T., SPARKS, A. D., CHILLAKURU, Y., STRUM, D., BENITO, D. A., & MONFARED, A. 2020. Pediatric head and neck rhabdomyosarcoma: An analysis of treatment and survival in the United States (1975–2016). *Int J Pediatr Otorhinolaryngol*, 139, 110403.

EL-MALLAWANY, N. K., ALEXANDER, S., FLUCHEL, M., HAYASHI, R. J., LOWE, E. J., GIULINO-ROTH, L., WISTINGHAUSEN, B., HERMISTON, M., & ALLEN, C. E. 2023. COG NHL Committee. Children's Oncology Group's 2023 blueprint for research: Non-Hodgkin lymphoma. *Pediatr Blood Cancer*, 70 (Suppl 6), e30565.

ESTILO, C. L., HURYN, J. M., KRAUS, D. H., SKLAR, C. A., WEXLER, L. H., WOLDEN, S. L., & ZLOTOLOW, I. M. 2003. Effects of therapy on dentofacial development in long-term survivors of head and neck rhabdomyosarcoma: The Memorial Sloan-Kettering Cancer Center experience. *J Pediatr Hematol Oncol*, 25(3), 215–22.

FERRARI, A., VENNARINI, S., FIORE, M., BERGAMASCHI, L., CHIARAVALLI, S., MOROSI, C., COLOMBO, C., PECORI, E., PUMA, N., LUKSCH, R., TERENZIANI, M., SPREAFICO, F., MEAZZA, C., PODDA, M., BIASSONI, V., SCHIAVELLO, E., MASSIMINO, M., & CASANOVA, M. 2024. Local treatment in initially unresected non-rhabdomyosarcoma soft-tissue sarcomas of children and adolescents: A retrospective single-center experience. *Pediatr Blood Cancer*, 71(4), e30901.

FERRAZ C. 2024. Molecular testing for thyroid nodules: Where are we now? *Rev Endocr Metab Disord*, 25(1), 149–59.

FIGAJI, A. 2023. An update on pediatric traumatic brain injury. *Childs Nerv Syst*, 39(11), 3071–81.

FORCE, L. M., ABDOLLAHPOUR, I., ADVANI, S. M., et al., 2019. The global burden of childhood and adolescent cancer in 2017: An analysis of the Global Burden of Disease Study 2017. *Lancet Oncol*, 20, 1211–25.

FOSTER-THOMAS, E., AZNAR, M., INDELICATO, D., PAN, S., HWANG, E., SITCH, P., HORNER, K., SMITH, E., & GAITO, S. 2022. Late dental toxicities after proton chemoradiation for rhabdomyosarcoma: A pediatric case report. *Int J Particle Ther*, 9(3), 50–7.

FOUCHE, P. E., JENKINS, L. S., & VERMEULEN, A. 2021. Appropriateness of computed tomography and magnetic resonance imaging scans in a rural regional hospital in South Africa: A 6-year follow-up study. *S Afr Med J*, 111(1), 46–51.

FRANKART, A. J., BRENEMAN, J. C., & PATER, L. E. 2021. Radiation therapy in the treatment of head and neck rhabdomyosarcoma. *Cancers*, 13(14), 3567.

GERGES, A., & CANNING, U. 2024. Neuroblastoma and its target therapies: A medicinal chemistry review. *ChemMedChem*, 19(9), e202300535.

GIOVANELLA, L., MILAN, L., ROLL, W., WEBER, M., SCHENKE, S., KREISSL, M., VRACHIMIS, A., PABST, K., MURAT, T., PETRANOVIĆ OVČARIČEK, P., CAMPENNI, A., GÖRGES, R., & CERIANI, L. 2024. Thyroglobulin measurement is the most powerful outcome predictor in differentiated thyroid cancer: A decision tree analysis in a European multicenter series. *Clin Chem Lab Med*. doi:10.1515/cclm-2024-0405

GONG, C., HUANG, Y., LUO, M., CAO, S., GONG, X., DING, S., YUAN, X., ZHENG, W., & ZHANG, Y. 2024. Channel-wise attention enhanced and structural similarity constrained cycleGAN for effective synthetic CT generation from head and neck MRI images. *Radiat Oncol*, 19(1), 37.

GUO, M., SUN, Y., WEI, Y., XU, J., & ZHANG, C. 2024. Advances in targeted therapy and biomarker research in thyroid cancer. *Front Endocrinol* (Lausanne), 15, 1372553.

HADLEY, L. G., ROUMA, B. S., & SAAD-ELDIN, Y. 2012. Challenge of pediatric oncology in Africa. *Semin Pediatr Surg*, 21(2), 136–41.

HARRISON, D. J., QUMSEYA, A., XUE, W., ARNOLD, M., LAUTZ, T. B., HINIKER, S. M., THOMAS, S. M., VENKATRAMANI, R., WEISS, A. R., & MASCARENHAS, L. 2024.

Adolescents and young adults with rhabdomyosarcoma: A report from the Soft Tissue Sarcoma Committee of the Children's Oncology Group. *Pediatr Blood Cancer*, 71(4), e30847.

HASHIM, D., GENDEN, E., POSNER, M., HASHIBE, M., & BOFFETTA, P. 2019. Head and neck cancer prevention: from primary prevention to impact of clinicians on reducing burden. *Ann Oncol*, 30(5), 744–56.

HSU, C. L., CHANG, Y. S., & LI, H. P. 2024. Molecular diagnosis of nasopharyngeal carcinoma: Past and future. *Biomed J*, 23, 100748.

HUH, W. W., & SKAPEK, S. X. 2010. Childhood rhabdomyosarcoma: New insight on biology and treatment. *Curr Oncol Rep*, 12, 402–10.

JOHNSEN, J. I., & KOGNER, P. 2024. Recent advances in neuroblastoma research. *Cancers (Basel)*, 16(4), 812.

KELLER, F. G., KAHL, B., & FRIEDBERG, J. W. 2023. Current directions in the treatment of classical Hodgkin lymphoma. *EJHaem*, 4(4), 908–11.

KLIMENTOVA, M., PERMINOVA, M., SHELIKHOVA, L., ABUGOVA, Y., KOBYZEVA, D., PERSHIN, D., BALASHOV, D., MYAKOVA, N., MASCHAN, A., & MASCHAN, M. 2024. Allogeneic hematopoietic stem cell transplantation for mature T/NK-cell lymphomas in children. *Transplant Cell Ther*, 30(4), 437.e1–11.

KOZAK, K. R., ADAMS, J., KREJCAREK, S. J., TARBELL, N. J., & YOCK, T. I. 2009. A dosimetric comparison of proton and intensity-modulated photon radiotherapy for pediatric parameningeal rhabdomyosarcomas. *Int J Radiat Oncol Biol Physics*, 74(1), 179–86.

KUCHARSKA, E., RZEPAKOWSKA, A., ŻUREK, M., PIKUL, J., DANIEL, P., OLESZCZAK, A., & NIEMCZYK, K. 2024. Oncologic outcomes of the most prevalent major salivary gland cancers: Retrospective cohort study from single center. *Eur Arch Otorhinolaryngol*. doi:10.1007/s00405-024-08650-9

LI, X. F., MA, R. Q., WU, X., GAN, L., PENG, Z. Y., & QIAN, J. 2023. Adjuvant therapy for orbital non-rhabdomyosarcoma soft tissue sarcoma: Comparison of long-term outcome between radiotherapy and chemotherapy. *Int J Ophthalmol*, 16(3), 402–10.

LILJA-FISCHER, J. K., ULHØI, B. P., ALSNER, J., STOUGAARD, M., THOMSEN, M. S., BUSK, M., LASSEN, P., STEINICHE, T., NIELSEN, V. E., & OVERGAARD, J. 2019. Characterization and radiosensitivity of HPV-related oropharyngeal squamous cell carcinoma patient-derived xenografts. *Acta Oncol*, 58(10), 1489–94.

LOPEZ, F., AGAIMY, A., FRANCHI, A., SUÁREZ, C., VANDER POORTEN, V., MÄKITIE, A. A., HOMMA, A., EISBRUCH, A., OLSEN, K. D., SABA, N. F., NUYTS, S., SNYDERMAN, C., BEITLER, J. J., CORRY, J., HANNA, E., HELLQUIST, H., RINALDO, A., & FERLITO, A. 2024. Update on olfactory neuroblastoma. *Virchows Arch*, 484(4), 567–85.

LOPEZ, J., & TUFARO, A. P. 2024. Head and neck malignancies in children. *Oral Maxillofac Surg Clin North Am*, 21, S1042–3699(24)00029-3.

MCDONALD, M. W., ESIASHVILI, N., GEORGE, B. A., KATZENSTEIN, H. M., OLSON, T. A., RAPKIN, L. B., & MARCUS JR, R. B. 2008. Intensity-modulated radiotherapy with use of cone-down boost for pediatric head-and-neck rhabdomyosarcoma. *Int J Radiat Oncol Biol Physics*, 72(3), 884–91.

MILGROM, S. A., MILLION, L., MANDEVILLE, H., SAFWAT, A., ERMOIAN, R. P., & TEREZAKIS, S. 2021. Non-rhabdomyosarcoma soft-tissue sarcoma. *Pediatr Blood Cancer*, 68 Suppl 2, e28279.

MIWA, S., YAMAMOTO, N., HAYASHI, K., TAKEUCHI, A., IGARASHI, K., & TSUCHIYA, H. 2020. Recent advances and challenges in the treatment of rhabdomyosarcoma. *Cancers*, 12(7), 1758.

MOGENSEN, N., CANANAU, C., RANTA, S., KARLÉN, J., KWIECINSKA, A., & BAECKLUND, F. 2024. Successful treatment of paediatric refractory Hodgkin lymphoma with immunotherapy: A case report and literature review. *Acta Paediatr*, doi:10.1111/apa.17235

MORARU, L., MITRANOVICI, M. I., CHIOREAN, D. M., COROŞ, M., MORARU, R., OALĂ, I. E., & TURDEAN, S. G. 2023. Immature teratoma: Diagnosis and management – A review of the literature. *Diagnostics (Basel)*, 13(9), 1516.

NGUYEN, N. C., ANIGATI, E. M., DESAI, N. B., & ÖZ, O. K. 2024. Radioactive iodine therapy in differentiated thyroid cancer: An update on dose recommendations and risk of secondary primary malignancies. *Semin Nucl Med*, 20, S0001-2998(24)00042-4.

NGUYEN, Q. T., LEE, E. J., HUANG, M. G., PARK, Y. I., KHULLAR, A., & PLODKOWSKI, R. A. 2015. Diagnosis and treatment of patients with thyroid cancer. *Am Health Drug Benefits*, 8(1), 30–40.

NIKIFOROV, Y. E., YIP, L., & NIKIFOROVA, M. N. 2013. New strategies in diagnosing cancer in thyroid nodules: Impact of molecular markers. *Clin Cancer Res*,19, 2283–8.

NIMODIA, D., PARIHAR, P., NAGENDRA, V., GOWDA, H., & DESALE, P. 2024. Emergent management of growing teratoma syndrome: A case presentation. Cureus, 16(4), e59335.

NING, Z., LIU, X., QIN, G., WEI, L., LI, X., & SHEN, J. 2020. Evaluation of clinical efficacy of chemotherapy for rhabdomyosarcoma in children. *Pakistan J Med Sci*, 36(5), 1069.

ORR, C. J., MCCARTHA, E., VINCI, R. J., MINK, R. B., LEONARD, M. B., BISSELL, M., GAONA, A. R., & LESLIE, L. K. 2024. Projecting the future pediatric subspecialty workforce: Summary and recommendations. *Pediatrics*, 153(Suppl 2), e2023063678T.

OWOSHO, A. A., BRADY, P., WOLDEN, S. L., WEXLER, L. H., ANTONESCU, C. R., HURYN, J. M., & ESTILO, C. L. 2016. Long-term effect of chemotherapy-intensity-modulated radiation therapy (chemo-IMRT) on dentofacial development in head and neck rhabdomyosarcoma patients. *Pediatr Hematol Oncol*, 33(6), 383–92.

PATEL, J., KLOPPER, J., & COTTRILL, E. E. 2023. Molecular diagnostics in the evaluation of thyroid nodules: Current use and prospective opportunities. *Front Endocrinol (Lausanne)*, 14, 1101410.

PELUSO, E., FOWLER EDWARDS, W., & MARIE TRAN JANCO, J. 2024. Metastatic squamous cell carcinoma arising from mature teratoma of the ovary: Description of multimodality treatment including incorporation of adjuvant immunotherapy and maintenance PARP inhibitor therapy. *Gynecol Oncol Rep*, 52, 101371.

PFISTER, D., NÚÑEZ, N. G., PINYOL, R., GOVAERE, O., PINTER, M., SZYDLOWSKA, M., et al., 2021. NASH limits anti-tumour surveillance in immunotherapy-treated HCC. *Nature*, 592(7854), 450–6.

RADZIKOWSKA, J., KUKWA, W., KUKWA, A., CZARNECKA, A. M., KAWECKI, M., LIAN, F., SZCZYLIK, C., & KRZESKI, A. 2016. Management of pediatric head and neck rhabdomyosarcoma: A case-series of 36 patients. *Oncol Lett*, 12(5), 3555–3562.

RAISER, P., SCHLEIERMACHER, G., GAMBART, M., DUMONT, B., DEFACHELLES, A. S., THEBAUD, E., TANDONNET, J., PASQUALINI, C., PROUST, S., ENTZ-WERLE, N., AERTS, I., NDOUNGA-DIAKOU, L. A., PETIT, A., PUISEUX, C., KHANFAR, C., ROUGER, J., MANSUY, L., BENADIBA, J., MILLOT, F., PLUCHART, C., LAGHOUATI, S., GEOERGER, B., VASSAL, G., VALTEAU-COUANET, D., & BERLANGA, P. 2024. Chemo-immunotherapy with dinutuximab beta in patients with relapsed/progressive high-risk neuroblastoma: Does chemotherapy backbone matter? *Eur J Cancer*, 202, 114001.

RAYMOND, P., KLEIN, M., & BORSON-CHAZOT, F. 2024. Summary and update on the management of differentiated thyroid cancer in 2023. *Ann Endocrinol (Paris)*, 85(2), 110–117.

REILLY, B. K., KIM, A., PEÑA, M. T., DONG, T. A., ROSSI, C., MURNICK, J. G., & CHOI, S. S. 2015. Rhabdomyosarcoma of the head and neck in children: Review and update. *Int J Pediatr Otorhinolaryngol*, 79(9), 1477–83.

SAANI, I., RAJ, N., SOOD, R., ANSARI, S., MANDVIWALA, H. A., SANCHEZ, E., & BOUSSIOS, S. 2023. Clinical challenges in the management of malignant ovarian germ cell tumours. *Int J Environ Res Public Health*, 20(12), 6089.

SALOUS, T., & ADRA, N. 2024. Current outstanding challenges in germ cell tumors. *Curr Opin Oncol*, 36(3), 169–173.

SAPKOTA, S., & SHAIKH, H. (2023, February 24). Non-Hodgkin lymphoma. StatPearls. Treasure Island (FL): StatPearls Publishing, PMID: 32644754. https://www.ncbi.nlm.nih.gov/books/NBK559328/

SCHÄFER, J. F., GASSENMAIER, S., WARMANN, S., URLA, C., FRAUENFELD, L., FLAADT, T., CHAIKA, M., ESSER, M., TSIFLIKAS, I., TIMMERMANN, B., & FUCHS, J. 2023. Local MRI before and after tumor resection in neuroblastoma: Impact of residual disease on event free survival. *J Clin Med*, 12(23), 7297.

SCHOEMAN, S., BAGATELL, R., CAHILL, A. M., MARIS, J., MATTEI, P., MOSSE, Y., POGORILER, J., SRINIVASAN, A., & ACORD, M. 2024. Percutaneous biopsy for the diagnosis, risk stratification, and molecular profiling of neuroblastoma: A single-center retrospective study. *Pediatr Blood Cancer*, 71(4), e30887.

SERCARZ, J. A., MARK, R. J., NASRI, S., WANG, M. B., & TRAN, L. M. 1995. Pediatric rhabdomyosarcoma of the head and neck. *Int J Pediatr Otorhinolaryngol*, 31(1), 15–22.

SHAH, A. B., & NAGALLI, S. 2024, March 15. Nasopharyngeal carcinoma. 2024 Mar 15. StatPearls. Treasure Island (FL): StatPearls Publishing, PMID: 32119475. https://pubmed.ncbi.nlm.nih.gov/32119475/

SHENG, J., LI, T. T., ZHANG, H. H., XU, H. F., CAI, X. M., XU, R., JI, Q. Q., WU, Y. M., HUANG, T., & YANG, X. J. 2023. CT and MR imaging features of soft tissue rhabdoid tumor: Compared with rhabdomyosarcoma in children. *Front Pediatr*, 11, 1199444.

SINGH, H. K., KILPATRICK, S. E., & SILVERMAN, J. F. 2004. Fine needle aspiration biopsy of soft tissue sarcomas: Utility and diagnostic challenges. *Adv Anat Pathol*, 11(1), 24–37.

TANZAWA, A., SAITO, K., OTA, M., TAKAHASHI, K., OHNO, I., HANAZAWA, T., UZAWA, K., & TAKIGUCHI, Y. 2024. Salivary gland-type cancers: Cross-organ demographics of a rare cancer. *Int J Clin Oncol*, 29(6), 755–63.

TERWISSCHA VAN SCHELTINGA, S., ROGERS, T., SMEULDERS, N., DECORTI, F., GUERIN, F., CRAIGIE, R., BURRIEZA, G. G., SMEELE, L., HOL, M., VAN RIJN, R., FUCHS, J., SEITZ, G., SCHMIDT, A., TIMMERMANN, B., TUNN, P. U., CHARGARI, C., DÁVILA FAJARDO, R., SLATER, O., GAINS, J., & MERKS, H. 2023. Developments in the surgical approach to staging and resection of rhabdomyosarcoma. *Cancers (Basel)*, 15(2), 449.

TIAN, J., WEI, A., WANG, B., YANG, J., ZHENG, H., & QIN, M. 2024. Allogeneic hematopoietic stem cell transplantation for pediatric acute lymphoblastic leukemia. *Ann Hematol*, 103(1), 297–305.

TINKLE, C. L., FERNANDEZ-PINEDA, I., SYKES, A., LU, Z., HUA, C. H., NEEL, M. D., BAHRAMI, A., SHULKIN, B. L., KASTE, S. C., PAPPO, A., SPUNT, S. L., & KRASIN, M. J. 2017. Nonrhabdomyosarcoma soft tissue sarcoma (NRSTS) in pediatric and young adult patients: Results from a prospective study using limited-margin radiotherapy. *Cancer*, 123(22), 4419–29.

UTSUMI, Y., NAKAGURO, M., TADA, Y., & NAGAO, T. 2024. High-grade salivary carcinomas: A current insight on diagnostic pathology and the key to clinical decision making. *Semin Diagn Pathol*, 17, S0740–2570(24)00031-5.

VENNARINI, S., COLOMBO, F., MIRANDOLA, A., ORLANDI, E., PECORI, E., CHIARAVALLI, S., MASSIMINO, M., CASANOVA, M., & FERRARI, A. 2024. Proton therapy in non-rhabdomyosarcoma soft tissue sarcomas of children and adolescents. *Cancers (Basel)*, 16(9), 1694.

VIEIRA, L. S., ZHANG, Y., LÓPEZ QUIÑONES, A. J., HU, T., SINGH, D. K., STEVENS, J., PRASAD, B., PARK, J. R., & WANG, J. 2023. The plasma membrane monoamine transporter is highly expressed in neuroblastoma and functions as an mIBG transporter. *J Pharmacol Exp Ther*, 387(3), 239–48.

VOLEGOVA, M. P., BROWN, L. E., BANERJEE, U., DRIES, R., SHARMA, B., KENNEDY, A., PORCO, J. A. Jr., & GEORGE, R. E. 2024. The MYCN 5' UTR as a therapeutic target in neuroblastoma. *Cell Rep*, 43(5), 114134.

VON MEHREN, M., KANE, J. M., BUI, M. M., CHOY, E., CONNELLY, M., DRY, S., GANJOO, K. N., GEORGE, S., GONZALEZ, R. J., HESLIN, M. J., & HOMSI, J. 2020. NCCN guidelines insights: Soft tissue sarcoma, version 1.2021: Featured updates to the NCCN guidelines. *J Nat Comp Cancer Netw*, 18(12), 1604–12.

WAI, K. C., OKHOLM, T. L. H., HA, P. K., MARQUEZ, D. M., TENVOOREN, I., JONES, K. B., & SPITZER, M. H. 2024. The tumor microenvironment of benign and malignant salivary gland tumors. *Head Neck*. doi:10.1002/hed.27716

WARD, E., DESANTIS, C., ROBBINS, A., KOHLER, B., & JEMAL, A. 2014. Childhood and adolescent cancer statistics, 2014. *CA Cancer J Clin*, 64(2), 83–103.

WEI, X., YU, S., WANG, J., XIANG, Z., LIU, L., & MIN, Y. 2024. Association between time from diagnosis to treatment and survival of patients with nasopharyngeal carcinoma: A population-based cohort study. *Curr Probl Cancer*, 48, 101060.

WEN, Y., HUANG, D., ZHANG, W., ZHANG, Y., HU, H., & LI, J. 2020. Radiation therapy is an important factor to improve survival in pediatric patients with head and neck rhabdomyosarcoma by enhancing local control: A historical cohort study from a single center. *BMC Pediatr*, 20, 1–10.

XIA, X., ZHANG, J. W., ZHAO, B., ZHANG, M., CHEN, Z. R., ZHANG, B. F., JI, Y. L., WANG, X., XIONG, W. M., LI, J. W., & LV, Q. L. 2024. Progress of engineered bacteria for tumour therapy. *Int Immunopharmacol*, 132, 111935.

YOUNG, A., & OKUYEMI, O. T. 2023, January 12. Malignant salivary gland tumors. StatPearls. Treasure Island (FL): StatPearls Publishing; 2024 Jan–. PMID: 33079504. https://www.ncbi.nlm.nih.gov/books/NBK563022/

ZARRABI, A., PERRIN, D., KAVOOSI, M., SOMMER, M., SEZEN, S., MEHRBOD, P., BHUSHAN, B., MACHAJ, F., ROSIK, J., KAWALEC, P., AFIFI, S., BOLANDI, S. M., KOLEINI, P., TAHERI, M., MADRAKIAN, T., ŁOS, M. J., LINDSEY, B., CAKIR, N., ZAREPOUR, A., HUSHMANDI, K., FALLAH, A., KOC, B., KHOSRAVI, A., AHMADI, M., LOGUE, S., ORIVE, G., PECIC, S., GORDON, J. W., & GHAVAMI, S. 2023. Rhabdomyosarcoma: Current therapy, challenges, and future approaches to treatment strategies. *Cancers (Basel)*, 15(21), 5269.

ŻEBROWSKA, U., BALWIERZ, W., WECHOWSKI, J., & WIECZOREK, A. 2024. Survival benefit of myeloablative therapy with autologous stem cell transplantation in high-risk neuroblastoma: A systematic literature review. *Target Oncol*, 19(2), 143–59.

ZHANG, K., WANG, X., WEI, T., LI, Z., ZHU, J., & CHEN, Y. W. 2024. Radioactive iodine therapy improves overall survival outcome in oncocytic carcinoma of the thyroid by reducing death risks from noncancer causes: A competing risk analysis of 4641 patients. *Head Neck*. doi:10.1002/hed.27758

16
Prevention Strategies for Head and Neck Cancer

Shobana Sampath, Nkhensani Chauke-Malinga, Arun Mankan, Dunja Mihajlovic, Kamal S. Saini, and Zodwa Dlamini

16.1 Introduction

Head and neck cancers (HNCs) account for about 5% of all cancers. In absolute terms, globally, around 887,649 emerging cancer-related cases and 453,307 cancer deaths occurring in 2018 can be attributed to HNCs (Gormley et al., 2022). The increase in the number of cases of oropharyngeal carcinoma is primarily responsible for the rising incidence of HNC, which is expected to continue. *Head and neck squamous cell carcinoma* (HNSCC) is the common term for the majority of head and neck malignancies; these originate from the epithelial tissue of the mucosal layer of the pharynx, oral cavity, and larynx. The general phrase "HNC" includes a wide range of epithelial malignancies originating from the paranasal sinuses, nasal cavity, oral cavity, larynx, pharynx, and salivary glands. The majority of these epithelial malignancies are carcinomas of squamous cells of the head and neck, for which drinking alcohol and smoking and other tobacco use are the biggest risk factors (Kawashita et al., 2020; Liu et al., 2021).

Pharynx cancers are becoming more commonly associated with human papillomavirus (HPV), including HPV16. By contrast, oral cavity and larynx cancers typically correspond with the use of tobacco, alcohol abuse, or both (Johnson et al., 2020). While this disease seems to be becoming more common, and given the drop in smoking especially in high-income nations, there have been suggestions of possible alterations in its etiology (Gormley et al., 2022). While the incidence of HNSCC varies across nations and areas, exposure to carcinogens from tobacco smoke, alcohol, or both has generally been associated with it. Literature data showed that people who have had oropharyngeal tumors have also had infections with cancer-causing strains of HPV, mostly HPV16 but also HPV18 and some other variants. The number of cases of HPV-linked or HPV-positive HNSCC has significantly increased worldwide (Muzaffar et al., 2021). Geographic variation and variations in incidence between men and women have been linked the disparities in risk factor exposure between the sexes (Baijens et al., 2021).

Oral cancers account for 48% of HNCs, thereby ranking as the sixth most common cancer in humans. Of these, based on histology, oral SCCs (OSCCs) account for 90% of cases. In most countries, the 5-year survival rate for oral cancer is < 50%, even with the use of innovative management regimens. Since HNCs are heterogeneous tumors, devising a treatment plan can be difficult. Prevention is essential since oral cancer has such dismal results (Irani, 2020). Due to their complexity and multiple subsites, HNCs necessitate an integrated strategy with trimodal therapy to cure them. This approach includes support teams that include speech and swallowing treatment, physical therapy, occupational therapy, nutrition, and smoking cessation programs (Anderson et al., 2021). The disease's destruction of important structures, treatment side effects, and the long-term effects or toxicity of systemic treatments like radiation and chemotherapy can all contribute to lower quality of life (Loewen et al., 2021).

Reports suggest that lip, oral cavity, and pharyngeal cancers may have caused the 529,500 new cancer reports (approximately 3.8% of all cancer cases) and 292,300 cancer-related deaths (approximately 3.6% of all cancer deaths) that occurred globally in 2012. By 2035, Huang and Pan expect the incidence to rise by 62% to 856,000 cases. The patient's geographic location and the tumor's anatomical region have an impact on the occurrence and treatment of HNSCC, respectively. The most prevalent HNSCCs worldwide are laryngeal and oral cancers, with greater incidence and fatality rates in Europe than in the United States. HNSCC affects men far more frequently than it does women, with a prevalence ratio of 2:1 to 4:1 (Sabatini & Chiocca, 2020). It has long been believed that alcohol and tobacco use are the primary causes of HNCs. According to reports, alcohol consumption and/or tobacco use account for 72% of HNCs. Despite the recognition of alcohol and tobacco as separate risk factors, alcohol alone accounts for 4% of the 72%, tobacco for 33%, and both for 35%. Men are between three and five times more likely than women to have HNC, although the gender-related incidence varies depending on the location of the tumor.

Although more precisely focused radiation and immunotherapeutic drugs offer promise for decreasing long-term damage, current therapies for head and neck malignancies are effective (Cramer et al., 2019). For many years, surgery has been the primary therapeutic option for HNC, but new information suggests that HNC surgery is not always the best choice. It is vital to reexamine HNC treatment strategies for the benefit of patients, healthcare professionals, healthcare organizations, and society at large (Day et al., 2020). This chapter discusses various prevention strategies as well as methodologies allowing for the early detection of HNC.

16.2 Head and Neck Squamous Cell Carcinoma Prevention

The discovery of novel genes with a role in HNSCC, along with the identification of genetic pathways like tumor suppressor genes and oncogenes, nuclear genetic alterations, and mitochondrial genetic alterations, has allowed us to understand better the formation and progression of HNSCC. In this regard, researchers have identified several proven risk factors, such as HPV infection, smoking, and significant genetic abnormalities in epidermal growth factor receptor (EGFR), TP53, p16, and p14. To prevent or delay the development of HNSCC, some effective primary measures in the current context include quitting smoking, limiting alcohol consumption, avoiding tobacco chewing, avoiding exposure to secondhand smoke from cigarettes and environmental carcinogens, testing for HPV, sustaining good oral health, adopting healthy eating habits, and managing anxiety. It may also be advantageous to detect erythroplakia or leukoplakia lesions early on and remove them surgically to stop HNSCC from developing (Dasgupta et al., 2012). Figure 16.1 illustrated the different strategies that can be used to monitor and detect cases of HNC as well as some precautionary measures to prevent HNC.

Hong et al. studied patients who remained disease-free after primary treatment for squamous cell cancers of the larynx, pharynx, or oral cavity. After completion of surgery or radiotherapy (or both), these patients were randomly assigned to receive either isotretinoin (13-*cis*-retinoic acid) (50–100 $mg/m^2/day$ of body surface area) or placebo, to be taken daily for 12 months. The number of local, distant, or regional recurrences of the initial malignancies did not knowingly differ among the two groups. As well, there were noticeably fewer second primary tumors in the isotretinoin group. After following for a median of 32 months, only two patients (4%) in the isotretinoin category developed second primary malignancies, while 12 patients (24%) in the placebo group experienced the same outcome ($P = 0.005$).

In the placebo group, four patients developed multiple second primary tumors. The esophagus, lung, head, and neck accounted for 13 (93%) of the 14 second tumors. The conclusion of this study was that regular administration of large doses of isotretinoin is successful in preventing the development of additional primary tumors in patients who have undergone therapy for HNSCC. However, isotretinoin does not prevent the reappearance of the initial tumor (Hong et al., 1990).

In addition to preventing cancer recurrence, tertiary prevention also attempts to avoid or manage the morbidity brought on by cancer therapy. Even though HPV-positive oropharyngeal SCC (OPSCC) patients have a far better prediction than their HPV-negative counterparts as many as 25% of these individuals will experience a recurrence within 24 months of starting treatment.

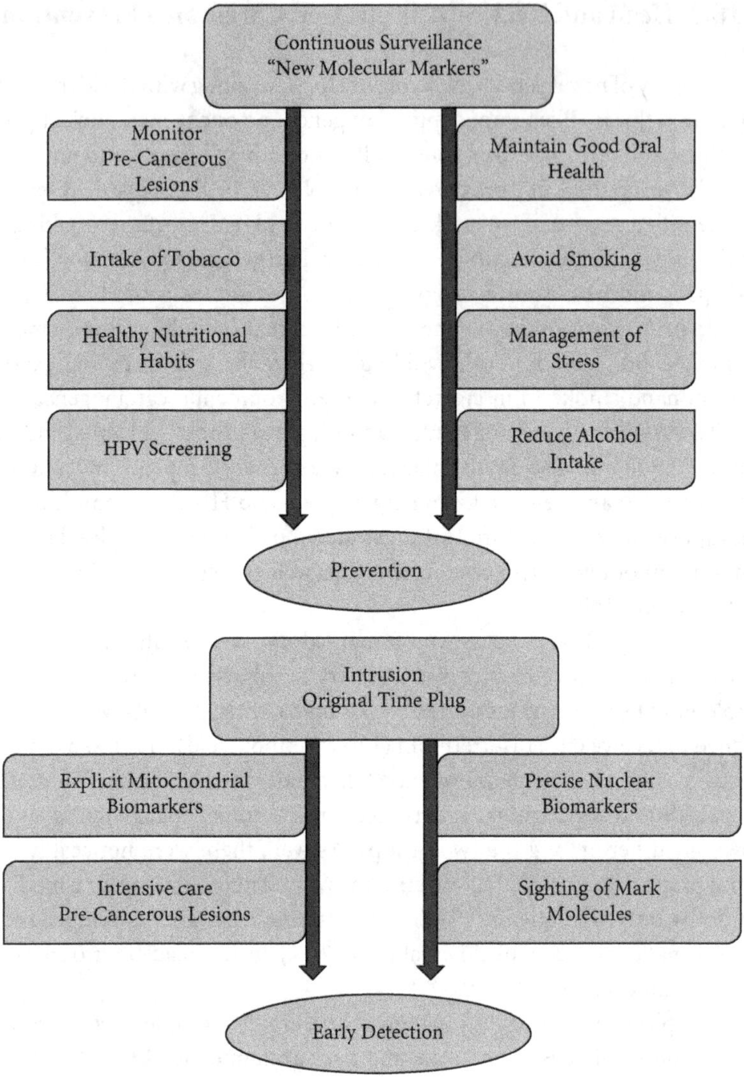

Figure 16.1 Strategies for the prevention and early detection of head and neck cancer (HNC). The comprehensive approach highlights the importance of combining early detection methods with preventive measures to effectively manage and reduce the incidence of HNC.

Blood-based biomarkers are effective in cancer identification; HPV16 E6 serology and the identification of circulating HPV16 DNA are very useful methods in cancer detection. Mirghani et al. showed that, prior to therapy, the oral rinses of HPV-positive OPSCCs revealed detectable HPV DNA. Of the 34 individuals without persistent HPV16 DNA, there were only two illness recurrences, compared to three in the four individuals who had HPV16 DNA and received post-treatment oral rinses (Mirghani et al., 2017). Understanding the needs of SCC patients not only provides an opportunity to develop prevention plans, but also provides valuable insights into human carcinogenesis. The current 13-cis-retinoic acid SPT prevention protocol closely links to various scientific projects that aim to gain basic knowledge of retinoids in cancer development and chemotherapy prevention (Benner et al., 1992).

16.2.1 Vaccine-Driven Prevention of Head and Neck Cancer

The current strategy to reduce the incidence of uterine cervical cancer, the archetypal HPV-driven malignancy, involves preventive HPV vaccines and screening programs for the early detection and treatment of premalignant lesions. Prophylactic vaccination and screening initiatives show potential for lowering the prevalence of cervical cancer. However, HPV-driven oropharyngeal malignancies necessitate novel and targeted preventive measures. Before they can improve post-treatment follow-up, viral biomarkers require further validation (Mirghani et al., 2017). HR-HPV vaccines most likely have the potential to prevent HPV-driven OPSCCs as well. Immunizations should protect against HPV16/18 oral infections, the root cause of nearly all HPV-positive OPSCCs. Animal models have revealed that immunization provides defense against canine oral papillomavirus lesions and mouth infections. Researchers have found that, following vaccination against HPV, high levels of type-specific antibodies are found in oral fluids like saliva from the salivary glands and oral mucosal transudation from vessels throughout the gingival mucosa (Mirghani et al., 2017). Another approach entails utilizing gene therapy to reverse the cancerous phenotype. Additionally, the adenovirus ONYX-015, which does not replicate and which kills cancer cells, shows promise when used with chemotherapy to treat HNSCC (Saba et al., 2007).

16.2.2 Immune-Based Prevention Strategies

Patients with HNC have impaired antitumor responses, as evidenced by recent discoveries of functional abnormalities and the death of circulating as well as tumor-infiltrating T cells. To better control the growth of the tumor, strategies for immunological competence restoration and tumor escape prevention are required for patients with HNC to better control the tumor's growth. Novel immunotherapeutic strategies include vaccines made from dendritic cells (DCs) and cytokines that try to protect immune cells from tumor-induced apoptosis and bring back responses that are specific to the tumor (Whiteside, 2005). From an immune perspective we know that HPV-positive malignant cells express viral DNA categorizations, particularly those associated with the E6 and E7 viral oncogenes. Their exterior, visible viral antigens trigger a tailored immune response. These distinctive features of HPV-positive malignancies can be identified and hence serve as tumor biomarkers. More specifically, patients with HPV-related malignancies frequently exhibit antibodies targeting the viral cancer-causing proteins E6 and E7, particularly in the oropharyngeal and anal regions. Conversely, healthy individuals rarely exhibit these antibodies (Mirghani et al., 2017).

Bioadjuvant therapy, which combines retinoids, α-tocopherol, interferon, molecularly targeted medicines, and oncolytic viruses, can prevent HNC, but retinoid resistance and toxicity limit the clinical promise of retinoid-based chemoprevention. It is believed that solid tumors acquire intrinsic resistance to retinoids throughout the carcinogenesis process through a number of still to be fully understood mechanisms. The downregulation of retinoic acid receptor-b, which typically takes place during epithelial carcinogenesis, is considered one important cause. To overcome these challenges, a novel type of receptor-specific synthetic retinoid and combination regimens that can induce long-lasting inhibition of epithelium cancerization across the upper aerodigestive tract will be needed. Researchers are conducting a thorough preclinical and clinical assessment of nonclassical retinoids with retinoid receptor-independent qualities to reduce retinoid resistance, minimize toxicity, and improve bioavailability (Saba et al., 2007).

Animal experiments have provided further support for the epidemiologic evidence indicating that dietary retinoids offer protection against cancer. For example, after the use of isotretinoin in a Syrian hamster cancer model, researchers saw a big drop in lingual and buccal cancers caused by 7,12-dimethylbenz[a]anthracene (DMBA) (Benner et al., 1992). Researchers also have conducted explorations of T-cell transfer with engineered chimeric receptors for antigens (CAR-T cells) in various tumor types, suggesting potential applications in the therapy of HNCs. And, despite the current lack of data on HNCs, it is likely that we can engineer T cells specifically targeting EGFR. Ninety percent of HNCs contain EGFR, and studies have shown that cetuximab, a monoclonal antibody that targets EGFR, enhances survival in these malignancies.

Research in the field of tumor immunotherapy, from preventive vaccination for viral-related cancers to the use of PD-1 checkpoint inhibitors in the treatment of metastatic disease, has demonstrated considerable potential (Schoenfeld, 2015). Cancer immunotherapy depends on the immune system's capacity to identify cancer cells and initiate a targeted immunological response resulting in long-lasting control of the illness through immunologic memory. Immunotherapy has demonstrated efficacy in treating both HPV-related and HPV-unrelated HNSCC (Carlisle et al., 2020).

16.2.3 Prevention through Natural Compounds

A wealth of evidence from various studies indicates the potential cancer-fighting properties of certain nutrients, including green and yellow vegetables and citrus fruits. Green tea is a nutritional compound that has shown potential for fighting cancer. In various tumor cell lines, including those from oral cavity cancers, use of green tea polyphenols has been shown to trigger apoptosis resulting from the activation of different cell cycle regulators. The anticancer properties of black raspberries' curcuminoid, which is similar to compounds found in green tea, are being actively investigated (Saba et al., 2007).

Oral mucositis is a notable issue for individuals diagnosed with HNC because it develops from an inflammatory response to the formation of ulcerative sores in the oropharynx and mouth. Combining radiation therapy (RT) and chemotherapy increases the vulnerability of the oral mucosa to harm (Dodd et al., 2022). Clinical studies in patients with radiation-induced oral mucositis, conducted to check the efficacy of granulocyte macrophage colony stimulating factor (GM-CSF) mouthwash compared to salt and soda mouthwash, have shown that the use of GM-CSF mouthwash did not aid in preventing or treatment of oral mucositis.

16.3 Shielding against Side Effects

16.3.1 Strategies to Prevent the Side Effects of Radiotherapy

Preventing osteoradionecrosis (ORN) is the goal of oral treatment preceding the initiation of RT. Even though ORN is rare, once it does arise, it seldom goes away on its own; in patients with severe lesions, jaw surgery is required. As a result, it is necessary to identify whether dental extractions are required and to evaluate the source of dental infections. If necessary, extractions should be completed at least 2 weeks prior to the start of radiation treatment (Kawashita et al., 2020). An ionizing radiation (IR) experiment using a 3D spheroid culture was conducted to understand the mechanism of IR-induced cellular death. The experiment demonstrated that combining human paratoid tissue-derived spheroids (hPTS) to form 3D structures resembling acinar accurately reflected how IR impairs salivary gland function in living organisms (Yoon et al., 2019).

Depending on risk factors, postoperative surgical care frequently recommends RT for patients with positive margins and/or extracapsular spread of tumors (ECE). There are currently trials looking into ways to make treatment for HPV-positive oropharyngeal cancers less intense. These strategies involve reducing the dosage and volume of RT and potentially reducing the intensity of concurrent systemic therapy (Anderson et al., 2021). Figure 16.2 shows radiation-induced damage to the salivary gland.

The symptoms of radiation dermatitis (RD) typically manifest for a limited number of weeks following the start of RT. Even with improvements in RT methods, impact on the skin is still unavoidable, and moderate to severe skin responses occur in about 85% of HNC patients who have received RT. When compared to standard care, olive oil is the most efficient topical regimen for avoiding radiation dermatitis in patients with HNC (Kao et al., 2022). RT to the head and neck causes hyposalivation and xerostomia. This leads to the entry of pathogens into the jaw and the development of severe dental caries. Researchers have identified the oral health state following RT as a significant contributing factor to the occurrence of ORN. Therefore, programs to prevent dental cavities

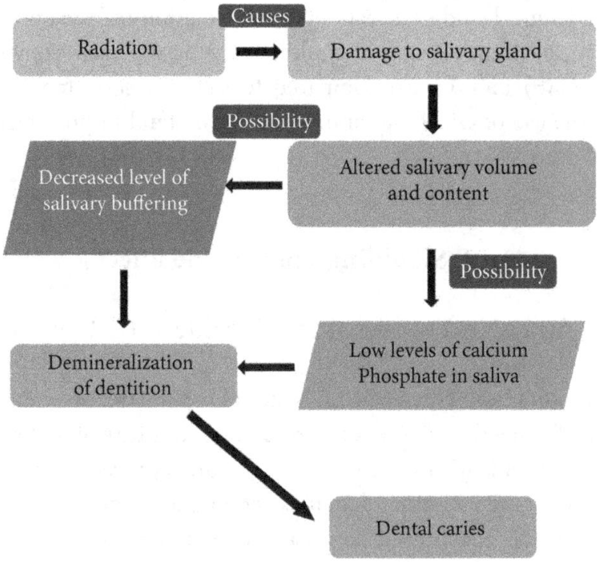

Figure 16.2 Radiation-induced salivary damage. Radiation-induced damage to the salivary glands is a significant complication of head and neck cancer (HNC) treatment. It leads to symptoms like xerostomia, dysphagia, and altered taste, significantly affecting the quality of life. Management strategies include advanced radiation techniques, pharmacological interventions, protective agents, and supportive care.

caused by radiation are essential to controlling ORN. Patients receiving head and neck RT have demonstrated a reduction in carcinogenic flora colonization when using chlorhexidine suspensions.

Furthermore, nutritional advice should be provided to minimize cariogenic meals and drugs to enhance salivary flow should be prescribed. These actions are crucial for reducing the incidence of dental caries brought on by RT (Kawashita et al., 2020). Salivary glands are extremely sensitive to radiation because of their specialized cells, which have a very low growth rate. Dealing with the damage and dysfunction caused by RT to the salivary glands is a complex situation. Conditions like autoimmune and chronic inflammatory illnesses can lead to permanent damage to the salivary glands (Ziyad, 2022). Administering basic fibroblast growth factor to the rat parotid gland before and immediately following radiation helped protect it (44%) (Thula et al., 2005). Targeted small interfering RNAs (siRNAs inhibited the expression of Pkcβ and Bax proteins, which ordinarily cause cell death in cultured glandular saliva. Successive irradiation dramatically lowered the quantity of cell death (Arany et al., 2012). Recombinant human hepatocyte growth factor treatment of irradiation-caused hyperparathyroidism restored salivary marker expression and secretory activity (Yoon et al., 2019).

Furthermore, it has been found that administering S-2-[3-aminopropylamino]-ethyl phosphorothioic acid WR-2721 before every dose of irradiation was feasible and did not result in significant toxicity at a dosage of 100 mg/m^2. In these patients, salivary gland function showed improvement over time following the completion of RT, with a notable focus on the parotid gland (McDonald et al., 1994). Amifostine effectively reduces the occurrence of acute xerostomia and mucositis (Vacha et al., 2003). Individuals suffering from hyposalivation have a higher susceptibility to dental caries and therefore require rigorous oral hygiene practices and regular dental monitoring. Swallowing abnormalities, such as difficulties swallowing, xerostomia (dry mouth), and poor dentition (bad teeth), can lead to changes in diet that may result in nutritional inadequacies. It is crucial to identify and handle unhealthy eating habits to maintain long-term good health (Murphy & Deng, 2015).

16.3.2 Preventing Adverse Reactions in Following Treatment

Tumor immunotherapy has shown promising results in improving outcomes and lowering side effects related to treatment for a variety of HNCs, including those caused by viruses and those linked to smoking. Immunotherapy using T cells is a promising approach for treating viral cancers. *Adoptive T-cell therapy* has shown promise in treating EBV-mediated posttransplant lymphoproliferative disorders (Schoenfeld, 2015).

16.4 Risk Factors

Tobacco: Tobacco usage is the main risk factor for HNSCC and several other malignancies. According to epidemiologic data, people who smoke have a five- to nine-fold higher risk of oral cancer than people who do not smoke; for very heavy smokers who smoke 80 or more cigarettes a day, this risk can rise to 17 times higher. Moreover, research has identified smokers receiving oral cancer therapy as having a two- to six-times higher chance of developing a second primary tumor of the upper aerodigestive tract compared to patients who quit smoking. Furthermore, evidence also shows that exposure to ambient tobacco smoke and marijuana smoking could potentially cause HNSCC (Day et al., 2005). The anatomic regions in direct contact with tobacco and tobacco smoke—the oral cavity, larynx, throat, esophagus, and outside of those in the neck and head regions, the lungs—are those most at risk for developing cancer as a result of tobacco use. There appears to be a slight correlation between the prevalence of pharyngeal and esophageal carcinomas and the use of smokeless tobacco in other head and neck regions. Tobacco users frequently combine multiple habits, further emphasizing the suggested dose-response link, but did not prove that smoking cigars and pipes increases the risk of developing lip cancer.

Lichen planus: Numerous studies have linked chronic oral lichen planus, an inflammatory condition that affects mucous membranes inside the mouth, particularly the erosive type, to an increased risk of developing SCC later (Day et al., 2005).

Alcohol: Information provided by National Cancer Institute has shown that moderate to heavy alcohol consumption is associated with higher risks of certain HNCs. Alcohol serves as both a solvent and an irritant. Alcohol toxicity is primarily triggered by ethanol itself and its metabolic byproducts. This toxicity is influenced by the oral microbiota and the effects of oxidative stress. Consumption of alcohol can also increase the risk of epithelial cells being exposed to carcinogens and DNA damage, leading to epigenetic changes and faulty DNA repair, resulting in the development of DNA adducts (Ferraguti et al., 2022). When consumed in greater quantities, alcohol and tobacco seem to work in concert. One study calculated a risk rise of 19 times when both factors were present compared to 3.6 times for alcohol by itself and 5.8 times for tobacco use alone (Schleper, 1989).

Human papillomavirus: Researchers have linked HPV16 to up to 45% of oropharyngeal cancers and 22% of oral cancers, and HPV18 with to up to 14% of cases. The majority of research has demonstrated evidence of a favorable prognosis for HPV-positive HNSCCs (Day et al., 2005; Schleper, 1989).

Sunlight: A history of persistent sun exposure strongly links to SCC of the lip, although other factors may be involved. Lip (and cutaneous) tumors are associated with a genetic susceptibility to skin cancer and excessive exposure to UV radiation from the sun through employment and/or leisure (Schleper, 1989).

Occupational exposures: Industries that produce manufactured wood products, textiles, and leather and nickel refining are all implicated in the pathogenesis of HNC. This is caused by the exposure of nasal passages and sinuses to mustard gas that can cause HNC (Schleper, 1989).

Nutrition: Consuming salted seafood and high nitrosamine consumption is known to cause HNC (Schleper, 1989). In contrast, the addition of β-carotene and/or vitamin A to the diet may offer protection against epithelial carcinoma.

Supportive Care: Modern developments in physical therapy and swallow therapy can assist HNC survivors in avoiding or treating long-term functional deficits and oral health issues (Murphy & Deng, 2015). Thus, absence of such supportive care impacts the quality of life of the HNC patient.

16.5 Early Detection of Head and Neck Cancer

The management of cancer greatly depends on early detection. It is widely known that benign hyperplastic to dysplastic alterations in the epithelial tissue are the first steps in the sequential histological phases that lead to HNSCC development. Surgical removal of nonmalignant epithelial cells, commonly identified as leukoplakia or erythroplakia, can occasionally halt the growth of HNSCC. However, it might not always be possible to find these spots at the earliest opportunity. Moreover, especially in smokers, HNSCC can advance quickly and occur without the identification of its nonmalignant counterparts.

The best primary detection methods for HNSCC involve identifying genetic abnormalities early on in the disease's development and combining this data with information on EGFR and TP53 mutations (Dasgupta et al., 2012). Furthermore, knowing that HNSCC is a malignancy characterized by epithelial cells that originate from the mucosa of the upper aerodigestive tract, patients with suspicious symptoms should be immediately assessed for abnormalities in this area (Chauhan et al., 2022). Figure 16.3 shows the various methods of prevention for human papillomavirus-driven HNC.

16.6 Social Awareness

Socioeconomic class significantly influences the incidence and mortality of HNCs, and quitting smoking and refraining from alcohol abuse can prevent

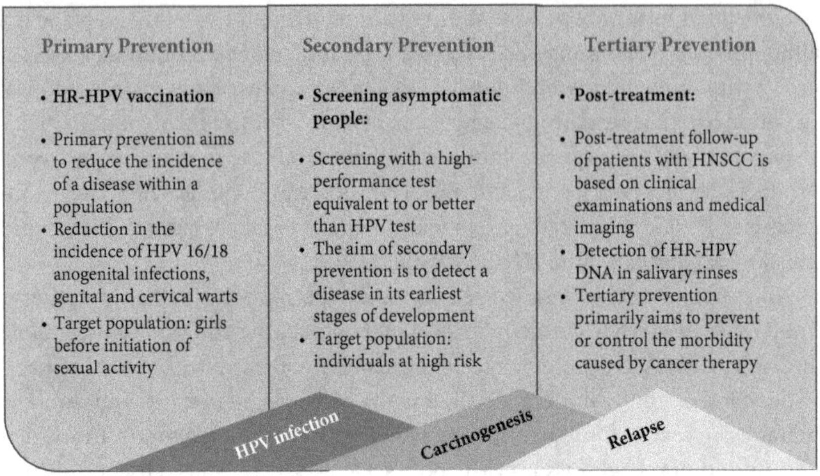

Figure 16.3 Different stages of prevention of human papillomavirus (HPV)-driven head and neck cancer (HNC). HPV is a significant risk factor for HNCs, particularly oropharyngeal cancers. Preventing HPV-driven HNC involves a multifaceted approach, including vaccination, education, and regular screening.

the majority of these diseases. Controlling HNCs is a top issue due to its widespread occurrence and rising frequency in developed nations. Given the well-established correlation between alcohol misuse, tobacco use, and HNCs, there is a significant chance that reducing alcohol use and curbing the smoking epidemic will prevent these malignancies (Whiteside, 2005).

It is imperative to persist in endeavors to raise social awareness about the detrimental effects of tobacco consumption. Chauhan et al. (2022) validated the widespread occurrence of tobacco use among patients with HNC. Hormonal differences may influence susceptibility to HPV-related carcinogenesis. Women may clear HPV infections differently than men, leading to a higher persistence of high-risk HPV strains in the oropharyngeal region. Indeed, numerous organizations have made it their mission to inform the general public, medical professionals, dentists, and others about the risk issues, therapies, and recovery associated with HNSCC. Since 1998, the Global Oral and Head and Neck Cancer Awareness Week, sponsored by the Yul Brynner Head and Neck Cancer Foundation, has effectively increased public and community awareness of this issue via media campaigns and free cancer screenings. Subsequent public education campaigns on HNSCC will eventually result in better health professional training and, hopefully, earlier detection of the illness (Day et al., 2005).

16.7 Bio Chemoprevention

Bio chemoprevention, a technique in which natural, synthetic, or biologic chemical agents are used to reverse, suppress, or prevent carcinogenic progression, is most useful for HNC because many carcinogens are known and there is a tendency for *field cancerization* (in which a large area of tissue becomes predisposed to cancer development) in the presence of carcinogens and a high rate of secondary primary tumors. Unfortunately, it is still unknown which specific medications ultimately increase disease-related survival. Patients who are in danger of recurrence and have a history of HNSCC may benefit from specialized treatments (such as retinoids) to reverse precancerous lesions and delay the emergence of new lesions (Day et al., 2005).

Gene transfer to increase fluid production and stem cell transfer to increase the chance of regeneration in radiation-damaged salivary glands are two promising ways to restore function and/or rejuvenate these tissues. It is still unclear how radiation causes tissue damage and malfunctions in the salivary glands; current therapeutic approaches offer temporary symptom alleviation, but they do not address lasting glandular damage. Alternative approaches to repairing radiation-damaged salivary glands are being investigated, with encouraging outcomes. These include gene transfer procedures and stem cell therapies, which enable the radiation-damaged salivary gland tissues to release water. Chemotherapy-induced hyposalivation is typically milder and more reversible than radiation damage to salivary gland tissue, which is mostly irreversible.

16.8 Use of Artificial Intelligence in Analysis of Medical Images

More recently, research involving histology has commonly employed conventional machine learning (ML) techniques to identify precancerous or cancerous tumors in the oral cavity. Mahmood and coworkers (2021) employed whole slide imaging (WSI) and deep learning (DL) techniques to identify HNSCC lesion in the larynx, oral cavity, nasopharynx, and other spots within the head and neck region. The DL approach incorporated in this study demonstrated promising results in accurately classifying thermal images from patients with HNSCC and mucositis. The categorization was determined by detecting tiny temperature fluctuations in the oral mucosa, which was found to be associated with changes in the severity of mucositis. The accuracy of the performance model confirmed its usefulness in arranging tasks. This suggested that the model had the potential to be useful in evaluating the effect of radiotherapy on the mucosa. Cohen and colleagues (2013) conducted pilot research that showed that thermal imaging has potential as a prediction technique for toxicity in individuals receiving therapy for localized HNSCC.

16.9 Limitations

Some HNCs have been associated with occupational carcinogen exposure. Effective oversight and implementation of occupational security can be difficult, especially in industries with little resources or monitoring. Policies relating to smoke exposure, alcohol regulation, and workplace safety are often inconsistently implemented and enforced, thus limiting their effectiveness in preventing HNC. Cultural assumptions and social norms may affect HNC risk-related behaviors; these include tobacco and alcohol use as well as attitudes toward immunization and healthcare utilization. To improve the efficacy of HNC preventive methods, a multimodal strategy is required to address these constraints, including enhanced public health efforts, education, legislative reforms, and healthcare access.

16.10 Conclusion

HNCs are a largely preventable disease. Using proactive intervention strategies that enable earlier diagnosis as well as implementing preventive measures will help reduce the incidence of this disease. There is a need for a multidisciplinary approach in treating this disease, and this depends on providing patients with access to a diverse team that can provide holistic therapy especially when a timely diagnosis is not achievable. However, many people are unable to access multidisciplinary care, and the survival rate for late-stage HNC is still low. To mitigate this, the most important actions that can be taken to prevent HNC include making the public aware of risk factors and of the importance of reducing or abstaining from smoking and drinking, emphasizing the importance of getting vaccinated against HPV, and making screening easier and more accurate.

References

ANDERSON, G., EBADI, M., VO, K., NOVAK, J., GOVINDARAJAN, A., & AMINI, A. 2021. An updated review on head and neck cancer treatment with radiation therapy. *Cancers*, 13(19), 4912.

ARANY, S., XU, Q., HERNADY, E., BENOIT, D. S. W., DEWHURST, S., & OVITT, C. E. 2012. Pro-apoptotic gene knockdown mediated by nanocomplexed siRNA reduces radiation damage in primary salivary gland cultures. *J Cell Biochem*, 113(6), 1955–65.

BAIJENS, L. W. J., WALSHE, M., AALTONEN, L.-M., ARENS, C., CORDIER, R., CRAS, P., CREVIER-BUCHMAN, L., CURTIS, C., GOLUSINSKI, W., GOVENDER, R., ERIKSEN, J. G., HANSEN, K., HEATHCOTE, K., HESS, M. M., HOSAL, S., KLUSSMANN, J. P., LEEMANS, C. R., MACCARTHY, D., MANDUCHI, B., & CLAVÉ, P. 2021. European white paper: Oropharyngeal dysphagia in head and neck cancer. *Eur Arch Oto-Rhino-Laryngol*, 278(2), 577–616.

BENNER, S. E., LIPPMAN, S. M., & HONG, W. K. 1992. Prevention of second head and neck cancers. *Semin Radiat Oncol*, 2(3), 206–12.

CARLISLE, J. W., STEUER, C. E., OWONIKOKO, T. K., & SABA, N. F. 2020. An update on the immune landscape in lung and head and neck cancers. *CA: Cancer Journal*, 70(6), 505–17.

CHAUHAN, R., TRIVEDI, V., RANI, R., & SINGH, U. 2022. A study of head and neck cancer patients with reference to tobacco use, gender, and subsite distribution. *S Asian J Cancer*, 11(01), 046–51.

COHEN, E. E. W., AHMED, O., KOCHERGINSKY, M., SHUSTAKOVA, G., KISTNER-GRIFFIN, E., SALAMA, J. K., YEFREMENKO, V., & NOVOSAD, V. 2013. Study of functional infrared imaging for early detection of mucositis in locally advanced head and neck cancer treated with chemoradiotherapy. *Oral Oncol*, 49(10), 1025–31.

CRAMER, J. D., BURTNESS, B., LE, Q. T., & FERRIS, R. L. 2019. The changing therapeutic landscape of head and neck cancer. *Nat Rev Clin Oncol*, 16(11), 669–83.

DASGUPTA, S., DASH, R., DAS, S. K., SARKAR, D., & FISHER, P. B. 2012. Emerging strategies for the early detection and prevention of head and neck squamous cell cancer. *J Cell Physiol*, 227(2), 467–73.

DAY, A. T., SHER, D. J., LEE, R. C., TRUELSON, J. M., MYERS, L. L., SUMER, B. D., STANKOVA, L., TILLMAN, B. N., HUGHES, R. S., KHAN, S. A., & GORDIN, E. A. 2020. Head and neck oncology during the COVID-19 pandemic: Reconsidering traditional treatment paradigms in light of new surgical and other multilevel risks. *Oral Oncol*, 105, 104684.

DAY, T. A., CHI, A., NEVILLE, B., & HEBERT, J. R. 2005. Prevention of head and neck cancer. *Curr Oncol Rep*, 7(2), 145–53. https://doi.org/10.1007/s11912-005-0041-x

DODD, M. J., CHO, M. H., COOPER, B. A., MACPHAIL, L., & MIASKOWSKI, C. 2022. A randomized clinical trial of granulocyte macrophage colony stimulating factor mouthwash for oral mucositis in head and neck cancer. *Eur J Oncol Nurs*, 56, 102093.

FERRAGUTI, G., TERRACINA, S., PETRELLA, C., GRECO, A., MINNI, A., LUCARELLI, M., AGOSTINELLI, E., RALLI, M., DE VINCENTIIS, M., RAPONI, G., POLIMENI, A., CECCANTI, M., CARONTI, B., DI CERTO, M. G., BARBATO, C., MATTIA, A., TARANI, L., & FIORE, M. 2022. Alcohol and head and neck cancer: Updates on the role of oxidative stress, genetic, epigenetics, oral microbiota, antioxidants, and alkylating agents. *Antioxidants*, 11(1), 145.

GORMLEY, M., CREANEY, G., SCHACHE, A., INGARFIELD, K., & CONWAY, D. I. 2022. Reviewing the epidemiology of head and neck cancer: Definitions, trends and risk factors. *Br Dent J*, 233(9), 780–6.

HONG, W. K., LIPPMAN, S. M., ITRI, L. M., KARP, D. D., LEE, J. S., BYERS, R. M., SCHANTZ, S. P., KRAMER, A. M., LOTAN, R., PETERS, L. J., DIMERY, I. W., BROWN, B. W., & GOEPFERT, H. 1990. Prevention of second primary tumors with isotretinoin in squamous-cell carcinoma of the head and neck. *N Engl J Med*, 323(12), 795–801.

IRANI, S. 2020. New insights into oral cancer – Risk factors and prevention: A review of literature. *Int J Prevent Med*, 11(1), 202.

JOHNSON, D. E., BURTNESS, B., LEEMANS, C. R., LUI, V. W. Y., BAUMAN, J. E., & GRANDIS, J. R. 2020. Head and neck squamous cell carcinoma. *Nat Rev Dis Primers*, 6(1), 92.

KAO, Y.-S., MA, K. S.-K., WU, M.-Y., WU, Y.-C., TU, Y.-K., & HUNG, C.-H. 2022. Topical prevention of radiation dermatitis in head and neck cancer patients: A network meta-analysis. *In Vivo*, 36(3), 1453–60.

KAWASHITA, Y., SOUTOME, S., UMEDA, M., & SAITO, T. 2020. Oral management strategies for radiotherapy of head and neck cancer. *Japan Dent Sci Rev*, 56(1), 62–7.

LIU, S., ZHAO, Q., ZHENG, Z., LIU, Z., MENG, L., DONG, L., & JIANG, X. 2021. Status of treatment and prophylaxis for radiation-induced oral mucositis in patients with head and neck cancer. *Front Oncol*, 11, 642575.

LOEWEN, I., JEFFERY, C. C., RIEGER, J., & CONSTANTINESCU, G. 2021. Prehabilitation in head and neck cancer patients: A literature review. *J Otolaryngol Head Neck Surg*, 50(1), 2.

MAHMOOD, H., SHABAN, M., RAJPOOT, N., & KHURRAM, S. A. 2021. Artificial Intelligence-based methods in head and neck cancer diagnosis: An overview. *Br J Cancer*, 124(12), 1934–40.

MCDONALD, S., MEYEROWITZ, C., SMUDZIN, T., & RUBIN, P. 1994. Preliminary results of a pilot study using WR-2721 before fractionated irradiation of the head and neck to reduce salivary gland dysfunction. *Int J Radiat Oncol Biol Physics*, 29(4), 747–54.

MIRGHANI, H., JUNG, A. C., & FAKHRY, C. 2017. Primary, secondary and tertiary prevention of human papillomavirus-driven head and neck cancers. *Eur J Cancer*, 78, 105–15.

MURPHY, B. A., & DENG, J. 2015. Advances in supportive care for late effects of head and neck cancer. *J Clin Oncol*, 33(29), 3314–21.

MUZAFFAR, J., BARI, S., KIRTANE, K., & CHUNG, C. H. 2021. Recent advances and future directions in clinical management of head and neck squamous cell carcinoma. *Cancers*, 13(2), 338.

SABA, N. F., HAMMOND, A., SHIN, D. M., & KHURI, F. R. 2007. Moving toward bioadjuvant approaches to head and neck cancer prevention. *Int J Radiat Oncol Biol Physics*, 69(2), S132–5.

SABATINI, M. E., & CHIOCCA, S. 2020. Human papillomavirus as a driver of head and neck cancers. *Br J Cancer*, 122(3), 306–14.

SCHLEPER, J. R. 1989. Prevention, detection, and diagnosis of head and neck cancers. *Semin Oncol Nurs*, 5(3), 139–49. https://doi.org/10.1016/0749-2081(89)90086-7

SCHOENFELD, J. D. 2015. Immunity in head and neck cancer. *Cancer Immunol Res*, 3(1), 12–17.

THULA, T. T., SCHULTZ, G., TRAN-SON-TAY, R., & BATICH, C. 2005. Effects of EGF and bFGF on irradiated parotid glands. *Ann Biomed Engineer*, 33(5), 685–95.

VACHA, P., FEHLAUER, F., MAHLMANN, B., MARX, M., HINKE, A., SOMMER, K., RICHTER, E., & FEYERABEND, T. 2003. Randomized phase III trial of postoperative radiochemotherapy ± amifostine in head and neck cancer: Is there evidence for radioprotection? *Strahlentherapie Und Onkologie*, 179(6), 385–9.

WHITESIDE, T. L. 2005. Immunobiology of head and neck cancer. *Cancer Metastasis Rev*, 24(1), 95–105.

YOON, Y. J., SHIN, H.-S., & LIM, J.-Y. 2019. A hepatocyte growth factor/MET-induced antiapoptotic pathway protects against radiation-induced salivary gland dysfunction. *Radiother Oncol*, 138, 9–16.

ZIYAD, S. H. 2022. Radiation-induced salivary gland damage/dysfunction in head and neck cancer: Nano-bioengineering strategies and artificial intelligence for prevention, therapy and reparation. *J Radiol Oncol*, 6(3), 027–44.

17

Psychosocial Impact of Head and Neck Cancer

Onyemaechi O. Azu, Innocent A. Edagha, Samuel O. Olojede, Charles A. Maimela, Sylvester L. Lyantagaye, Lloyd Mabonga, and Zodwa Dlamini

17.1 Introduction

Head and neck cancers (HNCs) constitutes a broad range of malignancies that implicates divergent subsites, including the oronasal cavities, pharyngolarynx, hypopharynx, and associated salivary glands (Hashim & Boffetta, 2020). Therefore, HNCs principally affect anatomical sites and structures of head and neck region. Squamous cell carcinoma (SCC) is the most routinely diagnosed histologically typed tumor in HNCs, with an estimated >90% occurrence (Muzaffar et al., 2021). HNCs constitute an anatomically local but phenotypically divergent tumor type commonly associated with viral or environmental risk factors.

In 2020, cancer was responsible for causing about 10 million deaths worldwide, ranking it as the second most common cause of death that year. The burden of this disease is mainly borne by low- and middle-income countries (LMICs), with 70% of an approximately 10 million cancer-related mortalities mainly localized in LMICs as of 2020 (WHO International Agency for Research on Cancer, 2020). World Health Organization (WHO) projects a 77% increase in cancer cases by 2050, an elevated incidence associated with population aging, growth, and changes in risk factors linked to socioeconomic development. Tobacco and alcohol use, along with obesity, are major health risks for cancer, while pollution remains a crucial potentiator of ecological hazard factors (WHO, 2024). Impediments to diagnosis and treatment may result in a surge in the advanced stage of this disease, leading to higher mortality rates (Yabroff et al., 2022).

Current healthcare systems are primarily focused on acute diseases and largely unaware of these growing cancer threats. The most common cancer incidence report in the WHO/AFRO region for females and males is presented and summarized in Figure 17.1. Unique features exist for cancers characterized

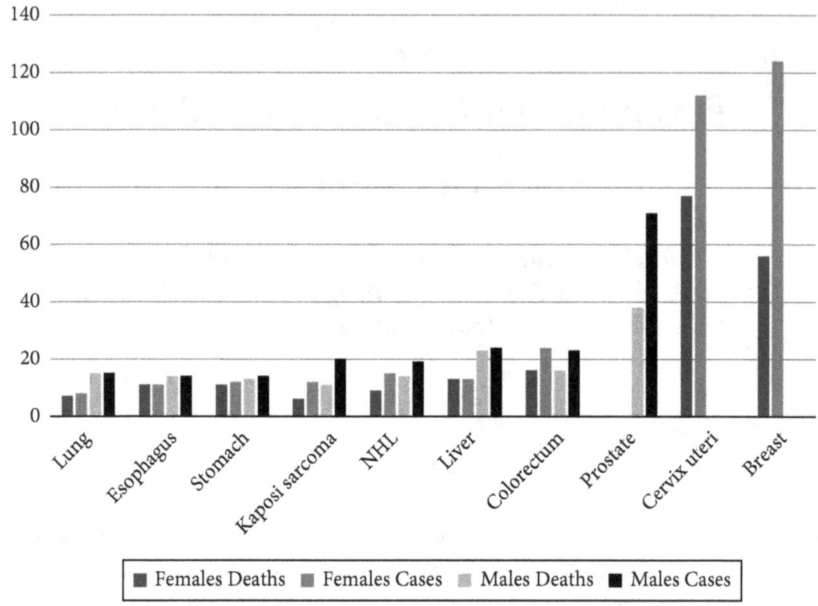

Figure 17.1 Most common cancers WHO/AFRO region (cases deaths: thousands). Data on incidence and mortality for esophageal cancers remains very high across both genders.

in sub-Saharan Africa and conflict with reported cancer incidence in other regions globally. Notably, an estimated 80% of all cancer-related deaths occur in populations < 60 years (American Cancer Society, 2018). This significantly impacts families, communities, and nations' socioeconomic dynamics because this age group is responsible for the national workforce, and mothers taking care of families and young children are equally affected. Additionally, the prevalence of pediatric cancers in African countries is estimated at around 6%, more elevated than in other regions of the world (Stefan & Harif, 2017). With increasing life expectancy, a corresponding upsurge in cancer prevalence is expected in the elderly population (Pilleron et al., 2021).

Some regions of the world, including parts of Africa, have higher rates of cancer than the global average throughout a lifetime. For instance, African women may face a greater risk of cumulative cancer mortality (Nwagwu & Ogoke, 2024). In sub-Saharan Africa, it has been found that up to one-third of cancer cases can be linked to infectious diseases like hepatitis B and C, human papillomavirus (HPV), Epstein-Barr virus, *Helicobacter pylori*, and HIV. These infectious agents have been associated with cervical cancer, gastric cancer, hepatic carcinomas, Burkitt lymphoma, and Kaposi sarcoma (Figure 17.2) (Parkin, 2019).

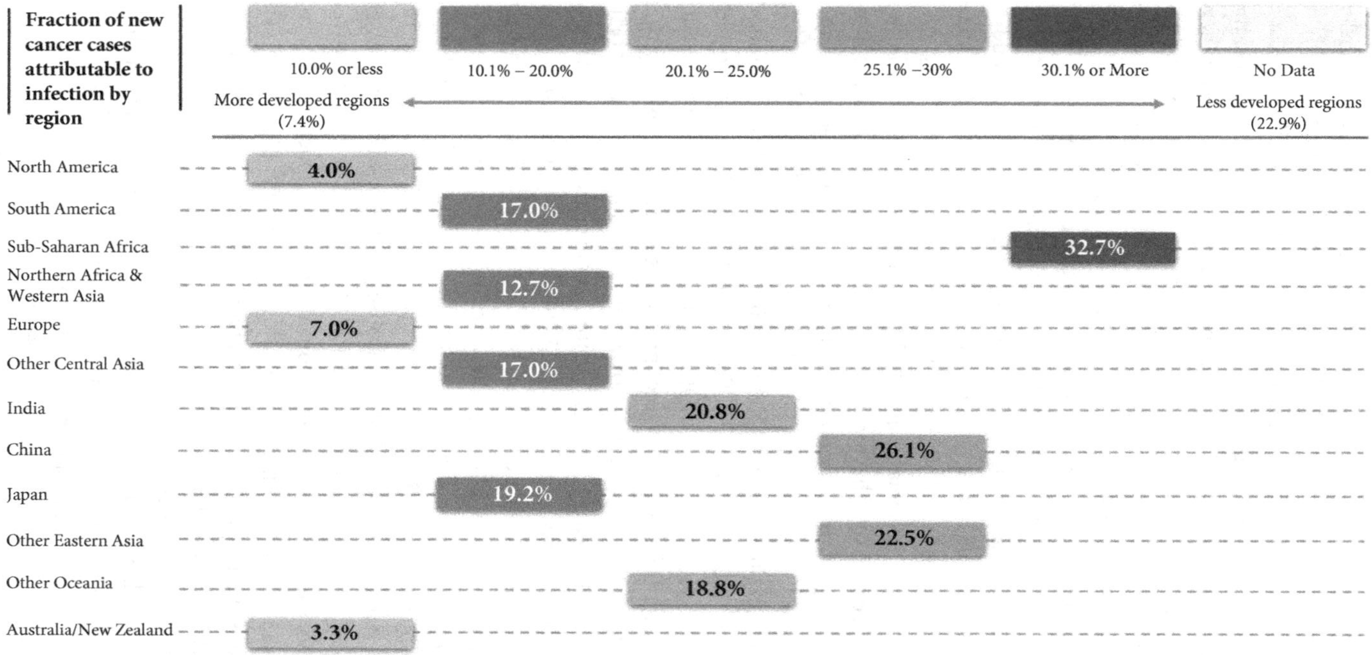

Figure 17.2 Cancer cases attributable to infection by region. The bulk of infection-driven cancers can be seen in sub-Saharan Africa and some parts of China.

Efforts aimed at promoting overall well-being and preventing cancer may demonstrate a significant contribution in the decline of disease burden for both the general population and high-risk cohorts, including sexually active individuals. Additionally, campaigns focused on reducing smoking and alcohol consumption and promoting healthy lifestyle choices can help mitigate the risk of associated cancers among the population (Hashim et al., 2019). It is worth noting that while there are notable genetic differences among sub-Saharan Africa populations and other ethnic groups, insufficient scrutiny has been focused on cancer biology as it affects African patients (Rotimi et al., 2021).

Improved knowledge and implementation strategies can better guide therapy recommendations (Rotimi et al., 2021). African patients often inhabit relatively unique sociocultural and demographic settings (e.g., the number and distribution of healthcare facilities, way of life, traditional beliefs, and a hierarchy of decision-making in families) that can negatively affect their ability to access and adhere to care (Tessema et al., 2022). Thus it is important to better understand the patterns of behavior, biology, and responses to treatment as well as the socioeconomic dynamics of women and men diagnosed with cancer in African settings, and particularly against the backdrop of HNCs. Multilateral organizations increasingly recognize the existing and future health implications of noncommunicable diseases (NCDs) in LMICs, and, in this regard, the Sustainable Development Goals (SDGs) of the United Nations for 2030 have stipulated an ambitious target to reduce premature mortality caused by NCDs.

Many HNCs are relatively rare in occurrence, leading to underreporting of the disease. Worldwide, HNCs rank eighth in cancer frequency, with approximately 660,000 new cases and about 325,000 fatalities yearly (Gormley et al., 2022). HNCs account for an estimated 3–10% of all cancer cases and are more frequent in older patients, although there has been an increase in its incidence among younger patients and females (Gupta et al., 2016; Marur & Forastiere, 2008). The incidence of HNC differs according to WHO geographic region, with certain types being more frequently observed in specific areas (Mishra & Meherotra, 2014). The timely identification of HNC can be problematic, often due to a tumor's location and delayed consultation with a medical professional (Schutte et al., 2020). Treatment modalities frequently applied in HNC usually integrate surgery, chemotherapy, radiation therapy, and targeted therapy (Anderson et al., 2021; Kitamura et al., 2020).

Head and neck malignancies are on the rise worldwide, particularly in developing countries where tobacco and alcohol intake primarily contribute to its development (Barsouk et al., 2023). In developed nations, HPV-related HNCs are becoming more prevalent, especially involving the oropharynx, hypopharynx, and larynx (Pinkiewicz et al., 2022). Preliminary management of HNCs involves assessing and staging the disease in accordance with the latest staging system (Pisani et al., 2020). Education on cancer risk, community engagement, smoking and alcohol cessation, HPV vaccination, and routine oral screening are effective strategies for its prevention and early detection (Barsouk et al., 2023; Kamaraju et al., 2020).

17.2 Diagnosis of Head and Neck Cancers

Cancer detection and determination of its spread often involve standard diagnostic tools such as endoscopy; magnetic resonance imaging (MRI), positron emission tomography (PET), and computed tomography (CT) scans of the head; chest imaging; panoramic dental x-rays; and/or cone beam CT. A cancer diagnosis is usually overwhelming and immediately causes challenges to the patient's physical and mental well-being, and these have implications for psychosocial and existential outcomes. The impact of HNC is even more profound due to its anatomical location and the extent of necessary treatment options, especially when a curative intent is being considered (Riechelmann et al., 2022).

An HNC diagnosis is premised on the genetic basis, phenotype, and location in which it occurs. The WHO Classification of Tumors (WHO, 2024) lists 16 different HNCs.

1. Nasal, paranasal, and skull base tumors
2. Nasopharyngeal tumors
3. Hypopharyngeal, laryngeal, tracheal, and parapharyngeal tumors
4. Salivary gland tumors
5. Oral cavity and mobile tongue tumors
6. Oropharyngeal tumors
7. Odontogenic and maxillofacial bone tumors
8. Ear tumors
9. Soft tissue tumors
10. Hematolymphoid proliferations and neoplasia
11. Melanocytic tumors
12. Tumors and tumor-like lesions of the neck and lymph nodes
13. Germ cell tumors
14. Metastasis
15. Neuroendocrine neoplasms and paraganglioma
16. Genetic tumor syndromes involving the head and neck

Side effects of HNC and its treatment may present outcomes that impact diverse functions and anatomic structures; these are typified by difficulty in speaking (Riechelmann et al., 2022), breathing challenges (Hunter et al., 2020;

Riechelmann et al., 2022), chewing problems, pain, swallowing dysfunction, and xerostomia (Crowder et al., 2018), to mention a few. In addition, HNC patients may develop heightened self-consciousness about their altered physical appearance, depressed mood, loss of independence, fatigue, worry about caregiver burden/overdependence, and compromised personal relationships, all of which eventually negatively influence their quality of life (QOL; Stenhammar et al., 2017; Van Beek et al., 2020) and are related to the psychosocial dynamics of HNC patient management.

HNCs present a substantial public health issue owing to their elevated occurrence and death rates (Gormley et al., 2022). Early diagnosis improves outcomes, but current screening methods are inadequate. There is a lack of strict criteria for triggering physical examinations by ear, nose, and throat (ENT) specialists, and the frequency of screening in at-risk populations is unknown (Juster & Page, 2023). Implementing a screening program for heightened-risk individuals, such as smokers and alcohol users, can aid in quicker detection of HNCs (Zabala & Santaolalla, 2023). This screening program includes ENT exploration, CT scans or biopsies, and follow-up visits for patients with potential malignant lesions (Boscolo Nata et al., 2022). Human β-defensins (hBDs) have shown potential as diagnostic markers for HNCs because their expression profiles are altered during tumor progression (Kompuinen et al., 2023). A noninvasive diagnostic approach using circulating tumor HPV DNA (ctHPVDNA) coupled with routine physical examination and image diagnostics has proved to improve accuracy, lower cost, and shorten the duration to diagnosis for HPV-associated head and neck squamous cell carcinoma (HNSCC; Kuhs et al., 2023; Siravegna et al., 2022).

17.2.1 Emotional Reactions in Head and Neck Cancers

Emotional distress is prevalent in patients with HNCs and can have a significant impact on their well-being. Studies have shown that 60% or more of HNC patients report emotional distress before radiotherapy (Al-Salool et al., 2023; Lewis et al., 2021). Emotional distress in this population is associated with physical complaints and female gender (McDowell et al., 2022). People who have been diagnosed with cancer affecting the head and neck region have an elevated risk of experiencing emotional complaints as compared to patients with other cancer types (Hammermüller et al., 2021). Distress screening tools like the Patient Health Questionnaire-9 (PHQ-9) and Generalized Anxiety Disorders-7 (GAD-7) can help identify patients with significant emotional distress (Gascon et al., 2022). Negative impacts of HNC on affective and sexual relationships have also been observed, highlighting the need for comprehensive care that addresses emotional and sexual aspects (Saghafi et al., 2023). Furthermore, the psychological impact of HNC treatment, including post-treatment pain and disfigurement, can lead to high levels of anxiety and stigma in sufferers (Albert et al., 2022). Couples-based interventions that encourage emotional disclosure may be beneficial in enhancing cognitive processing and relieving distress in HNC patients and their spouses (Bakhshaie et al., 2020).

17.2.2 Societal and Family Issues Related to Head and Neck Cancers

Frequently HNC patients encounter various societal and familial issues. Psychosocial factors such as household size and mental health outcomes significantly affect the QOL of HNC patients (Qamar et al., 2024). Oncologists face ethical challenges in screening, diagnosing, treating, and the general management of HNC patients, especially those from rural areas (Baliga et al., 2023). Patients with low socioeconomic status experience inequality in their cancer treatment owing to different perceptions and challenges in their interactions with healthcare professionals (Allen et al., 2021). Family caregivers of patients with HNC experiences challenging processes, face life changes, and require external support to provide better care (Zeng et al., 2023). HNC patients also experience interrelated cancer stigma, anxiety, and depression, and reducing stigma is crucial for mental health improvement efforts (Zheng et al., 2024).

17.3 Psychosocial Impact in Disease and Well-Being: The Ripple Effect

"Psychosocial" refers to the relationship between an individual's behavior and the social elements that surround them. The term "psychosocial impact" refers to the influence of environmental and biological factors on a person's psychological and social well-being (Stenhammar et al., 2017; Van Beek et al., 2020; Vizzotto et al., 2020). "Psychosocial attributes" represent the impact of social elements on a person's mental well-being and conduct (Vizzotto et al., 2020). The term "general well-being" pertains to an individual's overall emotional state, encompassing their feelings of happiness, contentment, or sadness. It can be broken down into two categories: feeling sad or happy. The distinction between these categories has been studied and described (Alexander et al. 2020; Arias., 2020; McDowell, 2006).

The psychosocial well-being of HNC patients is of significant concern (Elaldi et al., 2021). The ailment and its therapies impact physical and functional capabilities while eliciting psychological suffering, thus producing a decline in the general QOL (Covrig et al., 2021). Research has indicated that persons diagnosed with head and neck tumors tend to experience intense feelings of anxiety and sadness, which are linked to a decline in their overall well-being (Hortense et al., 2020; Patterson et al., 2022). The weight of HNC on the psychosocial dynamics of a person's QOL, including mental health, emotional stability, social encounters, and relationships, requires more research (Covrig et al., 2021). Utilizing psychoeducational interventions and support groups can be beneficial for patients to enhance their general well-being and help them cope with their illness (Malik et al., 2021). It is of utmost importance to comprehend and focus on the psychosocial requirements of individuals with HNC to ensure all-inclusive treatment and enhanced patient results.

17.3.1 Psychosocial Dimensions of Head and Neck Cancer Patients

Several reports have also interrogated the psychosocial dimensions of HNC patients (Chen et al., 2021; McDowell et al., 2022). HNC patients face unique challenges that affect their psychosocial health. The origins of psychosocial distress in HNC patients are diverse, including irksome symptoms, distressing physical disability, social inquisitiveness, and distressing thoughts concerning the future (Nayak et al., 2023). The disease course of HNC can negatively affect a patients' QOL, and psychosocial factors such as ongoing cancer treatment, tracheostomy, and adjuvant chemoradiotherapy are associated with poorer global QOL (Assas, 2020; Zebralla et al., 2021). Reports are replete showing that HNC patients receiving radiotherapy experience high levels of psychosocial distress, including depression and anxiety, with a prevalence ranging from 9.8% to 83.8% (Nayak et al., 2022, 2024). Predictive factors for depression in patients with HNC revolve around physical manifestations, appearance, decreased social support, fatigue, and unique radiotherapy interventions (Miller, 2020). These findings highlight the need for interventions and supportive therapy to address the psychosocial dimensions of patients with HNC during treatment. We have therefore compiled a comprehensive list of tools adopted in different parts of the globe that are relevant in improving overall management and care and thus improving psychosocial well-being in patients with HNCs (Table 17.1).

Table 17.1 Some psychosocial tools in the management of head and neck cancers

S/N.	Tool	Functional assessment	References
1.	Distress Thermometer (DT)	DT is a self-reported tool using a 0-to-10 rating scale (0 showing no distress and 10 indicating extreme distress). The patient is encouraged to list and recognize the things that cause them distress using a Problem List tool.	Ownby, 2019
2.	Modified Head and Neck Cancer Specific Problem List (HNC-specific PL)	The HNC-specific PL is a list of 28 items divided into four categories: "Practical," "Family," "Physical," and "Spiritual/Religious." Patients must indicate if they have experienced a problem in the past week by selecting "Yes" or "No."	Brauer et al., 2021
3.	Patient Health Questionnaire-4 (PHQ-4)	The PHQ-4 has replaced the "Emotional" category of the standard Patient Health Questionnaire (PL) to lessen patient burden. The responses for each item range from 0 ("not at all") to 3 ("nearly every day"). A score of ≥ 3 on either tool indicates a positive screening result.	Brauer et al., 2021
4.	Patient Health Qustionnaire-9 (PHQ-9)	The PHQ-9 is a tool consisting of nine questions that evaluate the severity of depression. Each question can be rated on a scale from 0 (indicating no depression) to 3 (indicating severe depression). A higher overall score, ranging from 0 to 27, suggests a more severe case of depression.	Degefa et al., 2020
5.	The Patient Health Questionnaire-8 (PHQ-8)	An 8-item questionnaire was used to assess depression. Scores are rated as usual (0 - 2), mild (3-5), moderate (6-8), and severe (9 - 12). A total score ≥3 for the first 2 questions suggests anxiety. A total score ≥ 3 for the last two questions suggests depression. Higher scores indicate the presence of more significant symptoms of depression.	Kroenke et al., 2009
6.	Generalized Anxiety Disorder-7 (GAD-7)	This assessment evaluates if you are experiencing symptoms of anxiety, such as feeling nervous, anxious, or on edge; inability to stop worrying; worrying too much about different things; having trouble relaxing; feeling restless; becoming easily annoyed or irritable; and feeling afraid as if something terrible might happen. You will be asked to rate each symptom on a scale of 0 to 3. The total score can range from 0 to 21, with higher scores indicating more severe anxiety. Scores above ten are considered to be in the clinical range.	Johnson et al., 2019

(*continued*)

Table 17.1 Continued

S/N.	Tool	Functional assessment	References
7.	Kessler Psychological Distress Tool (K10)	The K10 questionnaire comprises ten queries that relate to emotional states. Each query has five response levels, ranging from 'none of the time' to 'all of the time' on a scale of one to five. The sum of the scores for all ten questions results in a minimum score of 10 and a maximum score of 50. The lower the score, the lower the psychological distress, and the higher the score, the higher the psychological distress.	Kessler et al., 2003
8.	Brief Symptom Inventory (BSI-18)	The measurement tool comprises 53 items, which assess nine symptom dimensions, including Somatization, Obsession-Compulsion, Interpersonal Sensitivity, Depression, Anxiety, Hostility, Phobic anxiety, Paranoid ideation, and Psychoticism. Additionally, it includes three global indices of distress: Global Severity Index, Positive Symptom Distress Index, and Positive Symptom Total. The global indices measure the present or past level of symptomatology, the intensity of symptoms, and the number of reported symptoms, respectively.	Derogatis, 1975
9.	Hospital Anxiety and Depression scale (HADS)	This assessment tool comprises 14 items rated using a Likert scale with four points, ranging from 0 to 3. The primary aim of the tool is to evaluate the levels of depression and anxiety, with seven items dedicated to each subscale. The sum of all 14 items is taken to calculate the total score, while the sum of the respective seven items is collected for each subscale, resulting in scores ranging from 0 to 21. Higher scores indicate greater severity of anxiety and depression symptoms.	Michopoulos et al., 2008
10.	Cancer Worry Scale (CWS)	The total score for FCR ranges from 8 to 32. A higher score indicates a higher level of FCR. To differentiate between those with normal FCR and those with bothersome levels of FCR (referred to as high FCR), a cutoff score of 13 vs 14 has been established. In other words, a low FCR is considered 13 or less, while a high FCR is considered 14 or more.	Mirosevic et al., 2019
11.	Impact of Event Scale-Revised	The scale consists of 22 items and is divided into intrusion, sleep disturbance, hyperarousal, avoidance, and numbing subscales. Each item is scored on a 5-point scale, ranging from 0 (not at all) to 4 (extremely). For analysis, only the scores for the avoidance and intrusion subscales are used, including eight items for avoidance and 7 for intrusion.	Mirosevic et al., 2019

	Quality of Life Tools	The assessment comprises twelve domains and is evaluated based on two composite scores: A physical QOL score (computed by taking an average of chewing, swallowing, speech, taste, saliva, and appearance domains) and a social-emotional QOL score (computed by taking an average of anxiety, mood, pain, activity, recreation, and shoulder domains). The scores range from 0 to 100, where higher scores indicate better QOL.	
12.	University of Washington Quality of Life (UWQOL)	Includes 15 scales: five functional scales assessing physical functioning, role functioning, emotional functioning, cognitive functioning, and social functioning; nine multi- and single-item scales assessing fatigue, nausea and vomiting, pain, dyspnoea, insomnia, appetite loss, constipation, diarrhea, financial difficulties, and a global health status/QOL scale.	Kassir et al., 2021
13	European Organization for Research and Treatment of Cancer Quality of Life Questionnaire Core 30 (EORTC-QLQ -C30)	Includes 14 subscales, with each subscale consisting of two items. Those subscales are as follows: self-distraction (Items 1 and 19), active coping (Items 2 and 7), denial (Items 3 and 8), substance use (Items 4 and 11), use of emotional support (Items 5 and 15), use of instrumental support (Items 10 and 23), behavioral disengagement (Items 6 and 16), venting (Items 9 and 21), positive reframing (Items 12 and 17), planning (Items 14 and 25), humor (Items 18 and 28), acceptance (Items 20 and 24), religion (Items 22 and 27) and self-blame (Items 13 and 26). The score of each item ranged from 1 ('I usually do not do this at all') to 4 ('I usually do this often'). Higher scores indicated the more frequent use of the corresponding coping strategy.	Cocks et al., 2023
	Coping Scale Tools	Consists of 50 items assessing the patient's self-rated use of cognitive and behavioral strategies to cope with pain. It comprises six subscales for cognitive strategies (ignoring pain, reinterpreting pain, diverting attention, coping self-statements, catastrophizing, praying/hoping) and two for behavioral strategies (increasing activity levels and increasing pain behaviors). Each coping strategy subscale consists of six items with a numerical rating scale ranging from 0 (never do that) to 6 (always do that), indicating how frequently the strategy is used to cope with pain. Each subscale has a maximum score of 36 and a minimum score of 0.	

(*continued*)

Table 17.1 Continued

S/N.	Tool	Functional assessment	References
14.	Coping Orientation to Problems Experienced (COPE)	It contains 66 statements about coping with a stressful situation. Responses are given on a 4-point Likert scale, ranging from 0 to 3 (0 = does not apply and not used; 1 = used somewhat; 2 = used quite a bit; and 3 = used a great deal). Eight coping factors were identified using α and principal factoring with oblique rotation, which maps onto eight distinct coping strategies, including Confronting coping (6 items), Distancing (6 items), Self-controlling (7 items), Seeking Social Support (6 items), Accepting Responsibility (4 items), Escape Avoidance (8 items), Planful Problem Solving (6 items), and Positive Reappraisal (7 items). The remaining ten items are distractor items.	Cheng et al., 2022
15	Coping Strategy Questionnaire (CSQ)		Abbott, 2010
16.	Ways of Coping Questionnaire (WCQ)	The measurement tool comprises 53 items, which assess nine symptom dimensions, including Somatization, Obsession-Compulsion, Interpersonal Sensitivity, Depression, Anxiety, Hostility, Phobic anxiety, Paranoid ideation, and Psychoticism. Additionally, it includes three global indices of distress: Global Severity Index, Positive Symptom Distress Index, and Positive Symptom Total. The global indices measure the present or past level of symptomatology, the intensity of symptoms, and the number of reported symptoms, respectively.	Lars-Olov Lundqvist., 2006; Corti et al., 2018
17.	Coping Inventory for Stressful Situations (CISS)	The survey is meticulously designed with 48 items, each precisely describing people's behaviors in stressful situations. The respondents are guided to rate the frequency of their engagement in the suggested activities when facing complex, stressful, or upsetting situations on a 5-point Likert-type scale, ensuring a nuanced understanding of their coping mechanisms. The responses are then presented on three scales relating to the CISS's three dimensions: Task-oriented, emotion-oriented, and avoidance-oriented coping. The avoidance-oriented coping scale further delves into two subscales: distraction and social diversion, providing a comprehensive view of the respondents' coping strategies.	Michałowska et al., 2019

		Palliative (End-of-Life) Tools	
18.	Brief Fatigue Inventory (BFI)	The assessment comprises nine items, each rated using Likert scales ranging from 0 to 10. The average scores for these nine items are used to determine the global fatigue scores (GFSs). Scores from 1 to 3, 4 to 6, and 7 to 10 are classified as mild, moderate, and severe, respectively.	Iwase et al., 2015
19.	European Organization for Research and Treatment of Cancer Quality of Life Questionnaire-Core 15-Palliative (EORTC QLQ-C15-PAL)	The questionnaire is a comprehensive tool, comprising 15 items that assess the quality of life and health status. It includes a functioning subscale of 5 items that evaluate physical, emotional, cognitive, and social functioning, and a symptom subscale of 9 items that assess a wide range of symptoms including fatigue, nausea, vomiting, pain, dyspnea, insomnia, appetite loss, constipation, diarrhea, and financial difficulties. Each item's scores range from 0 to 100, providing a detailed picture of the respondents' health status. In the functioning subscale, higher scores of 60 and above indicate better functioning, whereas lower scores of 40 and below indicates better physical condition in the symptom subscale, ensuring a comprehensive assessment of the respondents' health.	Iwase et al., 2015
20.	Brief Pain Inventory	It consists of 15 items concerning presence (1 item), sites (1 item) and severity of pain (4 items), status (1 item) and effects of pain treatment (1 item), and interference of pain in QOL (7 items). In this study, item 3 (severity of the worst pain experienced in the previous 24 hours) was only used to consider the burden that pain placed upon patients;	Iwase et al., 2015
21.	Pain Management Index (PMI)	It measures the appropriateness of pharmacological strategies and compares the potency of prescribed analgesic medications using patient-reported pain levels. Analgesics were classified into four levels: 0: no analgesic; 1: nonopioid; 2: weak opioid; 3: potent opioid. Pain levels were scored as follows: 1–3: mild; 4–7: moderate; and 8–10: severe. PMI scores are calculated by subtracting patient-reported pain levels from analgesic levels, which produces a score range of -3 to 3. Negative scores (<0) indicate inadequate analgesia, and positive scores (≥ 0) indicate adequate analgesia.	Iwase et al., 2015

(continued)

Table 17.1 Continued

S/N.	Tool	Functional assessment	References
22.	Palliative Performance Scale (PPS)	The PPS is scored in increments of 10, from a high score of 100 (fully functional) to 0 (deceased) and uses branching logic to assess domains of functional capacity.	Anderson et al 1996; Olajide et al., 2007; Wharton et al., 2015
23.	Screening for Palliative Care Needs in the Emergency Department (SPEED)	The SPEED tool is a practical instrument, intended to assist emergency department providers with a brief comprehensive 'first-pass' assessment. It allows for the identification of palliative needs that likely require intervention either in the emergency department, as an in-patient, or in follow-up, ensuring timely and appropriate care. In particular, the social domain of SPEED is meant to assess deeper causal relationships between symptoms and care needs, providing valuable insights for effective intervention.	Richards et al., 2011
24.	Palliative Care Outcome Scale (POS)	Ten questions were chosen for inclusion based on those reliable and valid questions used in other measures that covered life's physical, psychological, and spiritual domains within the remit of palliative care.	Hearn & Higginson, 1999
25.	Memorial Symptom Assessment Scale (MSAS)	The MSAS questionnaire consists of 32 symptoms and has three dimensions: frequency, severity, and distress. There are shorter versions of the questionnaire, such as the MSAS form (which has one dimension and 32 symptoms) and the condensed MSAS (which includes one dimension and 14 symptoms). The questionnaire version is specially designed for children aged 7-12 years. The MSAS stands out due to its summary subscales for physical and psychological distress and the Global Distress Index. It has been utilized in various studies involving patients with cancer, AIDS, and other advanced medical conditions.	Chang et al., 2004

17.4 Coping Mechanisms for Patients with Head and Neck Cancer

Investigations have been conducted concerning the coping strategies adopted by HNC patients. One study found that different coping modalities can affect posttraumatic growth in HNC patients over a prolonged period (Nik Jaafar et al., 2021). Another study compared coping strategies of patients with alcohol-dependency with and without cancers of the oral cavity and oropharynx and found that patients with cancer relied more on disengaging/distancing coping strategies (Petrić et al., 2021). An investigation of HNC survivors revealed that, despite facing constraints in their everyday lives, they expressed contentment and a positive outlook toward their lives (Crowder et al., 2021).

One way to manage the negative effects of cancer on a person's life is to adjust to a new routine and participate more actively in cancer support groups and religious communities (Crowder et al., 2021; Semple et al., 2008). A review of empirical evidence found that disengagement coping mechanisms, such as avoidance, were consistently associated with increased psychological distress in patients with HNC (Morris et al., 2018). Hence, recommendations for patients to participate in supportive care groups with specialists like speech-language pathologists, physiotherapists, and nutritionists are essential for improving the level of care for cancer survivors prior, during, and following treatment. This helps them adjust their lives post-treatment and address any extended fitness issues that may arise due to their disease (Crowder et al., 2021). Overall, coping strategies in HNC patients can have an impact on their posttraumatic growth, psychological discomfort, and QOL.

17.4.1 Social Support in Head and Neck Cancer Patients

The support and motivation that an individual receives from their loved ones and general society are of utmost significance for the physical and emotional well-being of HNC patients from onset of diagnosis, over the course of treatment, and during the recovery or ambulatory/hospice phases. Reports indicate that HNC patients have changing supportive care needs over time, and these needs are influenced by various factors such as sex, tumor location, fear of recurrence, and social support (Molenaar et al., 2023; So et al., 2019). Improving social help can enhance the mental health and well-being of cancer patients because social support positively bolsters a patients' emotional capability to deal with cancer (Karnell et al., 2007). Furthermore, social support from healthcare workers and family members/friends is essential for HNC patients, with these patients often receiving more informational support from healthcare workers and more aid/

assistance and emotional support from family members/friends (Mayo et al., 2022). Delays in initiating postoperative radiotherapy in HNC patients have been linked to lower social support, notably lower tangible support (Ghazali, 2018; Popovtzer & Eisbruch, 2008). Overall, social support is crucial for patients with HNC and can remarkably influence their health and medical outcomes.

17.4.2 Quality of Life Impact for Head and Neck Cancer Patients

The QOL of HNC patients is affected by various factors. Genetic predisposition to depression, as measured by polygenic risk scores, and a previous medical background check hinting at suicidal ideation are associated with compromised QOL immediately post-treatment in patients with HNC (Litsas et al., 2022). A person's age, time interval to postoperative intervention, duration of surgery, duration of hospitalization, comorbidity, and approximate 10-year survival prognosis are outcomes linked to QOL in HNC patients (McDowell et al., 2022). Ongoing cancer treatment, tracheostomy, and adjuvant chemoradiotherapy are significantly associated with a below-par global QOL in HNC patients, while larger family household size is linked with enhanced global QOL (Shiraz, 2015). Sleep disturbances, psychological distress, and physical symptoms can affect sleep quality in patients with HNC, and screening for insomnia should commence post-diagnosis (Santoso, 2023; Santoso et al., 2021). QOL declines during radiotherapy but slowly improves after treatment completion, and sociodemographic and clinical variables, such as HPV status, gender, educational status, alcohol consumption, surgical intervention, age at diagnosis, employment level, and score on the Eastern Cooperative Oncology Group (ECOG) report, play a role in QOL outcomes (Viganò et al., 2023). Research indicates that lifestyle elements and demography alongside clinical features can positively influence biological aging (Xiao et al., 2021).

Additionally, Do Nascimento Santos Lima et al. (2020) reported that the QOL decreased approximately 1 month following the beginning of the HNC patients' treatment and stayed low until therapy termination. In addition, standard policies guiding early nutritional counseling and interventions can boost immunity and provide necessary micronutrients following treatment plans thus mitigating drug-associated toxicities and improving the overall outcomes of HNC patients.

17.4.3 Body Image and Self-Esteem Issues

Individuals diagnosed with HNCs frequently encounter challenges with self-image including decreases in their confidence levels and self-esteem as a result of the physical and emotional alterations arising from the illness and its therapy. (Cerea et al., 2022). These issues constitute a remarkable influence on patients and their families alike. It has been reported that body image distress can persist over extended periods in HNC survivors, with a significant proportion of patients reporting mild to moderate concerns or even a disturbed body image (Macias et al., 2021). Factors such as treatment modality, daily functioning, and symptoms such as oral and throat pain can contribute to these concerns (Shu-Ching, 2019). There is potential in using tele-cognitive behavioral therapy as a means to decrease body image distress and enhance the overall well-being of HNC survivors (Arring et al., 2023). Healthcare providers must offer appropriate interventions to support patients in dealing with self-esteem and body image challenges.

17.4.4 Communication Challenges for Patients with Head and Neck Cancers

HNC patients routinely encounter communication challenges owing to the influence of the disease and the rigors of medical interventions on their speech and swallowing abilities (Ringash et al., 2018). These complications can significantly alter QOL as well as psychological well-being. Speech and language therapists (SLTs) are crucial to addressing these impediments and optimizing patients' communication functions before, during, and after treatment (Hurren et al., 2023). Communication challenges can elicit elevated psychosocial difficulties, and SLTs have specialized skillsets to assist in managing patients with speech difficulties (Hancock et al., 2023). Additionally, breakdowns in communication between patients and the medical team can lead to feelings of being unheard, isolated, and lacking in individualized care (Grattan et al., 2018). Effective communication aids and strategies are essential to overcome these challenges and provide holistic care for HNC patients.

17.5 Financial and Legal Ramifications Affecting Head and Neck Cancer Patients

HNC patients commonly experience financial burdens arising from declining QOL and the expensive costs of treatment, including complications of treatment-induced disability, known as "financial toxicity" (FT) (Rosi-Schumacher et al., 2023). HNC treatment leads to higher medical expenses compared to other cancers, with major surgical procedures and hospitalizations in intensive care units increasing treatment costs (Jayakar et al., 2017; Wissinger et al., 2014). The loss of lifetime wages contributes significantly to the incidental costs of HNC treatment because > 50% of HNC patients are impaired in ways that affect their return to work (Rosi-Schumacher et al., 2023). Most HNC patients are at risk for severe depression, anxiety, and social seclusion, which are likely to further negatively affect their QOL and treatment compliance (Smith et al., 2017). The sole tools currently applied to determine FT in HNC patients include the Comprehensive Score for Financial Toxicity (COST) and the Financial Index of Toxicity (FIT) (Rosi-Schumacher et al., 2023). Financial hardship is more prevalent in HNC patients compared to other cancers, particularly with respect to the coping behaviors domain, and it is more common among inadequately insured or uninsured patients (Mott et al., 2022). Proton therapy, a curative treatment for HNC, also has financial implications that need to be addressed, and a cost-of-illness framework could help evaluate the value of proton therapy and measure its financial toxicity (Athiyamaan & Kamath, 2023). Informal caregivers of patients with HNC also experience FT, and screening for FT in both patients and caregivers is important (Nguyen et al., 2023).

17.6 Ethical Issues Affecting the Treatment and Care of Head and Neck Cancer Patients

The presence of HNC evokes a myriad of ethical complications for healthcare professionals saddled with the responsibility for screening, diagnosis, treatment, and management (Baliga et al., 2023). These challenges include the need for ethical decision-making in treatment selection, communication with patients, and provision of consistent care (Nguyen & Ringash, 2018). With respect to HNC, ethical challenges commonly encountered relate to communication, end-of-life care, and resource allocation (Mayland et al., 2021). However, healthcare professionals often lack institutional tools and strategies to address these ethical issues, leading to the need for the development of ethical support services (Deleemans et al., 2020; Leuter et al., 2018). An ideal support service should be fast, flexible, and adaptable to different clinical cases (van Overveld et al., 2018). It is important to enhance ethical awareness among healthcare professionals to effectively address ethical challenges in HNC care.

17.6.1 Caregiver Burden in the Management of Head and Neck Cancer Patients

There are currently few standard protocols for evaluating HNC caregiver needs, although there is evidence of increased healthcare utilization (Benyo et al., 2023). Generally, cancer patients undergo significant lifestyle alterations requiring considerable support from healthcare personnel (Patel et al., 2016). These caregivers are often responsible for the challenging duties of assisting with mobility, communication, finances, and everyday chores (Cohen et al., 2016; Miller et al., 2016). Notably, HNC patients also receive immense continuous care involving wound care, tracheotomy superintendency, and gastrostomy tube care. A myriad of severe complications may arise affecting caregiver duties, including psychosocial and financial worries. In addition, caregivers may neglect personal healthcare in pursuit of better health outcomes for the patients under their care during lengthy treatment and recovery periods (Nekhlyudov et al., 2017). Benyo and coworkers (2023) reported that the predominant group of caregivers for patients with HNC were partners and spouses, constituting 60–100% in their analyses of various reports.

Following the completion of a detailed and required diagnostic investigation such as a holistic head and neck physical inspection, radiological imaging, and surgical biopsy, the principal steps for HNC patient management revolve around the principal anatomic site, classification, and patient treatment modalities. An estimated 30–40% of HNC patients who represent early stages (I or II) of the disease may undergo single-treatment modalities such as surgery or radiation, while multimodality treatment may constitute an estimated 60% of HNC patients showing locally or regionally advanced disease (National Comprehensive Cancer Network, 2020).

While prognosis for advanced-stage HNC remain poor, there has been an increase in the United States of HNC survivors with HPV-positive tumors (Patel et al., 2016). As of 1985, Dr. Fitzhugh Mullan described his personal struggle with cancer and crucially altered the notion of cancer survivorship. He outlined three key phases of survival: "acute survival," a duration that comprises diagnosis and treatment; "extended survival," a time span that starts at treatment conclusion and comprises surveillance; and "permanent survival," a time frame ambiguously referred to as "cured" status (Mullan, 1985). During this voyage, encompassing many distinct experiences, HNC survivors may recount considerable medical, psychosocial, interpersonal, economic, and functional impediments (Miller & Shuman, 2016).

Thus, a specialized area of expertise for cancer survivorship has generated appreciable recognition in recent years, with increased attention being paid to continuing care for patients exceeding their treatment course (i.e., surgery, radiation therapy, and/or chemotherapy). In cognizance of these developments, the American Head and Neck Society (AHNS) assembled a HNC survivorship committee. Benyo and coworkers reviewed the concept of survivorship, outlining both current practice guides for HNC patients and gray areas requiring further attention. They formulated a standard policy document to act as a future implementation guide in the management of HNC survivorship. They did so by expanding on the guidelines laid down by the American Cancer Society (ACS) and the American Society of Clinical Oncology (ASCO), with special focus on the value of a multidisciplinary approach (Cohen et al., 2016; Nekhlyudov et al., 2017). The goal was to generate a working protocol for primary healthcare physicians and specialist head and neck oncologists, as well as for allied healthcare providers treating HNC survivors. These clinical guides are detailed in Tables 17.2 and 17.3, respectively.

Caring for patients with HNC is a major concern that affects both patients and their caregivers. Several studies have highlighted the prevalence and risk factors associated with caregiver burden in HNC survivors (Kudrick et al., 2023; Lu et al., 2019). Issues like a patient's daily mental health directly impinges on their QOL, and, together with the working status of their caregiver, have been found to be directly associated with increased caregiver burden (Kassir et al., 2021). Those caring for patients with advanced cancer frequently experience an elevated degree of care burden, with consequential depression and anxiety (Soto-Guerrero et al., 2023). However, caregivers of breast cancer patients with higher levels of spiritual intelligence experience less burden of care, suggesting that spiritual intelligence acts as a protective factor against caregiver burden (La, 2020). Unfulfilled expectations among those caring for HNC patients are also common, with economic challenges increasingly linked with those unmet needs over extended periods (van Hof et al., 2023). Overall, these discoveries put a spotlight on the need for interventions and support for those caring for HNC patients in order to alleviate untoward burdens on caregivers and improve their well-being.

17.6.2 Work/Professional Ethics for Caregivers of Patients with Head and Neck Cancer

Work ethics for caregivers to patients with HNC involves addressing the ethical challenges faced by healthcare professionals in screening, diagnosing, treating, and rehabilitating these patients (Baliga et al., 2023). It is important to screen patients with HNC for distress and provide appropriate psychosocial support to reduce suffering and improve overall well-being (Deleemans et al., 2020). Implementing screening practices for distress and psychosocial care is crucial for addressing the unmet psychosocial needs of these vulnerable patients (Deshields et al., 2021).

17.6.3 Support Needs for Caregivers and Patients with Head and Neck Cancers

Minimizing caregiver distress is essential to promoting the well-being of both caregivers and their patients (Kassir et al., 2021). Survivors of HNCs are about twice as likely to die by suicide compared with survivors of other cancers (Nugent et al., 2021), and a study reported that although suicide ideation is increased among HNC patients, it is considerably elevated for patients living in rural localities. Therefore, it is important to develop effective suicide prevention strategies for HNC patients living in rural areas owing to their elevated risk of suicide (Osazuwa-Peters et al., 2021).

Support needs for HNC patients alternate over time but remain high (Fang & Heckman, 2016). At baseline, 65% of HNC patients had at least one moderate/high supportive care need (SCN), which decreased to 42.8% at 24 months (Molenaar et al., 2023). Even those informally caring for HNC patients also had unfulfilled expectations, with 70.3% reporting at least one need at baseline (van Hof et al., 2023). These needs decreased over time, but 28.3% still reported unmet needs 2 years post-treatment. Caregivers of patients with too many unfulfilled expectations, an advanced tumor stage, or worsened comorbidities have significantly more unmet needs (Hart et al., 2022). Pretreatment, HNC patients do not perceive the relevance of supportive care and experience anxiety about diagnosis and treatment (Henry et al., 2020). Malnutrition is prevalent in patients with HNC and can occur at any stage of the treatment (Kubrak et al., 2020). Optimizing nutritional status is critical because malnutrition is connected with adverse therapy sequels and QOL (Silva et al., 2019).

Support groups and services for HNC patients are vital for enhancing QOL and providing coping mechanisms for patients. Peer support (PS) activities have been demonstrated to be effective in positively assisting individuals burdened by cancers and chronic conditions, including HNC (Hatton et al., 2022; Kristensen et al., 2019). PS permits patients to team up, pool their efforts, disseminate information, increase motivation, and share insights that can be conveyed through one-to-one interactions, web-based platforms, and support clusters (Hatton et al., 2022; Bingham et al., 2023). However, there is limited evidence on the variants of, durations of, and obstacles to PS for HNC patients (Hatton et al., 2022; Rocke et al., 2020). Healthcare professionals play a crucial role in providing support and removing obstacles to alleviatory care for HNC patients (Meredith et al., 2022). The COVID-19 pandemic further highlighted the challenges in delivering appropriate and effective support to HNC patients (Day et al., 2020; Yan et al., 2021). To address these challenges, various interventions, including group interventions led by psychotherapists and peers, have been developed to support HNC patients in their work ability, QOL, self-efficacy, and mental well-being (Howren et al., 2013; Ringash et al., 2018).

17.7 Survivorship and Long-Term Implications in Head and Neck Cancer

Tele-health survivorship care programs (De Ravin et al., 2023) are often feasible and cost-effective. These programs have shown positive outcomes in terms of patient enrollment, attrition rates, adherence, patient satisfaction, and cost savings. Additionally, survivorship care programs have been found to be effective in identifying and managing post-treatment side effects, such as hypothyroidism, in patients with HNC (Milas et al., 2022).

When laying out long-term management and assistance for survivors, it is vital to consider the psychosocial, economic, and emotional influence of these cancers. Furthermore, non–cancer-associated mortalities, including suicide and comorbidity-related mortality, are increasing among HNC survivors, which underscores the need for population-specific surveillance and survivorship plans (Jung et al., 2023). Routine screening for psychological conditions is recommended for HNC patients as they grapple with psychological challenges related to the disease and its treatment (Elaldi et al., 2021; Penner, 2009).

Psychosocial interventions have been shown to be effective in enhancing the mental health and QOL of HNC patients (Van der Meulen et al., 2014). A systematic review of randomized controlled trials (RCTs) found that psychological interventions led to a greater decrease in anxiety and depression scores as well as improved QOL scores for HNC patients (Richardson et al., 2019). Another study that specifically focused on a brief cognitive-behavioral intervention (CBI) found that it enhanced self-assurance in dealing with cancer, depressive symptoms, other psychological symptoms, and health-linked QOL among HNC patients (Thilges et al., 2023). However, more well-designed and better-qualified investigations are required to validate these results.

The US healthcare system following cancer management is piloted by specialist primary care physicians (Cohen et al., 2016); this is in contrast with healthcare systems in Europe where cancer treatment, recovery, and ongoing care are administered by a multidisciplinary team (Pfister et al., 2020). Adapting and updating the AHNS Guidelines to mirror study data as of 2015, Verdonck-de Leeuw et al. (2022) a proposed how survivorship care in European healthcare systems ought to be managed and recommended a standard protocol for management of European HNC patients, as shown in Table 17.2.

Globally, in the overall management of HNCs, experts have developed and tested validated scientific tools for the general psychosocial aspects of dealing with cancers irrespective of their domain. This tool (Table 17.3) could be relevant specifically for HNC patients and caregivers.

17.8 Digital Health as Psychosocial Interventions for Patients with Head and Neck Cancers

Patients with HNC and their families frequently undergo significant worries amid worsening QOL. Patients' and families' psychosocial needs were

Table 17.2 Head and neck cancer survivorship: American Head and Neck Society (AHNS) Committee Guidelines

Level of evidence	Topic	Recommendation
2A[a]	Surgical oncology evaluation	Evaluate every 1–3 months in the 1st year after treatment; every 2–6 months in the 2nd year after treatment; every 4–8 months in the 3rd–5th year after treatment; and every 12 months thereafter
		Follow closely for a complete head and neck examination, indirect mirror and/or flexible fiberoptic laryngoscopy, and nasal endoscopy for patients with sinonasal malignancies
2B[a]		Monitor with EBV DNA in the setting of nasopharyngeal carcinoma surveillance
2A[a]	Radiation oncology evaluation	Evaluate for thyroid dysfunction (TSH/T4) every 6–12 months, particularly with prior neck irradiation
2A[a]		Refer for regular dental examinations, especially if the patient received intraoral or salivary gland irradiation
		Follow in close, alternating intervals with surgical and medical oncology
2A[a]	Medical oncology evaluation	Follow in close, alternating intervals with surgical and radiation oncology with attention to adverse effects related to chemotherapy and immunotherapy
2A[a]	Radiographic imaging	Follow with radiographic imaging (CT, MRI, and/or PET/CT) based on worrisome signs or symptoms and areas inaccessible to clinical examination (i.e., salivary glands, nasopharynx, and skull base)
		Consider chest CT with or without contrast as clinically indicated for those with a smoking history
2A[a]	Survivorship clinic	Incorporate a multidisciplinary team including nurses, advanced practice providers, oncologists (medical, radiation, surgical) in close coordination with the patient's primary care provider on at least an annual basis
2A[a]	Dysphonia and dysphagia	Incorporate speech-language pathology evaluation and management for at risk patients
5b	Fatigue	Evaluate for underlying etiologies of fatigue

(continued)

Table 17.2 Continued

Level of evidence	Topic	Recommendation
2A[b]	Sexual dysfunction and intimacy	Screen for sexual and intimacy dysfunction
		Offer supportive care services for sexual function and intimacy issue
		Consider pituitary dysfunction if patients have received skull base irradiation
		Counsel regarding the risk of HPV transmission after treatment for HPV-related OPSCC
2A[a]	Chronic pain	Screen for chronic pain at routine intervals
		Assess for the quality and severity of their pain using pain assessment tools
		Evaluate for depressive symptoms in the presence of chronic pain
3B[b]		Consider ruling out recurrent disease as a cause of pain
2A[a]		Screen for opioid abuse
2C[b], 2A[a], 1A[b]		Offer nonopioid analgesics including nonsteroidal anti-inflammatory agents, acetaminophen, neuromodulators, and acupuncture
5[b]		Refer to palliative and/or pain management specialists for refractory or opioid-dependent pain
5[b]	Physical therapy	Screen for physical rehabilitation needs early in the post-treatment phase with objective assessments of upper limb dysfunction at regular intervals
2A[a]		Assess for objective measures of trismus at regular intervals prior to and following therapy
5[b]		Refer to exercise and physiotherapy professionals for structured rehabilitation after HNC treatment
1B[b]		Incorporate shoulder physiotherapy after completion of neck dissection
2A[a]	Lymphedema	Evaluate for lymphedema after HNC treatment
		Refer to certified lymphedema therapists for CDT
2A[a]	Psycho-oncology	Screen for BID concerns
2A[a]		Refer to psychology or psychiatry for the management of BID as indicated

Table 17.2 Continued

Level of evidence	Topic	Recommendation
1A[b]		Assess for distress, depression, and/or anxiety at regular intervals using a validated questionnaire
1B[b]		Consider referral to psychology or psychiatry if distress, depression, and/or anxiety is present
2A[a]	Hearing loss	Evaluate yearly, for first 2 years, for hearing loss via pure tone audiometry in at risk patients
5[b]	Respiratory therapy	Multidisciplinary team should be aware and versed in tracheostomy and laryngectomy stoma care
5[b]	Caregivers	Include caregivers in all aspects of HNC care provided by the oncology team and PCP
5[b]	Social support groups	Educate on social support groups and their impact on understanding the wide-ranging sequelae of oncologic treatment
5[b]	Return to work	Counsel on medical disability rights and protections afforded by federal law
5[b]	Financial burden	Refer to social workers and financial navigators to understand health care costs associated with HNC care
2A[b]	Primary care physician	Include PCP involvement for age-appropriate and gender-appropriate screening of other neoplasms and general health as well as well-being
1B[b]	Dental care	Counsel to maintain close follow-up with the dental professional
5[b]		Encourage to avoid tobacco and alcohol to minimize the risk of dental disease
1A[b]	Substance abuse	Refer for tobacco and alcohol cessation counseling and abstinence resources as needed
1B[b]	Physical activity/ exercise	Encourage regular physical activity and exercise
5[b]	HPV counseling	Counsel on the sequelae of HPV related oncologic disease and the potential value of vaccination

CT, computed tomography; HNC, head and neck cancer; HPV, human papillomavirus; PCP, primary care provider; BID, body image disturbance; CDT, complex decongestive therapy; OPSCC, oropharyngeal squa mous cell carcinoma; PET, positron emission tomography; MRI, magnetic resonance imaging; EBV, Epstein-Barr virus; TSH, thyroid-stimulating hormone.

Table 17.3 Overall guidelines related to the management of head and neck cancers (European Guidelines)

Guideline overview:

Target population: Adult post-treatment head and neck cancer (HNC) survivors

Target audience: Primary care clinicians, secondary care oncologists, and other clinicians caring for HNC survivors

Methods: An expert panel was convened to revise clinical practice guideline recommendations based on a systematic review of medical literature and the American Cancer Society (ACS) key recommendations for HNC survivorship.

Recommendation 1.1. (a) conduct a detailed cancer-related history and physical examination every 1–3 months for the first year after primary treatment, every 2–6 months in the second year, every 4–8 months in years 3–5, and annually after 5 years.

(b) individualize clinical follow-up care as suggested in (a) based on age, specific diagnosis, and treatment protocol as recommended by the treating oncology team; (c) confirm continued follow-up with an otolaryngologist or HNC specialist for head and neck (HN)-focused examination.

Surveillance education:

Recommendation 1.2. (a) educate and counsel all HNC survivors about the signs and symptoms of local recurrence and that this education should be considerate of the anxiety that possible recurrence causes in HNC survivors; (b) refer HNC survivors to an HNC specialist if signs and symptoms of local recurrence are present.

Screening and early detection of second primary cancers (SPCs):

Recommendation 2.1. (a) screen HNC survivors for other cancers as they would for patients in the general population by adhering to the ACS Early Detection Recommendations. (b) screen HNC survivors for lung cancer according to American Society of Clinical Oncology (ASCO) or National Comprehensive Cancer Network (NCCN) recommendations for annual lung cancer screening with low dose computed tomography (LDCT) for high-risk patients based on smoking history; (c) screen HNC survivors for another HNC and esophageal cancer as they would for patients of increased risk.

Assessment and management of physical and psychosocial long-term and late effects of HNC and its treatment:

Recommendation 3.1. assess for long-term and late effects of HNC and its treatment at each follow-up visit (LOE 5 0).

Recommendation 3.1.1. (a) assess the information and supportive care needs of the HNC survivor related to HNC and its treatment, adverse effects, speech pathology, other health concerns, and available support services; (b) provide or refer HNC survivors to appropriate resources to meet identified needs.

Spinal accessory nerve palsy:

Recommendation 3.2. Refer HNC survivors with spinal accessory nerve palsy occurring post-radical neck dissection to a rehabilitation specialist physical therapist to improve range of motion and ability to perform daily tasks.

Table 17.3 Continued

Shoulder dysfunction:

Recommendation 3.3. (a) conduct baseline assessment of HNC survivor shoulder function post-treatment for strength, range of motion, and impingement signs, and continue to assess as follow-up for ongoing complications or worsening condition; (b) refer HNC survivors to a rehabilitation specialist for improvement to pain, disability, and range of motion where shoulder morbidity exists.

Cervical dystonia/muscle spasms/neuropathies/pain:

Recommendation 3.4. (a) assess HNC survivors for cervical dystonia, which is characterized by painful dystonic spasms of the cervical muscles and can be caused by neck dissection, radiation, or both; (b) refer HNC survivors to a rehabilitation specialist for comprehensive neuromusculoskeletal management if cervical dystonia or neuropathy is found; (c) receive assessment and consultation for the management of pain as part of regular follow-up; (d) prescribe nerve-stabilizing agents, such as pregabalin, gabapentin, and duloxetine, or refer to a specialist for botulinum toxin type A injections into the affected muscles for pain management and spasm control as indicated; (e) expect that these can occur as some of the very late effects of treatment.

Trismus:

Recommendation 3.5. (a) refer HNC survivors to rehabilitation specialists and the appropriate dental/maxillofacial specialists to prevent trismus and to treat trismus as soon as it is diagnosed; (b) prescribe nerve-stabilizing agents to combat pain and spasms, which may also ease physical therapy and stretching devices; (c) provide patients with interactive self-management guidance where possible.

Dysphagia/aspiration/stricture:

Recommendation 3.6. (a) refer HNC survivors presenting with complaints of dysphagia, postprandial cough, unexplained weight loss, and/or pneumonia to an experienced speech-language pathologist for instrumental evaluation of swallowing function to assess and manage dysphagia and possible aspiration and oropharyngeal residue) recognize potential for psychosocial barriers to swallowing recovery and the need for psychosocial and psychological support and refer HNC survivors for appropriate clinical support; (c) refer patients to a speech-language pathologist for video fluoroscopy as the first-line test for HNC survivors with suspected stricture due to the high degree of coexisting physiological dysphagia; (d) refer HNC survivors with stricture to a gastroenterologist or head and neck surgeon for dilation; (e) provide patients with self-management tools and guidance.

Gastroesophageal reflux disease:

Recommendation 3.7. (a) monitor HNC survivors for developing or worsening gastroesophageal reflux disease, as it prevents healing of irradiated tissues and is associated with increased risk of HNC recurrence or SPCs; (b) counsel HNC survivors on the increased risk of esophageal cancer and the associated symptoms; (c) recommend proton-pump inhibitors or antacids, sleeping with a wedge pillow or 3-inch blocks under the head of the bed, not eating or drinking fluids for 3 h before bedtime, tobacco cessation, and avoidance of alcohol; (d) refer HNC survivors to a gastroenterologist if symptoms are not relieved by treatments listed in 3.7c.

(*continued*)

Table 17.3 Continued

Lymphedema:

Recommendation 3.8. (a) assess HNC survivors for lymphoedema using the National Cancer Institute Common Terminology Criteria for Adverse Events or refer for endoscopic evaluation of mucosal oedema of the oropharynx and larynx, tape measurements, sonography, or external photographs; (b) refer HNC survivors to a rehabilitation specialist for treatment consisting of manual lymphatic drainage and, if tolerated, compressive bandaging, or complete decongestion therapy.

Fatigue:

Recommendation 3.9. (a) assess for fatigue and investigate any routine causative factors for fatigue, including anemia, thyroid dysfunction, and depression; (b) offer treatment or referral for factors that may impact fatigue (e.g. mood disorders, sleep disturbance, pain) for those who do not have an otherwise identifiable cause of fatigue; (c) counsel HNC survivors to engage in regular physical activity and refer for psychosocial counselling or psychotherapy as appropriate.

Altered or loss of taste and smell:

Recommendation 3.10. (a) ensure all patients are assessed for possible taste and sense changes as part of their nutritional assessments; (b) refer HNC survivors with altered or loss of taste to a registered dietitian for dietary counselling and assistance in additional seasoning of food, avoiding unpleasant food, and expanding dietary options and; (c) encourage those with altered sense of smell to practice the nasal airflow-inducing maneuver; (d) offer psychosocial counseling or psychotherapy as appropriate.

Hearing loss, vertigo, vestibular neuropathy:

Recommendation 3.11. Refer HNC survivors to an otologist and/or neuro-otologist for loss of hearing, vertigo, or vestibular neuropathy related to treatment.

Sleep disturbance/sleep apnea:

Recommendation 3.12. (a) screen HNC survivors for sleep disturbance by asking HNC survivors and partners about snoring and symptoms of sleep apnea and about other forms of disturbed sleep (e.g., difficulties falling asleep, difficulties keeping asleep, changes of sleep-wake-rhythm, nightmares); (b) refer HNC survivors to a sleep specialist for more detailed assessment; (c) manage sleep disturbance similar to patients in the general population; (d) recommend nasal decongestants, nasal strips, and sleeping in the propped-up position to reduce snoring and mouth-breathing; room cool-mist humidifiers can aid sleep as well by keeping the airway moist; (e) refer patients to a dental professional to test the fit of dentures to ensure proper fit and counsel HNC survivors to remove dentures at night to avoid irritation; (f) assess whether patients are experiencing distress and, if so, refer to mental health specialists for psychotherapy.

Speech and voice:

Recommendation 3.13. It is recommended that clinical care teams should: (a) assess HNC survivors for speech pathology; (b) refer HNC survivors to an experienced speech language pathologist if communication disorder exists; (c) where appropriate provide patients with appropriate exercise to help self-manage their recovery; (d) provide support for the emotional and psychosocial issues surrounding speech difficulties.

Table 17.3 Continued

Oral and dental surveillance:

Recommendation 3.14. It is recommended that the post-cancer care team should: (a) counsel HNC survivors to maintain close follow-up with the dental professional and reiterate that proper preventive care can help reduce caries and gingival disease; (b) counsel HNC survivors to avoid tobacco, alcohol (including mouthwash containing alcohol), spicy or abrasive foods, extreme temperature liquids, sugar-containing chewing gum or sugary soft drinks, and acidic or citric liquids; (c) refer HNC survivors to a dental professional specializing in the care of oncology patients; (d) provide patients with advice to enable self-management of oral pain and the recommendations in 3.3 further apply here specifically for the management of oral pain.

Recommendation 3.15. Dental professionals should provide any dental reconstruction required, where prosthetics may be required to support functionality. Complex dental reconstruction may require the need for patients to be referred to specialists or specialist services where available.

Dental health and caries:

Recommendation 3.16. (a) counsel HNC survivors to seek regular professional dental care for routine examination and cleaning and immediate attention to any intraoral changes that may occur; (b) counsel HNC survivors to minimize intake of sticky and/or sugar-containing food and drink to minimize risk of caries; (c) counsel HNC survivors on dental prophylaxis, including brushing with re-mineralizing toothpaste, the use of dental floss, and fluoride use (prescription 1.1 % sodium fluoride toothpaste as a dentifrice or in customized delivery trays; (d) test fit dentures to ensure proper fit and counsel HNC survivors to remove them at night to avoid irritation; (e) counsel HNC survivors that nasal strips can reduce snoring and mouth-breathing and that room humidifiers and nasal saline sprays can aid sleep as well; (f) train HNC survivors to do at-home HN self-evaluations and be instructed to report any suspicions or concerns immediately.

Periodontitis:

Recommendation 3.17. (a) refer HNC survivors to a dentist or periodontist for thorough evaluation; (b) counsel HNC survivors to seek regular treatment from and follow recommendations of a qualified dental professional and reinforce that proper examination of the gingival attachment is a normal part of ongoing dental care.

Xerostomia:

Recommendation 3.18. (a) encourage use of alcohol-free rinses if an HNC survivor requires mouth rinses; (b) counsel HNC survivors to consume a low-sucrose diet and to avoid caffeine, spicy and highly acidic foods, and tobacco; (c) encourage HNC survivors to avoid dehydration by drinking fluoridated tap water, but explain that consumption of water will not eliminate xerostomia; (d) consider the use of anticholinergic drugs to increase saliva and reduce xerostomia symptoms if other methods fail; (e) be aware that this can be a very late symptom of HNC treatment and to be mindful of this during long-term follow-up; (f) provide psychological support for the potential impact of xerostomia on quality of life if required.

(continued)

Table 17.3 Continued

Osteonecrosis:

Recommendation 3.19. (a) monitor HNC survivors for swelling of the jaw and/or jaw pain, indicating possible osteonecrosis; (b) administer conservative treatment protocols, such as broad-spectrum antibiotics and daily saline or aqueous chlorhexidine gluconate irrigations, for early-stage lesions; (c) consider referral to HN surgeon for dental extractions particularly complex or surgical extractions to assess if needed to minimize the risk of osteonecrosis; (d) refer to an HN surgeon for consideration of hyperbaric oxygen therapy for early and intermediate lesions, for debridement of necrotic bone while undergoing conservative management, or for external mandible bony exposure through the skin.

Oral infections/candidiasis:

Recommendation 3.20. (a) refer HNC survivors to a qualified dental professional for treatment and management of complicated oral conditions and infections; (b) consider systemic fluconazole and/or localized therapy of clotrimazole troches to treat oral fungal infections.

Body and self-image:

Recommendation 3.21. (a) assess HNC survivors for body and self-image concerns; (b) refer for psychosocial care as indicated.

Psychosocial problems and resilience:

Recommendation 3.22. (a) assess HNC survivors for psychosocial problems, such as symptoms of distress, depression, anxiety and adjustment disorder, fear of cancer recurrence, loneliness, and financial and employment challenges, as well as protective factors as coping and meaning, periodically (3 months post-treatment and at least annually), ideally using a validated screening tool, with frequency dictated by HNC sequelae severity and patient need); (b) offer in-office counseling and/or pharmacotherapy and/or refer to appropriate psycho-oncology and mental health resources as clinically indicated if symptoms of fear of recurrence or other psychosocial problems are present; (c) refer HNC survivors to mental health specialists for specific QOL concerns, such as to social workers for issues, including financial and employment challenges, finding meaning in life and living, in adjusting to living beyond cancer.

Dyspnea:

Recommendation 3.23. (a) perform a complete dyspnea assessment on patients who report this symptom; (b) provide psychoeducational and self-management tools.

Concentration and memory:

Recommendation 3.24. (a) assess patients for cognitive function; (b) provide psychosocial support for cognitive difficulties; (c) refer patients for additional support in coping with cognitive changes.

Sexuality and intimacy:

Recommendation 3.25. (a) offer advice and support in managing changes in sexual relationships; (b) offer patients psychosocial support for the potential impact of these changes.

Table 17.3 Continued

Health promotion:

Healthy weight:

Recommendation 4.1. (a) counsel HNC survivors to achieve and maintain a healthy weight; (b) refer patients for clinical dietician support to counsel HNC survivors on nutrition strategies to maintain a healthy weight for those at risk for cachexia; (c) counsel HNC survivors if overweight or obese to limit consumption of high-calorie foods and beverages and increase physical activity to promote and maintain weight loss.

Physical activity:

Recommendation 4.2. Counsel HNC survivors to engage in regular physical activity consistent with the ACS guideline, and specifically to: (a) avoid inactivity and return to normal daily activities as soon as possible after diagnosis; (b) aim for at least 150 min of moderate or 75 min of vigorous aerobic exercise per week; (c) include strength training exercises at least 2 days/week

Return to work and financial toxicity:

Recommendation 4.3. Support survivors return to work and that patients are referred to occupational therapists, or the relevant social care services.

Recommendation 4.4. Evaluate patients for risk of financial toxicity and are referred to the relevant social support services.

Nutrition:

Recommendation 4.5. (a) counsel HNC survivors to achieve a dietary pattern that is high in vegetables, fruits, and whole grains, low in saturated fats, sufficient in dietary fiber (unless otherwise recommended by a dietician), and avoids alcohol consumption; (b) refer HNC survivors with nutrition related challenges (e.g. swallowing problems that impact nutrient intake) to a registered dietician or other specialist; (c) include assessments regarding taste and smell changes as part of dietary assessments.

Tobacco cessation and substance abuse:

Recommendation 4.6. (a) counsel HNC survivors to avoid tobacco products and offer or refer patients to cessation counselling and resources; (b) refer patients for counselling and support regarding broader substance abuse issues.

Care coordination and practice implications

Survivorship care plan:

Recommendation 5.1. Collaborate to develop and continue survivorship and rehabilitation care plans.

Communication with other providers:

Recommendation 5.2. (a) maintain communication with the oncology team throughout diagnosis, treatment, and post-treatment care to ensure care is evidence-based and well-coordinated; (b) refer HNC survivors to a dentist to provide diagnosis and treatment of dental caries, periodontal disease, and other intraoral conditions, including mucositis and oral infections, and communicate with the dentist on follow-up recommendations and patient education; (c) maintain communication with specialists referred to for management of comorbidities, symptoms, and long-term and late effects.

(*continued*)

Table 17.3 Continued

Inclusion of caregivers and patient support groups
Recommendation 5.3. Encourage the inclusion of caregivers and spouses in healthcare, and that they are provided with an understanding of symptoms, rehabilitation programs and how to manage these.
Recommendation 5.4. Patients be referred to patient and self-management support groups to help deal with the consequences of HNC survivorship.

Source: Verdonck-de Leeuw et al., 2022.

investigated using psychosocial interventions. Digital technologies are increasingly being used to deliver psychosocial interventions to patients with cancer and their families. The adoption and implementation of policies on specific digital technologies as effective tools to monitor HNC patients has become imperative, with their capabilities for altering the tide of patient outcomes, especially in rural settings. Rural dwellers experience increased cancer incidence rates and mortality, an inequality that the deployment of health technology interventions could mitigate. However, this apparent digital divide continues to be neglected. It should be the focus of any rural-based intervention strategies to improve the psychosocial well-being of HNC patients (Morris et al., 2022). eHealth is "an emerging field in the convergence of medical informatics, public health, and business, dealing with health services and information conveyed or enhanced through the internet and associated technologies" (Eysenbach, 2001; Pagliari et al., 2005).

Among eHealth approaches are various modes of delivery, such as by telephone (Krzyzanowska et al., 2021), website (Maguire et al., 2021), and telehealth messaging device (Pfeifer et al., 2015). Implementing and scaling up empirical digital technologies for common cancer care plans is still challenging. Examples are online platforms, digital apps, and wearable gadgets that may assist end users in tracking or altering the behaviors, cognitions, and emotional mindsets of HNC patients in rural areas. Such efforts may utilize varying formats, such as text messaging, audio, video, or games.

17.9 Limitations

In the holistic management of HNC toward achieving better prognostic indices in the psychosocial well-being of patients, we recognize that several limitations abound, partly reflecting difference in accessing optimal healthcare. It is also recognized that the greatest burdens and suicidal ideations are tilted more toward the socioeconomically deprived individuals with poor access to technology and healthcare screening services as well as other stressors that culminate in a negative outlook for psychosocial health.

17.10 Conclusion and Future Directions

Undoubtably, a cancer diagnosis impacts the patient, caregivers, and their workplace as well as healthcare systems with untoward negative implications that continue to generate unmet medical needs. Integrating available scientific evidence for implementable psychosocial tools is relevant for patient assessment and determination of QOL outcomes. The prolonged burden of patient care often impedes the sound judgment of caregivers, thus generating ethical concerns and a need for adequate supervision of their roles and mental well-being. New insights into increased mortality among rural dwellers who suffer from HNC require concerted efforts and policy adoptions toward mobilizing frontline care workers to engage against isolation tendencies and suicide ideations vigilantly. We agree that the need to include digital technologies as a toolkit to follow-up HNC patients, especially in light of alarming facts coming particularly from rural settings, requires top priority handling by all health systems.

References

ALEXANDER, R., ARAGON, O. R., BOOKWALA, J., CHERBUIN, N., GATT, J. M., KAHRILAS, I. J., KASTNER, N., LAWRENCE, A., LOWE, L., MORRISON, R. G., MUELLER, S. C., NUSSLOCK, R., PAPADELIS, C., POLNASZEK, K. L., RICHTER, S. H., SILTON, R. L., & STYLIADIS, C. 2020. The neuroscience of positive emotions and affect: Implications for cultivating happiness and wellbeing. *Neurosci Biobehav Rev* 121, 220–49.

AL-SALOOL, A., SOROR, T., YU, N. Y., IDEL, C., BRUCHHAGE, K. L., HAKIM, S. G., & RADES, D. 2023. Emotional distress in head-and-neck cancer patients scheduled for chemoradiation or radiotherapy alone. *Anticancer Res*, 43, 2227–33.

ALBERT, J. G., LO, C., ROSBERGER, Z., FRENKIEL, S., HIER, M., ZEITOUNI, A., KOST, K., MLYNAREK, A., BLACK, M., & MACDONALD, C. 2022. Biopsychosocial markers of body image concerns in patients with head and neck cancer: A prospective longitudinal study. *Curr Oncol*, 29, 4438–54.

ALLEN, S., ROGERS, S. N., BROWN, S., & HARRIS, R. V. 2021. What are the underlying reasons behind socioeconomic differences in doctor-patient communication in head and neck oncology review clinics? *Health Expect*, 24, 140–51.

AMERICAN CANCER SOCIETY. 2018. *Global cancer facts & figures*, 4th edition. https://www.cancer.org/content/dam/cancer-org/research/cancer-facts-and-statistics/global-cancer-facts-and-figures/global-cancer-facts-and-figures-4th-edition.pdf

ANDERSON, G., EBADI, M., VO, K., NOVAK, J., GOVINDARAJAN, A., & AMINI, A. 2021. An updated review on head and neck cancer treatment with radiation therapy. *Cancers*, 13, 4912.

ARIAS, D. L. C. 2020. Emotions associated with plastic packaging among college students. *Revista [IN] Genios*, 7(1), 1–17.

ARRING, N., BARTON, D. L., & REESE, J. B. 2023. Clinical practice strategies to address sexual health in female cancer survivors. *J Clin Oncol*, 41, 4927–36.

ASSAS, M. B. 2020. *The Methodological Quality of Patient-Reported Outcome Measures for Radiotherapy Induced Xerostomia in Head and Neck Cancer.* London: University College London.

ATHIYAMAAN, M., & KAMATH, A. 2023. A Systematic review of the economic burden of proton therapy in head and neck cancer. *Asian Pacific Journal of Cancer Prevention: APJCP*, 24, 3643.

BAKHSHAIE, J., BONNEN, M., ASPER, J., SANDULACHE, V., & BADR, H. 2020. Emotional disclosure and cognitive processing in couples coping with head and neck cancer. *J Behave Med*, 43, 411–25.

BALIGA, M. S., LASRADO, S., KRISHNA, A., GEORGE, T., MADATHIL, L. P., D'SOUZA, R. F., & PALATTY, P. L. 2023. Social, ethical and treatment related problems faced by healthcare workers in the care of head and neck cancer patients: A narrative review from the bioethics consortium from India. *Indian J Otolaryngol Head Neck Surg*, 75, 4137–47.

BARSOUK, A., ALURU, J. S., RAWLA, P., SAGINALA, K., & BARSOUK, A. 2023. Epidemiology, risk factors, and prevention of head and neck squamous cell carcinoma. *Med Sci*, 11, 42.

BENYO, S., PHAN, C., & GOYAL, N. 2023. Health and well-being needs among head and neck cancer caregivers—A systematic review. *Ann Otol Rhinol Laryngol*, 132(4), 449–59.

BINGHAM, S. L., SMALL, S., & SEMPLE, C. J. (2023). A qualitative evaluation of a multimodal cancer prehabilitation programme for colorectal, head and neck and lung cancers patients. *PLoS ONE*, 18(10), 1–22. Article e0277589. Advance online publication. https://doi.org/10.1371/journal.pone.0277589

BOSCOLO NATA, F., GARDENAL, N., GIUDICI, F., & TIRELLI, G. 2022. The role of NBI with flexible video-endoscope in the follow-up of head and neck cancer patients: A prospective study. *Eur Arch Oto Rhino-Laryngol*, 1–9.

CEREA, S., SANSONI, M., SCARZELLO, G., GROFF, E., & GHISI, M. 2022. Psychological variables associated with quality of life in patients with head and neck cancer: The role of body image distress. *Support Care Cancer*, 30, 9127–39.

CHANG, V. T., HWANG, S. S., KASIMIS, B., & THALER, H. T. 2004. Shorter symptom assessment instruments: The Condensed Memorial Symptom Assessment Scale (CMSAS). *Cancer Invest*, 22(4), 526–36

CHEN, Y.-J., LAI, Y.-H., LEE, Y.-H., TSAI, K.-Y., CHEN, M.-K., & HSIEH, M.-Y. 2021. Impact of illness perception, mental adjustment, and sociodemographic characteristics on return to work in patients with head and neck cancer. *Support Care Cancer*, 29, 1519–26.

COHEN, E. E., LAMONTE, S. J., ERB, N. L., et al. 2016. American Cancer Society head and neck cancer survivorship care guideline. *CA Cancer J Clin*, 66(3), 203–39.

COVRIG, V. I., LAZĂR, D. E., COSTAN, V. V., POSTOLICĂ, R., & IOAN, B. G. 2021. The psychosocial role of body image in the quality of life of head and neck cancer patients. what does the future hold? A review of the literature. *Medicina*, 57, 1078.

CROWDER, S. L., NAJAM, N., SARMA, K. P., FIESE, B. H., & ARTHUR, A. E. 2021. Quality of life, coping strategies, and supportive care needs in head and neck cancer survivors: A qualitative study. *Support Care Cancer*, 29, 4349–56.

DAY, A. T., SHER, D. J., LEE, R. C., TRUELSON, J. M., MYERS, L. L., SUMER, B. D., STANKOVA, L., TILLMAN, B. N., HUGHES, R. S., & KHAN, S. A. 2020. Head and neck oncology during the COVID-19 pandemic: Reconsidering traditional treatment paradigms in light of new surgical and other multilevel risks. *Oral Oncol*, 105, 104684.

DEGEFA, M., DUBALE, B., BAYOUH, F., AYELE, B., & ZEWDE, Y. 2020. Validation of the PHQ-9 depression scale in Ethiopian cancer patients attending the oncology clinic at Tikur Anbessa Specialized Hospital, *BMC Psychiatry*, 20(1), 1–7

DE FELICE, F., BELGIOIA, L., ALTERIO, D., BONOMO, P., MADDALO, M., PAIAR, F., DENARO, N., CORVO, R., MERLOTTI, A., & BOSSI, P. 2021. Survival and toxicity of weekly cisplatin chemoradiotherapy versus three-weekly cisplatin chemoradiotherapy for head and neck cancer: A systematic review and meta-analysis endorsed by the Italian Association of Radiotherapy and Clinical Oncology (AIRO). *Crit Rev Oncol Hematol*, 162, 103345.

DE RAVIN, E., ARMACHE, M., CAMPBELL, F., RISING, K. L., WORSTER, B., HANDLEY, N. R., FUNDAKOWSKI, C. E., COGNETTI, D. M., & MADY, L. J. 2023. Feasibility and cost of telehealth head and neck cancer survivorship care: A systematic review. *Otolaryngol Head Neck Surg*, 168, 1312–23.

DELEEMANS, J. M., MOTHERSILL, K., BULTZ, B. D., & SCHULTE, F. 2020. Ethical considerations in screening head and neck cancer patients for psychosocial distress. *Support Care Cancer*, 28, 617–24.

DESHIELDS, T. L., WELLS-DI GREGORIO, S., FLOWERS, S. R., IRWIN, K. E., NIPP, R., PADGETT, L., & ZEBRACK, B. 2021. Addressing distress management challenges: Recommendations from the consensus panel of the American Psychosocial Oncology Society and the Association of Oncology Social Work. *CA: Cancer J*, 71, 407–36.

DO NASCIMENTO SANTOS LIMA, E., FERREIRA, I. B., LAJOLO, P. P., PAIVA, C. E., DE PAIVA MAIA, Y. C., & DAS GRAÇAS PENA, G. 2020. Health-related quality of life became worse in short-term during treatment in head and neck cancer patients: A prospective study. *Health Quality Life Outc*, 18(1), 307.

ELALDI, R., ROUSSEL, L.-M., GAL, J., SCHELLER, B., CHAMOREY, E., SCHIAPPA, R., LASNE-CARDON, A., LOUIS, M.-Y., CULIÉ, D., & DASSONVILLE, O. 2021. Correlations between long-term quality of life and patient needs and concerns following head and neck cancer treatment and the impact of psychological distress. A multicentric cross-sectional study. *Eur Arch Oto-Rhino-Laryngol*, 278, 2437–45.

EYSENBACH, G. 2001. What is e-health? *J Med Internet Res*, 3 (2), 1–5.

FANG, C. Y., & HECKMAN, C. J. 2016. Informational and support needs of patients with head and neck cancer: Current status and emerging issues. *Cancers Head Neck*, 1, 1–9.

GASCON, B., PANJWANI, A. A., MAZZURCO, O., & LI, M. 2022. Screening for distress and health outcomes in head and neck cancer. *Curr Oncol*, 29, 3793–806.

GHAZALI, N. 2018. *Personalising Head and Neck Cancer Survivorship: Intervention with the Head and Neck Cancer Patients Concerns Inventory in Routine Head and Neck Cancer Outpatient Visits*. Liverpool: University of Liverpool Press.

GORMLEY, M., CREANEY, G., SCHACHE, A., INGARFIELD, K., & CONWAY, D. I. 2022. Reviewing the epidemiology of head and neck cancer: Definitions, trends and risk factors. *Br Dent J*, 233, 780–6.

GRATTAN, K., KUBRAK, C., CAINE, V., O'CONNELL, D. A., & OLSON, K. 2018. Experiences of head and neck cancer patients in middle adulthood: Consequences and coping. *Global Qual Nurs Res*, 5, 2333393618760337.

GUPTA, B., JOHNSON, N. W., & KUMAR, N. 2016. Global epidemiology of head and neck cancers: A continuing challenge. *Oncology*, 91, 13–23.

HAMMERMÜLLER, C., HINZ, A., DIETZ, A., WICHMANN, G., PIRLICH, M., BERGER, T., ZIMMERMANN, K., NEUMUTH, T., MEHNERT-THEUERKAUF, A., & WIEGAND, S. 2021. Depression, anxiety, fatigue, and quality of life in a large sample of patients suffering from head and neck cancer in comparison with the general population. *BMC Cancer*, 21, 1–11.

HANCOCK, A., NORTHCOTT, S., HOBSON, H., & CLARKE, M. 2023. Speech, language and communication needs and mental health: The experiences of speech and language therapists and mental health professionals. *Int J Lang Comm Dis*, 58, 52–66.

HART, N. H., CRAWFORD-WILLIAMS, F., CRICHTON, M., YEE, J., SMITH, T. J., KOCZWARA, B., FITCH, M. I., CRAWFORD, G. B., MUKHOPADHYAY, S., & MAHONY,

J. 2022. Unmet supportive care needs of people with advanced cancer and their caregivers: A systematic scoping review. *Crit Rev Oncol Hematol*, 176, 103728.

HASHIM, D., & BOFFETTA, P. 2020. Head and neck cancers. *Occupat Cancers*, 57–105.

HASHIM, D., GENDEN, E., POSNER, M., HASHIBE, M., & BOFFETTA, P. (2019). Head and neck cancer prevention: From primary prevention to impact of clinicians on reducing burden. *Ann Oncol: Off J Eur Soc Med Oncol*, 30(5), 744–56. https://doi.org/10.1093/annonc/mdz084

HATTON, R., CRANE, J., PATTERSON, J., & ROGERS, S. 2022. A survey to ascertain peer support models available in head and neck cancer across the United Kingdom. *Br J Oral Maxillofac Surg*, 60, 488–92.

HENRY, M., ALIAS, A., CHERBA, M., WORONKO, C., ROSBERGER, Z., HIER, M., ZEITOUNI, A., KOST, K., MLYNAREK, A., & RICHARDSON, K. 2020. Immediate post-treatment supportive care needs of patients newly diagnosed with head and neck cancer. *Support Care Cancer*, 28, 5557–67.

HORTENSE, F. T. P., BERGEROT, C. D., & DOMENICO, E. B. L. D. 2020. Quality of life, anxiety and depression in head and neck cancer patients: A randomized clinical trial. *Revista da Escola de Enfermagem da USP*, 54, e03546.

HOWREN, M. B., CHRISTENSEN, A. J., KARNELL, L. H., & FUNK, G. F. 2013. Psychological factors associated with head and neck cancer treatment and survivorship: Evidence and opportunities for behavioral medicine. *J Consult Clin Psychol*, 81, 299.

HUNTER, M., KELLETT, J., TOOHEY, K., D'CUNHA, N. M., ISBEL, S., & NAUMOVSKI, N. 2020. Toxicities caused by head and neck cancer treatments and their influence on the development of malnutrition: Review of the literature. *Eur J Investig Health Psychol Educ*, 10(4), 935–49. https://doi.org/10.3390/ejihpe10040066

HURREN, A., MCLACHLAN, K., & MILLER, N. 2023. *Communicating With People with Tracheostomies and Head and Neck Cancers: A Guide to Managing Atypical Communication in Healthcare*. London: Routledge.

IWASE, S., KAWAGUCHI, T., TOKORO, A., YAMADA, K., KANAI, Y., MATSUDA, Y., KASHIWAYA, Y., OKUMA, K., INADA, S., ARIYOSHI, K., MIYAJI, T., AZUMA, K., ISHIKI, H, UNEZAKI, S., & YAMAGUCHI, T. 2015. Assessment of cancer-related fatigue, pain, and quality of life in cancer patients at palliative care team referral: A multicenter observational study (JORTC pal-09), *PLOS ONE*, 10(8), 1–12.

JAYAKAR, R., CHOI, J., MACKINNON, C., & TAN, S. 2017. The cost of major head and neck cancer surgery. *N Zealand Med J (Online)*, 130, 111.

JOHNSON, S. U., ULVENES, P. G., ØKTEDALEN, T., & HOFFART, A. 2019. Psychometric properties of the General Anxiety Disorder 7-item (GAD-7) scale in a heterogeneous psychiatric sample. *Front Psychol*, 10, 1–8.

JUNG, Y.-S., LEE, D., JUNG, K.-W., & CHO, H. 2023. Long-term survivorship and non-cancer competing mortality in head and neck cancer: A nationwide population-based study in South Korea. *Cancer Res Treat*, 55, 50.

JUSTER, J., & PAGE, C. 2023. Possibilities for the early diagnosis of head and neck squamous cell carcinoma. *Cancer Screen Prevent*, 2, 130–7.

KAMARAJU, S., DROPE, J., SANKARANARAYANAN, R., & SHASTRI, S. 2020. Cancer prevention in low-resource countries: An overview of the opportunity. *Am Soc Clin Oncol Educ*, 40, 72–83.

KARNELL, L. H., CHRISTENSEN, A. J., ROSENTHAL, E. L., MAGNUSON, J. S., & FUNK, G. F. 2007. Influence of social support on health-related quality of life outcomes in head and neck cancer. *Head Neck*, 29, 143–6.

KASSIR, Z. M., LI, J., HARRISON, C., JOHNSON, J. T., & NILSEN, M. L. 2021. Disparity of perception of quality of life between head and neck cancer patients and caregivers. *BMC Cancer*, 21(1), 1127.

KITAMURA, N., SENTO, S., YOSHIZAWA, Y., SASABE, E., KUDO, Y., & YAMAMOTO, T. 2020. Current trends and future prospects of molecular targeted therapy in head and neck squamous cell carcinoma. *Int J Mol Sci*, 22, 240.

KOMPUINEN, J., KESKIN, M., YILMAZ, D., GÜRSOY, M., & GÜRSOY, U. K. 2023. Human β-defensins in diagnosis of head and neck cancers. *Cells*, 12, 830.

KRISTENSEN, M. B., MIKKELSEN, T. B., BECK, A. M., ZWISLER, A.-D., WESSEL, I., & DIEPERINK, K. B. 2019. To eat is to practice: Managing eating problems after head and neck cancer. *J Cancer Survivorship*, 13, 792–803.

KRZYZANOWSKA, M. K., A JULIAN, J., GU, C.-S., POWIS, M., LI, Q., ENRIGHT, K., HOWELL, D., EARLE, C.C., GANDHI, S., RASK, S., et al. 2021. Remote, proactive, telephone based management of toxicity in outpatients during adjuvant or neoadjuvant chemotherapy for early-stage breast cancer: Pragmatic, cluster randomised trial. *BMJ*, 375, e066588.

KUBRAK, C., MARTIN, L., GRAMLICH, L., SCRIMGER, R., JHA, N., DEBENHAM, B., CHUA, N., WALKER, J., & BARACOS, V. E. 2020. Prevalence and prognostic significance of malnutrition in patients with cancers of the head and neck. *Clin Nutrit*, 39, 901–9.

KUDRICK, L. D., BADDOUR, K., WU, R., FADEL, M., SNYDER, V., NEOPANEY, A., THOMAS, T. H., SABIK, L. M., NILSEN, M. L., & JOHNSON, J. T. 2023. Longitudinal analysis of caregiver burden in head and neck cancer. *JAMA Otolaryngol Head Neck Surg*, 149, 681–9.

KUHS, K. A. L., BRENNER, J. C., HOLSINGER, F. C., & RETTIG, E. M. 2023. Circulating tumor HPV DNA for surveillance of HPV-positive oropharyngeal squamous cell carcinoma: A narrative review. *JAMA Oncol.* 9(12), 1716–24. doi:10.1001/jamaoncol.2023.4042

LA, I. S. 2020. *Burden and Mental Health of Family Caregivers of Cancer Patients: The Impact of Spirituality.* University of Maryland, Baltimore.

LEUTER, C., PETRUCCI, C., CAPONNETTO, V., LA CERRA, C., & LANCIA, L. 2018. Need for ethics support in clinical practice and suggestion for an ethics consultation service: views of nurses and physicians working in Italian healthcare institutions. *Annali dell'Istituto Superiore di Sanità*, 54, 117–25.

LEWIS, S., PANDEY, S., SALINS, N., DEODHAR, J., PATIL, V., GUPTA, T., LASKAR, S. G., BUDRUKKAR, A., MURTHY, V., & JOSHI, A. 2021. Distress Screening in Head and Neck Cancer Patients Planned for Cancer-Directed Radiotherapy. *Laryngoscope*, 131, 2023–9.

LITSAS, D., ZISMAN-ILANI, Y., SIMINOFF, L. A., & NACE, T. 2022. Culturally appropriate patient-clinician communication methods for discussing mammography results among black American Women search strategy. Temple University Libraries.

LU, L., O'SULLIVAN, E., & SHARP, L. 2019. Cancer-related financial hardship among head and neck cancer survivors: Risk factors and associations with health-related quality of life. *Psycho-oncol*, 28, 863–71.

LUNDQVIST, L., & AHLSTRÖM, G. 2006. Psychometric evaluation of the Ways of Coping Questionnaire as applied to clinical and non-clinical groups, *J Psychosom Res*, 60(5), 485–93.

MACIAS, D., HAND, B. N., MAURER, S., BALLIET, W., ELLIS, M. A., PIPKORN, P., HUANG, A. T., NILSEN, M. L., RUGGIERO, K. J., & WILLIAMS, A. M. 2021. Factors associated with risk of body image–related distress in patients with head and neck cancer. *JAMA Otolaryngol Head Neck Surg*, 147, 1019–26.

MAGUIRE, R., MCCANN, L., KOTRONOULAS, G., KEARNEY, N., REAM, E., ARMES, J., PATIRAKI, E., FURLONG, E., FOX, P., GAIGER, A., et al. 2021. Real time remote symptom monitoring during chemotherapy for cancer: European multicentre randomised controlled trial (eSMART). *BMJ*, 374, n1647.

MALIK, N. H., MAGANTI, M., MCQUESTION, M., TJONG, M. C., KEILTY, D., MONTEIRO, E., HUANG, S. H., JANG, R. W.-J., GOMES, A., & PUN, J. 2021. Pretreatment psychoeducational intervention and outcomes in head and neck cancer patients undergoing radiotherapy. *Support Care Cancer*, 29, 1643–52.

MARUR, S., & FORASTIERE, A. A. 2008. Head and neck cancer: Changing epidemiology, diagnosis, and treatment. *Mayo Clin Proc*, 489–501.

MAYLAND, C. R., HO, Q. M., DOUGHTY, H. C., ROGERS, S. N., PEDDINTI, P., CHADA, P., MASON, S., COOPER, M., & DEY, P. 2021. The palliative care needs and experiences of people with advanced head and neck cancer: A scoping review. *Palliat Med*, 35, 27–44.

MAYO, A., LAM, J., MAGANTI, M., MCQUESTION, M., GOMES, A., CLUETT, S., LEE, Y., DEERING, J., DAVIES, M., & TOSONI, S. 2022. Getting back on track: A group psychoeducational intervention for patients and families living with head and neck cancer. *Support Care Cancer*, 1–10.

MCDOWELL, I. 2006. Psychological well-being. *Measuring Health: A guide to rating scales and questionnaires*, 3rd edn (New York, 2006; online edn, Oxford Academic, 1 Sept. 2009), https://doi.org/10.1093/acprof:oso/9780195165678.003.0005, accessed 2 Apr. 2025.

MCDOWELL, L., RISCHIN, D., GOUGH, K., & HENSON, C. 2022. Health-related quality of life, psychosocial distress and unmet needs in older patients with head and neck cancer. *Front Oncol*, 12, 834068.

MEREDITH, E., O'DONOVAN, J., ERRINGTON, L., MATHUR, M., & HAMILTON, D. 2022. The role of community healthcare workers in head and neck cancer: A systematic scoping review of the literature. *Global Public Health*, 17, 3283–302.

MICHAŁOWSKA, S., MATUSEWICZ, S., & SAMOCHOWIEC, A. 2019. Coping and anxiety in cancer patients. *Arch Psychiatry Psychother*, 2, 28–32.

MILAS, Z. L., NEELANDS, B., TRUFAN, S. J., BENBOW, J., CARRIZOSA, D., BRICKMAN, D. S., FRENKEL, C. H., SUMRALL, A. L., SUDHAKAR, S. M., & WARD, M. C. 2022. Survivorship care plans improve the identification of post-radiation hypothyroidism after head and neck cancer treatment. *Anticancer Res*, 42, 4429–37.

MILLER, J. L. 2020. *Predictors of Nonadherence to Radiation Therapy Schedules among Head and Neck Cancer Patients*. Tampa, FL: University of South Florida.

MILLER, M. C., SHUMAN, A. G., & AMERICAN HEAD AND NECK SOCIETY'S COMMITTEE ON SURVIVORSHIP. 2016. Survivorship in head and neck cancer: A primer. *JAMA Otolaryngol Head Neck Surg*, 142 (10),1002–8.

MIROSEVIC, S., THEWES, B., VAN HERPEN, C., KAANDERS, J., THIJS MERKX, T., HUMPHRIS, G., DE JONG, B. J. B., LANGENDIJK, J. A., LEEMANS, C. R., TERHAARD, C. H. J., VERDONCK-DE LEEUW, I. M., TAKES, R., PRINS, J., & THE NET-QUBIC CONSORTIUM. 2019. Prevalence and clinical and psychological correlates of high fear of cancer recurrence in patients newly diagnosed with head and neck cancer. *Head Neck*, 41(7), 3187–200.

MISHRA, A., & MEHEROTRA, R. 2014. Head and neck cancer: Global burden and regional trends in India. *Asian Pacific J Cancer Prevent*, 15, 537–50.

MOLENAAR, D., VERDONCK-DE LEEUW, I. M., LISSENBERG-WITTE, B. I., TAKES, R. P., TERHAARD, C. H., LANGENDIJK, J. A., LEEMANS, C. R., & JANSEN, F. 2023. Changes in supportive care needs over time from diagnosis up to two years after treatment in head and neck cancer patients: A prospective cohort study. *Oral Oncol Rep*, 6, 100047.

MORRIS, N., MOGHADDAM, N., TICKLE, A., & BISWAS, S. 2018. The relationship between coping style and psychological distress in people with head and neck cancer: A systematic review. *Psycho-oncol*, 27, 734–47.

MORRIS, B. B., ROSSI, B., & FUEMMELER, B. 2022. The role of digital health technology in rural cancer care delivery: A systematic review. *J Rural Health*, 38(3), 493–511.

MOTT, N. M., MIERZWA, M. L., CASPER, K. A., SHAH, J. L., MALLEN-ST CLAIR, J., HO, A. S., ZUMSTEG, Z. S., PRINCE, M. E., DOSSETT, L. A., & CHEN, M. M. 2022. Financial hardship in patients with head and neck cancer. *JCO Oncol Pract*, 18, e925–37.

MULLAN, F. 1985. Seasons of survival: Reflections of a physician with cancer. *N Engl J Med*. 313(4), 270–3.

MUZAFFAR, J., BARI, S., KIRTANE, K., & CHUNG, C. H. 2021. Recent advances and future directions in clinical management of head and neck squamous cell carcinoma. *Cancers*, 13, 338.

NATIONAL COMPREHENSIVE CANCER NETWORK. 2020. Head and neck cancer. Available at: https://www.nccn.org/professionals/physician_gls/pdf/headand-neck.pdf

NAYAK, S. G., GEORGE, A., SHARAN, K., NAYAK, B. S., & RAVISHANKAR, N. 2024. Effectiveness of comprehensive intervention programme on quality of life, fatigue, self-efficacy, and psychosocial distress among head and neck cancer patients receiving radiotherapy. *Support Care Cancer*, 32, 1–11.

NAYAK, S. G., SHARAN, K., CHAKRABARTY, J., DEVI, E. S., RAVISHANKAR, N., & GEORGE, A. 2022. Psychosocial distress of Head Neck Cancer (HNC) patients receiving radiotherapy: A systematic review. *Asian Pacific J Cancer Prevent*, 23, 1827.

NAYAK, S. G., SHARAN, K., & GEORGE, A. 2023. Attributes of psychosocial distress from the perspectives of head-and-neck cancer patients: A thematic analysis. *Indian J Palliat Care*, 29, 181.

NEKHLYUDOV, L., LACCHETTI, C., DAVIS, N. B., et al. 2017. Head and neck cancer survivorship care guideline: American Society of Clinical Oncology clinical practice guideline endorsement of the American Cancer Society guideline. *J Clin Oncol*, 35(14), 1606–21.

NGUYEN, N.-T. A., & RINGASH, J. 2018. Head and neck cancer survivorship care: A review of the current guidelines and remaining unmet needs. *Curr Treat Opt Oncol*, 19, 1–20.

NGUYEN, O. T., DONATO, U., MCCORMICK, R., REBLIN, M., KIM, L., HUME, E., OTTO, A. K., ALISHAHI TABRIZ, A., ISLAM, J. Y., & HONG, Y. R. 2023. Financial toxicity among head and neck cancer patients and their caregivers: A cross-sectional pilot study. *Laryngoscope Invest Otolaryngol*, 8, 450–7.

NIK JAAFAR, N. R., RAJANDRAM, R. K., & LEONG BIN ABDULLAH, M. F. I. 2021. Posttraumatic growth and coping strategies among patients with head and neck cancer: Do approach coping and avoidant coping predict posttraumatic growth over time? *Front Psychol*, 12, 716674.

NUGENT, S. M., MORASCO, B. J., HANDLEY, R., CLAYBURGH, D., HOOKER, E. R., GANZINI, L., KNIGHT, S. J., CHEN, J. I., SULLIVAN, D. R., & SLATORE, C. G. 2021. Risk of suicidal self-directed violence among US veteran survivors of head and neck cancer. *JAMA Otolaryngol Head Neck Surg*, 147(11), 981–9.

NWAGWU, C. C., & OGOKE, U. P. 2024. Cancer incidence, mortality, and survivorship in African women: A comparative analysis (2016–2020). *Front Glob Women's Health*, 4, 1173244. https://doi.org/10.3389/fgwh.2023.1173244

OSAZUWA-PETERS, N., BARNES, J. M., OKAFOR, S. I., TAYLOR, D. B., HUSSAINI, A. S., BOAKYE, E. A., SIMPSON, M. C., GRABOYES, E. M., & LEE, W. T. 2021. Incidence and risk of suicide among patients with head and neck cancer in rural, urban, and metropolitan areas. *JAMA Otolaryngol Head Neck Surg*, 147(12), 1045–52.

OWNBY, K. K. 2019. Use of the Distress Thermometer in clinical practice. *J Adv Pract Oncol*, 10(2), 175–9.

PAGLIARI, C., SLOAN, D., GREGOR, P., SULLIVAN, F., DETMER, D., KAHAN, J. P., et al. 2005. What is eHealth (4): A scoping exercise to map the field *J Med Internet Res*, 7(1), e9.

PATEL, M. A., BLACKFORD, A. L., RETTIG, E. M., RICHMON, J. D., EISELE, D. W., & FAKHRY, C. 2016. Rising population of survivors of oral squamous cell cancer in the United States. *Cancer*, 122 (9), 1380–7.

PATTERSON, J. M., LU, L., WATSON, L. J., HARDING, S., NESS, A. R., THOMAS, S., WAYLEN, A., PRING, M., WATERBOER, T., & SHARP, L. 2022. Associations between markers of social functioning and depression and quality of life in survivors of head and neck cancer: Findings from the Head and Neck Cancer 5000 study. *Psycho-Oncol*, 31, 478–85.

PENNER, J. L. 2009. Psychosocial care of patients with head and neck cancer. *Semin Oncol Nurs*, 231–41.

PETRIĆ, D., RAČKI, V., PEITL, M., ZUBOVIĆ, A., RAČKI, N., ROGIĆ, M., GOBIĆ, M., & TOVILOVIĆ, Z. 2021. Coping strategies in oral and oropharyngeal cancer patients with alcohol dependence. *Eur J Psychiatry*, 35, 99–106.

PFEIFER, M.P., KEENEY, C., BUMPOUS, J., SCHAPMIRE, T.J., STUDTS, J.L., MYERS, J., & HEAD, B. 2015. Impact of a telehealth intervention on quality of life and symptom distress in patients with head and neck cancer. *J Comm Support Oncol*, 13, 14–21.

PFISTER, D. G., SPENCER, S., ADELSTEIN, D., ADKINS, D., ANZAI, Y., BRIZEL, D. M., BRUCE, J. Y., BUSSE, P. M., CAUDELL, J. J., CMELAK, A. J., & COLEVAS, A. D. 2020. Head and neck cancers, version 2.2020, NCCN clinical practice guidelines in oncology. *J Natl Compr Cancer Netw*, 18(7), 873–98.

PILLERON, S., SOTO-PEREZ-DE-CELIS, E., VIGNAT, J., FERLAY, J., SOERJOMATARAM, I., BRAY, F., & SARFATI, D. 2021. Estimated global cancer incidence in the oldest adults in 2018 and projections to 2050. *Int J Cancer*, 148(3), 601–8.

PINKIEWICZ, M., DOROBISZ, K., & ZATOŃSKI, T. 2022. Human papillomavirus-associated head and neck cancers. Where are we now? A systematic review. *Cancer Manage Res*, 14, 3313.

PISANI, P., AIROLDI, M., ALLAIS, A., VALLETTI, P. A., BATTISTA, M., BENAZZO, M., BRIATORE, R., CACCIOLA, S., COCUZZA, S., & COLOMBO, A. 2020. Metastatic disease in head & neck oncology. *Acta Otorhinolaryngologica Italica*, 40, S1.

POPOVTZER, A., & EISBRUCH, A. 2008. Advances in radiation therapy of head and neck cancer. *Exp Rev Anticancer Ther*, 8, 633–44.

QAMAR, S., ROZI, S., SAWANI, S., AWAN, M. S., AKHTAR, S., SIDDIQUI, M. I., ABBAS, S. A., TAIMOOR, S., & RAZA KHAN, F. 2024. Oral health related quality of life in head and neck cancer survivors within the first year following treatment: A cross-sectional study in Karachi, Pakistan. *Sci Rep*, 14, 2560.

RICHARDSON, A. E., BROADBENT, E., & MORTON, R. P. 2019. A systematic review of psychological interventions for patients with head and neck cancer. *Support Care Cancer*, 27, 2007–21.

RIECHELMANN, H., DEJACO, D., STEINBICHLER, T. B., LETTENBICHLER-HAUG, A., ANEGG, M., GANSWINDT, U., GAMERITH, G., & RIEDL, D. 2022. Functional outcomes in head and neck cancer patients. *Cancers*, 14(9), 2135. https://doi.org/10.3390/cancers14092135

RINGASH, J., BERNSTEIN, L. J., DEVINS, G., DUNPHY, C., GIULIANI, M., MARTINO, R., & MCEWEN, S. 2018. Head and neck cancer survivorship: learning the needs, meeting the needs. *Semin Radiat Oncol*, 64–74.

ROCKE, J., MCLAREN, O., HARDMAN, J., GARAS, G., SMITH, M. E., ISHII, H., CONSTABLE, J., TIKKA, T., WIE LIU, Z., & WILLIAMS, R. 2020. The role of allied healthcare professionals in head and neck cancer surveillance: A systematic review. *Clin Otolaryngol*, 45, 83–98.

ROSI-SCHUMACHER, M., PATEL, S., PHAN, C., & GOYAL, N. 2023. Understanding financial toxicity in patients with head and neck cancer: A systematic review. *Clin Med Insights Oncol*, 17, 11795549221147730.

ROTIMI, S. O., ROTIMI, O. A., & SALHIA, B. 2021. A review of cancer genetics and genomics studies in Africa. *Front Oncol*, 10, 606400. https://doi.org/10.3389/fonc.2020.606400

SAGHAFI, E., ANDÅS, C. A., BERNSON, J., & KJELLER, G. 2023. Patients' experiences of adverse symptoms, emotions, and coping strategies in connection to treatment of head and neck cancer-an interview study. *BMC Oral Health*, 23, 641.

SANTOSO, A. M., JANSEN, F., LISSENBERG-WITTE, B. I., BAATENBURG DE JONG, R. J., LANGENDIJK, J. A., LEEMANS, C. R., SMIT, J. H., TAKES, R. P., TERHAARD, C. H., & VAN STRATEN, A. 2021. Poor sleep quality among newly diagnosed head and neck cancer patients: Prevalence and associated factors. *Support Care Cancer*, 29, 1035–45.

SANTOSO, A. M. M. 2023. *Sleep quality in head and neck cancer patients.* [PhD-Thesis—Research and graduation internal, Vrije Universiteit Amsterdam]. https://doi.org/10.5463/thesis.226

SCHUTTE, H. W., HEUTINK, F., WELLENSTEIN, D. J., VAN DEN BROEK, G. B., VAN DEN HOOGEN, F. J., MARRES, H. A., VAN HERPEN, C. M., KAANDERS, J. H., MERKX, T. M., & TAKES, R. P. 2020. Impact of time to diagnosis and treatment in head and neck cancer: A systematic review. *Otolaryngol Head Neck Surg*, 162, 446–57.

SEMPLE, C. J., DUNWOODY, L., GEORGE KERNOHAN, W., MCCAUGHAN, E., & SULLIVAN, K. 2008. Changes and challenges to patients' lifestyle patterns following treatment for head and neck cancer. *J Adv Nurs*, 63, 85–93.

SHIRAZ, F. 2015. *"We Got Cancer": A Mixed Methods Study of Quality of Life and Psychological Distress in Head and Neck Cancer Patients and Their Families.* London: Queen Mary University of London.

SHU-CHING, C. 2019. Oral dysfunction in patients with head and neck cancer: A systematic review. *J Nurs Res*, 27, e58.

SILVA, J. C., SILVEIRA, A., SACAU, A., MONTEIRO, E., & SEQUEIRA, T. 2019. Head and neck cancer early identification of malnutrition high risk patients and quality of life optimization. *Int J Otolaryngol Head Neck Surg*, 8, 204.

SIRAVEGNA, G., O'BOYLE, C. J., VARMEH, S., QUEENAN, N., MICHEL, A., STEIN, J., THIERAUF, J., SADOW, P. M., FAQUIN, W. C., & PERRY, S. K. 2022. Cell-free HPV DNA provides an accurate and rapid diagnosis of HPV-associated head and neck cancer. *Clin Cancer Res*, 28, 719–27.

SMITH, J. D., SHUMAN, A. G., & RIBA, M. B. 2017. Psychosocial issues in patients with head and neck cancer: An updated review with a focus on clinical interventions. *Curr Psychiatry Rep*, 19, 1–11.

SO, W. K., WONG, C.-L., CHOI, K.-C., CHAN, C. W., CHAN, J. C., LAW, B. M., WAN, R. W., MAK, S. S., LING, W.-M., & NG, W.-T. 2019. A mixed-methods study of unmet supportive care needs among head and neck cancer survivors. *Cancer Nurs*, 42, 67–78.

SOTO-GUERRERO, S., PALACIOS, J., LANGER, P., CARRASCO, C., TUPPER-SATT, L., GONZÁLEZ-OTAÍZA, M., RODRÍGUEZ-NÚÑEZ, A., & PÉREZ-CRUZ, P. E. 2023. Objective burden, caregiver psychological distress, and patient religion and quality of life are associated with high-intensity burden of care among caregivers of advanced cancer patients in a Latino population. *Palliat Support Care*, 1–9.

STEFAN, D. C., & HARIF, M. 2017. *Pediatric cancer in Africa: A case-based guide to diagnosis and management.* Springer International Publishing.

STENHAMMAR, C., ISAKSSON, J., GRANSTRÖM, B., LAURELL, G., & EHRSSON, Y. T. 2017. Changes in intimate relationships following treatment for head and neck cancer—A qualitative study. *J Psychosoc Oncol*, 35(5), 614–30.

TESSEMA, Z. T., WORKU, M. G., TESEMA, G. A., ALAMNEH, T. S., TESHALE, A. B., YESHAW, Y., ALEM, A. Z., AYALEW, H. G., & LIYEW, A. M. 2022. Determinants of accessing healthcare in Sub-Saharan Africa: A mixed-effect analysis of recent Demographic and Health Surveys from 36 countries. *BMJ Open*, 12(1), e054397. https://doi.org/10.1136/bmjopen-2021-054397

THILGES, S., MUMBY, P., SINACORE, J., CLARK, J., & CZERLANIS, C. 2023. Implementing a cognitive behavioral intervention for patients with head and neck cancer. *Support Care Cancer*, 31, 476.

VAN BEEK, F. E., JANSEN, F., MAK, L., LISSENBERG-WITTE, B. I., BUTER, J., VERGEER, M. R., VOORTMAN, J., CUIJPERS, P., LEEMANS, C. R., & VERDONCK-DE LEEUW, I. M. 2020. The course of symptoms of anxiety and depression from time of diagnosis up to 2 years follow-up in head and neck cancer patients treated with primary (chemo) radiation. *Oral Oncol*, 102, 104576.

VAN DER MEULEN, I., MAY, A., DE LEEUW, J., KOOLE, R., OOSTEROM, M., HORDIJK, G., & ROS, W. 2014. Long-term effect of a nurse-led psychosocial intervention on health-related quality of life in patients with head and neck cancer: A randomised controlled trial. *Br J Cancer*, 110, 593–601.

VAN HOF, K. S., HOESSEINI, A., DORR, M. C., VERDONCK-DE LEEUW, I. M., JANSEN, F., LEEMANS, C. R., TAKES, R. P., TERHAARD, C. H., DE JONG, R. J. B., & SEWNAIK, A. 2023. Unmet supportive care needs among informal caregivers of patients with head and neck cancer in the first 2 years after diagnosis and treatment: A prospective cohort study. *Support Care Cancer*, 31, 262.

VAN OVERVELD, L. F., TAKES, R. P., TURAN, A. S., BRASPENNING, J. C., SMEELE, L. E., MERKX, M., HERMENS, R., HEAD, D., GROUP, N. A., BAATENBURG DE JONG, R. J., & DE BOER, J. P. 2018. Needs and preferences of patients with head and neck cancer in integrated care. *Clin Otolaryngol*, 43, 553–61.

VERDONCK-DE LEEUW, I., DAWSON, C., LICITRA, L., ERIKSEN, J. G., HOSAL, S., SINGER, S., LAVERTY, D. P., GOLUSINSKI, W., MACHCZYNSKI, P., GOMES, A. V., & GIRVALAKI, C. 2022. European Head and Neck Society recommendations for head and neck cancer survivorship care. *Oral Oncol*, 133, 106047.

VIGANÒ, A., DE FELICE, F., IACOVELLI, N. A., ALTERIO, D., INGARGIOLA, R., CASBARRA, A., FACCHINETTI, N., ONETA, O., BACIGALUPO, A., & TORNARI, E. 2023. Quality of life changes over time and predictors in a large head and neck patients' cohort: Secondary analysis from an Italian multi-center longitudinal, prospective, observational study: A study of the Italian Association of Radiotherapy and Clinical Oncology (AIRO) head and neck working group. *Support Care Cancer*, 31, 220.

VIZZOTTO, A. D. B., DE OLIVEIRA, A. M., ELKIS, H., CORDEIRO, Q., & BUCHAIN, P. C. 2020. Psychosocial characteristics. In *Encyclopedia of behavioral medicine* (pp. 1794–95). Cham: Springer International Publishing.

WHARTON, T., MANU, E., & VITALE, C. A. 2015. Enhancing provider knowledge and patient screening for palliative care needs in chronic multimorbid patients receiving home-based primary care. *Am J Hospice Palliat Med*, 32(1), 78–83.

WORLD HEALTH ORGANIZATIÒN (WHO). 2024 Global cancer burden growing, amidst mounting need for services. Global cancer burden growing, amidst mounting need for services (who.int). Dostupno na: https://gco.iarc.fr/en [Accessed March 30, 2024.]

WHO INTERNATIONAL AGENCY FOR RESEARCH ON CANCER. 2020). Estimated number of deaths in 2020, all cancers, both sexes, all ages. *Cancer today*. Available at: https://gco.iarc.fr/today/online-analysis [Accessed January 14, 2022.]

WISSINGER, E., GRIEBSCH, I., LUNGERSHAUSEN, J., FOSTER, T., & PASHOS, C. L. 2014. The economic burden of head and neck cancer: A systematic literature review. *Pharmacoeconomics*, 32, 865–82.

XIAO, C., MILLER, A. H., PENG, G., LEVINE, M. E., CONNEELY, K. N., ZHAO, H., ELDRIDGE, R. C., WOMMACK, E. C., JEON, S., HIGGINS, K. A., SHIN, D. M., SABA, N. F., SMITH, A. K., BURTNESS, B., PARK, H. S., IRWIN, M. L., FERRUCCI, L. M., ULRICH, B., QIAN, D. C., BEITLER, J. J., & BRUNER, D. W. 2021. Association of epigenetic age acceleration with risk factors, survival, and quality of life in patients with head and neck cancer. Int J Rad Oncol Biol Physics, 111(1), 157–67.

YABROFF, K. R., WU, X. C., NEGOITA, S., et al. 2022. Association of the COVID-19 pandemic with patterns of statewide cancer services. *J Natl Cancer Inst*, 114 (6), 907–9.

YAN, F., RAUSCHER, E., HOLLINGER, A., CAPUTO, M. A., READY, J., NGUYEN, S. A., FAKHRY, C., NATHAN, C.-A. O., LEONARDIS, C., & YEAROUT, D. 2021. Concerns and needs of patients with head and neck cancer in the COVID-19 era. *OTO Open*, 5, 2473974X211047794.

ZABALA, A., & SANTAOLALLA, F. 2023. An evaluation of an innovative screening program based on risk criteria for early diagnosis of head and neck cancers. *Front Public Health*, 10, 1004039.

ZEBRALLA, V., WICHMANN, G., PIRLICH, M., HAMMERMÜLLER, C., BERGER, T., ZIMMERMANN, K., NEUMUTH, T., MEHNERT-THEUERKAUF, A., DIETZ, A., &

HINZ, A. 2021. Dysphagia, voice problems, and pain in head and neck cancer patients. *Eur Arch Oto Rhino Laryngol*, 1–10.

ZENG, Q., LING, D., CHEN, W., LIAO, Y., AN, R., & HE, L. 2023. Family caregivers' experiences of caring for patients with head and neck cancer: A systematic review and metasynthesis of qualitative studies. *Cancer Nurs*, 46, E41–61.

ZHENG, S., LIU, S., YANG, Q., CHAN, S., HUANG, W., JIANG, X., & ZHU, J. 2024. The effectiveness of interventions to reduce cancer-related stigma: An integrative review. *J Clin Nurs*, 33(7), 2438–55.

18

Holistic Approaches and Palliative Care in Head and Neck Cancer

Thabiso Victor Miya, Suzana Savkovic, and Zodwa Dlamini

18.1 Introduction

Many patients with head and neck cancer (HNC) have pessimistic beliefs regarding the prognosis of their disease. Approximately 10% of patients with advanced stages will be found to have metastasized disease, accounting for 40% of cases. About 20–30% of patients will experience local and/or regional recurrences with or without distant metastases despite current surgical, nonsurgical, and combination therapy. This has a poor prognosis, with a median survival of approximately 6 months (Roland & Bradley, 2014). Advanced head and neck tumors have a dismal prognosis and a high burden of symptoms. Quality of life (QOL), resource use, and treatment results can all be significantly impacted by the identification and management of symptoms and distress. The ideology of "if I am going to live, I might as well live well" and the "all other things being equal" paradigm puts more pressure on doctors to provide appropriate care and reduce side effects after surgery (McCammon, 2019). Achieving a balance between expectations and reality is crucial when treating cancer patients. Patients desire a treatment plan covering all bases, from the initial consultation to the clinical examination, biopsy, research, surgery, and postoperative monitoring.

In-depth conversations regarding QOL and postoperative survivorship should occur during the first visit, and the surgeon should either acquaint the patient with a group of HNC survivors or recommend that they see patients who have undergone surgery, radiation therapy, or both during different phases of their care. Engaging with patients helps them understand what to expect, determines what patients want from their treatment, and encourages a view of what outcomes are realistic. Patients now have a voice in their treatment planning thanks to advances in patient-centric care and longer life expectancies, and it is the surgeon's role to enlighten patients and utilize their expertise to help them make wise choices. The patient has the right to select the course of treatment that is best for them. However, patients must to make their choices only after extensive consultation with others and being fully aware of the risks and problems involved with each of their treatment options. Whether physicians like it or not, patient decisions are increasingly focused on QOL and supportive of the patient's capacity to live as a contributing member of society. Many patients will select a conservative approach to cancer care, and often this may be at odds with what is taught at medical schools and what is considered by the healthcare team as the best course of action. Most patients will weigh the risks and benefits of various treatment alternatives and make their decisions based on their preferences; it is important to note that these preferences may be swayed by information from unreliable sources like social media and the internet (Mali & Pradeep, 2023).

The expansion of patient-reported outcome measures has yielded a wealth of data across domains, from problems unique to HNC or function to general health-related QOL. When a patient decides on a conservative course of therapy, palliative care (PC) enters the picture (Rogers & Barber, 2017; Rogers et al., 2018). This chapter explores PC in HNC, providing an in-depth look at supportive care for all phases of the disease. It also examines the ideals and methods of PC, with a focus on enhancing QOL.

18.2 Definition of Palliative Care

PC refers to the full range of care provided to patients and their families when curative treatment is no longer effective for the patient's illness. It is a multidisciplinary strategy that prioritizes patient autonomy and can start as early as the diagnosis. According to the World Health Organization (WHO), PC should value life and accept that dying is a normal part of existence (Roland & Bradley, 2014). PC is becoming more widely accepted in the field of oncology; its objectives are to maximize patient access to supportive treatment and enhance the well-being of both patients and caregivers. PC aims to "anticipate, prevent, and reduce suffering and to support the best possible QOL for patients/families/caregivers, regardless of the stage of the disease or the need for other therapies," according to the National Comprehensive Cancer Network (NCCN) recommendations (NCCN, 2020). It is important to note that medications aimed at prolonging life and that are focused on the disease do not conflict with the goals of PC. PC provides a support structure to enable patients to live as fully as possible until death; integrates the psychological, physical, social, and spiritual aspects of patient care; and assists the family in coping with the patient's disease and their eventual loss (Civantos et al., 2021; Jacob et al., 2019).

18.3 A Brief History of Palliative Care in Africa

A timeline of PC history on the African continent from 2002 to 2010 is shown in Figure 18.1. In 2002, the Cape Town Declaration stated that pain alleviation was a human right and that PC was to be included in the national healthcare strategy. This marked the first time that PC had been given priority in Africa (Mpanga Sebuyira et al., 2003). This led to the creation of the African Palliative Care Association (APCA), which made it a mission to provide PC that is both reasonably priced and appropriate for their cultural backgrounds to all individuals with life-threatening illnesses. The World Health Assembly demanded, in 2005, that every member state establish a national policy for PC, guarantee that morphine is available in all medical settings, and gradually adopt minimal standards for PC and pain management (World Health Organization [WHO]##, 2005). The Declaration of Venice committed to creating a Global Palliative Care Research Initiative in 2006, one specifically recognizing the importance of research conducted in Africa. Four elements were definitively identified and documented in 2007 as being essential to achieving fair and comprehensive coverage across the globe. The introduction of PC in Africa was particularly impacted by suitable government regulations, health professional education, a way to provide PC, and a sufficient drug supply (Stjernswärd et al., 2007).

By 2010, PC was provided in 28 out of 57 African countries, compared to just 5 in 2004 (Wright et al., 2008b), at a time when it was only nationally integrated

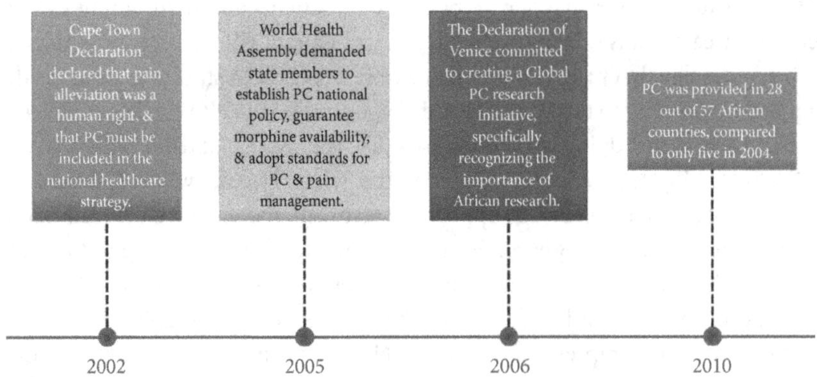

Figure 18.1 A timeline of palliative care history on the African continent between 2002 and 2010. Palliative care in Africa has made substantial strides since the establishment of the first hospice. While challenges remain, ongoing efforts of national and international organizations, coupled with increasing government support, continue to enhance the availability and quality of palliative care across the continent. These efforts are crucial in ensuring that patients with life-limiting illnesses receive compassionate and comprehensive care.

in 4 of those countries. PC providers increased from 8 in 2004 to 87 in 2010. PC is currently being financed by more than 141 donors, including 6 multinational, 19 bilateral, 54 humanitarian, 27 faith-based, 21 commercial, and 9 hospice support organizations (Wright et al., 2008a). As of 2010, 48 countries had access to morphine. However, only 7 of Kenya's 250 public hospitals had oral morphine available to treat severe chronic pain, according to research (Human Rights Watch, 2010). The fear of morphine being used illegally and the taxation of morphine powder were mentioned as obstacles. There were just 3 national Palliative Care Associations in Africa in 2001; today, there are 11, and more are being formed. Kenya, Malawi, South Africa, Tanzania, Uganda, and Zimbabwe also have all established some child-focused specialized PC services. However, a large portion of current care is provided outside of national health systems, and conventional PC receives little funding from governments (Grant et al., 2011).

18.4 The Significance of Palliative Care

PC is an interdisciplinary field that aims to enhance the well-being of individuals and their families dealing with a terminal disease. It has been demonstrated to enhance happiness with care, lower depression, and improve QOL, especially when started early in advanced cancers (Ferrell et al., 2017; Nilsen & Johnson, 2017). Considering its effects on breathing, eating, and speaking, HNC presents particular complications. There is an increased risk of suicide as well as psychological discomfort and social isolation as a result of symptoms. Pain, nausea, vomiting, constipation, psychological issues, weight loss, poor oral intake, and exhaustion are common PC issues. Oral health issues, airway obstruction/stridor, communication challenges, fungal wounds, ulcers and fistulae, bleeding, facial nerve palsy, nasal obstruction, and conductive deafness are among the issues specific to HNCs. Sometimes treatments intended to be curative instead make people sicker.

PC professionals can assist in clinically significant increases in patients' mood and QOL. But, starting early in the course of the disease, it is crucial to talk about the patient's preferences since surgical care of HNCs can change the larynx or mouth cavity in a way that makes it difficult for the patient to speak normally and easily (Ferrell et al., 2017; Mayland et al., 2021; Nilsen & Johnson, 2017; Roland & Bradley, 2014). Airway protection, feeding, tumor debulking, pain management, and symptom management are the main goals of palliative treatments, which include surgery, radiation, chemotherapy, and pharmaceutical therapies. *Surgical PC* refers to the process of diagnosing and treating patients with surgical diseases to maximize their QOL in the shortest amount of time. Hospice care, nutritional assistance, tumor removal, and airway maintenance are surgical palliation options (Begbie et al., 2019; Schenker et al., 2016).

18.4.1 The Importance of Early Palliative Care for Patients with Advanced Head and Neck Cancer

Creating a plan for the patient's cancer treatment is typically the main priority when an advanced cancer patient arrives at an oncology clinic. These individuals frequently have upsetting physical symptoms in addition to spiritual and emotional distress. These symptoms become more frequent and intense as a patient moves closer to the end of their life and can be exacerbated through chemotherapy and radiation treatments. Psychosocial-emotional discomfort is not usually systematically screened for in cancer patients. However, the PC team is qualified to offer psychosocial and spiritual support in addition to symptomatic therapy (Greer et al., 2013). The advantages of PC integration following an advanced cancer diagnosis are shown in Figure 18.2 (Davis et al., 2015; Greer et al., 2013; Salins et al., 2016).

Multiple visits between the PC team and patients are beneficial for difficult talks like sharing prognosis, providing clarification on treatment options, and identifying and managing patients' evolving symptomatic needs. Involving PC teams facilitates precise and realistic detailed communication between surgical and oncology teams (Satija et al., 2019).

18.5 Symptom Burden for Patients with Head and Neck Cancer

The main goal of PC is to help patients with life-threatening conditions by relieving their symptoms and enhancing their QOL (Gandhi et al., 2014). Patients with HNC have a significant symptom load, which can be attributed to either the tumor or to acute or long-term treatment-related consequences. Patients with HNCs suffer from a wide range of upsetting symptoms, some of which are typical of other carcinomas and some of which need further attention (Murphy et al., 2010). The classification of late effects in HNC patients by Murphy and Deng (2015) included musculoskeletal disability as well as general or particular functional abnormalities, such as frailty and problematic speech/swallowing, respectively. The literature shows that the prevalence of symptoms in HNC patients varies depending on the stage of the disease (Murphy & Deng, 2015). Pain, exhaustion, anxiety, and trouble sleeping were listed by Hanna et al. (2015) as serious symptoms during the pretreatment stage (Hanna et al., 2015). According

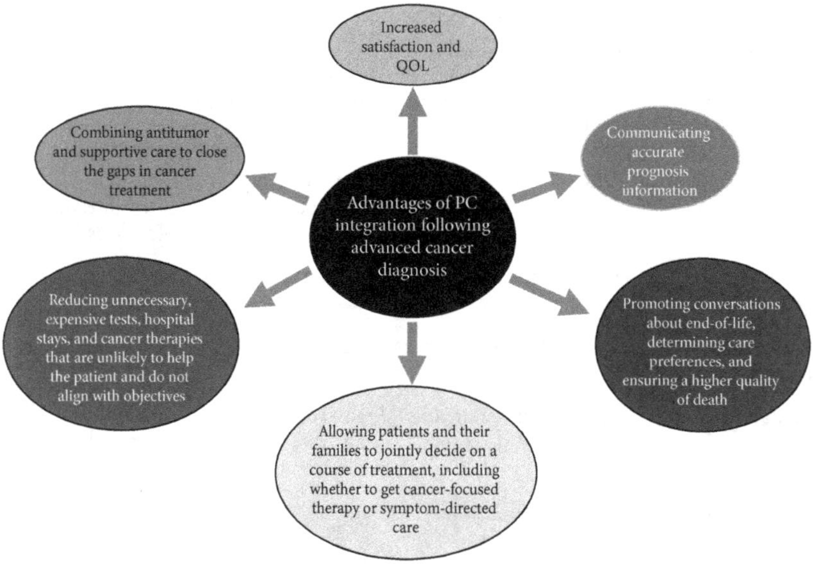

Figure 18.2 The advantages of palliative care integration following an advanced cancer diagnosis. The integration of palliative care in the treatment of advanced cancer is a holistic approach that not only improves the patient's quality of life and supports their families but also contributes to the efficiency and effectiveness of the healthcare system. This underscores the importance of incorporating palliative care early in the cancer treatment continuum to achieve optimal patient and healthcare outcomes.

to Gandhi et al. (2014), the most common symptoms among advanced HNC patients at their facility were pain, sleeplessness, lack of appetite, and exhaustion. Others noted that pain, dysphagia, anorexia, exhaustion, and dyspnea are symptoms that HNC patients experience in decreasing order of prevalence during the end-of-life phase (Price et al., 2009). Oral problems can develop from cancer treatment or from the disease itself; a summary of those resulting from cancer treatments is provided in Table 18.1 (Broadfield, 2006).

HNC patients have a significant burden of symptoms at every stage of the disease trajectory. This demonstrates unequivocally the function of PC in symptom alleviation (Satija et al., 2019).

18.6 Methods Used in Decision-Making

Guidelines for goals of care (GoC) conversations are important in patient–clinician communication. These include outlining treatment objectives,

Table 18.1 Oral complications induced by cancer therapies

Radiation		Hematopoietic stem cell transplantation	Chemotherapy
Chronic	**Acute**		
Osteoradionecrosis	Oral mucositis	Oropharyngeal mucositis	Oral and gastrointestinal Mucositis
Dysgeusia and ageusia	Salivary gland	Bleeding	Neuropathies
Mucosal fibrosis and atrophy	dysfunction-sialadenitis	Ulceration	Hemorrhage
Dental caries	Muscular or cutaneous fibrosis	Dental caries, gingivitis, periodontitis	Infection (bacterial, viral, or fungal)
Soft tissue necrosis	Infection (bacterial, viral or fungal)	Pain	Xerostomia
Infection (bacterial, viral, or fungal)	Xerostomia	Temporomandibular dysfunction	Taste dysfunction
Xerostomia	Taste dysfunction	Infection (bacterial, viral, or fungal)	
Taste dysfunction		Xerostomia	
		Taste dysfunction	

reviewing GoC when major changes are being considered, and starting GoC conversations with family caregivers. GoC talks have been demonstrated to help patients and their families achieve their objectives, increase healthcare usage, and improve QOL; however, because most of these conversations take place close to the end of life, their usefulness is limited. PC professionals use a collaborative decision-making process that culminates in a patient-centered, value-congruent treatment plan. They are skilled in eliciting patient values, determining acceptable tradeoffs, and establishing restrictions. PC clinicians are professionals in the ethics and practice of shared decision-making, which combines the knowledge of clinical experts concerning their patient's treatment options and associated risks with the lived experiences, anxieties, and suffering limitations of the individual patient (Cannon et al., 2023; Gilligan et al., 2018; Schulman-Green et al., 2018).

Unfortunately, PC is seen as "only necessary when all else is deemed to have failed," according to oncologic surgeons, and doctors in other specialties have historically failed to meet the palliative needs of critically ill surgical patients (Hua et al., 2021). Research has shown that patients with HNC typically see several consulting physicians in turn, each of whom may provide an index treatment (Davies et al., 2010; Deber et al., 2007). Patients' perception of engagement and control during an emergency room visit is influenced by various elements, including discourse, information sharing, attentiveness, and participation. Shared decision-making is a process in which patients and their healthcare professionals participate equally (Civantos et al., 2021; Roland & Bradley, 2014). To enhance the way PC is provided to advanced cancer patients, oncologists are essential stakeholders. Their opinions on the main obstacles and potential fixes for PC's shortcomings are crucial for activities aimed at enhancing QOL.

Occasionally, discussions concerning PC may be impeded by doctors' feelings, intimate bonds with their patients, and reluctance to deny them hope. It has been discovered that factors such as age, treatment alternatives, and patients' performance status affect doctors' decisions on the therapeutic objectives for a broader patient population than just cancer patients (Gidwani et al., 2017; Liao et al., 2017), and the decision to recommend PC to their patients is often based on such factors. Cannon et al. (2023) found that when physicians consulted with PC experts it resulted in improved physical pain and symptom management, patient-centered GoC talks, and holistic care for psychosocial and spiritual suffering (Cannon et al., 2023).

The findings of Gidwani et al. (2017) point to the need for increased access to specialized outpatient PC services as well as more organized communication regarding the objectives of consultation and prognostic data to prevent service fragmentation and duplication (Gidwani et al., 2017). The goal of PC is to improve the patient's QOL by putting their comfort and symptom management first as they near death. Because PC is linked to less drastic treatments near the end of life, advanced-stage patients who are receiving inpatient chemotherapy and/or radiation are less likely to receive it. Advanced HNC patients, according to Davies and colleagues, frequently perceive the medical information they receive from PC consultants as encouraging them to "decide to do something" as opposed to "choose a specific treatment" pathway (Davies et al., 2010). Upon reviewing the literature on PC interventions in surgical patients, Lilley and colleagues discovered that using PC principles reduced cost and resource consumption in 7 out of 25 trials. Early in the course of treatment, when the patient is still capable of having complex conversations about sources of deep meaning and values that will significantly influence their disease trajectory and coping, PC concepts can be applied (Lilley et al., 2016).

According to Esce and McCammon, patients with advanced HNC who experience substantial symptom loads and treatment-related morbidity are excellent candidates for concordant PC (Esce & McCammon, 2021). The Bow-Tie Model developed by Dr. Philippa Hawley is the 21st-century PC model, emphasizing the contemporaneous nature of PC used along with disease-directed therapy (Hawley, 2014).

Prolonged survival with deteriorating symptoms might be discouraging to those hoping for a good death. For patients with advanced cancer, early PC dramatically improves QOL, symptom load, mood, illness understanding, and QOL at the end of life. In 2017, the American Society of Clinical Oncology released a preliminary clinical opinion advocating for early PC integration to be standardized into all patient medical management. PC physicians prioritize recognizing patient concerns and building a supportive, personal relationship with patients and caregivers. By evaluating understanding and interpreting treatment information and prognosis, they foster trust and improve the relationship between patients, caregivers, and physicians. Additionally, they give patients concrete, helpful coping mechanisms so they may take an active role in controlling their conditions. According to this qualitative analysis, the early integrated PC paradigm is simultaneously practical, contemplative, and intimate (Ferrell et al., 2017; Thomas et al., 2019).

Decisional conflict measures assess patients' perceived effectiveness in decision-making, along with their level of uncertainty and the factors contributing to it. Satisfaction, regret, and hesitation in medical decision-making are evaluated using a validated decisional regret scale. The need for organized integration of PC in national cancer programs has been recognized by international professional organizations. To enable customized care, surgeons, oncologists, and PC specialists should work together. Decisions about palliation or intervention must be made using clinical instruments (McCammon, 2019; Shuman et al., 2017) such as the Holistic Needs Assessment (Rogers & Barber, 2017), the Patient Reported Outcome Measures, and the Patient Concerns Inventory (Rogers et al., 2020), which is an item prompt list. PC may be facilitated by customized needs-based referral systems for patients with advanced HNC.

18.7 Palliative Care Approach in Head and Neck Cancer

PC is defined by the WHO as a therapeutic approach that aims to enhance the QOL for patients and their families facing life-threatening illnesses. It does so by preventing and relieving suffering through early identification, assessment, and treatment of pain and other distressing symptoms. This is achieved through early patient condition assessment and the management of physical, psychosocial, and spiritual complaints (WHO, 2014). For patients with HNCs, supportive therapy often focuses on managing symptoms such as pain, ulceration, bleeding, dysphagia, and dyspnea because patient QOL is greatly impacted by these symptoms. Palliative therapy includes the administration of analgesics, tracheostomies to maintain airway patency, and the implantation of a nasogastric tube (NGT) to provide HNC patients with adequate nutrition (Begbie et al., 2019; Grewal et al., 2019; van der Velden et al., 2022).

PC considers the needs of both the patient and their caregivers. Patients and their family and friends may feel less afraid if they are given information about the illness and any consequences that may arise. Therefore, multidisciplinary teamwork involving otorhinolaryngology, surgery, radiology, radiotherapy (RT), medical rehabilitation, palliative medicine, medical oncology, pain management or anesthesiology, and psychiatry is required for the best management of patients with HNCs, especially those with advanced-stage disease (Begbie et al., 2019).

When it comes to patient management, medical teams are involved in deciding which patients are eligible for further treatment and which patients are considered incurable and thus eligible for PC. In cases of recurrent or later-stage HNC, radical therapy is deemed "futile" and may result in a reduced QOL. Determining what constitutes an effective decision-making process in PC settings is crucial. The prognosis and diagnosis of the illness must be well understood by the patient and their family. Patients who are fully aware and capable have the right to decide how their care is managed. Representatives may make medical choices for individuals who lack autonomy. The hierarchy of medical decision-making for individuals who lack autonomy varies across nations and cultures. While in many Western legal systems, spouses are typically granted the primary right to make medical decisions, followed by adult children and other family members, this is not a universal standard (Levy et al., 2009; Satija et al., 2019). Effective psychosocial functioning and symptom management play a crucial role in guiding the selection of appropriate treatments. Research has shown a correlation between palliative care and a reduction in aggressive cancer treatments (Cocks et al., 2016).

18.8 Targets of Palliative Care

A multidisciplinary and integrative approach is necessary for PC. Effective communication is necessary for every member of the PC team. PC's ultimate purpose is to address the patients' psychological and social issues in addition to treating their symptoms. Some forms of PC for people with advanced HNC include the following (Cocks et al., 2016).

18.8.1 Nonsurgical Palliative Therapy

Radiotherapy: There is still discussion on the ideal dosage schedule for palliative RT. The use of short-course RT with hypofractionation regimens is supported by low-level evidence. Benefits have also been shown by other procedures, such as those outlined by the Radiation Therapy Oncology Group. Up to 80% of carefully chosen individuals can experience symptom control, with a specific response in terms of pain management. While there is no solid evidence to favor one protocol over another, case series do show advantages to palliative RT. Reirradiation may be possible although it might come with a high risk of radiation poisoning. Up to 50% of patients show benefit from radiation therapy (RT) for painful bone metastases, according to a comprehensive evaluation (Wong & Wiffen, 2002). Evidence exists to support the use of bisphosphonates as a step-up after RT and traditional pharmacotherapy to help with bone pain management. The efficacy of the new monoclonal medications, such as RANK ligand inhibitors like denosumab, is still under investigation.

Chemotherapy: Palliative chemotherapy involves the use of platinum-based medications, such as methotrexate and 5-fluorouracil, either alone or in conjunction with RT. This approach shows promise in terms of improving QOL and controlling symptoms, but it may also increase toxicity, and, consequently, treatment side effects may be a problem. Each patient must have their unique set of circumstances carefully considered when weighing the benefits and risks. In the chosen circumstances, non–platinum-based medicines may provide symptom management (Cocks et al., 2016).

18.8.2 Palliative Surgery

End-stage HNC that is incurable results in debilitating symptoms. While attempting to manage pain, difficulty eating and breathing, and bleeding, patients may continue to be active and self-sufficient. In these situations, palliative surgery might be necessary. Although there is little high-level data to support palliative surgery, descriptive studies encourage its use in some circumstances. Surgery can lessen the bulk of the main tumor, lessen discomfort and bleeding, enhance feeding, and open the airway. For severe neck diseases, debulking surgery can help control symptoms, but substantial resections rarely provide benefits that outweigh the degree of surgical morbidity (Cocks et al., 2016).

In individuals at high risk of significant artery erosion, newer endovascular methods such as embolization and vessel stenting may provide symptom management for bleeding associated with major vascular erosion. A painful end-of-life occurrence is an acute hemorrhage due to a carotid "blow-out," or erosion of the carotid vessels. While quick surgical intervention can occasionally result in success, many patients die quickly. In these situations, efforts should be made to lower blood pressure directly while giving the right kind of fast-acting sedatives, including benzodiazepines. The patient needs ongoing verbal support to manage anxiety. Patients should not be left alone in this case, and dark towels and bed linens should be provided to lessen anxiety associated with blood loss. It is crucial to have a deliberate conversation and provide the patient—or their family members and caregivers if they choose to participate—with measured information if surgical intervention is deemed inappropriate. This should contain the expected clinical scenario, and a workable treatment plan should be created to handle these situations. This could affect the preferred place of care and may include anticipatory prescribing (Cocks et al., 2016).

18.8.3 Airway Palliation

In cases where there is a compromise in airway function, tracheostomy considerations are customary. However, in certain situations, tracheostomy might not be necessary if surgical debulking methods are considered. This depends on the knowledge and resources available locally (Wee & Hillier, 2008). Sometimes the best course of action is to avoid surgery. For instance, a patient who has had palliative RT and a tracheal tumor that has been repeatedly debulked is not a candidate for stenting. The compromise of the airway will eventually pose a hazard to life. In this case, a tracheostomy might not be an option. In such cases, the use of opioids for dyspnea, palliative sedation, and secretion decrease can assist a patient in moving toward a good death (Cocks et al., 2016).

Given the difficulty of these circumstances, information should be given tactfully to the patient. By talking about the pharmacological interventions that can be used to prevent any distress, one can help the patient regain control when they wish to talk about the expected scenario in detail. If the patient declines to engage in the conversation, this should be noted and shared with family and/or caregivers. The desired location of care may be impacted by this circumstance, and the patient and their family must be ready such a situation. The patient needs to be comfortable through the entire end-of-life process, and they need to know what measures will be taken to prevent the anxiety and dyspnea that come with it. If a tracheostomy is necessary, the patient, family, and community personnel should manage tracheostomy wound care and the upkeep of a clean, secure tube through the use of existing or newly established local protocols. To facilitate patient communication, voice attachments and heat-moisture exchange can be employed (Cocks et al., 2016).

18.8.4 Dysphagia Palliation

Dysphagia affects 40% of individuals with HNC. This is because of functional obstruction, mechanical obstruction, pain, fistula, and drug-induced adverse effects. In patients with HNC, evaluation of the swallow is crucial. Determining the safety and feasibility of oral ingestion is crucial. Because aspiration is widespread and might be silent in up to 40% of patients, bedside assessments are not very useful. Functional endoscopic evaluation of swallowing (FEES) is a simple, reproducible, portable procedure that can provide valuable insights into the cause of aspiration and provide the patient with feedback on the effectiveness of preventive measures. Additionally, it can help evaluate the patient's ability to swallow foods with a variety of textures and enhance data from videofluoroscopy (Cocks et al., 2016).

It is not always the case that aspiration equals no oral intake. Aspiration to a certain extent may be well tolerated, and techniques for opening the airway after swallowing can be used. In a similar vein, some textures might be easier to handle, and using thicker liquids can support oral intake. The patient may choose to continue swallowing despite the possible and actual risk of aspiration pneumonia; thus, it is crucial to respect their decisions. QOL is unchangeable. Hydration, nutrition, and medicine administration are made possible for individuals who are unable to swallow by using an enteral route through a gastrostomy or NGT. The ability to create a gastrostomy or pass an NGT depends on the patient's preference, and the perceived length of use all play a major role in the type of tube that is utilized. If the patient's need for enteral feeding by NGT exceeds 2–3 weeks, the possibility of a gastrostomy should be explored (Cocks et al., 2016).

There is no precise advice on when or if nutritional supplementation should be stopped. In this decision-making process, the patient's and their family's wishes are paramount, and comprehensive consultation is required. Palliating swallowing can benefit from conventional therapies. A hypopharyngeal tumor may benefit from surgical debulking, either with or without a laser or debrider, as well as RT treatment. Dilatation, which can be guided by radiography or surgery, can aid in easing a stricture. Stenting might be helpful, but frequently tumors of the head and neck are too high for a stent to be positioned comfortably and without interfering with other activities (Cocks et al., 2016).

18.8.5 Constipation

Half of the cancer patients who are admitted to a hospice because they are terminally sick experience constipation. Furthermore, constipation frequently occurs while a patient is receiving treatment. Dehydration, less physical activity, and the use of constipation-promoting medications—especially opioids and anticholinergic drugs—are to blame for this. The use of laxatives should begin as soon as an opioid prescription is issued. Other possible factors that are sometimes disregarded include hypothyroidism and hypercalcemia. Early detection and avoidance are the cornerstones of treatment. Early detection and prevention serve as the foundation of effective treatment. Additionally, assessing patient contact history is recommended. Stimulants like bisacodyl and senna, as well as softeners like lactulose, magnesium hydroxide, and docusate, are examples of laxative agents. Preparations of polyethylene glycol also are frequently utilized. These ought to be taken preventatively. Constipation can cause nausea, vomiting, and, in extreme cases, pseudobstruction if it persists. If a rectal examination reveals hard stool, enemas and suppositories may be beneficial. In the end, manual evacuation might be required (Cocks et al., 2016).

18.8.6 Nausea and Vomiting

The fact that a high proportion of patients are enterally fed must be considered in any strategy to prevent nausea and vomiting. For severe nausea and vomiting, injectable antiemetics are frequently required, either as continuous infusions or subcutaneous (SC) boluses, at least until initial control is achieved. Prokinetic medications like metoclopramide (tablet, oral solution, or injectable) or domperidone (tablet, suspension, or suppository) may be required to guarantee optimal function because enteral feeding presents unique challenges. Otherwise, the enteral feeding process follows standard practices, including the use of nasogastric (NG) tubes, nasojejunal (NJ) tubes, percutaneous endoscopic gastrostomy (PEG) tubes, or percutaneous endoscopic jejunostomy (PEJ) tubes, with administration via feeding pumps or gravity as appropriate. The nauseated patient should have access to a sizable bowl, tissues, and water, and caregivers should be ready to rehydrate them with intravenous or subcutaneous fluids if necessary (Cocks et al., 2016).

18.8.7 Confusion and Agitation

Distinguishing anxiety (agitated, terrified, panicked) from disorientation (especially delirium) is crucial. At some point in their lives, up to 75% of cancer patients experience confusion. Cognitive impairment is not uncommon in HNC patients because they are more likely to have a history of severe alcohol and tobacco use, which predisposes them to withdrawal symptoms. The cornerstone of pharmaceutical treatment for anxiety is benzodiazepines. Diazepam can be administered intravenously, orally, or via a NG tube when liquid formulations are required for patients receiving enteral feeding or those unable to take oral medications. The patient can either dissolve a lorazepam tablet under the tongue or swallow it. Midazolam is recommended if injections and/or infusions are required because it can be administered intravenously when a practically instantaneous effect is required, or subcutaneously (which is the most usual method). The main drawback to midazolam is quickly building tolerance. Benzodiazepines are helpful in the short term for controlling anxiety attacks, but they have their limitations in situations when anxiety is already present and well-established (Cocks et al., 2016).

Many organic factors, such as infection, dehydration, metabolic disturbance, respiratory failure, urine retention, constipation, brain metastases, etc., might contribute to delirium as a cause of disorientation. Drug side effects, especially from opioids, and drug withdrawal are frequently the reason for delirium. In the near term, symptom control is vital, even though the goal of treatment must be to address the inciting problem. While benzodiazepines certainly play a part and have a specific indication in drug withdrawal, haloperidol (tablet, liquid, or injection) or levomepromazine (tablet or injection) are frequently more effective in treating delirium when sedation is required (to treat paranoia, etc.). In certain situations, especially when a patient is dying and exhibits irreversible agitation or delirium, benzodiazepines and antipsychotics must be mixed. Syringe drivers are frequently used to administer these medications (Cocks et al., 2016).

18.8.8 Pain Management

Pain affects the majority of patients at some point. Pain may be caused by an illness or a course of therapy, and it can be acute, immediate, persistent, or lifelong. Pain that returns after a protracted period of painlessness is probably due to a recurring illness. The existence of "total pain," or the presence of emotional, psychological, spiritual, and bodily distress, must be considered during PC assessment. In HNC, the main types of physical pain are somatic, neuropathic, visceral, and mucosal; neuropathic pain is the most challenging. The WHO "pain ladder," which has three stages of increasing severity, is the best model for using analgesics; steps should be taken according to the degree of and patient's reaction to the pain. The pathophysiology determines the adjuvant employed, and the severity of the pain determines the strength of the analgesic (Cocks et al., 2016).

18.8.8.1 Somatic Pain

Apart from situations where an alternative is preferable due to renal impairment, morphine continues to be the strongest opioid of choice. Titrating oral solutions or tablets of immediate-release morphine is the first step in the process. Sustained-release preparations are utilized once responsiveness and dosage are established; immediate-release dosages for breakthrough pain are set at a sixth of the 24-hour sustained-release dosage. Sustained-release pills or capsules can be administered if the patient can swallow. A morphine suspension or opened capsules can be utilized if an NGT is in place. If this is not possible—usually due to vomiting—morphine or diamorphine may be infused subcutaneously at breakthrough doses. Since diamorphine is more soluble and requires considerably fewer dosages, it is recommended (Cocks et al., 2016).

As an option for stable background pain, transdermal fentanyl formulations have both theoretical and practical appeal, especially in cases of renal failure or morphine sensitivity (e.g., sedation and dysphoria). It is still possible to take oral opioids for breakthrough pain. On the other hand, under the guidance of a specialized service, novel formulations of buccal, sublingual, or intranasal fentanyl might be useful in certain circumstances. When swallowing is impaired, oxycodone can be used as an alternative to morphine in cases of intolerance, especially dysphoria. It is available as an injectable and in an instant-release solution, but its sustained-release oral formulation is only available as tablets. When swallowing is not possible, hydromorphone can be injected but is not helpful when taken orally. Both immediate- and sustained-release options are available in capsule form. Methadone has a long half-life, acts slowly, and has a quick onset. Because of this, it is best utilized by specialists because it can accumulate in the system and lead to unintentional overdose.

18.8.8.2 Neuropathic Pain

Neuropathic pain is a fairly prevalent side effect of treatment, especially radiation, as well as a presenting feature of HNC. The following adjuvant medications are usually employed:

1. *Amitriptyline* is a tricyclic antidepressant that is available as a tablet or liquid.
2. The most commonly used anticonvulsants, such as *gabapentin* and *pregabalin*, are only available as pills or capsules unless specific arrangements are made with a pharmacist. Gabapentin capsules can be opened and administered via a gastrostomy tube.
3. As an alternative, *carbamazepine* is available as a tablet, liquid, or suppository. *Sodium valproate* is available in a liquid solution.

First-line treatment involves using an antidepressant or an anticonvulsant titrated to the highest dose tolerated (sometimes combined with a traditional painkiller); second-line treatment involves using both. Some support the use of corticosteroids as the first-line treatment for acute neuropathic pain when there is thought to be a considerable inflammatory component (e.g., dexamethasone 8–16 mg/d). If dysphagia coexists, use is restricted by appetite stimulation. It is not intended for persistent or foreseeable long-term pain. Clonazepam can be helpful sometimes. Ketamine and methadone are helpful, but only in certain situations (Cocks et al., 2016).

18.8.8.3 Visceral Pain

The cause of visceral pain must be addressed while pain is controlled using the pain ladder and titrating medications. Adjuvants, such as dexamethasone (4–8 mg daily) to relieve pain from liver disease metastases or nerve compression, should be addressed early if the pain is not well responsive to opioids. The best way to ensure that all of these medications are used responsibly is to consult a specialist PC provider whenever there are any concerns. When systemic treatments are ineffective or the patient is unable to tolerate the high dosages of combination analgesics, interventional pain management approaches can be highly beneficial (Cocks et al., 2016).

18.8.8.4 Mucosal Pain

Mucosal pain may be the result of a tumor, infection, or therapy. It is critical to treat infections like herpes and candida. Sucralfate, benzydamine, chlorhexidine, steroids, and topical local anesthetics such as lignocaine preparations are useful supplementary topical medications. Depending on the patient, coating techniques like bioadherent oral gel may be preferred (Cocks et al., 2016).

18.8.9 Psychological Care

18.8.9.1 Psychiatric Mental Health Nurses/Doctors

Psychological distress symptoms like anxiety and depression are typical of all cancers but are more common in those with HNCs impacting up to 35% of patients (Holland et al., 2014; Zabora et al., 2001). Risk factors include a history of substance misuse and deformity following therapy (Callahan, 2005; El-Guebaly, 1990; Hammerlid et al., 1999; Humphris et al., 2003; Lydiatt et al., 2009). However, physicians frequently fail to identify patients who are at risk (Fallowfield et al., 2001; Greenberg, 2004; Kadan-Lottick et al., 2005; Newell et al., 1998; Söllner et al., 2001). Distress can lead to a lower QOL and a lower chance of survival if left untreated (de Graeff et al., 2000; Fangand & Schnoll,

2002; Hammerlid et al., 2001; Howren et al., 2010; Lazure et al., 2009; Misono et al., 2008; Pinquart & Duberstein, 2010, Prieto et al., 2002). The NCCN Clinical Practice Guidelines in Oncology (NCCN Guidelines) for Distress Management emphasize the significance of identifying individuals who are at risk and advise cancer centers to integrate stress screening into standard care (Holland et al., 2014). Consequently, to assist HNC patients with psychological concerns, healthcare providers worldwide should assign qualified psychiatric mental health nurses and doctors to these patients.

18.8.9.2 Faith-Based Support

Numerous studies have discovered a direct correlation between cancer patients' ability to effectively cope with their condition and their reliance on religious rituals and beliefs (Brady et al., 1999; Ferrell et al., 1998; Holland et al., 1999). A patient may find a framework for deriving perspective and meaning from a source higher than themselves through faith (McIntosh et al., 1993), and this can provide them with a sense of control over their emotions of powerlessness (Koenig, 2002). In times of severe need, religious practice can give access to established support systems and social networks, such as pastoral care (Weaver et al., 2004). Therefore, HNC patients need to receive faith-based support to improve their QOL.

18.9 Challenges and Limitations in Integrating Palliative Care with Conventional Oncology Care

Access to PC is limited because of scarcity in four areas: critical drugs, education/knowledge, resources for development, and government policies (Ward & Jackson, 2013). The hurdles to PC access are associated with the following domains (Aldridge et al., 2016):

1. *Education*: Insufficient training and instruction provided to residents and fellows, and the belief held by the public and healthcare providers that PC is end-of-life care
2. *Policy*: Insufficient funding and reimbursement, obstacles posed by regulations, and a disjointed healthcare system
3. *Implementation*: Cultural hurdles, a shortage of skilled PC experts, and a lack of common referral criteria for PC

According to Ahmed and colleagues, the two most important factors that prevent patients from being referred for PC therapy are the lack of standard screening criteria and the lack of education for medical personnel (Ahmed et al., 2004). Furthermore, Love and Liversage (2014) showed how communication abilities and the preference for curative treatment affect PC recommendations (Love & Liversage, 2014). The primary purpose of these referrals is the management of medical symptoms; psychosocial problems are typically disregarded (Johnson et al., 2008). Even though PC has been called a human right (Palliative Care Alliance & World Health Organization, 2014), HNC patients are not receiving enough services.

18.10 Models to Encourage the Integration of Palliative and Oncology Care

Conceptual models for integration (Hui & Bruera, 2015) are as follows:

1. *Time-based*: Emphasizes the integration of time
2. *Pallicentric (provider-based)*: Comprises primary, secondary, and tertiary PC teams/providers according to the complexity and situations of the patient
3. *Oncocentric (issue-based)*:
   a. Solo practice: Exclusively offered by oncologists
   b. Congress practice: Referral by oncologists of patients to specialist treatment tailored to their requirements
   c. Integrated care: Regular referrals made possible by oncology and PC teams working together.
4. *Patient-centric (system-based)*: Comprises modern, integrated models according to PC referral eligibility/screening standards

The application of conceptual models to many clinical contexts highlights strategies for fostering teamwork and communication in clinical practice, offers details on the results of integration in terms of clinical outcomes, and illustrates the practical difficulties (Hui & Bruera, 2015). Integration can additionally be categorized into the following groups based on the therapeutic structure:

1. Existence of an inpatient team, an outpatient clinic, and community-based support (Hui & Bruera, 2015)
2. Clinics that are embedded, colocated, and standalone (Greer et al., 2013)

18.11 Conclusion and Future Perspectives

Age, general health, comorbidity, patient preferences, motivation, support from family and caregivers, tumor type, clinician team, accessibility to healthcare, patient and treating surgeon bias, treatment complications, perceived treatment outcomes, and the clinician–patient relationship are some of the factors that affect patients' shared decision-making. Due to the unfavorable opinions of PC held by some patients and their families, the fragmented and walled organizational structure of the healthcare system, and provider perceptions of PC, it is difficult to provide early and integrated PC with cancer care. Knowledge of available PC services, the ease and clarity of referral procedures, the demands on clinicians' time and competing priorities, communication problems, and role confusion are some of the factors that affect whether or not doctors consider PC for their patients (Mali & Pradeep, 2023).

The most common perceived difficulties in providing PC in conjunction with cancer-modifying medicines are time constraints, conflicting priorities, patient perception worries, and physicians' social work skills. Palliative aims and values should be upstreamed to the diagnosis and initial decision-making stage for patients with HNCs. A comprehensive grasp of PC principles and aims, the natural history of the disease, health-related QOL concerns, and surgical procedures that may be addressed should all be part of the surgeon's skill set. It is recommended that oncologists be taught PC principles in undergraduate curricula, undergo rotations for fellows in the field, attend conferences, and finish medical education requirements for oncology practitioners. The clinical system should include outpatient clinics, inpatient consultation teams, palliative units, and community-based care. Particular training regarding the management of tracheotomies and feeding tubes may help reduce the need for hospital care by improving integration and coordination between various multidisciplinary teams, fostering greater team collaboration, and upskilling healthcare professionals supporting patients in the community. Models of care that emphasize better coordination and integration between interdisciplinary teams and various care venues may be able to better recognize patient requirements and better customize services to satisfy those needs (Mali & Pradeep, 2023).

References

AHMED, N., BESTALL, J., AHMEDZAI, S., PAYNE, S., CLARK, D., & NOBLE, B. 2004. Systematic review of the problems and issues of accessing specialist palliative care by patients, carers and health and social care professionals. *Palliat Med*, 18, 525–42.

ALDRIDGE, M. D., HASSELAAR, J., GARRALDA, E., VAN DER EERDEN, M., STEVENSON, D., MCKENDRICK, K., CENTENO, C., & MEIER, D. E. 2016. Education, implementation, and policy barriers to greater integration of palliative care: A literature review. *Palliat Med*, 30, 224–39.

BEGBIE, F., DOUGLAS, C., FINLAY, F., & MONTGOMERY, J. 2019. Palliative intent treatment for head and neck cancer: An analysis of practice and outcomes. *J Laryngol Otol*, 133, 313–17.

BRADY, M. J., PETERMAN, A. H., FITCHETT, G., MO, M., & CELLA, D. 1999. A case for including spirituality in quality of life measurement in oncology. *Psycho-Oncology*, 8, 417–28.

BROADFIELD, L. 2006. *Best Practice Guidelines for the Management of Oral Complications from Cancer Therapy*. Halifax, NS: Cancer Care Nova Scotia.

CALLAHAN, C. 2005. Facial disfigurement and sense of self in head and neck cancer. *Soc Work Health Care*, 40, 73–87.

CANNON, S. T., GABBARD, J., WALSH, R. C., STATLER, T. M., BROWNE, J. D., & MARTERRE, B. 2023. Concordant palliative care delivery in advanced head and neck cancer. *Am J Otolaryngol* 44, 103675.

CIVANTOS, A. M., PRASAD, A., CAREY, R. M., BUR, A. M., MADY, L. J., BRODY, R. M., RAJASEKARAN, K., CANNADY, S. B., HARTNER, L., & IBRAHIM, S. A. 2021. Palliative care in metastatic head and neck cancer. *Head Neck*, 43, 2764–77.

COCKS, H., AH-SEE, K., CAPEL, M., & TAYLOR, P. 2016. Palliative and supportive care in head and neck cancer: United Kingdom National Multidisciplinary Guidelines. *J Laryngol Otol*, 130, S198–207.

DAVIES, L., RHODES, L. A., GROSSMAN, D. C., ROSENBERG, M. C., & STEVENS, D. P. 2010. Decision making in head and neck cancer care. *Laryngoscope*, 120, 2434–45.

DAVIS, M. P., TEMEL, J. S., BALBONI, T., & GLARE, P. 2015. A review of the trials which examine early integration of outpatient and home palliative care for patients with serious illnesses. *Ann Palliat Med*, 4, 9921.

DEBER, R. B., KRAETSCHMER, N., UROWITZ, S., & SHARPE, N. 2007. Do people want to be autonomous patients? Preferred roles in treatment decision-making in several patient populations. *Health Expectations*, 10, 248–58.

DE GRAEFF, A., DE LEEUW, J. R. J., ROS, W. J., HORDIJK, G. J., BLIJHAM, G. H., & WINNUBST, J. A. 2000. Pretreatment factors predicting quality of life after treatment for head and neck cancer. *Head Neck*, 22, 398–407.

EL-GUEBALY, N. 1990. Substance abuse and mental disorders: The dual diagnoses concept. *Can J Psychiatry*, 35, 261–7.

ESCE, A., & MCCAMMON, S. 2021. Holding curative and palliative intentions. *AMA J Ethics*, 23, 766–71.

FALLOWFIELD, L., RATCLIFFE, D., JENKINS, V., & SAUL, J. 2001. Psychiatric morbidity and its recognition by doctors in patients with cancer. *Br J Cancer*, 84, 1011–15.

FANGAND, C. Y., & SCHNOLL, R. A. 2002. Impact of psychological distress on outcomes in cancer patients. *Exp Rev Pharmacoeconomics Outcomes Res*, 2, 495–506.

FERRELL, B. R., GRANT, M., FUNK, B., OTIS-GREEN, S., & GARCIA, N. 1998. Quality of life in breast cancer: Part II: Psychological and spiritual well-being. *Cancer Nurs*, 21, 1–9.

FERRELL, B. R., TEMEL, J. S., TEMIN, S., ALESI, E. R., BALBONI, T. A., BASCH, E. M., FIRN, J. I., PAICE, J. A., PEPPERCORN, J. M., & PHILLIPS, T. 2017. Integration of palliative care into standard oncology care: American Society of Clinical Oncology clinical practice guideline update. *J Clin Oncol*, 35, 96–112.

GANDHI, A. K., ROY, S., THAKAR, A., SHARMA, A., & MOHANTI, B. K. 2014. Symptom burden and quality of life in advanced head and neck cancer patients: AIIMS study of 100 patients. *Indian J Palliat Care*, 20, 189.

GIDWANI, R., NEVEDAL, A., PATEL, M., BLAYNEY, D. W., TIMKO, C., RAMCHANDRAN, K., KELLY, P. A., & ASCH, S. M. 2017. The appropriate provision of primary versus specialist palliative care to cancer patients: Oncologists' perspectives. *J Palliat Med*, 20, 395–403.

GILLIGAN, T., BOHLKE, K., & BAILE, W. F. 2018. Patient-clinician communication: American Society of Clinical Oncology consensus guideline summary. *J Oncol Pract*, 14, 42–6.

GRANT, L., DOWNING, J., NAMUKWAYA, E., LENG, M., & MURRAY, S. A. 2011. Palliative care in Africa since 2005: Good progress, but much further to go. *BMJ Support Palliat Care*, 1, 118–22.

GREENBERG, D. B. 2004. Barriers to the treatment of depression in cancer patients. *JNCI Monographs*, 2004, 127–35.

GREER, J. A., JACKSON, V. A., MEIER, D. E., & TEMEL, J. S. 2013. Early integration of palliative care services with standard oncology care for patients with advanced cancer. *CA: Cancer J*, 63, 349–63.

GREWAL, A. S., JONES, J., & LIN, A. 2019. Palliative radiation therapy for head and neck cancers. *Int J Radiat Oncol Biol Physics*, 105, 254–66.

HAMMERLID, E., AHLNER-ELMQVIST, M., BJORDAL, K., BIÖRKLUND, A., EVENSEN, J., BOYSEN, M., JANNERT, M., KAASA, S., SULLIVAN, M., & WESTIN, T. 1999. A prospective multicentre study in Sweden and Norway of mental distress and psychiatric morbidity in head and neck cancer patients. *Br J Cancer*, 80, 766–74.

HAMMERLID, E., SILANDER, E., HÖRNESTAM, L., & SULLIVAN, M. 2001. Health-related quality of life three years after diagnosis of head and neck cancer—a longitudinal study. *Head Neck*, 23, 113–25.

HANNA, E. Y., MENDOZA, T. R., ROSENTHAL, D. I., GUNN, G. B., SEHRA, P., YUCEL, E., & CLEELAND, C. S. 2015. The symptom burden of treatment-naive patients with head and neck cancer. *Cancer*, 121, 766–73.

HAWLEY, P. H. 2014. The bow tie model of 21st century palliative care. *J Pain Sympt Manage*, 47, e2–e5.

HOLLAND, J. C., ANDERSEN, B., BREITBART, W. S., BUCHMANN, L. O., COMPAS, B., DESHIELDS, T. L., DUDLEY, M. M., FLEISHMAN, S., FULCHER, C. D., GREENBERG, D. B., GREINER, C. B., HANDZO, G. F., HOOFRING, L., HOOVER, C., JACOBSEN, P. B., KVALE, E., LEVY, M. H., LOSCALZO, M. J., MCALLISTER-BLACK, R., MECHANIC, K. Y., & FREEDMAN-CASS, D. A. 2013. Distress management. *J Natl Compr Cancer Netw: JNCCN*, 11(2), 190–209. https://doi.org/10.6004/jnccn.2013.0027

HOLLAND, J. C., PASSIK, S., KASH, K. M., RUSSAK, S. M., GRONERT, M. K., SISON, A., LEDERBERG, M., FOX, B., & BAIDER, L. 1999. The role of religious and spiritual beliefs in coping with malignant melanoma. *Psycho-Oncology*, 8, 14–26.

HOWREN, M. B., CHRISTENSEN, A. J., KARNELL, L. H., & FUNK, G. F. 2010. Health-related quality of life in head and neck cancer survivors: Impact of pretreatment depressive symptoms. *Health Psychol* 29, 65.

HUA, M., FONSECA, L. D., MORRISON, R. S., WUNSCH, H., FULLILOVE, R., & WHITE, D. B. 2021. What affects adoption of specialty palliative care in intensive care units: A qualitative study. *J Pain Sympt Manage*, 62, 1273–82.

HUI, D., & BRUERA, E. 2015. Models of integration of oncology and palliative care. *Ann Palliat Med*, 4, 898.

HUMAN RIGHTS WATCH. 2010. Needless pain: Government failure to provide palliative care for children in Kenya. Human Rights Watch New York. https://www.hrw.org/report/2010/09/09/needless-pain/government-failure-provide-palliative-care-children-kenya

HUMPHRIS, G. M., ROGERS, S., MCNALLY, D., LEE-JONES, C., BROWN, J., & VAUGHAN, D. 2003. Fear of recurrence and possible cases of anxiety and depression in orofacial cancer patients. *Int J Oral Maxillofac Surg*, 32, 486–91.

JACOB, J., PALAT, G., VERGHESE, N., CHANDRAN, P., RAPELLI, V., KUMARI, S., MALHOTRA, C., TEO, I., FINKELSTEIN, E., & OZDEMIR, S. 2019. Health-related quality of life and its socio-economic and cultural predictors among advanced cancer patients: Evidence from the APPROACH cross-sectional survey in Hyderabad-India. *BMC Palliat Care*, 18, 1–12.

JOHNSON, C. E., GIRGIS, A., PAUL, C. L., & CURROW, D. C. 2008. Cancer specialists' palliative care referral practices and perceptions: Results of a national survey. *Palliat Med*, 22, 51–7.

KADAN-LOTTICK, N. S., VANDERWERKER, L. C., BLOCK, S. D., ZHANG, B., & PRIGERSON, H. G. 2005. Psychiatric disorders and mental health service use in patients with advanced cancer: A report from the coping with cancer study. *Cancer*, 104, 2872–81.

KOENIG, H. G. 2002. An 83-year-old woman with chronic illness and strong religious beliefs. *JAMA*, 288, 487–93.

LAZURE, K. E., LYDIATT, W. M., DENMAN, D., & BURKE, W. J. 2009. Association between depression and survival or disease recurrence in patients with head and neck cancer enrolled in a depression prevention trial. *Head Neck*, 31, 888–92.

LEVY, M. H., BACK, A., BENEDETTI, C., BILLINGS, J. A., BLOCK, S., BOSTON, B., BRUERA, E., DY, S., EBERLE, C., & FOLEY, K. M. 2009. NCCN clinical practice guidelines in oncology: Palliative care. *J Nat Comp Cancer Netw*, 7, 436–73.

LIAO, K., BLUMENTHAL-BARBY, J., & SIKORA, A. G. 2017. Factors influencing head and neck surgical oncologists' transition from curative to palliative treatment goals. *Otolaryngol Head Neck Surg*, 156, 46–51.

LILLEY, E. J., KHAN, K. T., JOHNSTON, F. M., BERLIN, A., BADER, A. M., MOSENTHAL, A. C., & COOPER, Z. 2016. Palliative care interventions for surgical patients: A systematic review. *JAMA Surg*, 151, 172–83.

LOVE, A. W., & LIVERSAGE, L. M. 2014. Barriers to accessing palliative care: A review of the literature. *Prog Palliat Care*, 22, 9–19.

LYDIATT, W. M., MORAN, J., & BURKE, W. J. 2009. A review of depression in the head and neck cancer patient. *Clin Adv Hematol Oncol*, 7, 397–403.

MALI, S. B., & PRADEEP, G. 2023. *Head Neck Cancer Care: Communication and Decision Making Regarding Palliative Care*. New York: Elsevier.

MAYLAND, C. R., HO, Q. M., DOUGHTY, H. C., ROGERS, S. N., PEDDINTI, P., CHADA, P., MASON, S., COOPER, M., & DEY, P. 2021. The palliative care needs and experiences of people with advanced head and neck cancer: A scoping review. *Palliat Med*, 35, 27–44.

MCCAMMON, S. D. 2019. Concurrent palliative care in the surgical management of head and neck cancer. *J Surg Oncol*, 120, 78–84.

MCINTOSH, D. N., SILVER, R. C., & WORTMAN, C. B. 1993. Religion's role in adjustment to a negative life event: Coping with the loss of a child. *J Personality Soc Psychol*, 65, 812.

MISONO, S., WEISS, N. S., FANN, J. R., REDMAN, M., & YUEH, B. 2008. Incidence of suicide in persons with cancer. *J Clin Oncol*, 26, 4731.

MPANGA SEBUYIRA, L., MWANGI-POWELL, F., PEREIRA, J., & SPENCE, C. 2003. The Cape Town palliative care declaration: Home-grown solutions for sub-Saharan Africa. *J Palliat Med*, 6, 341–3.

MURPHY, B. A., CMELAK, A., BAYLES, S., DOWLING, E., BILLANTE, C. R., RIDNER, S. H., HAMAN, K., BOND, S. M., FLORES, A. M., & WISAWATAPNIMIT, P. 2010. 11.2 Palliative issues in the care of patients with cancer of the head and neck. *In:* B. M. Andrews, ed. *Oxford Textbook of Palliative Medicine*. New York: Oxford University Press.

MURPHY, B. A., & DENG, J. 2015. Advances in supportive care for late effects of head and neck cancer. *J Clin Oncol*, 33, 3314–21.

NCCN. 2020. Palliative care. Available at: https://www.nccn.org/professionals/physician_gls/pdf/palliative.pdf [Accessed April 22, 2020.]

NEWELL, S., SANSON-FISHER, R. W., GIRGIS, A., & BONAVENTURA, A. 1998. How well do medical oncologists' perceptions reflect their patients' reported physical and psychosocial problems? Data from a survey of five oncologists. *Cancer*, 83, 1640–51.

NILSEN, M. L., & JOHNSON, J. T. 2017. Potential for low-value palliative care of patients with recurrent head and neck cancer. *Lancet Oncol*, 18, e284–9.

PALLIATIVE CARE ALLIANCE & WORLD HEALTH ORGANIZATION. 2014. *Global Atlas of Palliative Care at the End of Life*. London: Worldwide Palliative Care Alliance, 111.

PINQUART, M., & DUBERSTEIN, P. 2010. Depression and cancer mortality: A meta-analysis. *Psychol Med*, 40, 1797–810.

PRICE, K. A. R., MOORE, E. J., MOYNIHAN, T., & PRICE, D. L. 2009. Symptoms and terminal course of patients who died of head and neck cancer. *J Palliat Med*, 12, 117–18.

PRIETO, J. M., BLANCH, J., ATALA, J., CARRERAS, E., ROVIRA, M., CIRERA, E., & GASTÓ, C. 2002. Psychiatric morbidity and impact on hospital length of stay among hematologic cancer patients receiving stem-cell transplantation. *J Clin Oncol*, 20, 1907–17.

ROGERS, S., THOMSON, F., & LOWE, D. 2018. The Patient Concerns Inventory integrated as part of routine head and neck cancer follow-up consultations: Frequency, case-mix, and items initiated by the patient. *Ann R Coll Surg Engl*, 100, 209–15.

ROGERS, S. N., ALVEAR, A., ANESI, A., BABIN, E., BALIK, A., BATSTONE, M., BROCKMEYER, P., CARRASCO, C. C., CHIEN, C. Y., & CHIRILA, M. 2020. Variations in concerns reported on the patient concerns inventory in patients with head and neck cancer from different health settings across the world. *Head Neck*, 42, 498–512.

ROGERS, S. N., & BARBER, B. 2017. Using PROMs to guide patients and practitioners through the head and neck cancer journey. *Patient Related Outcome Measures*, 133–142.

ROLAND, N. J., & BRADLEY, P. J. 2014. The role of surgery in the palliation of head and neck cancer. *Curr Opin Otolaryngol Head Neck Surg*, 22, 101–8.

SALINS, N., RAMANJULU, R., PATRA, L., DEODHAR, J., & MUCKADEN, M. A. 2016. Integration of early specialist palliative care in cancer care and patient related outcomes: A critical review of evidence. *Indian J Palliat Care*, 22, 252.

SATIJA, A., LORENZ, K., DENATALE, M., SPRUYT, O., DEO, S., & BHATNAGAR, S. 2019. Role of early palliative care in advanced head-and-neck cancers patients. *Indian J Palliat Care*, 25, 153.

SCHENKER, Y., ARNOLD, R. M., BAUMAN, J. E., HERON, D. E., & JOHNSON, J. T. 2016. An enhanced role for palliative care in the multidisciplinary approach to high-risk head and neck cancer. *Cancer*, 122, 340–3.

SCHULMAN-GREEN, D., LIN, J. J., SMITH, C. B., FEDER, S., & BICKELL, N. A. 2018. Facilitators and barriers to oncologists' conduct of goals of care conversations. *J Palliat Care*, 33, 143–8.

SHUMAN, A. G., LARKIN, K., THOMAS, D., PALMER, F. L., FINS, J. J., BAXI, S. S., LEE, N., SHAH, J. P., FAGERLIN, A., & PATEL, S. G. 2017. Patient reflections on decision making for laryngeal cancer treatment. *Otolaryngol Head Neck Surg*, 156, 299–304.

SÖLLNER, W., DEVRIES, A., STEIXNER, E., LUKAS, P., SPRINZL, G., RUMPOLD, G., & MAISLINGER, S. 2001. How successful are oncologists in identifying patient distress, perceived social support, and need for psychosocial counselling? *Br J Cancer*, 84, 179–85.

STJERNSWÄRD, J., FOLEY, K. M., & FERRIS, F. D. 2007. The public health strategy for palliative care. *J Pain Sympt Manage*, 33, 486–93.

THOMAS, T. H., JACKSON, V. A., CARLSON, H., RINALDI, S., SOUSA, A., HANSEN, A., KAMDAR, M., JACOBSEN, J., PARK, E. R., & PIRL, W. F. 2019. Communication differences between oncologists and palliative care clinicians: A qualitative analysis of early, integrated palliative care in patients with advanced cancer. *J Palliat Med*, 22, 41–9.

VAN DER VELDEN, J., WILLMANN, J., SPAŁEK, M., OLDENBURGER, E., BROWN, S., KAZMIERSKA, J., ANDRATSCHKE, N., MENTEN, J., VAN DER LINDEN, Y., & HOSKIN, P. 2022. ESTRO ACROP guidelines for external beam radiotherapy of patients with uncomplicated bone metastases. *Radiother Oncol*, 173, 197–206.

WARD, D., & JACKSON, K. 2013. Ehospice: Palliative care news, views, and inspiration from around the world. *Int J Palliat Nurs*, 19, 109.

WEAVER, A. J., FLANNELLY, L. T., & PRESTON, J. D. 2004. *Counseling Survivors of Traumatic Events*. London: Abingdon Press.

WEE, B., & HILLIER, R. 2008. Interventions for noisy breathing in patients near to death. *Cochrane Database Syst Rev*, 2008(1), CD005177. https://doi.org/10.1002/14651858.CD005177.pub2

WONG, R., & WIFFEN, P. J. 2002. Bisphosphonates for the relief of pain secondary to bone metastases. *Cochrane Database Syst Rev*, 2002(2), CD002068. https://doi.org/10.1002/14651858.CD002068.

WORLD HEALTH ORGANIZATION (WHO). 2005. Cancer prevention and control. Available at: http://www.who.int/gb/ebwha/pdf_files/WHA58-REC1/english/A58_2005_REC1-en.pdf [Accessed July 27, 2011.]

WORLD HEALTH ORGANIZATION (WHO). 2014. World palliative care alliance. Global atlas of palliative care at the end of life Available at : http://www.who.int/cancer/publications/palliative-care-atlas/en/ [Accessed September 17, 2014.]

WRIGHT, M., LYNCH, T., & CLARK, D. 2008a. *A Review of Donor Organisations That Support Palliative Care Development in Five World Regions*. Lancaster: International Observatory on End of Life Care, Lancaster University.

WRIGHT, M., WOOD, J., LYNCH, T., & CLARK, D. 2008b. Mapping levels of palliative care development: A global view. *J Pain Sympt Manage*, 35, 469–85.

ZABORA, J., BRINTZENHOFESZOC, K., CURBOW, B., HOOKER, C., & PIANTADOSI, S. 2001. The prevalence of psychological distress by cancer site. *Psycho-oncology*, 10, 19–28.

19

Global Perspectives and Future Directions in Head and Neck Cancer

Zodwa Dlamini, Talent Chipiti, Solly Selahle, Rodney Hull, Demetra Demetriou, and Georgios Lolas

19.1 Global Perspectives on Head and Neck Cancer

Head and neck cancer (HNC) is the world's third most frequent cancer, accounting for 7.6% of all malignancies and 4.8% of cancer-related deaths (Zhou et al., 2025). Despite breakthroughs in therapy, our grasp of the global disease burden is limited due to various factors (Zhou et al., 2024). HNC presents a complex global health challenge, one characterized by significant variations in incidence, risk factors, and outcomes across different regions, age groups, and populations. In high-income countries, the epidemiology of HNC is evolving, with human papillomavirus (HPV)-related cancers on the rise, surpassing those caused by traditional risk factors such as tobacco and alcohol use (Gillison et al., 2015; Marur & Forastiere, 2016).

In contrast, low- and middle-income countries (LMICs) continue to face a high burden of HNC linked to tobacco and bidi smoking, areca or betel nut (*Areca catechu*)

quid chewing, and poor access to healthcare, which often leads to late-stage diagnoses and poorer outcomes (Bray et al., 2018; Shield & Ferlay, 2017). In managing HNC, Africa faces unique challenges such as limited healthcare infrastructure, shortages of trained healthcare professionals, and a lack of context-specific data to guide policy and clinical practice (Parkin et al., 2008). These challenges highlight the need for comprehensive public health initiatives aimed at reducing risk factors and improving access to early detection and treatment services. Similarly, in Asia, the high prevalence of betel quid use significantly contributes to HNC incidence, requiring targeted interventions (IARC Working Group, 2004).

19.2 Future Directions in Head and Neck Cancer Management

The future of HNC management lies in the integration of advanced diagnostic tools, precision medicine, and multidisciplinary care approaches. Innovations in molecular profiling and next-generation sequencing (NGS) are paving the way for more personalized treatment strategies. Identifying specific biomarkers associated with HNC can enhance early detection, predict treatment response, and tailor therapies to individual patient profiles, thereby optimizing outcomes and minimizing side effects (Leemans et al., 2018).

19.2.1 Diagnostic Innovations

The role of artificial intelligence (AI) in HNC diagnosis is increasingly significant, offering transformative potential in various aspects of patient care. AI algorithms can analyze complex datasets, such as imaging studies, histopathological slides, and genetic information, with precision and efficiency that exceeds traditional methods. These capabilities allow AI to identify patterns and provide accurate prognostic information, thereby assisting clinicians in making well-informed decisions (Esteva et al., 2017). This technology promises to revolutionize early diagnosis and improve the accuracy of cancer staging and treatment planning.

19.2.2 Precision Medicine

The advent of precision medicine has revolutionized HNC treatment. By leveraging molecular profiling, clinicians can develop personalized treatment plans that target specific genetic mutations and pathways involved in cancer progression. This approach not only enhances the efficacy of treatments but also reduces the toxicity associated with conventional therapies (Moreira et al., 2017; van Harten et al., 2021). Molecular profiling helps identify genetic mutations in tumors, guiding targeted therapies. For example, the presence of epidermal growth factor receptor (EGFR) mutations can lead to the use of cetuximab, a monoclonal antibody that targets the EGFR on cancer cells. By blocking EGFR, cetuximab inhibits cancer cell growth and survival, improving outcomes in patients with EGFR-positive HNC. Similarly, alterations in the *PIK3CA* gene or HPV presence can influence treatment decisions (Baumann et al., 2008; Leemans et al., 2018). Precision medicine enhances treatment effectiveness and reduces side effects compared to traditional therapies. Traditional therapies, such as chemotherapy and radiation, often affect both cancerous and normal cells, leading to significant adverse effects. In contrast, precision medicine tailors' treatments to an individual's unique genetic makeup, allowing for more specific interventions.

Targeted therapies specifically attack cancer cells by focusing on molecular targets associated with cancer, thereby sparing normal tissues and minimizing side effects. Immunotherapies, such as immune checkpoint inhibitors like pembrolizumab and nivolumab, enhance the body's immune response against cancer cells. These therapies have shown significant benefits in treating recurrent or metastatic HNC, offering a better safety profile compared to conventional chemotherapy (Ferris et al., 2016). Recent advancements in precision medicine include liquid biopsies, which are noninvasive tests used to monitor tumor dynamics and treatment response. These tests provide real-time insights into molecular changes within the tumor, allowing for prompt adjustments to treatment plans and personalized therapy. Additionally, the integration of AI and machine learning into precision medicine enables the development of more accurate and predictive models of treatment response, leading to improved patient outcomes (Siravegna et al., 2017; Topol, 2019).

Precision medicine has significantly transformed the approach to treating HNC. By harnessing molecular profiling and advanced technologies, clinicians can devise personalized treatment plans that target specific genetic and molecular irregularities, resulting in more effective and less toxic therapies. As research and technology continue to progress, the role of precision medicine in HNC is expected to expand further, offering new hope and improved outcomes for patients.

19.3 Immunotherapy and Targeted Therapies

Immunotherapy, particularly immune checkpoint inhibitors like pembrolizumab and nivolumab, has shown significant promise in treating advanced HNC. Combining immunotherapy with targeted therapies that disrupt specific oncogenic pathways can provide a synergistic effect, improving treatment outcomes. Ongoing research aims to overcome challenges such as drug resistance and treatment-related toxicities (Burtness et al., 2019; Cohen et al., 2019; Ferris et al., 2016). The combination of immunotherapy with targeted therapies can improve treatment outcomes for HNC. Targeted therapies disrupt specific oncogenic pathways, such as overexpressed EGFR and can be used in conjunction with immune checkpoint inhibitors to enhance the overall antitumor response (Burtness et al., 2019; Cohen et al., 2019; Ferris et al., 2016).

Research is focused on overcoming challenges such as drug resistance and treatment-related toxicities. Strategies include exploring combination therapies, managing immune-related adverse events, and identifying biomarkers to predict treatment response (Burtness et al., 2019; Cohen et al., 2019; Ferris et al., 2016). The integration of immunotherapy and targeted therapies represents a significant advancement in HNC treatment, offering better disease control and improved patient outcomes. Ongoing research aims to address resistance and toxicity challenges, promising a more effective future for treatment (Burtness et al., 2019; Cohen et al., 2019; Leemans et al., 2018; Postow et al., 2018).

19.4 Surgical Innovations

Advances in surgical techniques, including transoral robotic surgery (TORS) and minimally invasive procedures, have improved the precision of tumor resection while preserving function and reducing recovery times. Advancements in imaging technologies and intraoperative monitoring have further enhanced surgical precision and patient recovery, leading to better overall quality of life for HNC surgery patients (Hanna et al., 2018; Mella et al., 2023; Moore & Olsen, 2015; Moore et al., 2018; Pierik et al., 2021). The advent and innovation of free tissue transfer and perforator flaps have made it possible to reconstruct very large head and neck defects that are left after extirpative cancer surgery (Varadhan & Gardiner, 2013; Morani et al., 2009). These reconstructions can be tailored to improve a patient's function and form (cosmesis) and thereby improve the overall quality of life (Cordeiro, 2015; Hidalgo & Disa, 2015).

19.5 Radiation Therapy

Technological advancements in radiation therapy, such as proton therapy and stereotactic body radiotherapy (SBRT), have enabled more precise targeting of tumors, minimizing damage to surrounding healthy tissues (Lillo et al., 2024; Prezzano et al., 2019). Proton therapy and SBRT are advanced radiation treatment techniques for HNC. Proton therapy uses protons instead of x-rays to precisely target tumors with minimal damage to surrounding healthy tissues, thus reducing side effects like dry mouth and difficulty swallowing. SBRT delivers highly focused radiation beams to the tumor in fewer treatments, effectively controlling tumor growth and improving survival rates (Frank et al., 2014; Holtzman et al., 2019; Noel & Gondi, 2016).

Combining radiation therapy with immunotherapy agents, such as pembrolizumab and nivolumab, shows promise in enhancing antitumor immune responses and targeting metastatic sites. Additionally, combining SBRT with immunotherapy has demonstrated potential in enhancing systemic antitumor immunity. These advanced techniques and their combinations with immunotherapy hold great promise in significantly improving the prognosis and quality of life for HNC patients (Gillison et al., 2019; Ma et al., 2019; McBride et al., 2010; Ngwa et al., 2018; Scott et al., 2020; Siva et al., 2013).

19.6 Multidisciplinary Approaches

The integration of multidisciplinary teams (MDTs) in HNC care is essential for providing comprehensive, patient-centered care. MDTs facilitate collaboration among specialists, ensuring coordinated and continuous care from diagnosis through treatment and follow-up. One of the key benefits of MDTs is the improvement in treatment adherence (Maguire et al., 2005; Taylor et al., 2010). When experts from various disciplines such as oncologists, surgeons, radiation therapists, nutritionists, and speech and language therapists collaborate, they can develop and implement a cohesive treatment plan tailored to the individual patient's needs. This plan often includes a combination of surgery, radiation therapy, and chemotherapy, along with supportive care measures. The involvement of these specialists ensures that every aspect of the patient's care is addressed, reducing the likelihood of treatment interruptions and ensuring adherence to the prescribed therapeutic regimen (Taylor et al., 2010).

MDTs are essential in minimizing the long-term side effects associated with HNC treatments. For instance, the collaboration between oncologists and nutritionists can effectively manage and alleviate the severe nutritional deficits often experienced by HNC patients. Likewise, the involvement of speech and language therapists can effectively address the communication and swallowing difficulties that frequently arise from HNC treatments. By proactively addressing these side effects in a coordinated manner, MDTs significantly enhance the patient's quality of life and overall outcomes (Kelly et al., 2013; Taberna et al., 2020). Furthermore, MDTs improve overall patient satisfaction by offering a more comprehensive and patient-centered approach to care. Patients often feel more supported and understood when they receive care from a team of specialists who communicate effectively and work together seamlessly (Kelly et al., 2013).

The holistic approach not only addresses the physical aspects of the disease but also considers the emotional, psychological, and social impacts, leading to a more satisfactory healthcare experience for patients (Kelly et al., 2013). MDTs have been proved to enhance survival rates in HNC patients by providing more precise diagnoses, timely treatments, and improved management of complications. This holistic care model has been linked to better survival outcomes, emphasizing the crucial role of MDTs in HNC management (Taberna et al., 2020).

19.7 Addressing Disparities and Enhancing Global Collaboration

Efforts to address global disparities in HNC care must focus on enhancing healthcare infrastructure, training healthcare professionals, and implementing context-specific guidelines and policies. International collaborations and knowledge sharing can play a pivotal role in building capacity in LMICs, improving access to advanced diagnostic and treatment technologies, and promoting research that addresses the unique epidemiological and sociocultural contexts of different regions. Improving healthcare infrastructure requires not only expanding medical facilities and equipment but also making sure that these resources are distributed effectively to reach underserved populations. Training healthcare professionals is also crucial because it provides them with the necessary skills to diagnose and treat health issues effectively, even in areas with limited resources. Implementing guidelines and policies specific to each context ensures that prevention, diagnosis, and treatment approaches are tailored to the unique needs and circumstances of different regions, making them more effective (Bray et al., 2018; Parkin et al., 2008).

International collaborations and knowledge sharing can be extremely beneficial in helping to build capacity in LMICs. These collaborations can provide access to advanced diagnostic and treatment technologies, including modern imaging techniques, minimally invasive surgical tools, and state-of-the-art radiotherapy equipment that may otherwise be unavailable. Additionally, by supporting research that addresses the unique epidemiological and sociocultural contexts of different regions, these partnerships can aid in developing more effective and culturally appropriate interventions. This approach not only enhances the quality of care but also encourages innovation tailored to the specific challenges faced by LMICs (Parkin et al., 2008). Public health initiatives should prioritize the prevention of HNC through education and awareness campaigns targeting major risk factors such as tobacco, alcohol, and HPV. Expanding access to HPV vaccination and promoting safe sexual behaviors are critical in reducing HPV-related HNCs. Additionally, early detection and screening programs, particularly in high-risk populations, are vital for improving prognosis and survival rates (Gillison et al., 2015; Marur & Forastiere, 2016).

Programs that promote safe sexual behaviors can help reduce the incidence of HPV-related HNCs. Additionally, early detection and screening programs are crucial for improving prognosis and survival rates. These programs should focus on high-risk populations, such as individuals with a history of tobacco and alcohol use, as well as those with high rates of HPV infection. Early detection enables timely intervention, which can significantly improve outcomes (Marur & Forastiere, 2016). It is crucial to take a multifaceted approach to address global disparities in HNC care. This should include improving infrastructure, providing professional training, fostering international collaboration, and implementing strong public health initiatives. By embracing these strategies, we can make significant strides in ensuring that everyone worldwide has fair access to high-quality HNC care.

19.8 Conclusion

The landscape of HNC management is rapidly evolving, driven by technological advancements and a deeper understanding of tumor biology. As we look to the future, the integration of precision medicine, innovative surgical and radiation techniques, and multidisciplinary care approaches holds the promise of significantly improving patient outcomes, as illustrated by Figure 19.1. Addressing global disparities through targeted public health initiatives and international collaboration is essential for ensuring equitable access to high-quality care for all individuals affected by HNC. Many LMICs encounter significant challenges in delivering sufficient cancer care due to limited resources and healthcare infrastructure. International collaborations and targeted public health initiatives can help address these gaps by providing resources, education, and support to healthcare providers and patients in underserved regions. Programs that emphasize early detection, vaccination against HPV, and education on risk factors such as tobacco and alcohol use are crucial for reducing the incidence and improving the outcomes of head and neck cancer globally.

Through continued research, innovation, and a commitment to comprehensive, patient-centered care, we can make significant strides in reducing the burden of HNC worldwide. The ongoing research on the molecular and genetic foundations of HNC will lead to the discovery of new targets for therapy. Additionally, advancements in immunotherapy and combination treatments offer hope for better management of advanced disease. It is crucial to adopt a multidisciplinary approach involving oncologists, surgeons, radiologists, pathologists, and supportive care teams to address the complex needs of HNC patients and enhance their quality of life.

Diagnosis and screening have been improved due to advances such as liquid biopsies and the use of molecular biomarkers in screening as well as improvements in molecular imaging. Advances have been made in all fields of

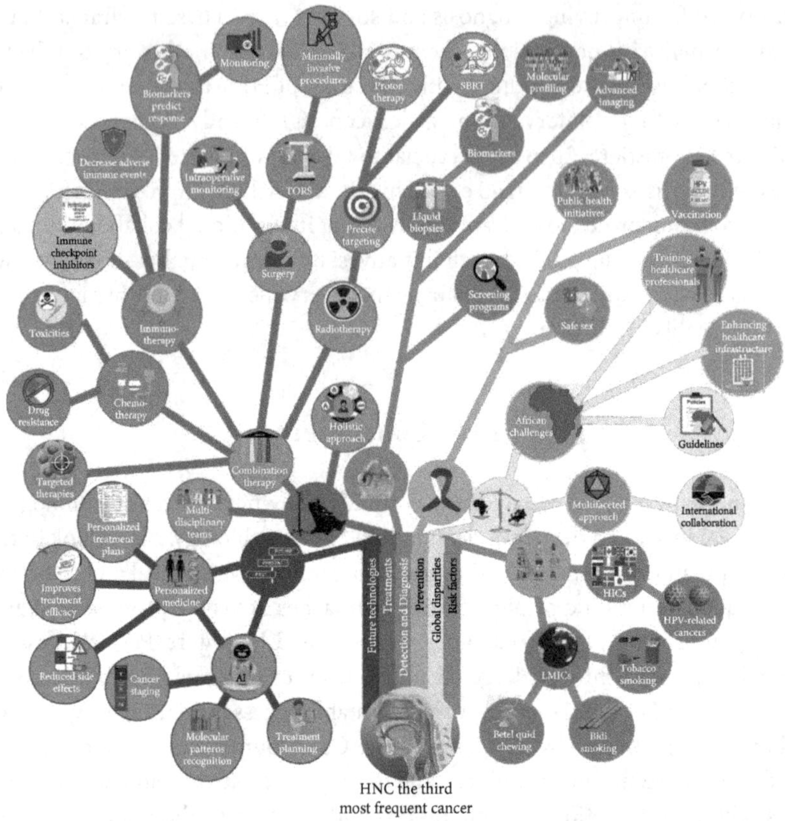

Figure 19.1 A roadmap of the advancements in the treatment and diagnosis of head and neck cancer (HNC). Improving the management of these cancers is an important goal since they are the third most frequent cancer and, as such, are a major public health burden. Improvements must be made to lower the exposure of patients to risk factors for the disease. Because these differ between high- and middle- to low-income countries, it is also important to address the worldwide disparities that are seen in the treatment of HNC, especially in Africa, which presents a unique set of challenges.
SBRT, stereotactic body radiotherapy; TORS, transoral robotic surgery; HICs, high-income countries; HPV, human papillomavirus; LMICs, low- and middle-income countries; AI, artificial intelligence.

treatment for HNC, including surgery and radiotherapy, the primary treatments for disease. These treatments have been further improved through the adoption of combination therapies and holistic approaches as well as the use of multidisciplinary teams. However, the most promising developments lie in the application of AI and the adoption of precision medicine, which impact treatment, screening, diagnosis, and disease management.

References

BAUMANN, M., KRAUSE, M., & HILL, R. 2008. Exploring the role of cancer stem cells in radioresistance. *Nat Rev Cancer*, 8(7), 545–54.

BRAY, F., FERLAY, J., SOERJOMATARAM, I., SIEGEL, R. L., TORRE, L. A., & JEMAL, A. 2018. Global cancer statistics 2018: GLOBOCAN estimates of incidence and mortality worldwide for 36 cancers in 185 countries. *CA Cancer J*, 68(6), 394–424.

BURTNESS, B., HARRINGTON, K. J., GREIL, R., SOULIÈRES, D., TAHARA, M., DE CASTRO, G. JR, PSYRRI, A., BASTÉ, N., NEUPANE, P., BRATLAND, Å., FUEREDER, T., HUGHES, B. G. M., MESÍA, R., NGAMPHAIBOON, N., RORDORF, T., WAN ISHAK, W. Z., HONG, R. L., GONZÁLEZ MENDOZA, R., ROY, A., ZHANG, Y., GUMUSCU, B., CHENG, J. D., JIN, F., RISCHIN, D.; KEYNOTE-048 INVESTIGATORS. 2019, November 1. Pembrolizumab alone or with chemotherapy versus cetuximab with chemotherapy for recurrent or metastatic squamous cell carcinoma of the head and neck (KEYNOTE-048): A randomised, open-label, phase 3 study. *Lancet*, 394(10212), 1915–28. doi:10.1016/S0140-6736(19)32591-7. Erratum in *Lancet*, 2020 Jan 25;395(10220), 272. Erratum in *Lancet*, 2020 Feb 22;395(10224), 564. Erratum in *Lancet*, 397(10291), 2252. PMID: 31679945.

COHEN, E. E. W., SOULIÈRES, D., LE TOURNEAU, C., DINIS, J., LICITRA, L., AHN, M. J., SORIA, A., MACHIELS, J. P., MACH, N., MEHRA, R., BURTNESS, B., ZHANG, P., CHENG, J., SWABY, R. F., & HARRINGTON, K. J. 2019. Pembrolizumab versus methotrexate, docetaxel, or cetuximab for recurrent or metastatic head-and-neck squamous cell carcinoma (KEYNOTE-040): A randomised, open-label, phase 3 study. *Lancet*, 393(10167), 156–67.

CORDEIRO, P. G. 2015. Microsurgical reconstruction of the head and neck: Current state and future directions. *J Surg Oncol*, 111(5), 472–7.

ESTEVA, A., et al. 2017. Dermatologist-level classification of skin cancer with deep neural networks. *Nature*, 542 (7639), 115–18.

FERRIS, R. L., BLUMENSCHEIN, G., FAYETTE, J., GUIGAY, J., COLEVAS, A. D., LICITRA, L., HARRINGTON, K., KASPER, S., VOKES, E. E., EVEN, C., WORDEN, F., SABA, N. F., IGLESIAS DOCAMPO, L. C., HADDAD, R., RORDORF, T., KIYOTA, N., TAHARA, M., MONGA, M., LYNCH, M., GEESE, W. J., KOPIT, J., SHAW, J. W., & GILLISON, M. L. 2016. Nivolumab for recurrent squamous-cell carcinoma of the head and neck. *N Engl J Med*, 375(19), 1856–66.

FRANK, S. J., COX, J. D., GILLIN, M., MOHAN, R., GARDEN, A. S., ROSENTHAL, D. I., GUNN, G. B., WEBER, R. S., KIES, M. S., LEWIN, J. S., MUNSELL, M. F., PALMER, M. B., SAHOO, N., ZHANG, X., LIU, W., & ZHU, X. R. 2014. Multifield optimization intensity modulated proton therapy for head and neck tumors: A translation to practice. *Int J Radiat Oncol Biol Phys*, 89(4), 846–53.

GILLISON, M. L., CHATURVEDI, A. K., ANDERSON, W. F., & FAKHRY, C. 2015. Epidemiology of human papillomavirus-positive head and neck squamous cell carcinoma. *J Clin Oncol*, 33(29), 3235–42.

GILLISON, M. L., TROTTI, A. M., HARRIS, J., EISBRUCH, A., HARARI, P. M., ADELSTEIN, D. J., JORDAN, R. C. K., ZHAO, W., STURGIS, E. M., BURTNESS, B., RIDGE, J. A., RINGASH, J., GALVIN, J., YAO, M., KOYFMAN, S. A., BLAKAJ, D. M., RAZAQ, M. A., COLEVAS, A. D., BEITLER, J. J., JONES, C. U., DUNLAP, N. E., SEAWARD, S. A., SPENCER, S., GALLOWAY, T. J., PHAN, J., DIGNAM, J. J., & LE, Q. T. 2019. Radiotherapy plus cetuximab or cisplatin in human papillomavirus-positive oropharyngeal cancer

(NRG Oncology RTOG 1016): A multicentre, non-inferiority, randomised trial. *Lancet*, 393(10166), 40–50.

HANNA, G. J., LIZOTTE, P., CAVANAUGH, M., KUO, F. C., SHIVDASANI, P., FRIEDEN, A., CHAU, N. G., SCHOENFELD, J. D., LORCH, J. H., UPPALURI, R., MACCONAILL, L. E., & HADDAD, R. I. 2018. Frameshift events predict anti–PD-1/L1 response in head and neck cancer. *J Clin Invest*, 128(6), 2339–50.

HIDALGO, D. A., & DISA, J. J. 2015. Reconstruction of the head and neck with free flaps: A 10-year experience. *Plastic Reconstruct Surg*, 105(3), 1078–86.

HOLTZMAN, A., ROTONDO, R., RUTENBERG, M., INDELICATO, D., MERCADO, C., RAO, D., TAVANAIEPOUR, D., MORRIS, C., LOUIS, D., FLAMPOURI, S., & MENDENHALL, W. 2019. Proton therapy for skull-base chondrosarcoma, a single-institution outcomes study. *J Neuro-Oncol.* 142. 10.1007/s11060-019-03129-8

IARC WORKING GROUP ON THE EVALUATION OF CARCINOGENIC RISKS TO HUMANS. 2004. Betel-quid and areca-nut chewing and some areca-nut-derived nitrosamines. *IARC Monographs on the Evaluation of Carcinogenic Risks to Humans*, 85, 1–243.

KELLY, S., JACKSON, J., HICKEY, B., SZALLASI, F., & BOND, C. 2013. Multidisciplinary clinic care improves adherence to best practice in head and neck cancer. *Am J Otolaryngol*, 34, 57–60. 10.1016/j.amjoto.2012.08.010.

LEEMANS, C. R., SNIJDERS, P. J. F., & BRAKENHOFF, R. H. 2018. The molecular landscape of head and neck cancer. *Nat Rev Cancer*, 18(5), 269–82.

LILLO, S., MIRANDOLA, A., VAI, A., CAMARDA, A. M., RONCHI, S., BONORA, M., INGARGIOLA, R., VISCHIONI, B., & ORLANDI, E. 2024. Current status and future directions of proton therapy for head and neck carcinoma. *Cancers*, 16(11), 2085.

MA, D. J., PRICE, K. A., MOORE, E. J., PATEL, S. H., HINNI, M. L., GARCIA, J. J., GRANER, D. E., FOSTER, N. R., GINOS, B., NEBEN-WITTICH, M., GARCES, Y. I., CHINTAKUNTLAWAR, A. V., PRICE, D. L., OLSEN, K. D., VAN ABEL, K. M., KASPERBAUER, J. L., JANUS, J. R., WADDLE, M., MILLER, R., SHIRAISHI, S., & FOOTE, R. L. 2019. Phase II evaluation of aggressive dose de-escalation for adjuvant chemoradiotherapy in human papillomavirus-associated oropharynx squamous cell carcinoma. *J Clin Oncol*, 37(22), 1909–18.

MAGUIRE, S., & GUISHARD-PINE, J. 2005. Parents' and clinicians' perception of severity of referral problems. *Child Adolesc Ment Health*, 10(4), 183–9. doi:10.1111/j.1475-3588.2005.00356.x. PMID: 32806853.

MCBRIDE, S., SHERMAN, E., TSAI, C. J., BAXI, S., AGHALAR, J., ENG, J., ZHI, W. I., MCFARLAND, D., MICHEL, L. S., YOUNG, R., LEFKOWITZ, R., SPIELSINGER, D., ZHANG, Z., FLYNN, J., DUNN, L., HO, A., RIAZ, N., PFISTER, D., & LEE N. 2021. Randomized Phase II trial of nivolumab with stereotactic body radiotherapy versus nivolumab alone in metastatic head and neck squamous cell carcinoma. *J Clin Oncol*, 39(1), 30–7.

MELLA, M. H., CHABRILLAC, E., DUPRET-BORIES, A., MIRALLIE, M., & VERGEZ, S. 2023. Transoral robotic surgery for head and neck cancer: Advances and residual knowledge gaps. *J Clin Med*, *12*(6), 2303.

MOORE, E. J., & OLSEN, K. D. 2015. Transoral robotic surgery for oropharyngeal squamous cell carcinoma. *Mayo Clin Proc*, 90(11), 1555–63.

MOORE, E. J., VAN ABEL, K. M., PRICE, D. L., LOHSE, C. M., OLSEN, K. D., JACKSON, R. S., & MARTIN, E. J. 2018. Transoral robotic surgery for oropharyngeal carcinoma: Surgical margins and oncologic outcomes. *Head Neck*, 40(4), 747–55.

MORAN, S. L. 2009. Chapter 16—Temporoparietal fascia flap. In *Flaps and Reconstructive Surgery*, WEI, F.-C., MARDINI, S., Eds.; W.B. Saunders: Edinburgh, 157–73.

MOREIRA, J., TOBIAS, A., O'BRIEN, M. P., & AGULNIK, M. 2017. Targeted therapy in head and neck cancer: An update on current clinical developments in epidermal growth factor receptor-targeted therapy and immunotherapies. *Drugs*, 77(8), 843–57.

NGWA, W., IRABOR, O. C., SCHOENFELD, J. D., HESSER, J., DEMARIA, S., & FORMENTI, S. C. 2018. Using immunotherapy to boost the abscopal effect. *Nat Rev Cancer*, 18(5), 313–22.

NOEL, G., & GONDI, V. 2016. Proton therapy for tumors of the base of the skull. *Chin Clin Oncol*, 5(4), 51.

PARKIN, D. M., BRAY, F., FERLAY, J., & PISANI, P. 2008. Global cancer statistics, 2002. *CA: Cancer Journal*, 55(2), 74–108.

PIERIK, A. S., LEEMANS, C. R., & BRAKENHOFF, R. H. 2021. Resection margins in head and neck cancer surgery: An update of residual disease and field cancerization. *Cancers, 13*(11), 2635.

POSTOW, M. A., SIDLOW, R., & HELLMANN, M. D. 2018. Immune-related adverse events associated with immune checkpoint blockade. *N Engl J Med*, 378(2), 158–68.

PREZZANO, K. M., MA, S. J., HERMANN, G. M., RIVERS, C. I., GOMEZ-SUESCUN, J. A., & SINGH, A. K. 2019. Stereotactic body radiation therapy for non-small cell lung cancer: A review. *World J Clin Oncol, 10*(1), 14–27.

SCOTT, S., BYRD, J. K., FIGUEROA, R., WILLIAMS, H., CHEN, J., LEE, J., & PUCAR, D. 2020. ^{18}F-fluorodeoxyglucose positron emission tomography/computed tomography in predicting overall survival of oral cavity squamous cell carcinoma: Ongoing controversy. *World J Nuclear Med, 19*(2), 111–17.

SHIELD, K. D., & FERLAY, J. 2017. The global incidence of lip, oral cavity, and pharyngeal cancers by subsite in 2012. *CA Cancer Journal*, 67(1), 51–64.

SIRAVEGNA, G., MARSONI, S., SIENA, S., & BARDELLI, A. 2017. Integrating liquid biopsies into the management of cancer. *Nat Rev Clin Oncol*, 14(9), 531–48.

SIVA, S., MACMANUS, M. P., MARTIN, R. F., & MARTIN, O. A. 2013. Abscopal effects of radiation therapy: A clinical review for the radiobiologist. *Cancer Lett*, 356(1), 82–90.

TABERNA, M., GIL MONCAYO, F., JANÉ-SALAS, E., ANTONIO, M., ARRIBAS, L., VILAJOSANA, E., PERALVEZ TORRES, E., & MESÍA, R. 2020. The multidisciplinary team (MDT) approach and quality of care. *Front Oncol*, 10, 85.

TAYLOR, C., MUNRO, A. J., GLYNNE-JONES, R., GRIFFITH, C., TREVATT, P., RICHARDS, M., & RAMIREZ, A. J. 2010. Multidisciplinary team working in cancer: What is the evidence? *BMJ*, 340, c951.

TOPOL, E. J. 2019. High-performance medicine: The convergence of human and artificial intelligence. *Nat Med*, 25(1), 44–56.

VAN HARTEN, A. M., & BRAKENHOFF, R. H. 2021. Targeted treatment of head and neck (pre)cancer: Preclinical target identification and development of novel therapeutic applications. *Cancers* 13 (11), 2774.

VARADHAN, K. K., & GARDINER, M. S. 2013. The evolution and application of perforator flaps in reconstructive surgery. *Arch Plast Surg*, 40(3), 242–8.

ZHOU, T., HUANG, W., WANG, X., ZHANG, J., ZHOU, E., TU, Y., ZOU, J., SU, K., YI, H., & YIN, S. 2024. Global burden of head and neck cancers from 1990 to 2019. *iScience*, 27(3), 109282.

Index

For the benefit of digital users, indexed terms that span two pages (e.g., 52–53) may, on occasion, appear on only one of those pages.

Tables and figures are indicated by an italic *t* and *f* following the page number.